Radiology of the Foot and Ankle

Second Edition

Radiology of the Foot and Ankle

Second Edition

Editor

Thomas H. Berquist, M.D.
Professor
Mayo Medical School
Mayo Clinic
Jacksonville, Florida

Director of Education
Mayo Foundation
Mayo Clinic
Rochester, Minnesota

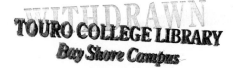

LIPPINCOTT WILLIAMS & WILKINS
A **Wolters Kluwer** Company
Philadelphia • Baltimore • New York • London
Buenos Aires • Hong Kong • Sydney • Tokyo

BS

Acquisitions Editor: James Ryan
Developmental Editor: Susan Rhyner
Production Editor: Jonathan Geffner
Manufacturing Manager: Tim Reynolds
Cover Designer: Patricia Gast
Compositor: Maryland Comp
Printer: Maple Press

© 2000 by Mayo Foundation. Published by LIPPINCOTT WILLIAMS & WILKINS
227 East Washington Square
Philadelphia, PA 19106-3780 USA
www.LWW.com

Printed in the USA

Library of Congress Cataloging-in-Publication Data

Radiology of the foot and ankle/editor, Thomas H. Berquist.—2nd ed.
    p. cm.
   Includes bibliographical references and index.
   ISBN 0-7817-2009-5
   1. Foot—Radiography. 2. Ankle—Radiography. 3. Foot—Diseases-
-Diagnosis. 4. Ankle—Diseases—Diagnosis. I. Berquist, Thomas H.
(Thomas Henry), 1945-   .
   [DNLM: 1. Foot—radiography. 2. Ankle—radiography. 3. Ankle
Injuries—radiography. 4. Foot Diseases—radiography. WE 880
R1292 1999]
RC951.R33 1999
617.5′850757—dc21
DNLM/DLC
for Library of Congress   99-30529
                                CIP

10 9 8 7 6 5 4 3 2 1

3/29/2000

*As time passes, the family grows
and relationships expand in heavenly fashion.
To my wife, Kay; sons, Aric, Matt, and Drew;
and our new daughter-in-law Gretchen,
who bring meaning and joy to my life.*

Contents

Contributing Authors

Laura Wasylenko Bancroft, M.D. *Instructor and Senior Associate Consultant, Department of Diagnostic Radiology, Mayo Clinic Jacksonville, 4500 San Pablo Road, Jacksonville, Florida 32224; Staff Radiologist, Department of Diagnostic Radiology, St. Luke's Hospital, 4201 Belfort Road, Jacksonville, Florida 32216*

Claire E. Bender, M.D. *Associate Professor, Department of Radiology, Mayo Clinic, 200 First Street Southwest, Rochester, Minnesota 55905*

Thomas H. Berquist, M.D. *Professor, Department of Diagnostic Radiology, Mayo Medical School, Mayo Clinic Jacksonville, 4500 San Pablo Road, Jacksonville, Florida 32224; Director of Education, Mayo Foundation, Mayo Clinic, 200 First Street Southwest, Rochester, Minnesota 55905*

Omer L. Burnett, Jr., M.D. *Director, Nuclear Medicine, Department of Diagnostic Radiology, Mayo Clinic Jacksonville, 4500 San Pablo Road, Jacksonville, Florida 32224; Director, Nuclear Medicine, Department of Diagnostic Radiology, St. Luke's Hospital, 4201 Belfort Road, Jacksonville, Florida 32216*

James Keith DeOrio, M.D. *Department Chairman and Assistant Professor, Department of Orthopaedics, Mayo Clinic Jacksonville, 4500 San Pablo Road, Jacksonville, Florida 32224; Consultant, St. Luke's Hospital, 4201 Belfort Road, Jacksonville, Florida 32216*

Gina A. Di Primio, M.D., F.R.C.P.C. *Musculoskeletal Fellow, Department of Diagnostic Radiology, Mayo Clinic Jacksonville, 4500 San Pablo Road, Jacksonville, Florida 32224*

Alan D. Hoffman, M.D. *Consultant, Department of Radiology, Mayo Clinic, 200 First Street Southwest, Rochester, Minnesota 55905*

Nolan Karstaedt, M.B., B.Ch. *Associate Professor of Radiology, Department of Diagnostic Radiology, Mayo Medical School, Mayo Clinic Jacksonville, 4500 San Pablo Road, Jacksonville, Florida 32224; Consultant, Department of Diagnostic Radiology, Mayo Clinic Jacksonville, 4500 San Pablo Road, Jacksonville, Florida 32224*

John M. Knudsen, M.D. *Instructor of Radiology, Department of Diagnostic Radiology, Mayo Medical School, Mayo Clinic Jacksonville, 4500 San Pablo Road, Jacksonville, Florida 32224; Consultant, Department of Diagnostic Radiology, Mayo Clinic Jacksonville, 4500 San Pablo Road, Jacksonville, Florida 32224*

Richard A. McLeod, M.D. *Emeritus Professor, Mayo Medical School, Mayo Clinic, 200 First Street Southwest, Rochester, Minnesota 55905*

Debbie J. Merinbaum, M.D. *Instructor, Department of Radiology, The Mayo Foundation, Mayo Medical School, 200 First Street Southwest, Rochester, Minnesota 55905; Staff Radiologist, Department of Radiology, Nemours Children's Clinic, 807 Nira Street, Jacksonville, Florida 32207*

W. Andrew Oldenburg, M.D. *Assistant Professor of Surgery, Mayo Medical School, Mayo Clinic Jacksonville, 4500 San Pablo Road, Jacksonville, Florida 32224; Consultant in Vascular Surgery, Mayo Clinic Jacksonville, 4500 San Pablo Road, Jacksonville, Florida 32224*

Hugh J. Williams, Jr., M.D. *Associate Professor, Department of Radiology, Mayo Clinic Jacksonville, Mayo Medical School, 4500 San Pablo Road, Jacksonville, Florida 32224*

Preface

The First Edition of this text, published in 1989, and this Second Edition have similar goals. Specifically, they both emphasize proper utilization of imaging techniques for evaluating foot and ankle disorders. In order to accomplish this goal multiple factors must be considered. First, one must have a thorough knowledge of the advantages and limitations of the numerous imaging techniques that are available. Secondly, the complex anatomy of the foot and ankle must be clearly understood. Finally, close communication between clinicians: internists, podiatrists, orthopedic surgeons, emergency room physicians, and radiologists is essential to select the most appropriate imaging approach for evaluating foot and ankle disorders. Communication is even more important today with the numerous, often costly, procedures that are available in a cost-conscious environment. The combined knowledge of the radiologist and clinician is essential to optimize patient care.

This edition, like the First Edition, is co-authored by radiologists and clinicians where appropriate to unify the clinical/imaging approach to foot and ankle disorders. Chapter One reviews anatomy and basic biomechanics which are essential for both clinicians and radiologists. Common normal variants and pitfalls are also reviewed.

Chapter Two discusses the principles and applications of current imaging procedures. This provides basic background information on technical aspects, applications, and limitations of imaging procedures. The chapter serves two purposes. First, to provide sufficient information, primarily for nonradiologists, to understand the technique in which patients may be appropriately examined using a given modality. Secondly, the information presented in this chapter can be referred to in later chapters to avoid redundancy when techniques are reviewed as they apply to specific pathologic conditions.

Chapters Three through Eight are pathologically oriented. Soft tissue trauma and overuse syndromes, fracture/dislocations, arthritis, bone and soft tissue tumors and tumor-like conditions, infection, and ischemic diseases are discussed. These chapters review clinical features and imaging approaches as they apply to these conditions.

Chapter Nine is devoted to pediatric disorders, with emphasis on congenital foot and ankle conditions. Chapter Ten discusses the pre- and postoperative imaging features that should be reviewed for surgical reconstructive procedures in the foot and ankle. Imaging of postoperative complications is also reviewed. Chapter Eleven covers a large variety of miscellaneous conditions such as metabolic disease, Paget's disease, and other less common disorders that may be encountered on foot and ankle images.

This text provides a comprehensive reference for radiologists, podiatrists, orthopedic surgeons, rheumatologists, emergency room physicians, and other clinicians or residents in training that deal with foot and ankle disorders. We hope the combined clinical and imaging information presented in this text will serve to emphasize the importance of communication between radiologists and clinicians in dealing with the imaging approach to foot and ankle disorders.

Thomas H. Berquist

Acknowledgments

Preparation of this text was facilitated by the efforts of many individuals in the department of Diagnostic Radiology. The numerous figures in the Second Edition were selected from case material at Mayo Clinic Jacksonville, Nemours Children's Clinic and affiliated institutions. I wish to thank the radiology recorders and technologists for their assistance in this regard. Lonnie Foster, Susan Ashley, Noel Bahr, Bobbi Maciaszek, and Pam Gordon were particularly helpful in saving selected cases needed to demonstrate features of pathological conditions discussed in this text.

The Department of Photographics provided quality prints of images for this edition. John Hagen, from the Department of Medical Graphics, provided the superb illustrations necessary to demonstrate anatomy, specific injuries, and classifications.

The manuscript and orchestration of the printed material was performed by Pam Chirico with assistance from Beverly Thompson, Betty Lee, and Laura Ulrich.

Finally, I wish to thank James Ryan and Christina Houston from Lippincott Williams & Wilkins for their support in preparing this text.

Radiology of the Foot and Ankle, Second Edition,
edited by Thomas H. Berquist.
© 2000 by Mayo Foundation.
Published by Lippincott Williams & Wilkins, Philadelphia.

CHAPTER 1

Anatomy, Normal Variants, and Basic Biomechanics

Thomas H. Berquist

New radiographic techniques, especially magnetic resonance imaging (MRI), provide significant diagnostic information because of improved tissue contrast and the ability to image in multiple planes (axial, sagittal, coronal, oblique). Therefore, a thorough knowledge of skeletal and soft tissue anatomy in multiple image planes is essential. Normal variants must also be mastered, to distinguish normal from pathologic changes in the foot and ankle.[7,25,55,61] A basic understanding of biomechanics is also essential for selecting the proper diagnostic techniques. Mastering the anatomy and basic functions of the foot and ankle is equally important to physicians involved in imaging procedures, clinical medicine, and surgery.

SOFT TISSUE ANATOMY

The lower extremity musculature develops from mesodermal tissues of the lower limb bud.[2] Functional muscle groups are organized in fascial compartments. Therefore, to sim-

T. H. Berquist: Mayo Medical School, Mayo Clinic Jacksonville, Jacksonville, Florida 32224; Mayo Foundation, Mayo Clinic, Rochester, Minnesota 55905.

plify the muscular anatomy of the foot and ankle, this discussion focuses on compartments or functional groups of muscles, including their origins, insertions, and actions. Normal variants are also discussed.

The muscles of the leg can be divided into anterior, posterior, and lateral compartments (Fig. 1-1). One of these muscles crosses only the knee, and two cross the knee and ankle. Most arise in the leg and act on both the foot and the ankle (Fig. 1-2).[19,55]

Posterior Musculature

The superficial and deep muscles of the calf are divided into compartments by the crural fascia (Fig. 1-3). The superficial muscle group includes the gastrocnemius, soleus, and plantaris (Fig. 1-4). The gastrocnemius has two heads arising from the medial and lateral femoral condyles (Fig. 1-5). The two heads unite to form the bulk of the muscle in the upper calf. At about the midpoint of the calf, the muscle ends in a wide, flat tendon (see Fig. 1-4A; Fig. 1-6). The soleus inserts into the anterior aspect of the gastrocnemius tendon (see Figs. 1-4B and 1-6D). Below this level, the tendon nar-

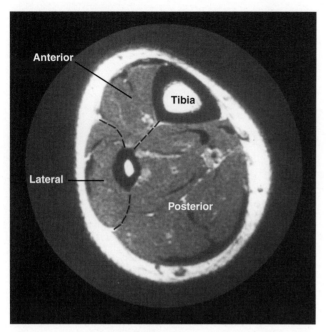

FIG. 1-1. Axial spin-echo 500/10 magnetic resonance image demonstrating the compartments of the leg.

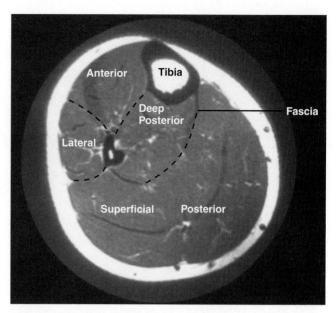

FIG. 1-3. Axial magnetic resonance image of the calf demonstrating the compartments with crural fascia separating the deep and superficial posterior muscle groups.

rows in transverse diameter and thickens, forming the Achilles tendon (tendo calcaneus), which inserts on the posterior calcaneus (see Figs. 1-4A and 1-6E). The gastrocnemius plantar flexes the foot and also assists in knee flexion during non-weight bearing. Innervation is by the tibial nerve, and the vascular supply is primarily derived from the posterior

tibial artery.[15,19,40,55] Reported variations of the gastrocnemius include absence of the lateral head and central origins from the posterior femur.[15,19]

The soleus lies deep to the gastrocnemius (see Figs. 1-2, 1-4B, and 1-6C) and also has two heads, one arising from the posterior superior fibula and the second from the popliteal line and posteromedial surface of the proximal tibia (see

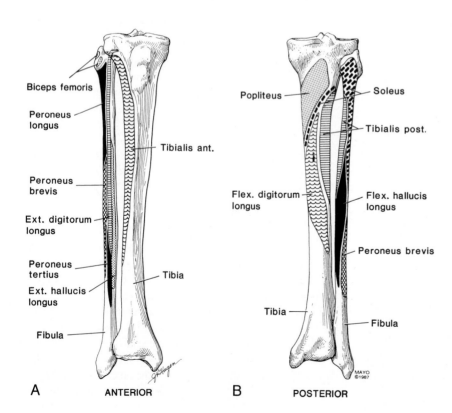

A   **ANTERIOR**

B   **POSTERIOR**

FIG. 1-2. Anterior (**A**) and posterior (**B**) illustrations of the tibia and fibula demonstrating the origins of muscles that insert on or affect the foot and ankle.

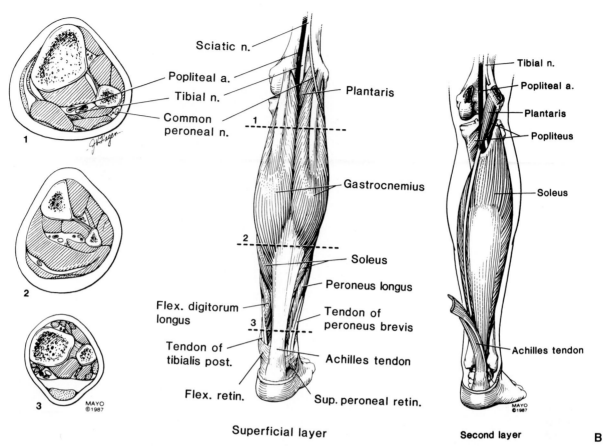

FIG. 1-4. Muscles of the posterior leg. **A:** Illustration of superficial musculature with cross sections at levels 1, 2, and 3. **B:** Illustration of soleus, popliteus, plantaris, and upper vascular relationships.

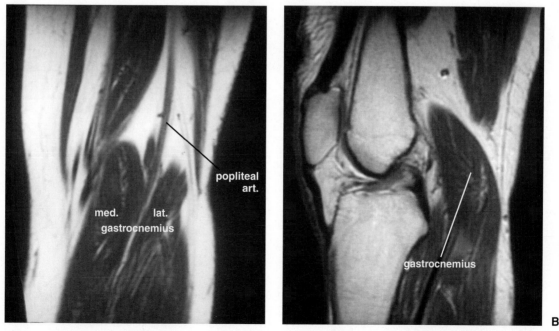

FIG. 1-5. Coronal (**A**) and sagittal (**B**) magnetic resonance images of the knee demonstrating the origins of the gastrocnemius muscles.

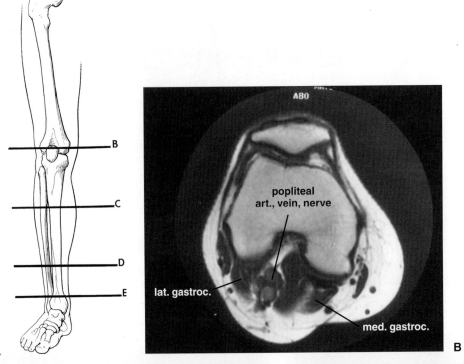

A

B

popliteal
art., vein, nerve

lat. gastroc.

med. gastroc.

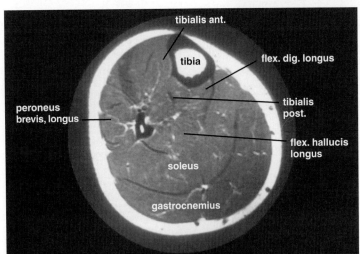

C

tibialis ant.

tibia

flex. dig. longus

tibialis
post.

flex. hallucis
longus

peroneus
brevis, longus

soleus

gastrocnemius

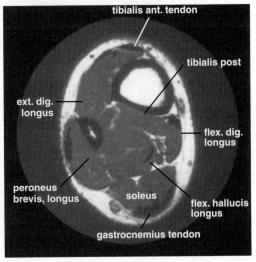

D

tibialis ant. tendon

tibialis post

ext. dig.
longus

flex. dig.
longus

peroneus
brevis, longus

soleus

flex. hallucis
longus

gastrocnemius tendon

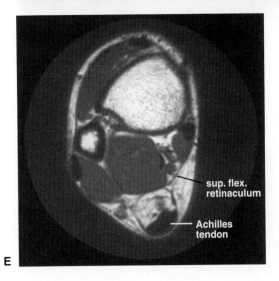

E

sup. flex.
retinaculum

Achilles
tendon

FIG. 1-6. A: Illustration demonstrating levels of axial magnetic reso-
nance images (MRI). **B:** Axial MRI at the level of the femoral condyles.
C: Axial MRI through the upper calf. **D:** Axial MRI through the lower leg.
E: Axial MRI just above the ankle joint.

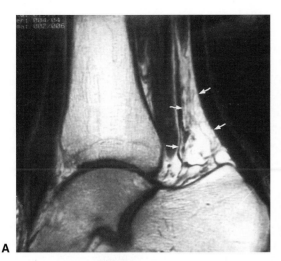
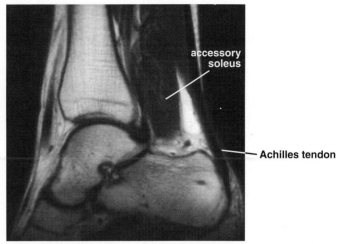

FIG. 1-7. A: Sagittal magnetic resonance image (MRI) of the ankle showing the normal pre-Achilles fat (*arrows*). **B:** Sagittal MRI showing an accessory soleus muscle that distorts the normally triangular configuration of the fatty tissue.

Fig. 1-2B). The popliteal vessels and tibial nerve pass deep to the body of the soleus (see Fig. 1-4B). The soleus inserts in the anterior aspect of the gastrocnemius tendon, forming the thicker Achilles tendon (see Fig. 1-6D and E).[15,19,55]

The soleus has no effect on the knee, but it serves as a plantar flexor of the foot. Innervation is via the tibial nerve, with vascular supply from the posterior tibial artery.[1,15,19,55]

An important, but uncommon, variable is the accessory soleus muscle. This accessory muscle bundle extends into Kager's fat triangle anterior to the Achilles tendon and inserts in the anterior aspect of this tendon, the calcaneus, or the flexor retinaculum (Fig. 1-7).[6,7,40,53] This muscle may be incidentally noted, but some patients may have clinical symptoms. The most common presenting complaints are soft tissue prominence and pain following exercise. Thus, it is important to differentiate this normal variant from a torn muscle remnant or a soft tissue mass.[6,7,53]

The plantaris is the third muscle included in the superficial compartment. This small muscle takes its origin from the lateral epicondyle of the femur and the oblique popliteal ligament (see Fig. 1-2).[15,19] The belly of the muscle is only several inches long and passes between the gastrocnemius and soleus in an oblique direction (see Fig. 1-4A and B). The long, thin tendon passes distally along the medial margin of the Achilles to insert in the calcaneus, Achilles, or flexor retinaculum.[19] Occasionally, the muscle is double, and it may be totally absent.[19,55]

The plantaris functions as a minor flexor of the knee and a plantar flexor of the foot. Innervation and blood supply are from the tibial nerve and the posterior tibial artery.[18,54]

The deep compartment of the calf contains the popliteus, tibialis posterior, flexor hallucis longus, and flexor digitorum longus (Fig. 1-8). The popliteus is a small triangular muscle forming a portion of the floor of the popliteal fossa (see Figs. 1-4B and 1-8).[15,19] Its origin is from the lateral femoral

epicondyle, the arcuate popliteal ligament, and the capsule of the knee. The insertion is the posterior surface of the upper tibia above the origin of the soleus (see Figs. 1-2 and 1-8).[1,19,55]

The popliteus acts on the knee and leg as a flexor and a

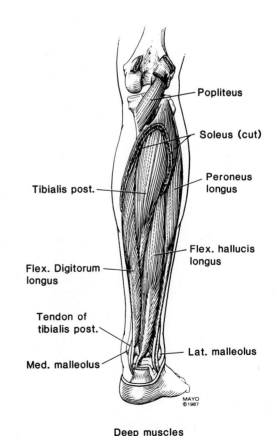

Deep muscles

FIG. 1-8. Illustration of the deep muscles of the posterior leg.

medial rotator. Neurovascular supply is by the tibial nerve and the posterior tibial artery.[15,19,55]

Variations may occur in the origins of the popliteus. In 14% of patients, this muscle arises from the inner aspect of the fibular head and inserts above the oblique tibial line.[15,19]

The flexor hallucis longus is the most lateral of the three remaining deep muscles of the leg (flexor hallucis longus, flexor digitorum longus, and tibialis posterior) (see Figs. 1-6C and D and 1-8). It arises from the lateral aspect of the middle half of the posterior fibula (see Fig. 1-2). Its tendon begins above the malleoli of the ankle and courses medially behind the ankle deep to the flexor retinaculum (see Fig. 1-8). The tendon is posterior to the tendons of the tibialis posterior (or posterior tibial tendon) and flexor digitorum longus behind the medial malleolus (Fig. 1-9). The tendon passes along the plantar aspect of the foot to insert in the distal phalanx of the great toe (see Figs. 1-18 and 1-19).[15,19,55]

The flexor hallucis longus is a flexor of the great toe and assists in ankle flexion. The muscle is innervated by the tibial nerve and receives its blood supply from the posterior tibial artery.[1,15,19,55]

Minor variations in the origin of the flexor digitorum longus are not uncommon. An accessory muscle, peroneocalcaneus internus, occurs in 1% of asymptomatic patients.[41] Up to 75% of these muscles are bilateral. The muscle arises from the lateral flexor hallucis longus and the posterior fibula. It lies posterolateral to the flexor hallucis longus as it courses inferiorly to the sustentaculum tali to insert on the calcaneus.[15,19] Both tendons may be visible on sagittal and axial MRI studies as they pass inferiorly to the sustentaculum tali

(Fig. 1-10).[41] The peroneocalcaneus internus muscle does not present as a soft tissue mass or cause neurovascular compression, which can occur with other accessory muscles.[6,7,41] However, in some cases, it may displace the flexor hallucis longus muscle and may cause indirect neurovascular compression.[41]

The flexor digitorum longus lies medially in the deep compartment of the calf (see Figs. 1-6D and 1-8). It arises from the upper half of the posteromedial aspect of the tibia (see Fig. 1-2). Along its caudad course, it passes posterior to the tibialis posterior so that, at the ankle, it lies between the flexor hallucis longus and the tibialis posterior (see Fig. 1-9). The tendon passes through the flexor retinaculum, posterior to the medial malleolus, and then divides into four slips, which insert in the distal phalanges of the lateral four digits (see Figs. 1-18 and 1-19). On the plantar aspect of the foot, these four tendon slips are associated with the lumbrical muscles and pass through the divided slips of the flexor digitorum brevis before inserting on the distal phalanges.[15,19,55]

The flexor digitorum longus flexes the lateral four toes and also plantar flexes the foot and supinates the ankle.[55] The muscle is innervated by branches of the tibial nerve and receives its vascular supply from posterior tibial artery branches.[15,19,55]

A fairly common accessory flexor muscle can be demonstrated. The flexor accessorius longus digitorum arises from the lower fibula, interosseous membrane, and tibia and passes beneath the flexor retinaculum to insert in the flexor digitorum longus tendon or quadratus plantae tendon.[15]

The tibialis posterior is the deepest and most centrally

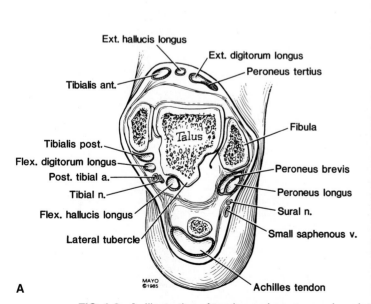

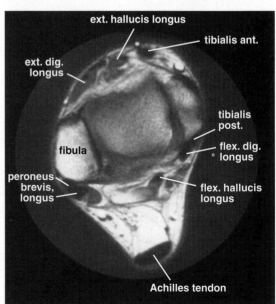

FIG. 1-9. A: Illustration of tendon and neurovascular relationships about the ankle. (From Berquist TH. MRI of the Musculoskeletal System. 3rd Ed. New York, Lippincott–Raven, 1996.) B: Axial magnetic resonance image with anatomy labeled.

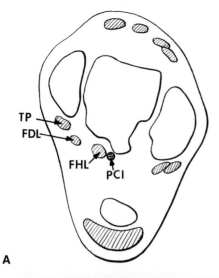

A

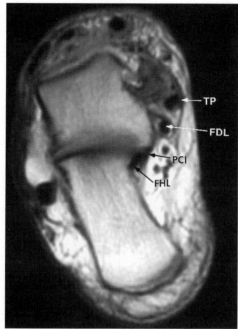

B

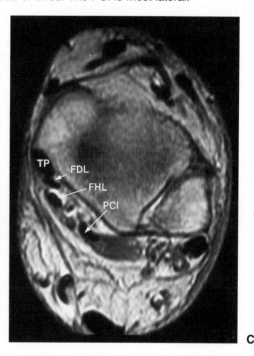

C

FIG. 1-10. A: Axial illustration of the ankle demonstrating four medial tendons instead of the usual three tendons: tibialis posterior (*TP*), flexor digitorum longus (*FDL*), flexor hallucis longus (*FHL*), peroneocalcaneus internus (*PCI*). **B:** Axial spin-echo 2000/20 magnetic resonance image just proximal to the sustentaculum tali demonstrating two tendons in the usual location of the flexor hallucis longus. **C:** Axial image at the tibiotalar junction shows four tendons instead of three. The PCI is most lateral.

located muscle in the deep posterior compartment (see Figs. 1-6C and D and 1-8). It arises from the upper posterior aspects of the tibia and fibula and the interosseous membrane (see Fig. 1-2). Thus, it is positioned between the flexor hallucis longus and the flexor digitorum longus. The tendon passes medially deep to the flexor retinaculum and the flexor digitorum longus (see Fig. 1-6E). Therefore, it is the most anterior of the three tendons as it passes behind the medial malleolus (see Fig. 1-9). The tendon flares (Fig. 1-11) to insert in the navicular, tarsal bones, and bases of the second to fourth metatarsals (see Fig. 1-21).[15,19,55]

The tibialis posterior aids in adduction, inversion, and plantar flexion of the foot. The muscle is innervated by branches of the tibial nerve and receives its blood supply from the posterior tibial artery.[15,19,55] Table 1-1 summarizes the muscles of the calf and their functions.

Neurovascular Anatomy of the Calf

The tibial nerve is a continuation of the sciatic nerve at the level of the popliteal fossa. As it passes inferiorly, it enters the calf between the heads of the gastrocnemius muscle, passing deep to the soleus to lie between the soleus and tibialis posterior in the deep compartment (Fig. 1-12).[19] The tibial nerve sends branches to all the superficial and deep muscles of the calf (see Table 1-1 and Figs. 1-8 and 1-12). At the ankle level, the nerve generally lies between the flexor hallucis longus and the flexor digitorum longus tendons (see Figs. 1-9 and 1-12). Distal to the flexor retinaculum, it divides, forming the medial and lateral plantar nerves.[15,19,55]

The popliteal artery is a direct continuation of the superficial femoral artery as it passes through the adductor canal (see Fig. 1-12). It divides into anterior and posterior tibial

TABLE 1-1. *Muscles of the leg, foot and ankle*[a]

Location	Muscle	Origin	Insertion	Action	Innervation (Segment)	Blood Supply
Calf Superficial compartment	Gastrocnemius	Femoral condyles	Posterior calcaneus	Flexor of foot and knee	Tibial nerve (S1, S2)	Posterior tibial artery
	Soleus	Upper tibia and fibula	Gastrocnemius tendon	Plantar flexor of foot	Tibial nerve (S1, S2)	Posterior tibial artery
	Plantaris	Lateral femoral condyle and oblique popliteal ligament	Posteromedial calcaneus	Plantar flexor of foot, flexor of leg	Tibial nerve (L4-S1)	Posterior tibial artery
Deep compartment	Popliteus	Lateral femur and capsule of knee		Flexor and medial rotator of leg	Tibial nerve (L5, S1)	Posterior tibial artery
	Flexor hallucis longus	Posterior midfibula	Distal phalanx great toe	Flexor of great toe and ankle	Tibial nerve (L5-S2)	Posterior tibial artery
	Flexor digitorum longus	Posterior tibia	Distal phalanges 2–5 toes	Flexor of toes and foot and supinator of ankle	Tibial nerve (L5, S1)	Posterior tibial artery
	Tibialis posterior	Posterior tibia, fibula, and interosseous membrane	Navicular, cuneiform, calcaneus, 2–4 metatarsals	Adductor of foot, invertor, plantar flexor	Tibial nerve (L5, S1)	Posterior tibial artery
Lateral compartment	Peroneus longus	Lateral fibula	First metatarsal and medial cuneiform	Evertor and weak plantar flexors	Superficial and deep nerve (L4-S1)	Peroneal artery
	Peroneous brevis	Lateral fibula	Base fifth metatarsal		Superficial peroneal (L4-S1)	Peroneal artery
Anterior compartment	Extensor digitorum longus	Upper tibia, fibula, and interosseous membrane	Lateral 4 toes	Dorsiflexor of toes, evertor of foot	Deep peroneal nerve (L4-S1)	Anterior tibial artery
	Peroneus tertius	Distal fibula, interosseous membrane	Base fifth metatarsal	Dorsiflexor and evertor of foot	Deep peroneal nerve	Anterior tibial artery
	Extensor hallucis longus	Distal fibula and interosseous membrane	Distal phalanx great toe	Extensor of great toe, weak invertor and dorsiflexor of foot	Deep peroneal nerve (L4-S1)	Anterior tibial artery
	Tibialis anterior	Lateral tibia and interosseous membrane	Medial cuneiform and first metatarsal	Strong dorsiflexor and invertor of foot	Deep peroneal nerve (L4-S1)	Anterior tibial artery

[a] Data from references 1, 19, and 26.

branches at the level of the popliteus muscle. The anterior tibial artery enters the anterolateral leg above the upper margin of the interosseous membrane, whereas the posterior tibial artery joins the tibial nerve in the deep compartment of the calf (see Figs. 1-12 and 1-16B). In the leg, it provides muscular branches to all the calf muscles and a nutrient artery to the tibia. Its largest branch, the peroneal artery, arises high in the leg and passes deep to the flexor hallucis longus near the interosseous membrane and the fibula (see Figs. 1-12 and 1-16B). At the ankle level, it forms anastomotic branches with the posterior tibial artery and perforates the interosseous membrane to supply the dorsal aspect of the foot. Generally, paired veins accompany the arteries. These veins are more variable and enter the popliteal vein superiorly.[15,19,55]

Anterolateral Musculature

The peroneus longus and brevis are the two muscles of the lateral compartment. Both arise from the superior lateral surface of the fibula. The origin of the peroneus longus is more superior, with the muscle passing superficial to the peroneus brevis (see Fig. 1-2). The muscles progress caudad in the lateral compartment (see Figs. 1-1, 1-6, and 1-9), with their tendons entering a common tendon sheath above the ankle (see Fig. 1-9; Fig. 1-13). The tendons pass posterior to the lateral malleolus and deep to the superior and inferior peroneal retinacula (Fig. 1-14). The tendons diverge on the lateral surface of the foot with the peroneus brevis inserting on the base of the fifth metatarsal. The peroneus longus takes an inferior course, passing under the lateral aspect of the

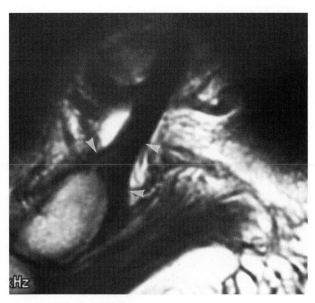

FIG. 1-11. Sagittal magnetic resonance image demonstrating the normal flare or widening (*arrowheads*) of the tibialis posterior tendon as it inserts onto the navicular.

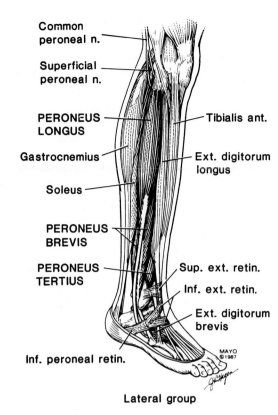

Lateral group

FIG. 1-13. Illustration of the lateral muscles of the leg and their tendinous relationships at the ankle.

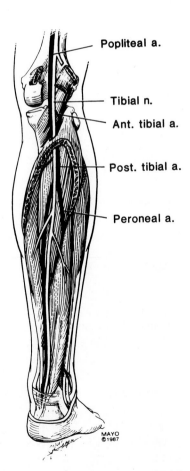

FIG. 1-12. Illustration of the major neurovascular structures of the posterior compartment.

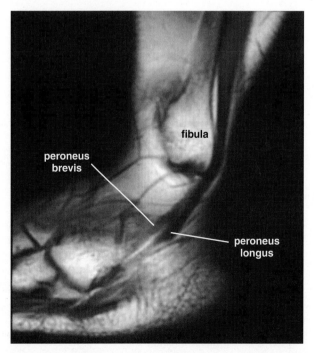

FIG. 1-14. Sagittal spin-echo 500/10 image demonstrating the peroneus brevis and longus as they separate after passing inferior to the lateral malleolus.

foot, where it inserts on the base of the first metatarsal and the medial cuneiform (see Fig. 1-21).[1,15,19,55]

These muscles serve as evertors of the foot and assist in plantar flexion. Innervation is from the superficial peroneal nerve with branches of the common or deep peroneal nerve supplying a portion of the peroneus longus. Vascular supply is via the peroneal artery.[1,19,55]

Multiple peroneal variations may cause confusion on MRI or computed tomography (CT) images. The muscles (longus and brevis) may fuse to form one unit, and occasionally the peroneus longus insertion expands to include the bases of the third to the fifth metatarsals. An accessory peroneal muscle may arise from the fibula between the peroneus longus and brevis. Its tendon generally inserts in the peroneus longus tendon on the plantar aspect of the foot.[15,19,55]

The peroneus quadratus is present in about 10 to 13% of patients.[5,19,55] This anomalous muscle is three times as common in males compared with females.[5] Three variations of the peroneus quadratus have been described, based on their insertions. One of this subgroup inserts on the calcaneus (peroneocalcaneus externum), one on the cuboid (peroneocuboideus), and the third variation inserts on the peroneal tendon (long peroneal).[18] The peroneus quadratus has been associated with clinical symptoms (pain and instability), and it is associated with peroneal tendon subluxation, which is discussed in detail in Chapter 3.[5] On MRI (Fig. 1-15), the peroneus quadratus tendon is posterior to the brevis and longus tendons.[5]

The peroneus digiti minimi is rare. It arises from the lower fibula and inserts on the extensor surface of the fifth toe.[4,5]

Anterior Compartment Musculature

The anterior compartment has four muscles. These are the extensor digitorum longus, the peroneus tertius, the extensor hallucis longus, and the tibialis anterior (Fig. 1-16).

The extensor digitorum longus is the most lateral muscle in the anterior compartment (see Fig. 1-16).[1,19] It arises from the lateral tibial condyle, the anterior fibula, and the interosseous membrane (see Fig. 1-2). The tendon passes deep to the superior and inferior extensor retinacula (see Fig. 1-9) before dividing into four slips that insert on the dorsal aspects of the four lateral toes (see Fig. 1-16A). The insertions are divided such that portions insert in the middle and distal phalanges.[1,15,19]

This muscle dorsiflexes the toes and also assists in eversion of the foot. It is innervated by the deep peroneal nerve and receives its vascular supply from the anterior tibial artery (see Fig. 1-16B). Variations in its origin and distal insertions are not uncommon, but these rarely cause confusion on CT or MRI.[15,19]

The peroneus tertius is closely associated with the extensor digitorum longus, and it may be considered a portion of the latter.[15,19] It arises from the distal anterior fibula, the interosseous membrane, and the membrane of the peroneus

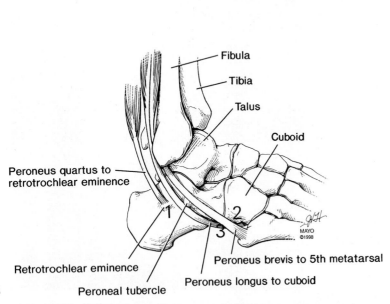

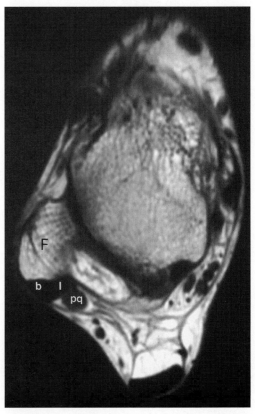

FIG. 1-15. A: Illustration of the peroneus quadratus, which may insert on the retrotrochlear eminence (*1*), cuboid (*2*), or longus tendon (*3*). **B:** Axial magnetic resonance image demonstrating peroneus quadratus (*pq*) medial and posterior to the peroneal brevis (*b*) and longus (*l*) tendons. *F,* fibula.

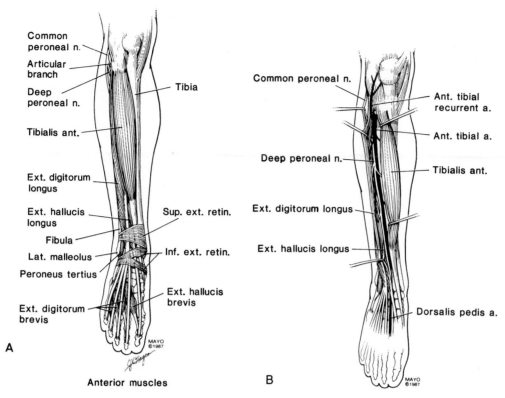

FIG. 1-16. Illustrations of the muscles (**A**) and neurovascular anatomy (**B**) in the anterior leg.

brevis (see Fig. 1-2). Its tendon passes deep to the extensor retinacula to insert on the dorsal aspect of the base of the fifth metatarsal (see Fig. 1-16A). It is supplied by the deep peroneal nerve and the anterior tibial artery. This muscle varies in size and may be absent.[15,19]

The extensor hallucis longus lies deep to the extensor digitorum longus and the tibialis anterior. It arises from the midfibula and the interosseous membrane and becomes superficial in the lower leg (see Fig. 1-2). Its tendon passes deep to the extensor retinacula to insert on the distal phalanx of the great toe (see Figs. 1-9 and 1-16A). This muscle extends the great toe and is a weak dorsiflexor and invertor of the foot. It is supplied by the deep peroneal nerve and the anterior tibial artery.[1,15,19,55]

Occasionally an accessory muscle, the extensor ossis metatarsi hallucis arises from the extensor digitorum longus, the tibialis interior, or the extensor hallucis longus. Unlike the accessory soleus, this muscle is generally too small to be confused with a soft tissue mass.[7,15,19]

The tibialis anterior arises from the lateral tibia surface, the deep fascia, and the interosseous membrane (see Fig. 1-2). It passes inferiorly, becoming tendinous in the lower leg (see Figs. 1-6, 1-9, and 1-16A). It is the most medial tendon as it passes deep to the extensor retinacula. It passes along the medial foot to insert in the medial cuneiform and plantar portion of the first metatarsal (see Fig. 1-16A).[15,19,55]

This muscle is a strong dorsiflexor and inverter of the foot.[19] Neurovascular supply is via the deep peroneal nerve and the anterior tibial artery.[15,19,55]

Neurovascular Anatomy of the Anterolateral Muscles

The common peroneal nerve is a branch of the sciatic nerve and courses laterally in the popliteal fossa. It is subcutaneous and is relatively unprotected just below the fibular head (see Fig. 1-16B). Therefore, it is susceptible to direct trauma in this area.[3,15,19] As it descends between the fibula and the peroneus longus, it divides into two or three branches. These are the superficial, deep, and articular branches of the peroneal nerve (see Fig. 1-16B). The superficial peroneal nerve lies between the peroneus longus and brevis and supplies these muscles and the subcutaneous tissues. The deep peroneal nerve courses anteriorly, deep to the peroneus longus, to supply the anterior muscles of the leg (see Table 1-1 and Fig. 1-16B). It joins the anterior tibial artery on the anterior aspect of the interosseous membrane.[15,19,55]

The anterior tibial artery passes superior to the interosseous membrane in the upper leg and then lies with the deep peroneal nerve along the anterior aspect of the interosseous membrane (see Figs. 1-12 and 1-16B). It supplies the anterior muscles and continues as the dorsalis pedis artery on the dorsum of the foot.[15,19,55] Table 1-1 summarizes the muscles of the leg, their functions, and neurovascular supply.

Foot Musculature

The muscles of the foot are discussed by layer, rather than by compartments as in the leg, to facilitate anatomic

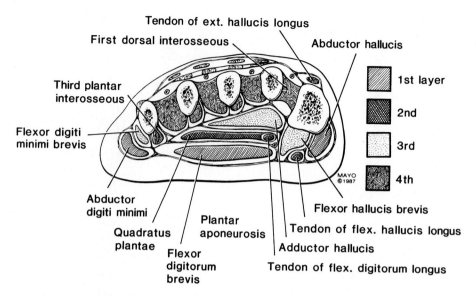

FIG. 1-17. Axial illustration of the muscle layers of the foot.

discussion (Fig. 1-17).[14,15,19] The compartment concept is included later in this section. The superficial layer of plantar muscles includes the abductor hallucis, the flexor digitorum brevis, and the abductor digiti minimi.[15,19]

The abductor hallucis arises from the medial process of the calcaneal tubercle, the flexor retinaculum, and the plantar aponeurosis. Its insertion is the medial side of the flexor surface of the proximal phalanx of the great toe (Figs. 1-18 and 1-19).[15,19,55] The medial and lateral plantar vessels and nerves pass deep to the proximal position of the muscle as

they enter the foot.[19] The muscle is supplied by branches of the medial plantar nerve and artery. The abductor hallucis functions weakly as an abductor of the metatarsophalangeal joint of the great toe.[15,19]

The flexor digitorum brevis is the most central of the superficial plantar muscles (see Figs. 1-17 and 1-18). It arises from the medial tubercular process of the calcaneus and the plantar fascia. Four tendons pass distally and divide into two slips at the level of the proximal phalanx. The tendons of

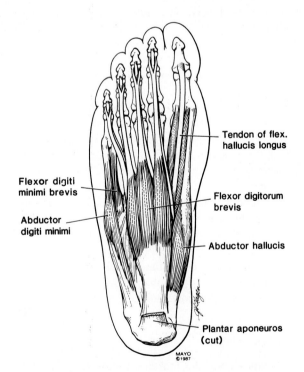

FIG. 1-18. Superficial plantar muscles of the foot.

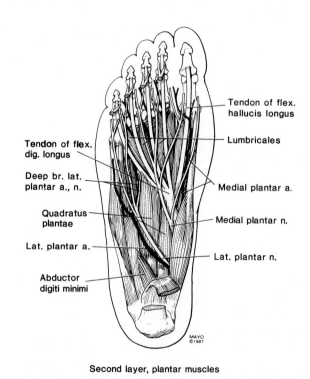

Second layer, plantar muscles

FIG. 1-19. Illustration of the second muscle layer of the foot.

the flexor digitorum longus pass through the divided brevis tendons. The divided tendon slips insert on the middle phalanges.[15,19,55]

The muscle flexes the lateral four toes. It is supplied by the medial plantar nerve and artery, with the lateral plantar nerve and artery passing deep to this muscle. It is not uncommon for the tendon to the fifth toe to be absent (38%).[1,15,18,54]

The abductor digiti minimi is the most lateral muscle in the superficial layer (see Figs. 1-17 through 1-19). It arises from the lateral process of the calcaneal tubercle and the distal portion of the medial process. It inserts in the lateral aspect of the base of the proximal phalanx of the fifth toe and serves to flex and abduct the toe at the metatarsophalangeal joint. It is supplied by the lateral plantar nerve and artery.[1,15,19]

The second layer of the foot is composed of the tendons of the flexor hallucis longus and flexor digitorum longus plus the quadratus plantae and lumbrical muscles (see Fig. 1-19).[19] The quadratus plantae has two heads that arise from the medial and lateral plantar aspects of the calcaneal tuberosity (see Figs. 1-17 and 1-19). The muscle inserts in the lateral and posterior margin of the flexor digitorum longus just before it divides into its four tendon slips (see Fig. 1-19).[15,19] The muscle assists the flexor digitorum longus in flexing the lateral four toes. It is supplied by the lateral plantar nerve and artery. Occasionally, the lateral head or, in certain cases, the entire muscle may be absent.[19]

The four lumbrical muscles arise from the flexor digitorum longus tendon. They pass distally to insert on the medial side of metatarsophalangeal joints of the four lateral toes (see Fig. 1-19). They act as flexors of the metatarsophalangeal joints. The most medial muscle is innervated by the medial plantar nerve, whereas the lateral plantar nerves supply the lateral three muscles. Blood supply is via the medial and lateral plantar arteries. Absence of one or more of the lumbricals has been reported. Occasionally, two muscles insert on the fourth and fifth toes.[1,15,19]

The third layer of plantar muscles includes the flexor hallucis brevis, the adductor hallucis, and the flexor digiti minimi brevis (see Fig. 1-17; Fig. 1-20). The flexor hallucis brevis has two bellies arising from the plantar aspect of the cuboid and adjacent cuneiform (see Fig. 1-20). The tendons insert at the sides of the base of the great toe and the sesamoids. The muscle serves as a flexor of the great toe and is supplied by the medial plantar nerve and artery.[15,18,55]

The adductor hallucis has oblique and transverse heads (see Fig. 1-20). The oblique head arises from the long plantar ligament and the second through fourth metatarsals bases.[19] The smaller transverse head arises from the capsules of the third through fifth metatarsophalangeal joints and the deep transverse ligaments. The two heads join lateral to the great toe to insert with the lateral head of the flexor hallucis brevis.[1,15,19]

The adductor hallucis adducts and flexes the great toe. In addition, it assists in flexion of the proximal phalanx and in

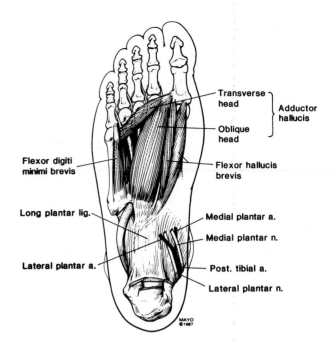

FIG. 1-20. Illustration of the third muscle layer of the foot.

maintaining the transverse arch. It is supplied by the lateral plantar arteries and nerve.[15,19]

The flexor digiti minimi brevis arises from the cuboid and base of the fifth metatarsal and inserts in the lateral base of the proximal phalanx of the fifth toe (see Fig. 1-20). The muscle serves as a flexor of the small toe and is supplied by branches of the lateral plantar nerve and artery.[15,19]

The fourth and deepest layer of plantar muscles consists of seven interosseous muscles—three plantar and four dorsal (see Fig. 1-17; Fig. 1-21). The four dorsal interossei arise with two heads from the adjacent aspects of the metatarsal bases (see Fig. 1-21). The tendons insert into the bases of the proximal phalanges with the two medial bellies inserting on the medial and lateral side of the second and the third and fourth inserting on the lateral sides of the third and fourth proximal phalanges. The three plantar interosseous muscles arise from the bases of the third through fifth metatarsals and insert on the medial sides of the proximal phalanges of the thirrd, fourth, and fifth toes. Thus, the dorsal interossei are abductors and the plantar interossei adductors. All interossei muscles are supplied by branches of the lateral plantar artery and nerve.[15,18,55]

The extensor digitorum brevis (see Figs. 1-13 and 1-16A) is the dorsal muscle of the foot. This broad, thin muscle arises from the superior calcaneus, the lateral talocalcaneal ligament, and the extensor retinaculum. It takes a medial oblique course ending in four tendons that insert in the lateral aspect of the proximal phalanx of the great toe and the lateral extensor digitorum longus tendons of the second to fourth toes.[15,19]

The muscle extends the great toe and second through fourth toes. It is supplied by the deep peroneal nerve and

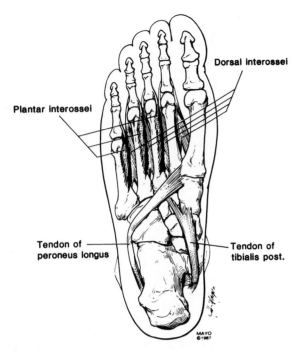

FIG. 1-21. Illustration of the fourth muscle layer of the foot.

dorsalis pedis artery. The muscles of the foot are summarized in Table 1-2.

Soft tissue contrast provided by MRI and, to a lesser degree, CT has popularized the compartment concept for evaluating soft tissue infection and neoplasms in the foot.[12,14,73] Although this concept is controversial, most clinicians consider that the plantar compartments of the foot are di-

vided by intermuscular septa that extend dorsally from the plantar aponeurosis (Fig. 1-22).[12–14] The medial septum (Fig. 1-22A) courses dorsally from the aponeurosis to attach to the navicular, the medial cuneiform, and the lateral plantar aspect of the first metatarsal. The lateral septum (see Fig. 1-22A) extends from the aponeurosis to the medial aspect of the fifth metatarsal. Thus, the lateral, central or intermediate, and medial compartments are created (see Fig. 1-22).[14,73] The medial compartment (see Figs. 1-17 and 1-22) contains the abductor hallucis and flexor hallucis brevis muscles and the flexor hallucis longus tendon. The lateral compartment (see Figs. 1-17 and 1-22) contains the flexor digiti brevis and abductor digiti minimi. The central compartment contains three layers described earlier including the flexor digitorum brevis, the flexor digitorum longus tendon, the quadratus plantae, the lumbrical muscles, and the adductor hallucis.[14,15,19,55] Infections tend to follow these compartments.[14]

Neurovascular Supply of the Foot

The anterior tibial artery continues over the midanterior aspect of the tibia passing deep to the extensor tendons and retinacula of the ankle (see Fig. 1-16B). At the ankle, the anterior tibial artery anastomoses with the perforating branch of the peroneal artery, both supplying the periarticular structures of the ankle.[15,19,55] As the anterior tibial artery emerges from the extensor retinaculum, it becomes the more superficial dorsalis pedis artery. After giving off the deep plantar artery, it becomes the first dorsal metatarsal artery. This ves-

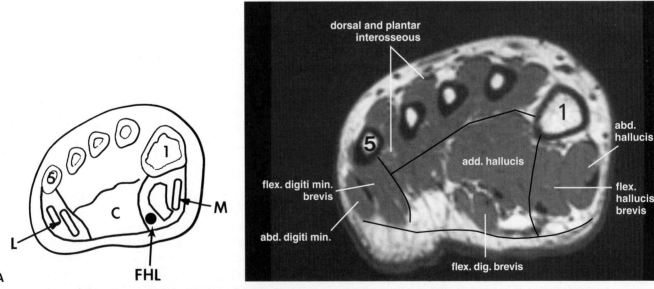

FIG. 1-22. A: Axial illustration through the proximal metatarsals demonstrating the lateral compartment (*L*), central compartment (*C*), and medial compartment (*M*). The medial compartment contains the flexor hallucis longus tendon (*FHL*). **B:** Axial magnetic resonance image demonstrating the compartments of the foot with muscular anatomy.

TABLE 1-2. *Muscles of the foot*[a]

Location	Muscle	Origin	Insertion	Action	Innervation (Segment)	Blood Supply
Plantar Superficial first layer	Abductor hallucis	Medial calcaneus, plantar aponeurosis, and flexor retinaculum	Proximal phalanx great toe	Flexor and abductor of MTP joint great toe	Medial plantar nerve (L5, S1)	Medial plantar artery
	Flexor digitorum brevis	Medial calcaneus plantar fascia	Middle phalanges 2–5 toes	Flexor of toes	Medial plantar nerve (L5, S1)	Medial plantar artery
	Abductor digiti minimi	Lateral process calcaneal tubercle	Lateral base proximal phalanx small toe	Abductor and flexor of small toe	Lateral plantar nerve (S1, S2)	Lateral plantar artery
Second layer	Quadratus plantae	Medial and lateral calcaneal tuberosity	Flexor digitorum longus tendon	Flexor of terminal phalanges 2–5	Lateral plantar nerve (S1, S2)	Lateral plantar artery
	Lumbricals	Flexor digitorum longus tendon	MTP joints 2–5	Flexor of MTP joints	Medial and lateral plantar nerve (S1, S2)	Medial and lateral plantar arteries
Third layer	Flexor hallucis brevis	Cuboid, cuneiform	Great toe	Flexor of great toe	Medial plantar nerve (L5, S1)	Medial and lateral plantar artery
	Adductor hallucis	2–4 metatarsal bases and 3–5 capsules transverse leg	Great toe	Adductor of great toe, maintains transverse arch	Lateral plantar nerve (L5, S1)	Lateral plantar artery
	Flexor digiti minimi brevis	Cuboid and fifth metatarsal base	Proximal phalanx fifth toe	Flexor of fifth toe	Lateral plantar nerve (S1, S2)	Lateral plantar artery
Fourth layer	Interossei dorsal	Metatarsal bases	Bases 2–4 proximal phalanges	Abductor of toes	Lateral plantar nerve (S1, S2)	Lateral plantar artery
	Plantar	Metatarsal bases	Bases of 3–5 proximal phalanges	Abductor of toes	Lateral plantar nerve (S1, S2)	Lateral plantar artery
Dorsal	Extensor digitorum brevis	Superior calcaneus, lateral talocalcaneal ligament, extensor retinaculum	Lateral 1–4 toes	Extensor of toes 1–4	Deep peroneal nerve (L5, S1)	Dorsalis pedis artery

MTP, Metatarsophalangeal.
[a] Data from references 1, 12, 19, and 21.

sel courses distally, ending in digital branches of the first and second toes. Dorsal branches of the foot include medial and lateral tarsal arteries and the arcuate artery with its dorsal metatarsal branches (Fig. 1-23).[15,19,36,55]

The deep peroneal nerve accompanies the anterior tibial, dorsalis pedis, and first dorsal metatarsal arteries. It supplies the anterior muscles of the foot and leg. The superficial peroneal nerve courses over the anterior aspect of the fibula and supplies the peroneal muscles and the lateral aspect of the foot (see Fig. 1-23).[1,15,19]

The posterior tibial artery divides into medial and lateral plantar branches deep to the flexor retinaculum.[15,19,36] It is accompanied by similarly named nerves and veins. The neural branches (medial and lateral plantar nerves) are branches of the tibial nerve (Fig. 1-24).[15,19,55,74]

The medial plantar artery is the smaller of the two branches of the posterior tibial artery and ends in digital branches to the first toe. The lateral plantar artery is larger and forms an arch at the midfoot level, which gives off four metatarsal arteries with their distal digital branches (see Fig.

1-24).[1,15,19] The lateral plantar artery also gives off perforating muscular branches that anastomose with the dorsal arteries. Numerous minor variations in the digital arteries have been described.[15,33,36]

The peroneal artery passes inferior to the lateral malleolus and ends on the calcaneal surface in the lateral calcaneal artery.[15,19,55] Table 1-2 summarizes the neurovascular supply to the muscles of the foot.

SKELETAL AND ARTICULAR ANATOMY

Developmental Anatomy

The limb buds appear during the fourth week of gestation.[2] With normal development, the cartilaginous model becomes well formed in 7 to 8 weeks or at the 21st fetal stage.[8,61] Normally, the proximal structures of the extremity develop before the distal structures. Abnormal progression or failure of the limbs to develop can occur. The following terms are frequently used to define abnormalities in limb development:

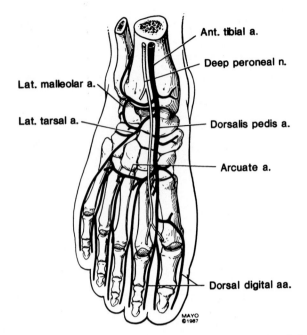

FIG. 1-23. Illustration of the dorsal vascular supply of the foot.

Amelia: congenital absence of a limb or limbs.

Hemimelia: absence of all or part of the distal limb; the proximal limb is normal.

Phocomelia: congenital absence of the proximal limbs such that the feet or hands are attached to the trunk by an anomalous segment.

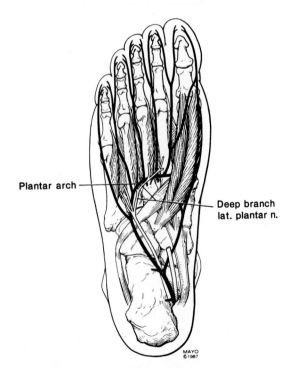

FIG. 1-24. Plantar neurovascular anatomy of the foot.

Sympodia: fusion of the lower extremities.

Polydactyly: supernumerary digits on the hands or feet.

Syndactyly: fusion or fleshy webbing between the digits of the hands or feet.

Brachydactyly: abnormal shortness of the fingers or toes.

Hyperphalangism: increased number of phalanges in a given digit.

Bone begins as a fibrous or cartilage model and develops by intramembranous or endochondral ossification.[2,19,51,61] Endochondral ossification is most common in the extremities. Ossification begins in primary and secondary ossification centers, which vary with the specific anatomic site. In tubular bones, the primary center is generally in the central diaphysis, with secondary centers appearing later in the epiphysis.[8,51]

The tibia develops from a central or diaphyseal ossification center and secondary epiphyseal centers proximally and distally. The diaphysis begins to ossify in the seventh fetal week, the proximal epiphysis just before birth, but the distal epiphyses may not appear for 2 years. Fusion of the epiphyseal centers to the tibial shaft occurs proximally at 19 to 20 years and distally at approximately 18 years of age.[8,19,51]

The fibula begins ossification in the eighth fetal week and the proximal and distal epiphyseal centers at 4 and 2 years, respectively. The growth plates close proximally at 19 to 25 years and distally at 18 to 20 years.[8,19,51,55]

The only tarsal bones that are consistently ossified at birth are the talus and calcaneus.[44,45] Table 1-3 summarizes the appearance time of ossification centers and closure of the growth plates in the foot.

Diarthrodial joint structures develop by segmentation of the cartilage model in the central region of chondroblastic transformation.[2,63] This is followed by formation of a joint cavity and the development of intra-articular structures. In the foot and ankle, both fibrous and cartilaginous joints are present. The interosseous membrane is an example of a fibrous joint or syndesmosis. This structure joins the distal tibia and fibula. The remaining joints of the foot and ankle are synovial joints. These joints have articular cartilage on the opposed bony surfaces with a synovial lined capsule.[19,51,50,63] An in-depth discussion of bone and joint formation and histochemical mechanisms of bone growth is available in other sources.[8,19,51,50,63,64] These topics are not discussed here, but from an imaging standpoint, it is important to be aware of developmental changes in bones and joints of the foot and ankle. This helps to prevent errors in interpretation during the growth years and adulthood.

Many anatomic variants can mimic more serious pathologic conditions.[39,46,61,71] These changes are most common in the metaphyseal and epiphyseal areas adjacent to the growth plates. The growth plates of the distal tibia are often irregular, with both sides often visible on anteroposterior and lateral radiographs. Occasionally, small ossification centers are evident adjacent to the growth plates simulating fractures (Fig. 1-25).[47,61] In primary ossification centers, the rate

TABLE 1-3. *Ossification center of the lower extremity*[a]

Site	Appearance		Closure
Leg	Female	Male	
Proximal tibia	Birth–6 mo	2 mo	19 yr
Distal tibia	1–6 mo	2–7 mo	18 yr
Proximal fibula	20–50 mo	27–65 mo	19 yr
Distal fibula	5–13 mo	7–21 mo	18 yr
Foot	Primary Center	Secondary Center	Closure
Calcaneus	3 fetal mo–1 mo		
Posterior tubercle		5–12 yr	12–22 yr
Talus	3.5 fetal mo–2 mo		
Navicular	3 mo–5 yr		
First cuneiform	9 mo–4 yr		
Second cuneiform	9 mo–5 yr		
Third cuneiform	9 fetal mo–3.5 yr		
Cuboid	6 fetal mo–1 yr		
First metatarsal	2–4 fetal mo		
Proximal epiphysis		6–24 mo	13–22 yr
Second–Fifth metatarsals	2–4 fetal mo		
Distal epiphysis 2–5		6–24 mo	13–22 yr
Phalanges			
Great toe	2–4 fetal mo		
Epiphysis proximal phalanx		6–24 mo	12–22 yr
Epiphysis distal phalanx		9–24 mo	12–22 yr (average, 18)
Phalanges 2–5			
Proximal	2–4 fetal mo		
Proximal epiphysis		6–24 mo	12–22 yr
Middle	10 fetal wk–7 yr		
Proximal epiphysis		9–24 mo	12–22 yr (average, 18)
Distal	2–3.5 fetal mo		
Proximal epiphysis		1–2 yr	11–22 yr

[a] Data from references 5, 9, 14, 25, and 44.

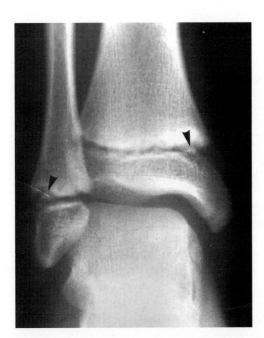

FIG. 1-25. Anteroposterior view of the ankle in a young child. Note the irregularity of the distal tibial and fibular growth plates with small areas of ossification in the growth plates. This appearance should not be confused with growth plate fracture.

of ossification may be irregular, so the ossification center can appear dramatically abnormal. Ossicles are also commonly noted near the medial and lateral malleoli. These frequently cause confusion in patients with recent injury (Figs. 1-26 and 1-27). Ossicles occur medially in 17 to 24% of females and up to 47% of males. Most are bilateral, and they are commonly seen from 6 to 12 years of age.[46] Ossicles are easily detected and characterized on routine radiographs (see Fig. 1-26) and CT. However, they may cause confusion on MRI (see Fig. 1-27). This is one of several reasons why it is important to compare MRI with routine radiographs before interpreting MRI studies.

Normal variants are also common in the tarsal bones.[44,45] The epiphyses of the calcaneus are often irregular, fragmented, and sclerotic. These are normal findings. On the oblique projection, the lucent lines in the epiphysis often project over the calcaneus and simulate a fracture (Fig. 1-28). The calcaneus may develop from two separate ossification centers, in which case a fracture may be simulated.[25,61] This finding is noted in anatomically normal patients, in patients with Hurler's syndrome, and in patients with Down's syndrome.[61]

Nearly 40 accessory ossicles have been described in the foot and ankle.[57] Most are asymptomatic; however, if they are large enough, symptoms from pressure on local struc-

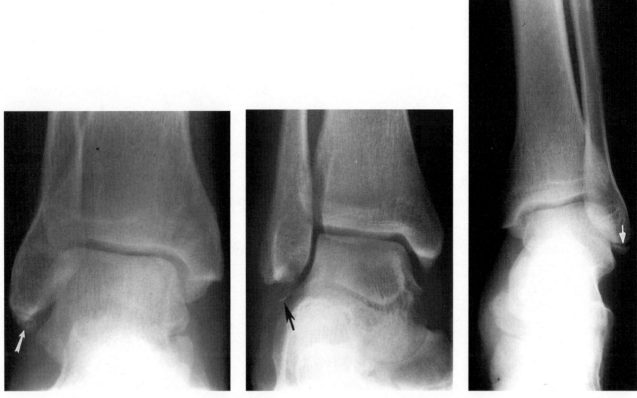

FIG. 1-26. A: Anteroposterior view of the ankle showing the os subfibulare (*arrow*). This normal variant has a well-defined cortical margin and should not be confused with an avulsion fracture. Compare this to avulsion fractures in two different patients. **B:** The first case has several flake avulsions (*arrow*). **C:** The fracture is more difficult to differentiate from an ossicle, except for the irregularity of the fracture margin (*arrow*).

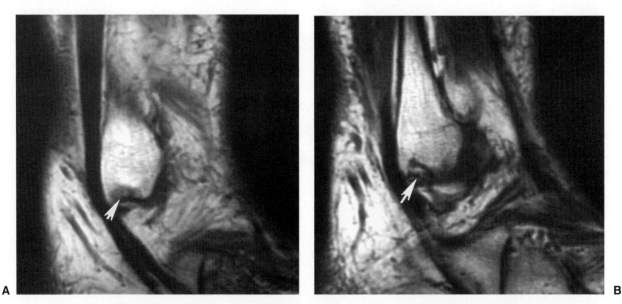

FIG. 1-27. A and **B:** Sagittal spin-echo 500/10 magnetic resonance images demonstrating a small os subfibulare (*arrow*). Determining whether an abnormality or an ossicle is present can be difficult, depending on the size and marrow content.

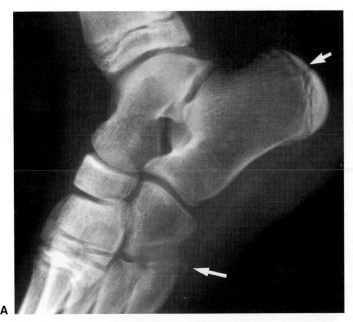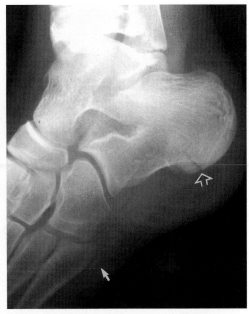

A

B

FIG. 1-28. Lateral (**A**) and oblique (**B**) views of the calcaneus in a 13-year-old boy. The calcaneal apophysis is sclerotic and segmented (*white arrow* in **A**). **B:** On the oblique view, the lucent area between the ossified portions mimics a fracture (*open arrow*). Note also the parallel orientation of the epiphysis at the base of the fifth metatarsal (*white arrows* **A** and **B**).

tures or decreased range of motion may develop. The accessory calcaneus is rare. This ossicle is usually located laterally near the talocalcaneal articulation. Special views or CT may be required to identify this ossicle.[29]

About 10% of children have a well-marginated lucent area in the midcalcaneus (Fig. 1-29) because of a lack of trabecular bone in this region. This should not be confused with a neoplasm.[61,62] This lucent area results from reduced trabecular bone surrounded a trabecular pattern emphasized by the calcaneal stress pattern.[62] Sclerotic bone islands are also common in the calcaneus, and these are of no clinical significance.[25,61,62]

Posterior to the talus, the flexor hallucis longus tendon

normally passes between the medial and lateral tubercles. The lateral tubercle may be prominent (Fig. 1-30). In this setting, the lateral process may be referred to as Stieda's process.[71] A small bone fragment may be present adjacent to the lateral tubercle that is termed the os trigonum. It appears at 8 to 11 years and normally fuses at 16 to 20 years of age. This somewhat controversial ossification center is the posterior part of the talar tubercle located lateral to the flexor hallucis longus tendon. If this center does not fuse to the talus, it is called the os trigonum tarsi. The unfused ossification center may be asymptomatic or may actually represent a fracture. Impingement of this ossicle in plantar flexion may result in os trigonum syndrome

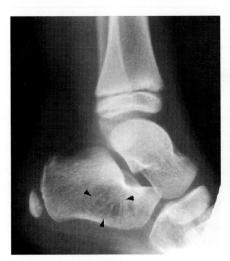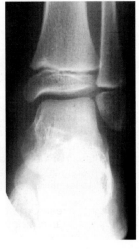

FIG. 1-29. Normal lucent area in the calcaneus (*arrows*).

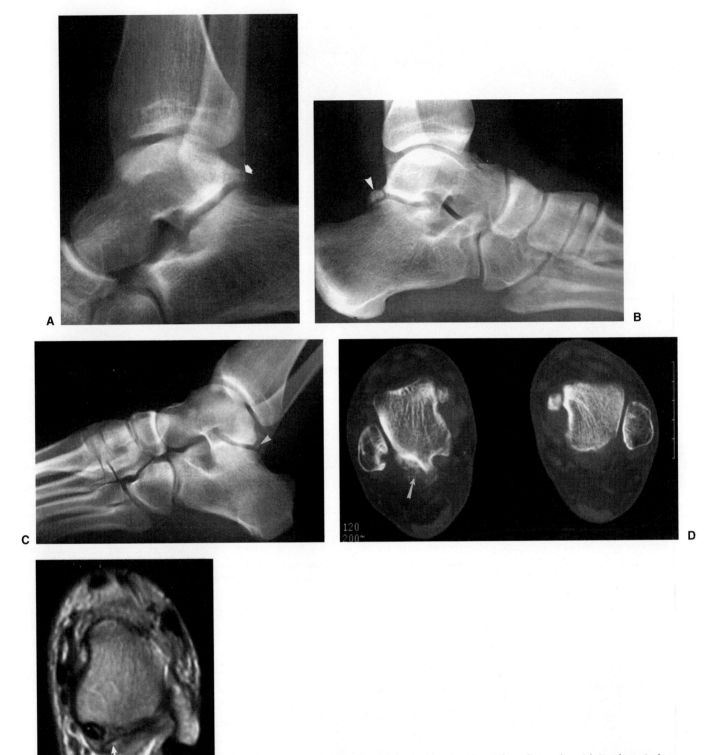

FIG. 1-30. A: Lateral view of the ankle showing a fused prominent lateral posterior talar process (*arrow*). **B** and **C:** The variation in appearance of the os trigonum (*arrow-heads*). **C:** The smaller ossicles may be more difficult to differentiate from fractures because the cortical margins are less obvious. **D:** Axial computed tomography image demonstrating fragmentation of the os trigonum (*arrow*) in a patient with os trigonum syndrome. **E:** Axial spin-echo 2000/20 magnetic resonance image. The os trigonum (*arrow*) may be difficult to identify if too little marrow exists.

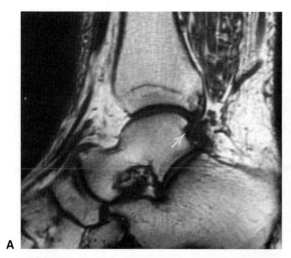 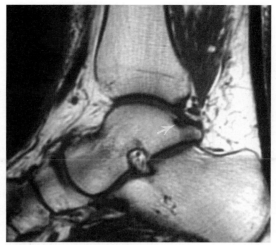

FIG. 1-31. A and **B:** Sagittal spin-echo 500/10 images demonstrating the low-intensity pseudodefect near the posterior articular margin of the talus (*arrow*).

(see Fig. 1-30).[25,39,43,71] The os supratalar near the anterior superior margin of the talus may also be mistaken for a fracture.[25,61]

Another talar variant has been described which may cause confusion on MRI (Fig. 1-31).[34,42] A pseudodefect seen as low intensity on T1- and T2-weighted sequences near the posterior articular surface of the talus is a common finding. This pseudodefect is not visible radiographically. On MRI, both tali are involved in 86% of patients. This signal abnormality should not be confused with an erosion, osteochondral fracture or avascular necrosis.[42]

The navicular mineralizes in an irregular fashion. This appearance may persist for years mimicking osteonecrosis (Fig. 1-32). Another common finding is the accessory navic-

ular or os tibiale externum (Fig. 1-33).[25,32,61] This lies in the posterior tibial tendon just proximal to the medial margin of the navicular. This ossicle may effect tendon function, especially during puberty when growth is accelerated.[35,61] Resection may be required to relieve the painful symptoms. The os supranaviculare (Fig. 1-34) is located at the proximal dorsal margin of the navicular distal to the joint space. This is more distal than the os supratalare, which is located proximal to the talonavicular joint.[25,32] The cuboid also develops from multiple ossification centers and may have an irregular appearance in childhood.[25,44]

Multiple normal variants have also been described in the forefoot (Figs. 1-35 and 1-36). Conical epiphyseal ossification centers can be seen in the phalanges of asymptomatic

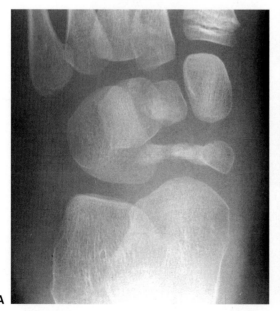 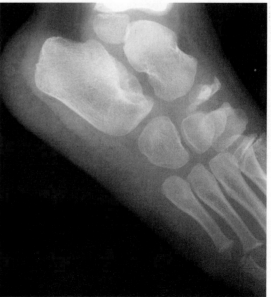

FIG. 1-32. Anteroposterior (**A**) and oblique (**B**) views of the foot in an asymptomatic child. Note the flat and irregular appearance of the partially ossified navicular. The space between the talus and the cuneiforms is normal.

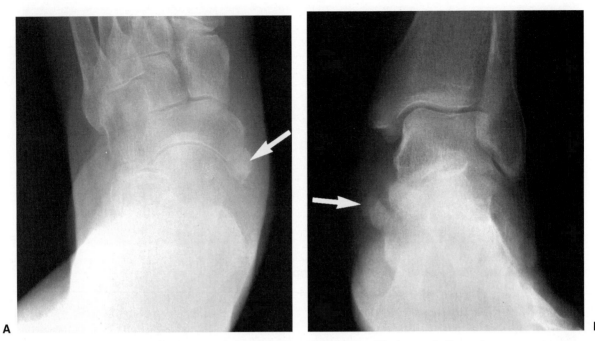

A   B

FIG. 1-33. Anteroposterior views of the foot (**A**) and the ankle (**B**) demonstrating a large accessory navicular (*arrow*) or os tibiale externum.

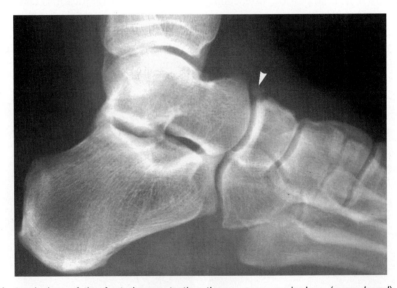

FIG. 1-34. Lateral view of the foot demonstrating the os supranaviculare (*arrowhead*). The cortical margins of this large ossicle are easily seen, thus allowing it to be easily differentiated from an avulsion fracture.

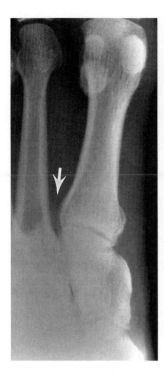 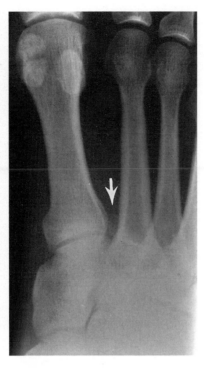

FIG. 1-35. Normal ossicle, os intermetatarsareum (*arrows*), located proximally between the first and second metatarsals of both feet.

children (Fig. 1-37). In a study of 1,800 anatomically normal children, these changes were noted in 4 to 26% of children 4 to 15 years old.[22] These epiphyseal changes are usually bilateral and may fuse earlier than the normal epiphysis. Involvement of only the third toe has been reported.[22,61]

Normal dysplastic splitting of the epiphysis and metaphyseal margin clefts are not uncommon. These findings can also be mistaken for a fracture. These changes have been noted more commonly in the distal phalanx of the great toe (Figs. 1-38 and 1-39).[25,70]

The secondary ossification center at the base of the proximal lateral fifth metatarsal is usually a flat, sliver-like structure with the growth plate parallel to the shaft (see Fig. 1-28B). This may ossify laterally first giving the appearance of an avulsed or displaced epiphysis. Comparison with the opposite foot assists in excluding this uncommon problem.

Fractures of the fifth metatarsal base are usually perpendicular to the shaft (Fig. 1-40).[46]

The most frequently noted ossicles in the foot are summarized in Figure 1-41. More thorough discussions of normal variants can be found in Silverman and Kuhn,[61] Keats,[25] O'Rahilly,[44] and Schmidt and Freyschmidt.[58]

Osseous and Ligamentous Structures of the Ankle

The ankle is composed of three bones; the tibia, the fibula, and the talus (Fig. 1-42).[13,15,19,43] The tibia is the second longest bone in the skeleton. It is expanded proximally and distally. The body of the tibia (diaphysis) has three surfaces (anterior, medial, and posterior). The anterior surface ends in the medial malleolus. The medial margin is subcutaneous.

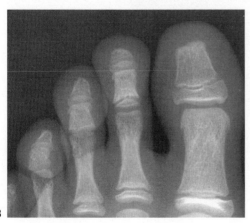 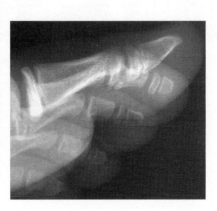

A,B

FIG. 1-36. Anteroposterior (**A**) and lateral (**B**) views of the phalanges demonstrating normal flattening of the tufts of the distal phalanges.

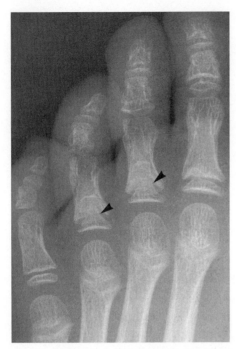

FIG. 1-37. Anteroposterior view of the forefoot showing a cone-shaped epiphysis in the third and fourth proximal phalanges.

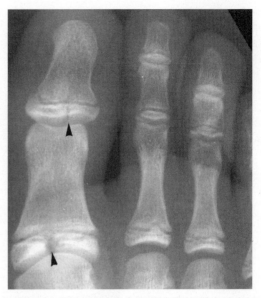

FIG. 1-38. Anteroposterior view of the forefoot with split epiphyses (*black arrowheads*) in the proximal and distal phalanges of the great toe.

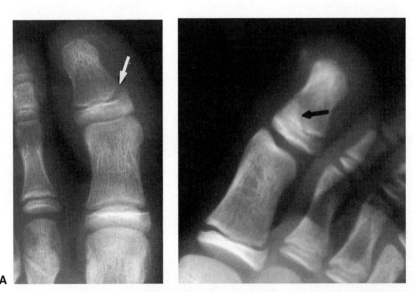

FIG. 1-39. Anteroposterior (**A**) and oblique (**B**) views of the great toe showing normal metaphyseal clefts (*arrows*).

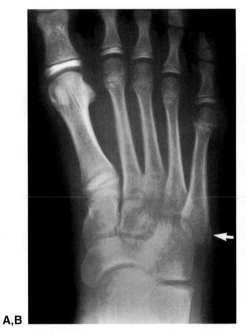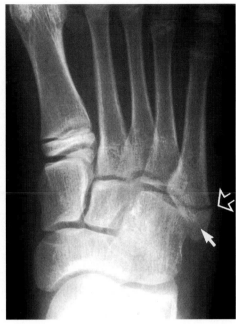

A,B

FIG. 1-40. A: Anteroposterior view of the foot demonstrating the normal epiphysis parallel to the fifth metatarsal base (*arrow*). **B:** Partially fused epiphyses (*arrow*) and transverse fracture (*open arrow*) of the fifth metatarsal base.

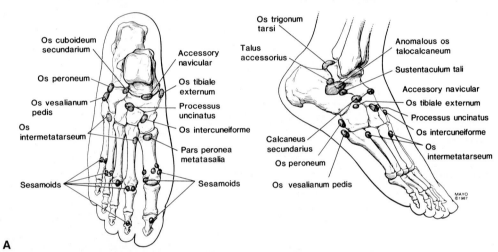

Os cuboideum secundarium

Accessory navicular

Os peroneum

Os tibiale externum

Os vesalianum pedis

Processus uncinatus

Os intermetatarseum

Os intercuneiforme

Pars peronea metatasalia

Sesamoids

Sesamoids

A

Os trigonum tarsi

Talus accessorius

Anomalous os talocalcaneum

Sustentaculum tali

Accessory navicular

Os tibiale externum

Processus uncinatus

Os intercuneiforme

Calcaneus secundarius

Os intermetatarseum

Os peroneum

Os vesalianum pedis

MAYO ©1987

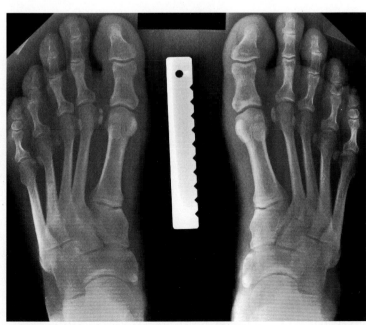

B

FIG. 1-41. A: Illustration of ossicles in the foot. **B:** Standing posteroanterior views of the feet demonstrating sesamoids at all metatarsophalangeal joints.

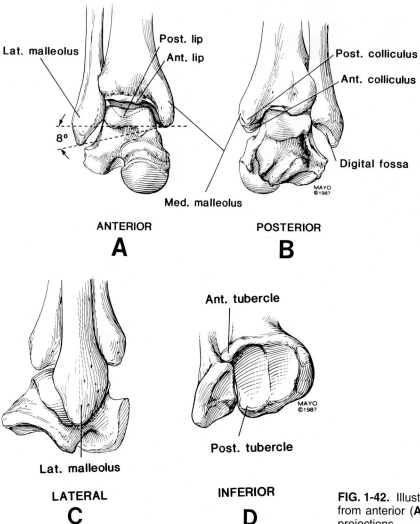

Lat. malleolus

Post. lip
Ant. lip

8°

Med. malleolus

ANTERIOR
A

Post. colliculus
Ant. colliculus

Digital fossa

MAYO
©1987

POSTERIOR
B

Lat. malleolus

LATERAL
C

Ant. tubercle

Post. tubercle

MAYO
©1987

INFERIOR
D

FIG. 1-42. Illustration of the bony anatomy of the ankle seen from anterior (A), posterior (B), lateral (C), and inferior (D) projections.

The interosseous membrane attaches to the lateral margin (see Fig. 1-2).[55]

Distally, the tibia expands at the metaphysis, forming the medial malleolus and the articular surface for the talus (see Fig. 1-42).[19,55] The inferior or articular surface is biconcave and articulates with the talar dome.[3] Hyaline cartilage covers the articular surface of the tibia and extends medially to the articular portion of the medial malleolus. The articular cartilage does not completely cover the posterior tibia (posterior malleolus) (Fig. 1-43). This is significant because if only small segments of the posterior malleolus are fractured, the articular portion may be excluded.[3,55]

The anterior surface of the tibia is smooth, except at the anterior inferior margin, where it is more irregular at the site for attachment of the anterior ankle capsule. The posterior tibia has grooves for the flexor hallucis longus (lateral) and flexor digitorum longus and tibialis posterior tendons (medial). The lateral surface articulates with the fibula. This articular surface is bounded anteriorly and posteriorly by ridges for insertion of the anterior and posterior distal tibiofibular ligaments (see Fig. 1-42). The strong medial exten-

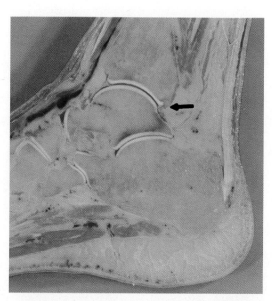

FIG. 1-43. Frozen anatomic section through the tibiotalar joint demonstrating the articular cartilage and posterior tibia (*arrow*), which is incompletely covered by cartilage.

sion (medial malleolus) articulates with the talus and forms the medial portion of the ankle mortise.[3,15,19,55]

The fibula is thin and flat and does not have a direct weight-bearing surface (see Fig. 1-2). The lateral malleolus is the expanded distal portion of the fibula. The fibula is irregular along its medial margin at the point of attachment for the interosseous ligament. Hyaline cartilage covers the articular surface on the inferomedial aspect. Irregular areas are noted anteriorly and posteriorly for insertions of the tibiofibular ligaments. The fibula (lateral malleolus) is more posterior than the medial malleolus and its distal extent is below the level of the medial malleolar tip.[3] Thus, an angle of approximately 8° is formed by a line drawn from the tips of the malleoli (see Fig. 1-42).[21] The posterior position of the lateral malleolus results in an angle of 20° between the malleoli in the axial plane. For this reason, the mortise view of the ankle is taken with the foot internally rotated approximately 20° (see Chapter 2) (Fig. 1-44).[3,15]

The hyaline cartilage trochlear surface of the talus is usually 2 to 3 mm wider anteriorly than posteriorly. It articulates with the weight-bearing surface of the tibia and the medial and lateral malleoli. Thus, the ankle mortise is formed by the tibial and fibular components of the ankle that roofs the talus (Fig. 1-45).[3,19,24,26] The tibial portion of the mortise is termed the plafond.[3,21,26] Forces on the talus that result in position changes of this structure in the mortise are responsible for many osseous or ligamentous ankle injuries.[3,21,26,30,31]

The supporting structures of the ankle include the joint capsule, the medial and lateral ligaments, and the interosseous ligament (Fig. 1-46). In addition, 13 tendons cross the ankle, and there are 4 retinacula.[3,26] Four ligaments support the distal tibia and fibula.[15,26] The interosseous ligament, with its oblique fibers, joins the tibia and fibula to a level just above the joint. The interosseous ligament is the thickened distal portion of the interosseous membrane. The tibial and fibular attachments of this ligament form a triangular configuration that is weakened at its base by the syndesmotic recess (Fig. 1-47). This recess is an extension of the joint into the tibiofibular space. The distal anterior and posterior tibiofibular ligaments join the tibia and fibula just proximal to the tibiotalar joint (see Fig. 1-46). The anterior ligament is weaker than the posterior. This explains the increased incidence of avulsion fractures posteriorly, compared with ligament disruptions.[3,21,26] The transverse ligament is the fourth ligament of the syndesmotic group. This ligament lies anterior to the posterior tibiofibular ligament and extends from the lateral malleolus to the posterior articular margin of the tibia just lateral to the medial malleolus.[12,13,18,61,67] The ligament actually forms part of the posterior articulation with the talus (see Fig. 1-46).

The posterior intermalleolar ligament is a normal variant that lies between the posterior tibiofibular ligament and the posterior talofibular ligament (see Fig. 1-46E; Fig. 1-48). The posterior intermalleolar ligament has received some attention in the orthopedic literature because of its association with posterior impingement syndrome.[21,26,54] Rosenberg and colleagues[54] studied MRI features of this ligament and found that it was most easily detected on axial or coronal images. The ligament was identified on 19% of clinical MRI studies (see Fig. 1-48).[54] The ligaments may be more easily studied using three-dimensional gradient-echo images.

The deltoid ligament provides medial stability.[3,12,13,19] This ligament is a strong triangular group of fibers with its apex at the medial malleolus. The ligament fans out as it progresses inferiorly and divides into superficial and deep fibers.[3,19] The superficial fibers insert in the navicular tuberosity. Progressing posteriorly, the remaining superficial fi-

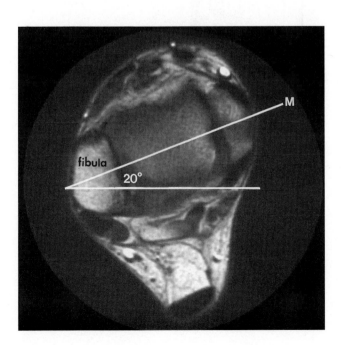

FIG. 1-44. Axial magnetic resonance image through the ankle mortise. The malleoli align (line *M*) 20° externally because of the posterior position of the fibula.

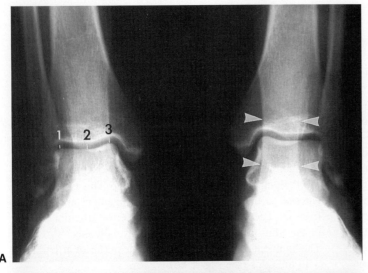

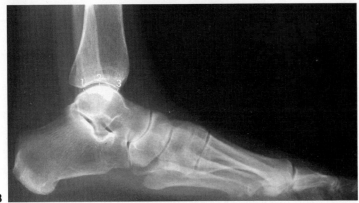

FIG. 1-45. Anteroposterior (**A**) and lateral (**B**) standing views demonstrate the width of the ankle joint measured at three sites: males, 3.5 ± 0.6 mm; females, 2.9 ± 0.4 mm; or females 15% less width than males.[23] The Achilles tendon (*arrowheads* in **A**) projects over the ankle.

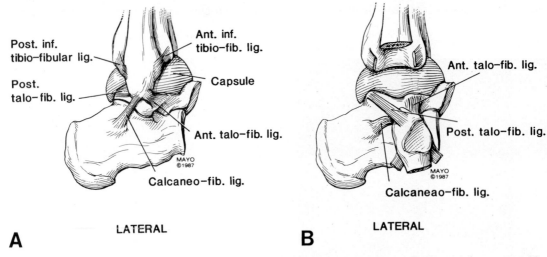

FIG. 1-46. Illustrations of the ligaments of the ankle. **A:** Lateral ligaments. **B:** Lateral ligaments with fibula displaced. *(continued)*

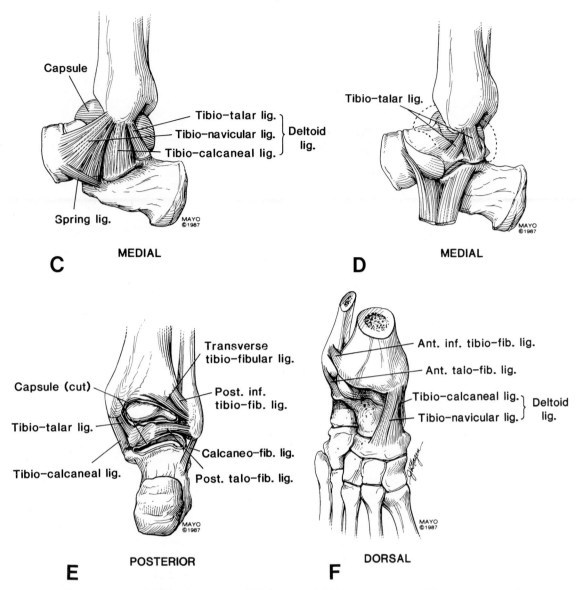

C MEDIAL

Capsule

Tibio-talar lig.
Tibio-navicular lig. ⎫ Deltoid
Tibio-calcaneal lig. ⎭ lig.

Spring lig.

MAYO
©1987

D MEDIAL

Tibio-talar lig.

MAYO
©1987

E POSTERIOR

Transverse
tibio-fibular lig.

Capsule (cut)

Post. inf.
tibio-fib. lig.

Tibio-talar lig.

Tibio-calcaneal lig.

Calcaneo-fib. lig.

Post. talo-fib. lig.

MAYO
©1987

F DORSAL

Ant. inf. tibio-fib. lig.

Ant. talo-fib. lig.

Tibio-calcaneal lig. ⎫ Deltoid
Tibio-navicular lig. ⎭ lig.

MAYO
©1987

FIG. 1-46. *Continued.* **C:** Medial ligaments. **D:** Medial ligaments with superficial fibers retracted inferiorly. **E:** Posterior view of ligaments. **F:** Dorsal view of ligaments.

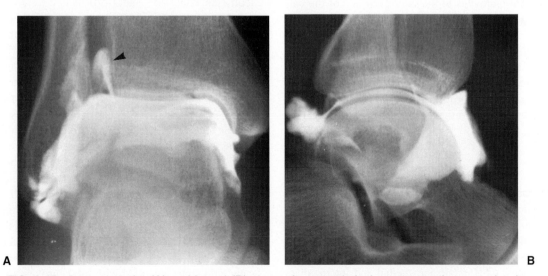

FIG. 1-47. Anteroposterior (**A**) and lateral (**B**) views of a normal single contrast arthrogram showing the configuration of the ankle capsule and syndesmotic recess (*black arrowhead*).

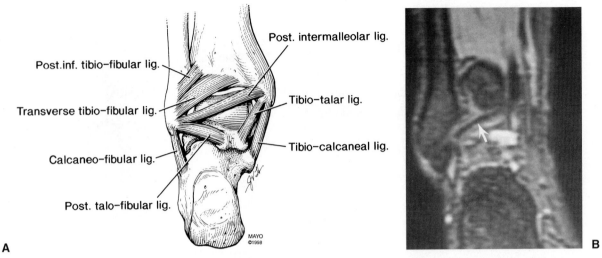

FIG. 1-48. Posterior intermalleolar ligament. **A:** Posterior illustration. **B:** Three-dimensional gradient-recalled echo coronal image demonstrating the posterior intermalleolar ligament (*arrow*).

bers insert in the sustentaculum tali and the talus. The deep fibers attach to the medial surface of the talus (see Fig. 1-46).[15,21,26,30,31] The deltoid ligament prevents excessive abduction and eversion of the ankle and subtalar joints. In addition, eversion, pronation, and anterior displacement of the talus are restricted.[12]

Three ligaments are present laterally. The anterior talofibular ligament is the weakest and most frequently injured.[3] It passes anteriorly from the fibula to insert anterior to the lateral talar articular facet.[15,19] This ligament restrains the anterior talar motion.[12] The posterior talofibular ligament is much stronger and courses transversely from the posterior aspect of the lateral malleolus to the posterior talar tubercle. The ligament prevents posterior talar motion (see Fig. 1-46). The calcaneofibular ligament (see Fig. 1-46) is the longest of the three ligaments and takes a nearly vertical course from the lateral malleolus to the lateral surface of the calcaneus. The calcaneofibular ligament prevents excessive inversion.[3,12] The peroneal tendons are just superficial to the calcaneofibular ligament.

The synovial-lined capsule of the ankle is attached to the acetabular margins of the tibia, the fibula, and the talus. The anterior and posterior portions of the capsule are thin and provide much less support than the foregoing ligaments (see Fig. 1-47).[3,15,19,21,26]

Foot

For purposes of discussion, the foot can be divided into three segments: the hindfoot (talus and calcaneus), the midfoot (remaining five tarsal bones), and the forefoot (metatarsals and phalanges) segments.[3,12] Three longitudinal columns have also been described. The medial column consists of the calcaneus, talus, navicular, medial and intermediate cuneiforms, and the first and second metatarsals and phalanges. The tibialis posterior tendon acts as a supporting sling for the medial arch along with the spring ligament.[56] The middle column consists of the lateral cuneiform and third metatarsal and phalanges. The lateral column is made up of the hindfoot (talus and calcaneus) and the fourth and fifth metatarsal with their phalanges.[3,12] All articulations are synovial joints that are supported by strong plantar and weaker dorsal ligaments.[3,15,19,55]

Hindfoot

The hindfoot includes the talus and calcaneus (Figs. 1-49 and 1-50).[3,15,46] The talus is the second largest of the tarsal bone and articulates with the tibia, medial and lateral malleoli, and calcaneus inferiorly (see Figs. 1-42 and 1-46). The talar head articulates with the navicular.[15,19,55]

Superiorly, the trochlear articulates with the tibia and malleoli (see Figs. 1-49 and 1-50). It is covered with hyaline cartilage and makes up the upper portion of the body of the talus.[3,4] The inferior surface of the talus has three articular facets (see Figs. 1-48 through 1-50).[1,3,15,16,19,55] The anterior and posterior facets articulate with similarly named calcaneal facets. The middle facet is just posterior to the anterior calcaneal articular facet. The middle facet articulates with the sustentaculum tali.[3,15] The talar sulcus lies between the middle and anterior facets. This structure, with its calcaneal counterpart, forms the tarsal sinus that contains the interosseous talocalcaneal ligament. The tarsal canal and sinus (see Figs. 1-49 and 1-50) can be identified radiographically. However, optimal imaging with CT or MRI in multiple image planes is preferred.[10,15,28] The cone-shaped region is located between the posterior subtalar joint and the talocalcaneonavicular joint (see Fig. 1-50).[28] The sinus is larger laterally and angles about 45° to the calcaneal axis. The canal and sinus are filled with fat, neurovascular structures (branches of posterior tibial and peroneal arteries), and five ligaments. Ligaments include the interosseous talocalcaneal

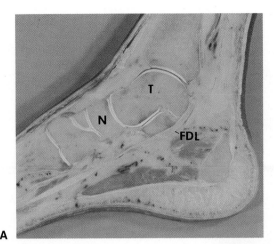

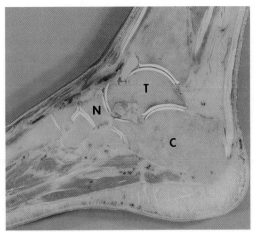

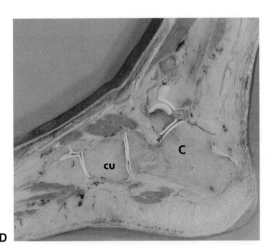

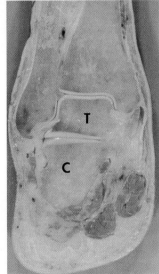

FIG. 1-49. Anatomic sections of the hindfoot and midfoot. **A:** Sagittal section medially at level of the flexor digitorum longus (*FDL*). *T,* talus; *N,* navicular. **B:** Sagittal section demonstrating talo-calcaneal and talonavicular articulations. **C:** Sagittal (*N,* navicular; *C,* calcaneus; *T,* talus) section through the calcaneocuboid articulation. (*C,* calcaneus; *cu,* cuboid). **D:** Coronal section through posterior ankle demonstrating the mortise and posterior subtalar joint. (*T,* talus; *c,* calcaneus). **E:** Coronal section anterior to the fibula in the tarsal canal and sinus region (*arrow*). **F:** Coronal section through the sustentacular (*s*) articulation. **G:** Axial image through the talonavicular and navicular cuneiform articulations (*T,* talus; *N,* navicular).

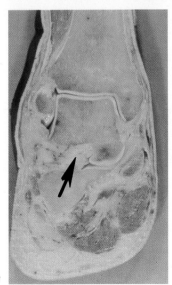

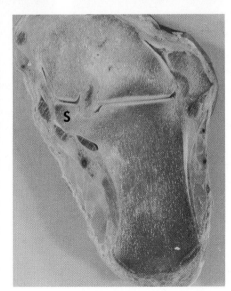

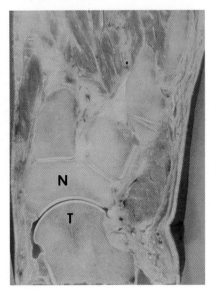

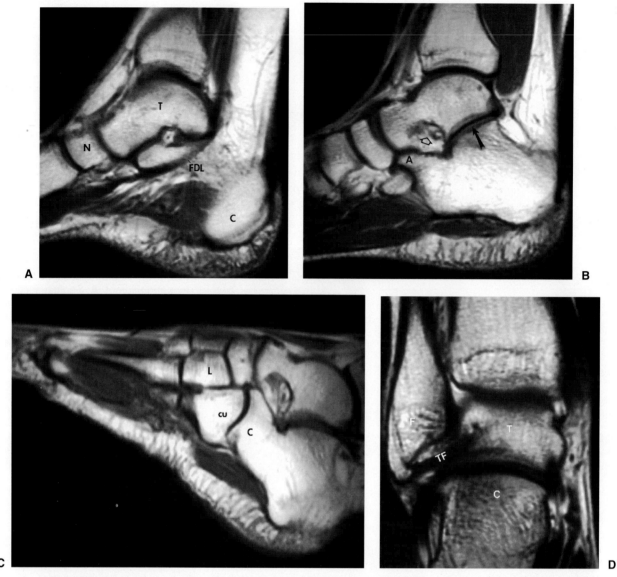

FIG. 1-50. Magnetic resonance images (spin-echo 500/10) demonstrating hindfoot and midfoot anatomy. **A:** Sagittal image at the flexor digitorum longus level (*FDL*). *T,* talus; *N,* navicular; *C,* calcaneus. **B:** Sagittal image at talonavicular level demonstrating the posterior talocalcaneal joint (*arrow*), the tarsal sinus (*open arrow*), and the anterior calcaneal process (*A*). **C:** Sagittal image at the level of the calcaneocuboid articulation. *C,* calcaneus; *cu,* cuboid; *L,* lateral cuneiform. **D:** Coronal image at the level of the posterior talocalcaneal joint. *T,* talus; *C,* calcaneus; *F,* fibula; *TF,* talofibular ligament. *(continued)*

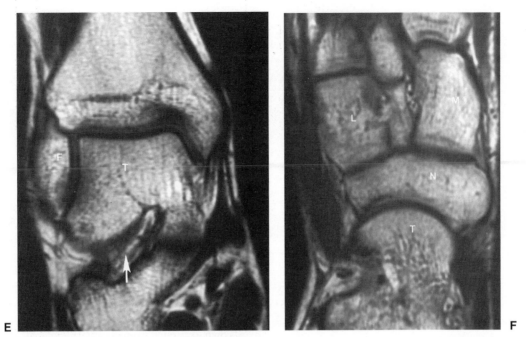

FIG. 1-50. *Continued.* **E:** Coronal image through the tarsal canal and sinus (*arrow*). *T,* talus; *F,* fibula. **F:** Axial oblique image through the talonavicular and navicular cuneiform articulations. *T,* talus; *N,* navicular; *M,* medial cuneiform; *L,* lateral cuneiform.

ligament, the cervical ligament, and three roots (medial, lateral and intermediate) of the extensor retinaculum laterally.[10,15,19,28,65]

The head of the talus articulates with the navicular. The talonavicular joint is at a 30° angle medial to the midpoint of the talar dome (Fig. 1-51A). The talocalcaneal relationship is also important. On the lateral radiograph of a normal foot, the talus and calcaneus form an angle of 50° (see Fig. 1-51B). On the anteroposterior view, this angle is normally 35° (see Fig. 1-51A). These values vary by as much as 20°. The angles are generally smaller in the immature foot.[3,66] The talus articulates with 75% of the navicular in pronation

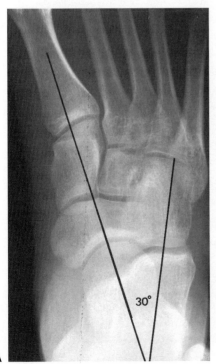

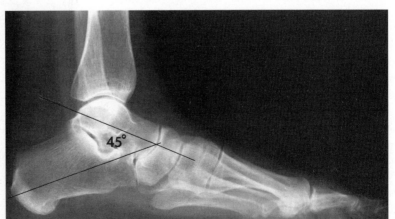

FIG. 1-51. Anteroposterior (**A**) and lateral (**B**) views of the foot showing the talonavicular and talocalcaneal relationships.

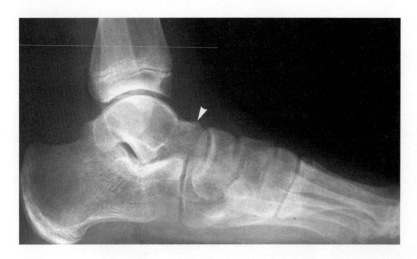

FIG. 1-52. Lateral view of the foot showing a normal ridge (*arrow*) in the dorsal aspect of the talus.

and 100% in supination. The normal talonavicular axis extends into the shaft of the first metatarsal (see Fig. 1-51B). During pronation, this axis is medial and during supination lateral to the first metatarsal head.[72]

Several osseous growths have been described on the talus. These are usually of no clinical significance. A normal ridge is present distal to the trochlear surface on the dorsal lateral aspect of the talus.[49,50] This can be seen on the lateral view of the ankle and should not be confused with a pathologic process. This ridge is the site of attachment of the dorsal talonavicular ligament and anterior tibiotalar joint capsule. Therefore, hypertrophy can occur in patients engaged in activities that require extremes of plantar flexion such as football and ballet dancing (Fig. 1-52).[49] The posterior aspect of the talus contains an oblique groove (Fig. 1-53) for the flexor hallucis longus tendon.[55]

The calcaneus, the largest tarsal bone, contains three superior articular facets.[3,15,16,19] The middle, most medial facet is on the sustentaculum tali. The calcaneal sulcus lies between the middle and anterior facets and forms the floor of the tarsal canal. The distal or plantar surface of the calcaneus contains two grooves. The lateral groove is for the peroneus longus tendon. More medially, the flexor hallucis longus runs in the groove beneath the sustentaculum tali (see Fig. 1-49A)[3,15,19,50]

The posterior aspect of the calcaneus forms the prominence of the heel.[3,15,19] It contains irregular areas superiorly for insertion of the Achilles tendon (superior tuberosity) and medially for the plantar aponeurosis, the flexor digitorum brevis and abductor hallucis, and the lateral inferior processes (abductor digiti minimi) for muscle attachments. The calcaneus articulates with the cuboid anteriorly (see Figs. 1-49 and 1-50).[3,15,19,55]

Two ligaments directly support the talocalcaneal joint. These are the interosseous talocalcaneal ligament that is located in the sinus tarsi and the smaller lateral talocalcaneal ligament (see Figs. 1-49 and 50).[10] In addition, the ligaments of the ankle and adjacent tendons provide stabilization. The latter include the peroneal tendons, the flexor hallucis lon-

gus, the flexor digitorum longus, and the tibialis posterior tendons.[3,15,19]

The posterior talocalcaneal joint has a synovial cavity of its own, separated from the anterior talocalcaneal articulation by the interosseous ligament. The posterior subtalar joint communicates with the ankle in 10% of patients.[3] The anterior joint may communicate with the talonavicular joint or the talocalcaneonavicular joint.[3,15,19]

Midfoot

The remaining tarsal bones make up the midfoot. These include the cuboid, navicular, and three cuneiforms (see Fig. 1-50).[15,19,52]

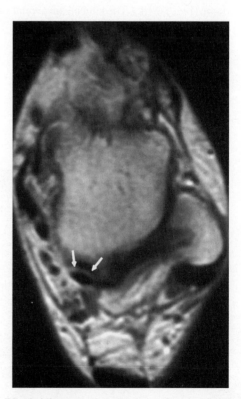

FIG. 1-53. Axial magnetic resonance image demonstrating the talar groove for the flexor hallucis longus tendon (*arrows*).

The cuboid articulates with the calcaneus proximally and distally with the fourth and fifth metatarsals (see Fig. 1-50). Dorsally, the cuboid is roughened at the points of ligament attachment. On the plantar surface, the cuboid contains a groove for the peroneus longus tendon (see Fig. 1-21). The medial cuboid surface contains a facet for articulation with the lateral cuneiform.[1,15,48]

The navicular is on the medial side of the foot anterior to the talus. It articulates proximally with the talus, anteriorly with the cuneiforms, and occasionally with the cuboid laterally (see Figs. 1-49 and 1-50).[3,13,17]

The spring ligament is contiguous with the deltoid ligament of the ankle (see Fig. 1-46C). It extends from the calcaneus to the navicular tuberosity. The cuboideonavicular ligament runs dorsally from the cuboid to the navicular. Proximally, the bifurcated ligament originates on the anterior superior calcaneus and sends medial fibers to the lateral navicular and lateral fibers to the cuboid. The calcaneonavicular ligament is on the plantar aspect of the capsule.[3,15,19,56]

Three cuneiform bones are located distal to the navicular and medial to the cuboid (see Figs. 1-49 and 1-50). The medial cuneiform is the largest and articulates with the navicular proximally, the intermediate cuneiform laterally, and the first and second metatarsals distally (see Fig. 1-50).[3,15] The intermediate cuneiform is the smallest cuneiform and lies between the medial and lateral cuneiforms. It articulates with the latter bones, the navicular, and the second metatarsal. The lateral cuneiform lies between the intermediate cuneiform and the cuboid and articulates with both. It also articulates with the navicular and the second through fourth metatarsals.[1,3,15,19,52]

The five metatarsals articulate proximally with the foregoing tarsal bones (see Fig. 1-23), and each, except the first (great) toe, typically has three phalanges distally. The metatarsals have similar configuration, except the first is broader from the proximal articular surface distally to its head. The fifth metatarsal has a broad base compared with the second through fourth metatarsals.[11,15,19,48]

Dorsal, plantar, and interosseous ligaments support the tarsometatarsal joints and bases of the metatarsals (Fig. 1-54). Distally, the transverse metatarsal ligament connects the heads of the metatarsals. Each of the metatarsophalangeal joints is supported by collateral and plantar ligaments. The extensor tendons replace the usually dorsal ligaments in these joints.[3,15,57]

Arches of the Foot

The foot has three arches, one transverse and two longitudinal arches (Fig. 1-55). The lateral longitudinal arch is formed by the calcaneus, cuboid, and fourth and fifth metatarsals. In a patient with normal gait, this arch normally receives the weight of the body before the medial longitudinal arch.[15,27] The peroneus longus tendon runs through the midpoint of this arch. The medial longitudinal arch is formed by the calcaneus, talus, navicular, cuneiforms, and first through third metatarsals. The vertical height of the medial arch is

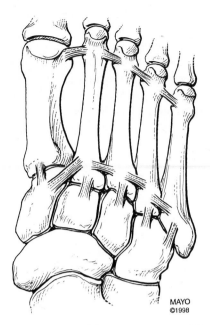

FIG. 1-54. Illustration of the tarsometatarsal ligaments.

greater than that of the lateral arch (see Fig. 1-55). The apex of the arch is more posteriorly located at the talocalcaneonavicular joint. The posterior tibial tendon inserts on the navicular and sends plantar fibers below the arch to add additional support.[3,15,19,27]

The transverse arch is completed when the feet are adjacent such that the two medial longitudinal arches are approximated. Thus, the bases of the metatarsals and midtarsal

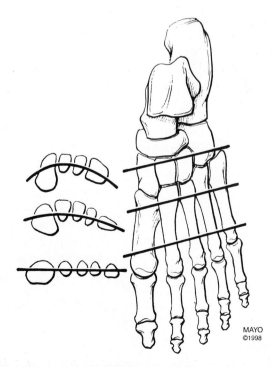

FIG. 1-55. Illustration of the arches of the foot seen at three axial levels.

bones form the arch with support from the peroneus longus and posterior tibial tendons.[3,9,12,15,19,20,21,23,26]

Weight-bearing radiographs (see Chapter 2 and Fig. 1-55) are important for evaluating arch disorders. Kitaoka and colleagues[27] demonstrated motion in all tarsal joints with physiologic loading. Therefore, in clinical conditions that affect motion in one joint such tarsal coalition, it is not unusual for other joints to be affected as well.

BASIC BIOMECHANICS

Terms used to describe the movements in the foot and ankle are often misused. This results in some confusion when using descriptive terms such as supination, eversion, and pronation. Definitions of these commonly used terms are listed in this discussion as they apply during physiologic motion of the foot and ankle (Fig. 1-56).

Plantar Flexion

The hinge motion at the tibiotalar joint allows the foot to plantar flex (sole of foot depressed). Several other motions and position changes occur with plantar flexion. During plantar flexion the gastrocnemius muscle pulls the calcaneus upward which shifts the calcaneus into a slight varus (posterior heel rotated medially) position. The head of the talus turns in and downward during plantar flexion which causes the foot to move inward.[19-21,55]

Dorsiflexion

The hinge motion of the ankle allows the foot to be elevated or dorsiflexed (the foot lifted toward the anterior leg) (see Fig. 1-56). The gastrocnemius muscle is relaxed and the heel shifts into valgus (heel rotated laterally). The talus turns upward and outward and the foot, therefore, also turns outward during dorsiflexion.[19-21,26,27,55]

Inversion

During inversion the sole of the foot is turned inward. In European literature the terms supination and/or adduction (see below) are often used interchangeably. The foot tends to dorsiflex slightly during inversion.[19-21,26,55]

Eversion

During eversion, the sole of the foot is turned outward. The terms pronation or abduction have been used interchangeably with eversion. The foot tends to plantar flex slightly during eversion (see Fig. 1-56).[19-21,26]

Adduction

By definition, adduction means movement of a part toward the axis or midline.[26] The term is most frequently used to describe forces acting on the foot or ankle. Inversion has been used as a term equated to adduction in the literature.

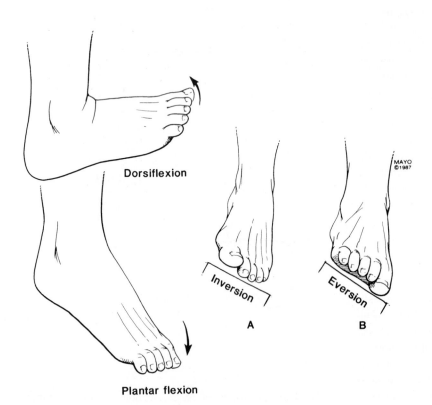

FIG. 1-56. Illustration of common positions of the foot.

I prefer to use the term adduction when describing forces applied to the foot and ankle.[3,19,20,26,30,31]

Abduction

This term indicates motion of a given part away from the midline. Again, terms such as eversion have been used interchangeably. I believe that it is best to use abduction when describing forces moving the foot or ankle outward.[3,19,20,26,30,31]

Supination and Pronation

Supination and pronation are commonly used terms for describing the rotation that occurs at the wrist.[26] Technically, the foot is pronated when the sole is flat. Pronation can occur to a minimal degree with the forefoot abducted and dorsiflexed. Limited supination is possible. Typically, the literature has used pronation and eversion and supination and inversion interchangeably.[26,30,31] I prefer to reserve the terms supination and pronation for the upper extremity. Eversion and inversion are less confusing when describing foot and ankle position.

External Rotation

This term is typically used to define outward rotation of the foot in relation to the longitudinal axis of the leg. With many athletic injuries, the leg actually rotates medially with the foot fixed. Therefore, the foot is actually rotated in an outward (external) position compared with the leg.[19,30,31,49]

Varus

Varus indicates rotation, bending, or positioning inward or toward the midline axis. The term should be used to describe position, not motion.

Valgus

Valgus is used to denote rotation, bending, or positioning away from the axis of the midline. Like varus, the term valgus denotes position. When standing, the weight of the body is distributed through the foot and ankle in a manner that distributes half of the body weight to each extremity. For example, if a person weighs 150 pounds, 75 pounds would be distributed to each side. The contact points of the foot share the weight in a fairly equal fashion. Therefore, the calcaneus shares 75/2 (36.5%) at its posterior contact point, and the other 36.5% is absorbed by the forefoot. The forefoot contact points are the first metatarsal and sesamoids and the lateral four metatarsal heads (see Fig. 1-55).[37,49] The axis is also medial to the foot and ankle, resulting in osseous loading. The ligaments in the normal foot support the normal arches with assistance from the evertor and invertor muscles.[19,23]

MECHANICS OF THE FOOT AND ANKLE MOTION

Ankle motion is essentially limited to flexion and extension. These terms, as noted earlier, are often confusing, and therefore anatomists and surgeons generally prefer the terms dorsiflexion and plantar flexion.[15,16,19,26,54] In the dorsiflexed position, the dorsum of the foot is elevated toward the leg (see Fig. 1-56). In plantar flexion, the heel is toward the posterior portion of the leg, and the sole of the foot is depressed (see Fig. 1-56).[15,19] The talus has no muscle attachments, and its motion is affected only by surrounding osseous and tendinoligamentous structures. During plantar flexion, it rotates inferiorly (see Fig. 1-56) 35° compared with 60° for the foot. Similarly, in dorsiflexion, the talus rotates superiorly 15°, whereas the foot rotates 30°.[26] The head of the talus also rotates medially during plantar flexion and laterally during dorsiflexion.[12,15,26]

The gastrocnemius and soleus are the muscles primarily involved in plantar flexion. Minor assistance is provided by the peroneus longus and brevis laterally and the flexor digitorum longus, flexor hallucis longus, and tibialis posterior medially (Fig. 1-57).[15,19,55] The gastrocnemius rotates the calcaneus into slight varus during plantar flexion.[26] During the stance and push-off phases of gait, the fibula is pulled distally by the foot flexors.[59] This causes tightening of the

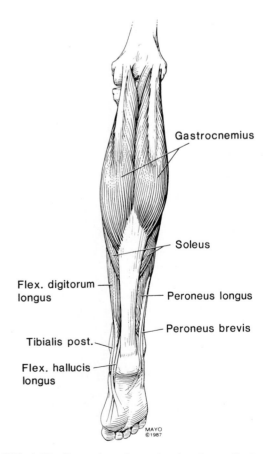

FIG. 1-57. Illustration of muscles for plantar flexion.

interosseous ligament and provides increased lateral stability.[26,37,38,68]

Dorsiflexion is assisted by all muscles crossing the anterior ankle but primarily the tibialis anterior (Fig. 1-58). In the dorsiflexed position, the calcaneus is in slight valgus position and the talus is rotated laterally.[26,37,38] The fibula also rotates laterally, creating some widening of the anterior syndesmoses.[26,37,38,69]

Inversion of the foot occurs when the medial aspect of the foot is elevated and the lateral aspect is depressed (see Fig. 1-56; Fig. 1-59).[26,37,38] The motion occurs in the subtalar joint and also in the calcaneocuboid and talonavicular joints (predominantly the talocalcaneonavicular).[12,26,27]

Muscles involved in inversion of the foot include the tibialis posterior, the flexor digitorum longus, and the flexor hallucis longus (see Fig. 1-59). The tibialis anterior and the extensor hallucis longus are involved to a lesser degree.[12,15,37,38]

Eversion of the foot occurs when the medial plantar surface is depressed and the lateral surface is elevated (Fig. 1-60).[26,37] Muscles involved in eversion include the peroneus longus, the peroneus brevis, the peroneus tertius, and the extensor digitorum longus.[6,15] The degree of motion that can be achieved with inversion exceeds that of eversion. This is largely because of the increased motion of the subtalar and

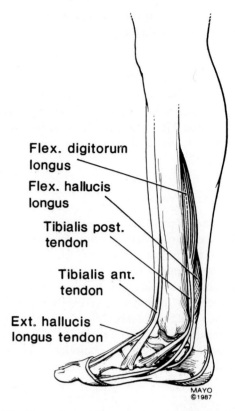

FIG. 1-59. Illustration of the muscles used during inversion.

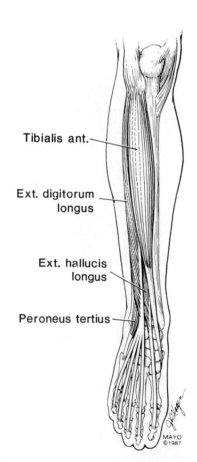

FIG. 1-58. Muscles used during dorsiflexion of the foot.

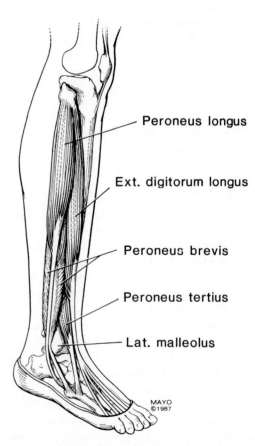

FIG. 1-60. Illustration of the muscles used during eversion.

talonavicular joints medially compared with the calcaneocuboid and tibiofibular articulations laterally.[26,27,49] Adduction indicates medial and abduction lateral motion of the forefoot.[12,26,37,38] Eversion generally accompanies significant abduction movements and inversion is associated with adduction of the foot. Ankle motion is also generally associated, so that plantar flexion accompanies inversion-adduction and dorsiflexion accompanies eversion abduction movements.[26] Tables 1-1 and 1-2 summarize muscles involved in abduction and adduction.

The terms supination and pronation are generally applied to the wrist and forearm (see the foregoing definitions). During supination, the radius rotates around the ulna so that the palm of the hand faces superiorly. In pronation, the hand and forearm are rotated so that the palm of the hand is directed inferiorly. Lauge-Hansen[30,31] applied these terms to the foot as well. Supination is combined adduction of the hindfoot and inversion of the forefoot. Pronation was defined as abduction of the hindfoot and eversion of the forefoot.[26,30,31] Kelikian and Kelikian[26] stated that active pronation is difficult unless the forefoot is abducted and the ankle dorsiflexed. This is because of the lateral articulations of the calcaneus and midfoot, which do not permit intercalary motion. Limited supination of the foot is more easily accomplished owing to the rotatory motion possible in the medial articulations. This motion is similar to inversion.[26] Thus, supination and pronation are combined motions that, although strictly incorrect, are most similar, and these terms are often interchangeably used with inversion and eversion, respectively.

A complete discussion of the phases of gait is beyond the scope of this text. These data are available in other sources.[21,26,37,38,59,60,68,69] The normal gait evolves rapidly with heel strike and reciprocal upper extremity swing by 18 months of age.[66,67] The adult gait is achieved as early as 3 years of age.[26]

The basic gait cycle and forces on the foot and ankle are walking, running, and sprinting, with the phases of the cycle having different lengths. With normal gait, the walking cycle begins with the calcaneus or heel striking the ground and reaches completion when the same heel strikes the ground a second time.[38,39] The cycle has stance and swing phases with double limb support during the initial 10% of the stance phase and single limb support for approximately 50%. The swing phase makes up 40% of the gait cycle.[38,67] Stability during gait is provided by the subtalar joint, the transverse tarsal joint, the talonavicular joint, the plantar aponeurosis, and the foot muscles (see Table 1-2).

The subtalar joint acts as a link between the foot and the lower extremity. When abnormalities such as tarsal coalition are present, the normal motion of the subtalar joint is restricted, increasing the stresses on the foot and ankle.[27] Similar stresses occur in patients with pes planus and pes cavus deformities.[37,38]

The transverse tarsal joint consists of the talonavicular and calcaneocuboid articulations. Its function also depends on normal subtalar motion.[38,67] Stability of these joints is important in allowing one to maintain the toe-to-ground relationship with the toes dorsiflexed during gait.[37,38]

The talus is engaged in the navicular during the lift-off phase of motion when the ball of the foot is in contact with the ground. The plantar aponeurosis that extends from the calcaneus to the proximal phalanges also plays an important stabilizing function during this portion of the gait cycle. The muscles of the foot assist in stabilization during both phases of the cycle, playing a complementary role with the aponeurosis in elevating the longitudinal arch.[38,67]

REFERENCES

1. Anderson JE. Grant's Atlas of Anatomy. 8th Ed. Baltimore, Williams & Wilkins, 1983.
2. Arey LB. Developmental Anatomy. Philadelphia, W.B. Saunders, 1974.
3. Berquist TH, Morrey BF, Cass JR. Foot and ankle in Berquist TH Ed. Imaging of Orthopedic Trauma. 2nd Ed. New York, Raven Press, 1992; pp. 453–578.
4. Burman MS, Lapidus PW. The functional disturbances caused by inconstant bones and sesamoids of the foot. Arch. Surg. 1931; 22: 936–975.
5. Cheung YY, Rosenberg ZS, Ramsinghavi R, Beltran J, Jahss MH. Peroneus quadratus muscle. MR imaging features. Radiology 1997; 202:745–750.
6. Dokter G, Linclau LA. The accessory soleus muscle. Symptomatic soft tissue tumor or accidental finding. Neth. J. Surg. 1981; 33(3):146–149.
7. Dunn AW. Anamolous muscles simulating soft tissue tumors in the lower extremities. J. Bone Joint Surg. Am. 1965; 47:1397–1400.
8. Edeiken J, Dalinka MK, Karasick D. Roentgen Diagnosis of Diseases of Bone. 4th Ed. Baltimore, Williams & Wilkins, 1990.
9. Edwards ME. The relation of the peroneal tendons to the fibula, calcaneus, cuboideum. Am. J. Anat. 1928; 42:213–253.
10. Erickson SJ, Quinn SF, Kneeland JB, Smith JW, Johnson JE, Carrera GF, Shereff MJ, Hyde JS, Jesmanowicz A. MR imaging of the tarsal tunnel and related spaces. Normal and abnormal findings with anatomic correlation. AJR Am. J. Roentgenol. 1990; 155: 323–328.
11. Erickson SJ, Rosengarten JL. MR imaging of the forefoot. Normal anatomic findings. AJR Am. J. Roentgenol. 1993; 160:565–571.
12. Fetto JF. Anatomy and physical examination of the foot and ankle. In Nicholas JA, Hershman EB, eds. The Lower Extremity and Spine in Sports Medicine. Vol. I. St. Louis, C.V. Mosby, 1986; pp. 371–395.
13. Goergen TG, Danzig LA, Resnick D, Owen CA. Roentgen evaluation of the tibiotalar joint. J. Bone Joint Surg. Am. 1977; 59:874–877.
14. Goodwin DW, Salonen DC, Yu JS, Brossman J, Trudell DJ, Resnick DL. Plantar compartments of the foot. MR appearance in cadavers and diabetic patients. Radiology 1995; 196:623–630.
15. Gray H, Williams PL, eds. Anatomy of the Human Body. 38th Ed. New York, Churchill-Livingstone, 1995.
16. Hamilton WC. Traumatic Disorders of the Ankle. New York, Springer Verlag, 1984.
17. Harper MC. The lateral ligamentous support of the subtalar joint. Foot Ankle 1991; 11:354–358.
18. Hecker P. Study on the peroneus of the tarsus. Anat. Rec. 1923; 26: 79–82.
19. Hollinshead WH. Anatomy for Surgeons. Vol 3. 3rd Ed. Philadelphia, Harper & Row, 1982.
20. Inkster RQ. Inversion and eversion of the foot and the transverse tarsal arch. J. Anat. 1938; 72:612–613.
21. Jahss MH. Disorders of the Foot. Philadelphia, W.B. Saunders, 1982.
22. Jenning P. Radiologic studies of variation in ossification of the foot. III. Cone-shaped epiphyses of the proximal phalanges. Am. J. Phys. Anthropol. 1961; 19:131–136.
23. Jones RL. The human foot. The role of its muscles and ligaments in the support of the arch. Am. J. Anat. 1941; 68:1–40.
24. Jonsson K, Fredin HO, Cederlund CG, Bauer M. Width of the normal ankle joint. Acta Radiol. 1984; 25:147–149.
25. Keats TE. Atlas of Normal Roentgen Variants that May Simulate Disease. 5th Ed. St. Louis, C.V. Mosby, 1992; pp. 615–693.

26. Kelikian H, Kelikian AS. Disorders of the Ankle. Philadelphia, W.B. Saunders, 1985.
27. Kitaoka HB, Lundberg A, Luo ZP, An K-N. Kinematics of the normal arch of the foot and ankle under physiologic loading. Foot Ankle 1995; 16:492–499.
28. Klein MA, Spreitzer AM. MR imaging of the tarsal sinus and canal. Normal anatomy, pathologic findings and features of sinus tarsi syndrome. Radiology 1993; 186:233–240.
29. Krause JO, Rouse AM. Accessory calcaneus. A case report and review of the literature. Foot Ankle 1995; 16:646–650.
30. Lauge-Hansen N. Fractures of the ankle. II. Combined experimental-surgical and experimental-roentgenological investigation. Arch. Surg. 1950; 60:959–985.
31. Lauge-Hansen N. Fractures of the ankle. Analytical historical survey as basis of new experimental, roentgenologic and clinical investigation. Arch. Surg. 1948; 56:259–317.
32. Lawson JP. Symptomatic radiographic variants in the extremities. Radiology 1985;157:625–631.
33. Leung RC, Wong WL. The vessels of the 1st metatarsal web space. An operative and radiographic study. J. Bone Joint Surg. Am. 1983; 65:235–238.
34. Lewis OJ. The joints of the evolving foot. I. The ankle joint. J. Anat. 1980; 13:527–543.
35. Link SC, Erickson SJ, Timins ME. MR imaging of the ankle and foot. Normal structures and anatomic variants that may simulate disease. AJR Am. J. Roentgenol. 1993; 161:607–612.
36. Loeffler RD, Ballard A. Plantar fascial spaces of the foot and a proposed surgical approach. Foot Ankle 1980; 1:11–14.
37. Mann RA. Biomechanics of running. In Nicholas JA, Hershman EB, eds. The Lower Extremity and Spine in Sports Medicine. Vol. I. St. Louis, C.V. Mosby, 1986; pp. 396–411.
38. Mann RA. Surgery of the foot. 5th Ed. St. Louis, C.V. Mosby, 1986.
39. McDougall A. The os trigonium. J. Bone Joint Surg. Br. 1955; 37: 256–265.
40. Mellado JM, Rosenberg ZS, Beltran J. Low incorporation of soleus tendon. A potential diagnostic pitfall on MR imaging. Skeletal Radiol. 1998; 27:222–224.
41. Mellado JM, Rosenberg ZS, Beltran J, Colon E. The peroneocalcaneus internus muscle. MR imaging features. AJR Am. J. Roentgenol. 1997; 169:585–588.
42. Miller TT, Bucchieri JS, Joshi A, Staron RB, Feldman F. Pseudodefect of the talar dome. An anatomic pitfall of ankle MR imaging. Radiology 1997; 203:857–858.
43. Mukherjee SK, Pringle RM, Baxter AD. Fracture of the lateral process of the talus. J. Bone Joint Surg. Br. 1974; 56:263–273.
44. O'Rahilly R. A survey of tarsal and carpal anomalies. J. Bone Joint Surg. Am. 1953; 35:626–641.
45. O'Rahilly R. The pseudocystic triangle in the normal os calcis. Acta Radiol. 1953; 36:516–520.
46. Ozonoff MB. Pediatric Orthopedic Radiology. 2nd Ed. Philadelphia, W.B. Saunders, 1992.
47. Powell HDW. Extra center of ossification for the medial malleolus in children. Incidence and significance. J. Bone Joint Surg. Br. 1961; 43: 107–113.
48. Preidler KW, Wang Y, Brossman J, Trudell D, Daenen B, Resnick D. Tarsometatarsal joint. Anatomic details on MR images. Radiology 1996; 199:733–736.
49. Resnick D. Talar ridges, osteophytes and beaks. A radiologic commentary. Radiology 1984; 151:329–332.
50. Resnick D. Radiology of the talocalcaneal articulations. Radiology 1974; 111:581–586.
51. Resnick D, Niwayama G. Articular anatomy and histology. In Resnick D, Niwayama G, eds. Diagnosis of Bone and Joint Disorders. 3rd Ed. Philadelphia, W.B. Saunders, 1995; pp. 652–672.
52. Rhea JT, Salvatore DA, Sheahan J. Radiographic anatomy of the tarsal bones. Med. Radiogr. Photogr. 1983; 59(1):28.
53. Romanus B, Lindahl S, Stener B. Accessory soleus muscle. A clinical and radiographic presentation of 11 cases. J. Bone Joint Surg. Am. 1986; 68:731–734.
54. Rosenberg ZS, Cheung YY, Beltran J, Sheskier S, Leong M, Jahss M. Posterior intermalleolar ligament of the ankle. Normal anatomy and MR imaging features. AJR Am. J. Roentgenol. 1995; 165:387–390.
55. Rosse C, Rosse PG. Hollinshead's Textbook of Anatomy. Philadelphia, Lippincott–Raven, 1997.
56. Rule J, Yas L, Seeger LL. Spring ligament of the ankle. Normal MR anatomy. AJR Am. J. Roentgenol. 1993; 161: 1241–1244.
57. Sarrafian SK. Osteology. In Anatomy of the Foot and Ankle. 2nd Ed. Philadelphia, J.B. Lippincott, 1993; pp. 89–112.
58. Schmidt H, Freyschmidt J. Köhler/Zimmer's Borderlines of Normal and Early Pathology in Skeletal Radiology. 4th Ed. New York, Thieme Medical Publishers, 1993.
59. Scranton PE, McMaster JH, Kelly E. Dynamic fibular function. A new concept. Clin. Orthop. 1976; 118:76–81.
60. Shereff MJ, Bejjani FJ, Kummer FJ. Kinematics of the first metatarsophalangeal joint. J. Bone Joint Surg. Am. 1986; 68:392–398.
61. Silverman FN, Kuhn JP, eds. Caffey's Pediatric X-ray Diagnoses. 9th Ed. St. Louis, C.V. Mosby, 1993.
62. Sirry A. The pseudocystic triangle in the normal os calcis. Acta Radiol. 1951; 36:516–520.
63. Sledge CB. Structure, development, and function of joints. Orthop. Clin. North Am. 1975; 6:619–628.
64. Sledge CB. Biochemical events in the epiphyseal plate and their physiologic control. Clin. Orthop. 1968; 61:37–47.
65. Smith JW. The ligamentous structures in the canalis and sinus tarsi. J. Anat. 1958; 92:616–620.
66. Steel M, Johnson KA, Pewitz MA. Radiographic measurements of the normal adult foot. Foot Ankle 1980; 1:151–158.
67. Stiehl JB. Inman's The Joints of the Ankle. Baltimore, Williams & Wilkins, 1991.
68. Sutherland DH, Cooper L, Daniel D. The role of plantar flexors in normal walking. J. Bone Joint Surg. Am. 1980; 62:354–363.
69. Sutherland DH, Olshen R, Cooper L, Woo SLY. The development of mature gait. J. Bone Joint Surg. Am. 1980; 62:336–353.
70. Venning P. Radiologic studies of variation in ossification of the foot. III. Cone shaped epiphyses of the proximal phalanges. Am. J. Phys. Anthropol. 1961; 19:131–136.
71. Wakeley CT, Johnson DP, Watt I. The value of MR imaging in diagnoses of the os trigonum syndrome. Skeletal Radiol. 1996; 25:133–136.
72. Weissman SD. Radiology of the Foot. Baltimore, Williams & Wilkins, 1989.
73. Wood Jones F. Structure and function as seen in the foot. Baltimore, Williams & Wilkins, 1944.
74. Zanetti M, Strehle JK, Zollinger H, Hodler J. Morton neuroma and fluid in the intermetatarsal bursae on MR images of 70 asymptomatic volunteers. Radiology 1997; 203:516–520.

Radiology of the Foot and Ankle, Second Edition,
edited by Thomas H. Berquist.
© 2000 by Mayo Foundation.
Published by Lippincott Williams & Wilkins, Philadelphia.

CHAPTER 2

Diagnostic Techniques

Thomas H. Berquist, John M. Knudsen, Omer L. Burnett, Jr., Claire E. Bender, Nolan Karstaedt, and Hugh J. Williams, Jr.

Proper application of imaging procedures is essential to obtain needed information for diagnosis and therapy planning in patients with suspected foot and ankle disorders. Appropriate selection and utilization of imaging techniques are especially important in today's cost-conscious environment. This chapter provides the basic background data for imaging techniques. These basic discussions include applications and limitations and serve as a reference source for subsequent chapters in which various imaging procedures are discussed as they apply to specific foot and ankle conditions.

ROUTINE RADIOGRAPHY

The structure and function of the foot and ankle are not only confusing and complicated, but are also poorly understood by most radiologists. Overlapping structures, multiplicity of normal variants and accessory ossicles (see Chapter 1), and variability of patient positioning add to the difficulty in interpretation of radiographs.[6,7,22,46]

Routine radiographs remain the primary screening examination for evaluating foot and ankle disorders. Standard views readily demonstrate the major areas of interest (bony architecture, soft tissues, fat planes) of the foot and ankle. Suspicious findings can be further evaluated with additional special views or fluoroscopically positioned spot views. If

T. H. Berquist: Mayo Medical School, Mayo Clinic Jacksonville, Jacksonville, Florida 32224; Mayo Foundation, Mayo Clinic, Rochester, Minnesota 55905.

J. M. Knudsen, N. Karstaedt, and H. J. Williams, Jr.: Mayo Medical School, Mayo Clinic Jacksonville, Jacksonville, Florida 32224.

O. L. Burnett, Jr., Mayo Clinic Jacksonville, Jacksonville, Florida 32224; St. Luke's Hospital, Jacksonville, Florida 32216.

C. E. Bender: Mayo Medical School, Mayo Clinic Rochester, Rochester, Minnesota 55905.

TABLE 2-1. *Exposure factors for anteroposterior and lateral views[a]*

Factors	Foot	Ankle
Film type	Kodak TML	Kodak TML
Screen	Kodak Lanex fine	Kodak Lanex medium
Source to image distance	48 inches	48 inches
mA	200	200
sec	0.033 sec	0.016
kVp	54(AP) 63(LAT)	60(AP) 58(LAT)

[a] Exposure factors are for an average-sized patient.

the latter are inconclusive, additional studies may be warranted.[6,7]

Radiographic Techniques for the Foot and Ankle

Standard exposure factors are described in Table 2-1. Film screen imaging technique differs from the foot to the ankle. A high-definition imaging system is required for the foot because of the bony detail needed. This is obtained by using high-definition film screen combinations. The ankle requires an imaging system with less detail; thus, a double-screen medium-speed film-screen combination is used that still provides adequate detail but with less patient X-ray exposure. Today, computed radiography is beginning to replace conventional screen-film techniques, at least in larger imaging centers.

Ankle

Ankle radiographs are commonly requested, especially in the emergency room setting. Up to 10% of patients present to emergency centers with a history of ankle sprain.[6,7] Should radiographs be obtained? If so, which views are necessary? Ankle radiographs result in costs of about $500,000 per year to our health systems. Therefore, the debate over when to request radiographs and which views are necessary is not surprising. Using clinical examination, the Ottawa rules may reduce the number of radiographs required. The likelihood of fracture can be more accurately predicted using this approach (see Chapter 4).[1,2]

O'Mary and colleagues[39] found that diagnosis and treatment were changed in about 37% of patients based on radiographic findings. Most radiologists consider the anteroposterior (AP), mortise, and lateral views essential.[1,6,7] Some authors suggest that lateral and mortise views are adequate for fracture diagnosis in 95% of cases.[53] Our standard trauma series includes both oblique views.[6,7] This discussion is not intended to solve the controversy regarding when to obtain radiographs or which views are needed. Instead, we emphasize proper technique and utility of radiographs that are commonly requested by orthopedic surgeons, podiatrists, and other clinicians.

Routine evaluation of the ankle includes the AP, lateral, and mortise (15° to 20° internal oblique) views. The external oblique view is added in our trauma series.[4–7,14,33,38]

Anteroposterior View

The patient is supine, with the foot placed vertically and centered on one-half of a divided 24 × 30 cm cassette (Fig. 2-1A). In ensure the true AP position, it may be necessary to slightly dorsiflex the ankle and pronate the foot. The central beam is perpendicular to the cassette and is centered to tibiotalar joint (1 to 2 cm proximal to the malleolar eminences, which should be palpable).[4–6] The radiograph (see Fig. 2-1B) demonstrates the normal tibiotalar joint and the medial mortise. Neither the lateral mortise nor the inferior tibiofibular articulation is well demonstrated because the fibula overlaps the tibia and talus on the AP view.[6,33] However, the osseous anatomy in the tibiofibular syndesmotic region can still provide valuable information regarding integrity of the ligaments.[21,41]

Figure 2-2 demonstrates the relationships of the distal tibia and fibula on the AP view. Measurements are made 1 cm above the tibial plafond (see Fig. 2-2B).[41] Normally, the tibia and fibula should overlap more than 5 mm when the distal ligaments are intact.[21,41]

Lateral (Mediolateral) View

With the patient on the affected side, the ankle is placed on the other half of the 24 × 30 cm cassette. The central beam is perpendicular to the cassette and is centered 1 to 2 cm proximal to the medial malleolar tip (Fig. 2-3A). To ensure a true lateral view, it may be necessary to place a support under the knee to keep the patella perpendicular to the horizontal plane. Slight dorsiflexion of the foot may also be necessary.[4,6]

Alternate views include the cross-table lateral and reverse lateral (lateromedial) with the medial malleolus next to the cassette.[4,5] The latter view is obtained with the tibiotalar joint closer to the film and thus resulting in a film with better detail. In addition, improved consistency in exact positioning of the ankle is obtained by placing the lower extremity on its relatively flat medial surface. This view is more difficult to obtain in the injured patient.

Structures identified on the lateral view (see Fig. 2-3B) include the AP dimensions of the tibiotalar joint, the lower third of the tibia and fibula, the posterior subtalar joint, and the posterior malleolus. The base of the fifth metatarsal should also be included on the film.[4–6,33] An inversion injury can result in fracture of the base of the fifth metatarsal. Clinical history and the location of ankle swelling may mimic an ankle sprain.[6,7]

Careful observation of the soft tissue structures on the lateral view can assist in detecting subtle injuries. The pre-Achilles fat pad is a large, triangular collection of fat anterior to the large tendon (see Fig. 2-3B). Hemorrhage in this area can occur with Achilles injury. Distortion of this fat pad can also be seen following ankle or calcaneal fractures.[20,24] Ankle effusion is demonstrated as a teardrop-shaped soft tissue mass anterior to the tibiotalar joint (see Fig. 2-3C).[13,20,52]

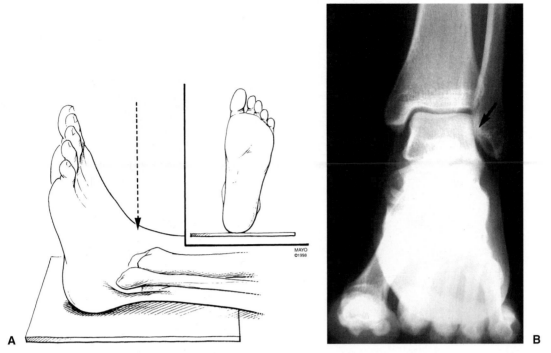

FIG. 2-1. **A:** Illustration of a patient positioned for the AP view with slight dorsiflexion of the ankle and pronation of the foot. **B:** AP radiograph demonstrates overlap of the fibula, tibia and fibula and talus (*black arrowhead*).

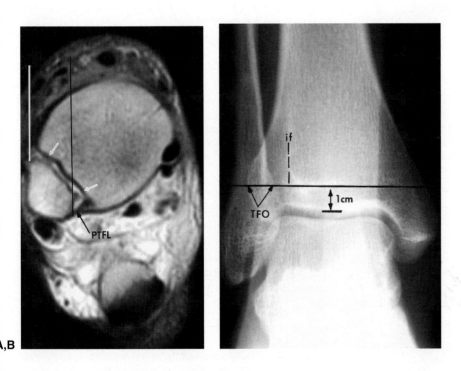

FIG. 2-2. Tibiofibular syndesmotic relationship on the AP view of the ankle. **A:** Axial MRI, with *vertical lines* indicating overlap at the level of the incisura fibularis tibiae (*arrows*). *PTFL.* Posterior tibiofibular ligament. **B:** AP radiograph demonstrating measurements made 1 cm above the tibial plafond. The *vertical broken line* marks the incisura fibularis on the tibia. The tibiofibular overlap (*TF0*) noted by the *black arrows* is normally greater than 2.1 mm in women and greater than 5.7 mm in men. The *left arrow* indicates the lateral tibial margin, and the *right arrow,* the medial fibular margin. The overlap is diminished with ligament injuries, and the distance from the incisura fibularis to the medial tibia is increased.[22,41]

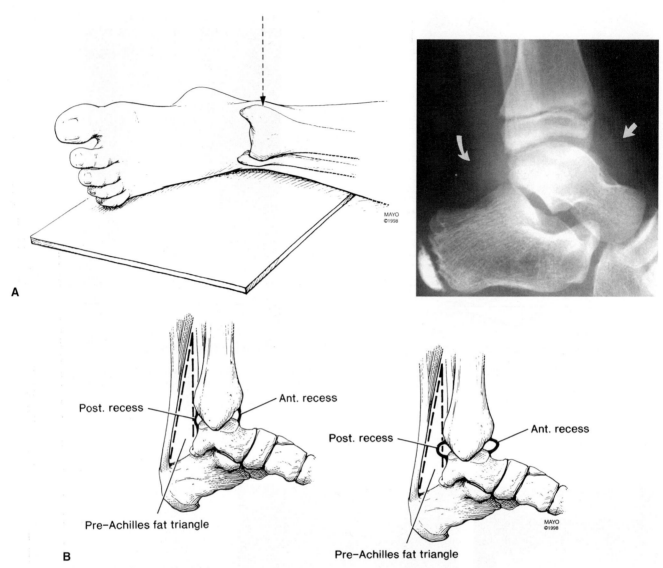

FIG. 2-3. A: Illustration of a patient positioned for the lateral view of the ankle. The central ray is perpendicular and is centered 1 to 2 cm above the malleolar tip. **B:** Lateral illustration demonstrating the pre-Achilles fat pad, marked with *broken lines,* and fluid distending the anterior and posterior recesses. **C:** Severe ankle sprain with a large effusion with anterior teardrop (*arrow*) and posterior soft tissue density owing to effusion (*curved arrow*).

Elevation of the pretalar fat pad also occurs.[51] Similar, but less obvious changes can be demonstrated posteriorly (see Fig. 2-3C). The presence of an effusion suggests intact capsule and ligaments in the immediate postinjury period. Small capsular or ligamentous tears can seal after 48 hr, thus reducing the reliability of this sign.[6,7,36]

Using the AP or lateral views, the average normal joint space (talar dome to tibial weight-bearing surface) in men is 3.4 mm and 2.9 mm in women. The medial aspect of the joint space may be slightly wider on the AP view (see Fig. 2-1B).[24,27]

Mortise View (Internal Oblique)

To evaluate the entire joint space and distal talofibular articulation, the ankle (leg) must be internally rotated 15° to 20° with the central beam perpendicular to the ankle joint (Fig. 2-4A).[4–7] Dorsiflexion of the foot may be necessary to prevent superimposition of the posterior calcaneus and the lateral malleolus. This view demonstrates the talar dome. The posterior portion of the lateral talar facet is also seen tangentially (see Fig. 2-4B).[4,5,38]

Oblique Views

Standard oblique views of the ankle are obtained by rotating the ankle 45° externally and internally.[4–6] The entire extended lower extremity is also rotated in the same direction for ease of X-ray examination. The beam is directed perpendicular to the cassette and is centered on the ankle joint. These projections better demonstrate the medial malleolus

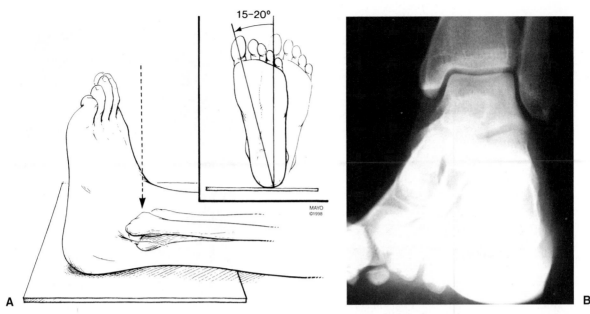

FIG. 2-4. A: Illustration of a patient positioned for the mortise view with the leg and ankle (internally) rotated 15° to 20°. **B:** Mortise view demonstrating the symmetric position of the talus and tibial and fibular articulations.

(external oblique) (Fig. 2-5) and the distal fibula (internal oblique) (Fig. 2-6). Additional anatomy of the hindfoot can also be obtained on the oblique views. In our trauma ankle series, the mortise view (15° to 20° internal rotation) replaces the standard internal oblique view.[7,14]

Stress Views

Assessment of ligamentous injury following ankle trauma can be obtained with carefully performed stress views. The presence of malleolar fractures often indicates the degree of soft tissue injury.[3,7,15,25,32,34,35] Stress views may be indicated if clinical findings suggest ligament injury when osseous structures are normal.[6,9,26] Focal soft tissue swelling is readily detected on properly exposed radiographs.[6,7,10]

In the acute postinjury period, stress views are often difficult to obtain because of pain and swelling. Local anesthetic injection into the painful site or joint may improve the accuracy of the examination. An experienced physician should apply the stress to the injured ankle. Some centers use me-

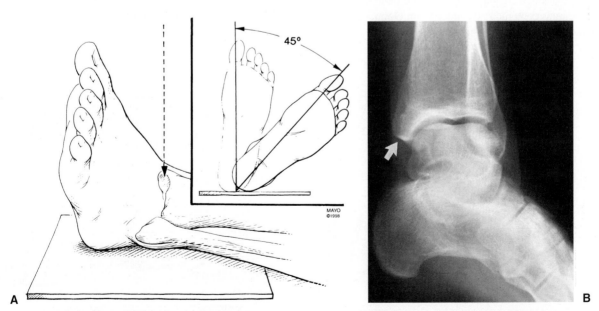

FIG. 2-5. A: Illustration of a patient positioned for the external oblique view. The ankle is rotated 45°, and the beam is centered on the ankle joint. **B:** External oblique view provides better visualization of the medial malleolus (*arrow*).

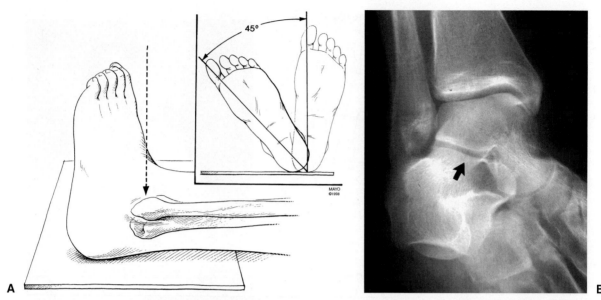

FIG. 2-6. A: Illustration of a patient positioned for the internal oblique view. The ankle is rotated 45° internally, and the beam is centered on the ankle joint. **B:** Internal oblique view demonstrates the lateral malleolus, lateral and posterior talus, and subtalar joint (*arrow*).

chanical stressing devices to ensure consistency and to allow the degree of stress applied to be more accurately assessed.[24,26]

Varus and Valgus Stress Views

Varus and valgus stress views evaluate the medial and lateral stability of the ankle joint (Fig. 2-7). With the lower leg stabilized, the foot is examined in neutral and plantar-flexed positions to assist in separating anterior talofibular and calcaneofibular ligament injuries. The patient is supine, and the beam is centered to the ankle joint. Optimal positioning is facilitated by using fluoroscopic guidance with spot films. Comparison testing of both ankles is mandatory. Olson[40] described a normal talar tilt up to 25° in the asymptomatic hypermobile ankle.

In varus stress (Fig. 2-8), the distance from the most lateral aspect of the talar dome to the lateral tibial articular surface is measured. The respective distance between the medial articular surfaces is measured with valgus stress (Fig. 2-9). The orthopedic literature provides a variety of criteria for instability. A 3-mm difference between the injured side and the normal side indicates ligament injury.[19,26,40] Using the angle measurement technique, a 5° difference of the talar tilt angle between injured and uninjured ankles suggests injury. If the difference between the normal side and the in-

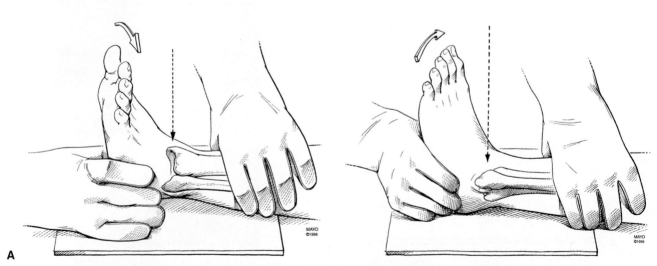

FIG. 2-7. Illustration of a patient positioned for valgus (**A**) and varus (**B**) stress views. The image is centered on the ankle joint (*arrow*). Fluoroscopic positioning is optimal.

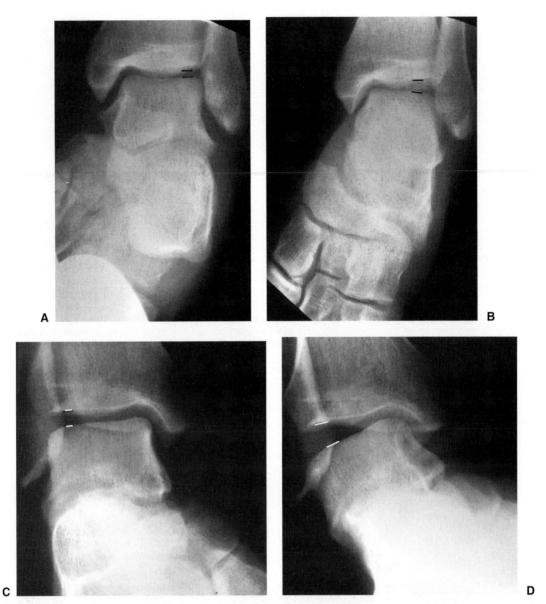

FIG. 2-8. Stress views of the ankle. **A:** AP view of the normal ankle positioned for varus stress with the foot plantar flexed. Note the lateral joint space (*lines*). **B:** AP varus stress view demonstrates slight lateral joint space widening (*lines*). **C:** Stress view with the foot in neutral shows slight widening (*lines*) on the injured side. **D:** Varus stress view with the foot plantar flexed shows more obvious widening, greater than 3 mm different from the normal side (see Fig. 2-7), indicating anterior talofibular ligament injury.

volved side is 10° or more, a ligamentous injury is usually present (see Fig. 2-9).[9,26]

AP stability of the ankle can be evaluated using the lateral double-exposure technique (Fig. 2-10) or two separate exposures (Fig. 2-11). The patient is supine, with the lower leg placed on separate supports so that the knee and ankle are parallel to the tabletop (see Fig. 2-10). The cassette is positioned perpendicular to the table using a cross-table technique. The foot is held in neutral position to prevent inadvertent motion. Exposures are made before and after stress is applied to the distal tibia. The double-exposure technique allows easy comparison measurement.[7,27] Both injured and

uninjured ankles are measured. A difference of 2 mm or more between the uninvolved side and the involved side indicates anterior talofibular ligament injury (positive drawer sign).[7] Stress views are discussed in more detail in the soft tissue injury section of Chapter 3.

Foot

Routine radiographs of the foot include AP, lateral, and oblique views. In some situations, specialized views or fluoroscopically positioned spot films may be required.

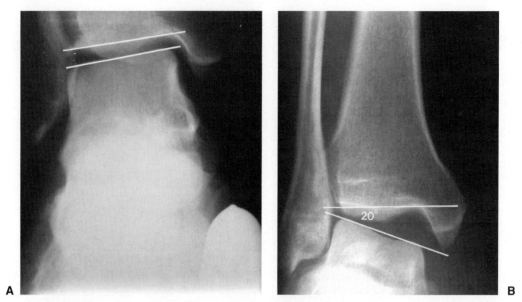

FIG. 2-9. Valgus stress views. **A:** Normal valgus stress view with lines along the tibial and talar surfaces. There is no opening of the medial joint. **B:** Medial ligament tear. Valgus stress view shows medial opening with a 20° angle formed by the tibial and talar articular lines.

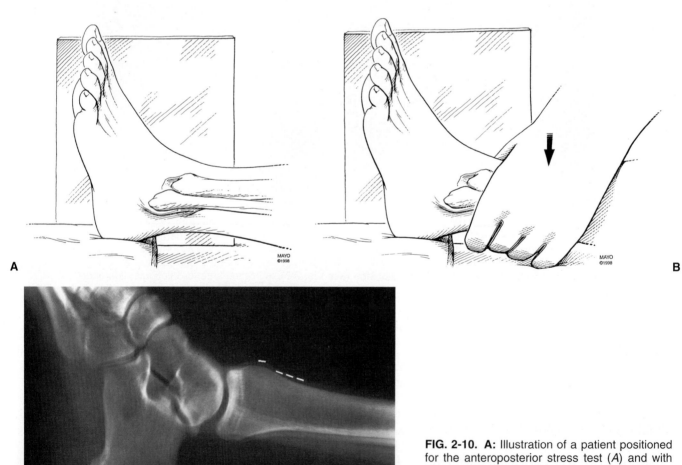

FIG. 2-10. A: Illustration of a patient positioned for the anteroposterior stress test (*A*) and with film double exposed when pressure is applied to the distal tibia (*B*). **B:** Double-exposed image allows the shift (*white broken lines*) to be measured accurately at multiple sites.

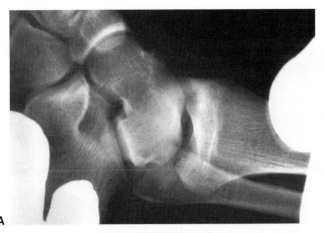
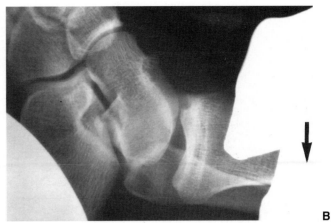

FIG. 2-11. Anteroposterior stress views using conventional two-film technique. In this case, the shift between the normal (**A**) and the abnormal (**B**) side is obvious.

Anteroposterior View

Two views of the foot are obtained to visualize the forefoot (metatarsals and toes) and midfoot (tarsals) adequately. The patient sits or lies on the table with the knee flexed. For the forefoot, the plantar surface of the foot is placed on a divided 8 × 10 inch cassette with the heel resting on the table (Fig. 2-12A and B). The central beam is perpendicular to the cassette and is centered on the distal third metatarsal.[4,5,33] The midfoot view is then taken with the entire foot on the remaining unused half of the cassette (see Fig. 2-12C and D), with the central beam directed either perpendicular to the table with the foot on a 17° angle board or with the foot placed on the cassette and the beam angled 17° cephalad. The angled view better visualizes the tarsometatarsal joints.[3] For either projection, the central beam is centered on the base of the third metatarsal.[4,6,33]

The radiographs demonstrate the osseous structures and articular relationships of the tarsometatarsal, metatarsophalangeal, and phalangeal joints. Care should be taken in evaluating the uniformity and parallel alignment, especially of the tarsometatarsal joints. The distance between the bases of the first and second metatarsals should be scrutinized. Subtle widening of the space may be the only clue to subluxation or dislocation (Lisfranc's injury) (Fig. 2-13).[17,18,37]

Oblique View

Multiple techniques have been described for obtaining oblique views of the foot.[4,6,33] We use the medial oblique projection for trauma or in immobilized patients. The patient is supine with the knee flexed and internally rotated. The lateral aspect of the foot is elevated 30° off the cassette. A radiolucent 30° wedge may be used for support. The central beam is perpendicular to the cassette and is centered at the base of the third or fourth metatarsal (Fig. 2-14). This view separates the third through fifth tarsometatarsal joints, which are overlapped on the AP view (see Fig. 2-12). The talonavi-

cular and calcaneocuboid joints are also well seen. The sinus tarsi can also be demonstrated on this view (see Fig. 2-14).[4-6]

Our routine, the reverse (lateral) oblique view of the foot, can visualize the interspaces between the first and second metatarsals as well as the joint space between the first and second cuneiform. With the patient toward the affected side, knee flexed and externally rotated, a 17° angle board is placed under the foot (with the film-screen placed between the foot and board). The central beam is perpendicular to the table and is centered on the bases of the third and fourth metatarsals.[6]

Lateral View

The lateral view is most frequently taken with the patient on the injured side (mediolateral projection). The lateral aspect of the foot is placed against the cassette (8 × 10 inches or 24 × 30 cm). If possible, the plantar surface of the foot should be perpendicular to the lower edge of the cassette. When the patient can tolerate it, the foot should be dorsiflexed so the lateral aspect of the foot rests on the cassette. The central beam is perpendicular to the cassette and is centered on the midfoot (Fig. 2-15A).

The radiograph visualizes the tibiotalar, subtalar, and proximal tarsal joints. There is overlapping of the metatarsal bases. The unique relationships between the midfoot and the hindfoot are well seen (see Fig. 2-15B).

Phalanges

Although most phalangeal disorders can be detected on the AP view of the foot, oblique and lateral views can provide improved visualization of the interphalangeal and metatarsophalangeal joints and the phalanges.[6,7]

Oblique Phalangeal View. With the patient in the recumbent position on the unaffected side, a sandbag is placed under the ankle. The foot is plantar flexed and positioned at

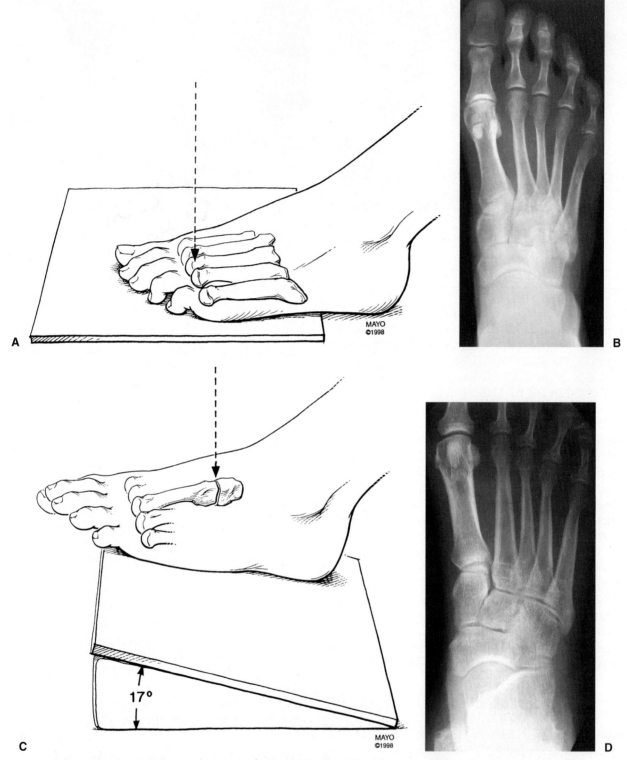

FIG. 2-12. A: Illustration of a patient positioned for the AP view of the forefoot. **B:** AP radiograph of the forefoot demonstrates the distal osseous and articular anatomy. **C:** Illustration of a patient positioned for AP view of the midfoot using a 17° angled board. **D:** Radiograph of the midfoot osseous and articular anatomy. Tarsal overlap still exists laterally.

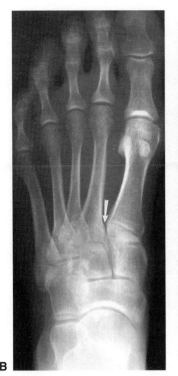
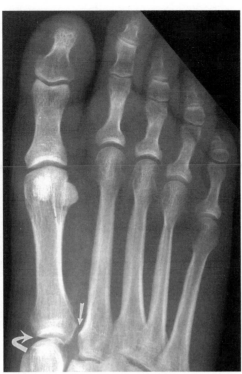

A,B

FIG. 2-13. Radiographs of normal (**A**) and abnormal (**B**) first and second metatarsal base relationships. Note the space between the metatarsal bases in (**A**) (*arrow*) compared with the widened metatarsal space (*arrow*) and the cuneiform first metatarsal space (*curved arrow*) in **B**. The patient in *B* has an acute ligament injury.

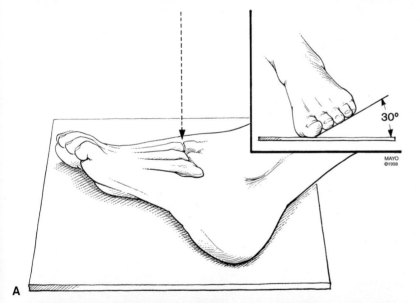

A

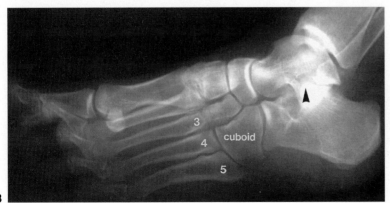

B

FIG. 2-14. A: The patient is positioned for the medial oblique view of the foot. The lateral portion of the foot is elevated 30° off the cassette. **B:** Oblique radiograph of the foot. The subtalar joint (*black arrowhead*) is not well demonstrated. The third to fifth tarsometatarsal joints, calcaneocuboid, talonavicular, and proximal tarsal relationships are well demonstrated.

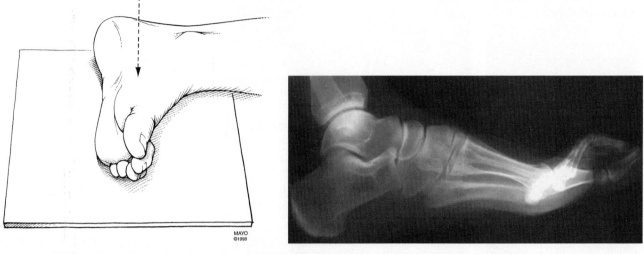

FIG. 2-15. **A:** Illustration of a patient positioned for the lateral view of the foot. **B:** Lateral, non–weight-bearing view demonstrates the ankle, subtalar, and proximal tarsal joints. The phalanges and metatarsals overlap.

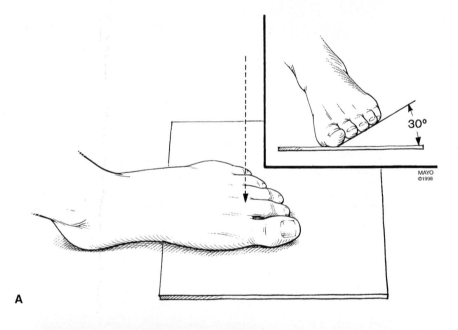

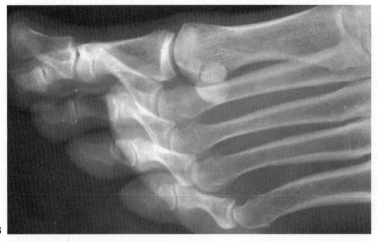

FIG. 2-16. **A:** Illustration of a patient positioned for the oblique view of the phalanges and metatarso-phalangeal joints. **B:** Radiograph demonstrates the metatarsophalangeal and phalangeal articulations.

an angle of approximately 30° with the cassette. The central beam is vertical to the cassette and is directed to the second metatarsophalangeal joint (Fig. 2-16).

Lateral Phalangeal Views. Each toe can be clearly evaluated on this view. The patient is placed in the lateral decubitus position on the unaffected side. To examine a particular toe, the remaining toes are flexed. Padding or tape may be used to separate or immobilize the unaffected toes. The toe being radiographed should be clearly marked on the film (Fig. 2-17).

With a collimated 8 × 10 inch cassette, and industrial or dental film placed under or between the toes, the central beam is directed perpendicular to the film and is centered on the corresponding proximal interphalangeal joint (see Fig. 2-17B through D).

Special Views

Complex anatomy of the hindfoot articulations may require additional views for further evaluation.[4,6,31,33] Fluoroscopically positioned spot views and complex (multidirec-

tional) or computed tomography (CT) may also be indicated to delineate the region of interest better.

Axial Calcaneal View. If a disorder of the calcaneus is suspected, localized lateral and axial views should be obtained. If there is no history of trauma, the patient is positioned prone on the table. The ankle is supported so the foot can be kept in neutral position (Fig. 2-18A). An 8 × 10 inch cassette is placed flat against the plantar surface of the foot. The cassette and its holder are perpendicular to the table. The central beam is angled 45° caudad and is centered through the talocalcaneal joint. The trochlear process, sustentaculum tali, calcaneocuboid articulation, and tuberosity are clearly seen (see Fig. 2-18C).[4,5]

If fracture is suspected, the patient may be studied in the supine position. An 8 × 10 inch cassette is placed under the ankle. A patient who cannot dorsiflex the ankle may use a long strip of gauze to hold the ankle gently in a dorsiflexed position. In severe injuries, it may be necessary to support the leg with sandbags to obtain the correct position.[4,6] The central beam is angled 40° cephalad and is centered on the plantar surface of the fifth metatarsal base (see Fig. 2-18B).

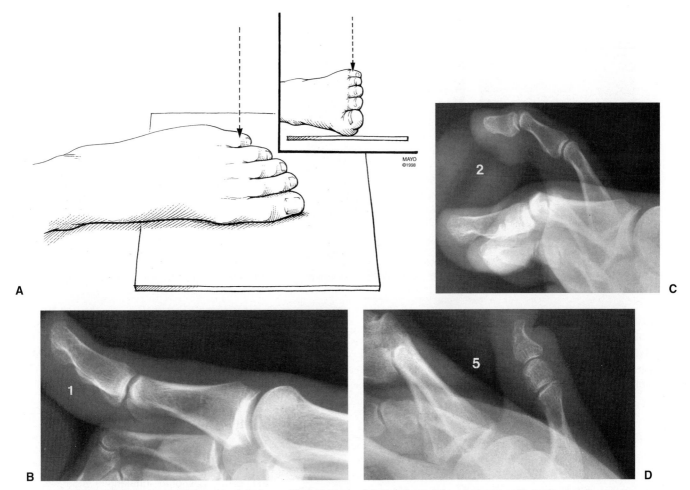

FIG. 2-17. A: Illustration of a patient positioned for the lateral view of the phalanges. **B:** Lateral radiograph of the great toe. Note digital separation by a gauze roll. **C:** Lateral radiograph of the second toe. **D:** Lateral radiograph of the fifth toe.

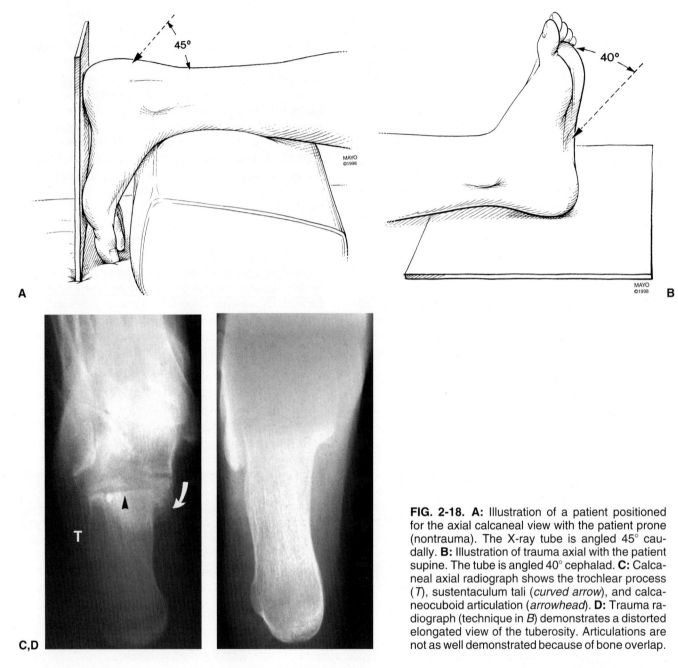

A

B

C,D

FIG. 2-18. **A:** Illustration of a patient positioned for the axial calcaneal view with the patient prone (nontrauma). The X-ray tube is angled 45° caudally. **B:** Illustration of trauma axial with the patient supine. The tube is angled 40° cephalad. **C:** Calcaneal axial radiograph shows the trochlear process (*T*), sustentaculum tali (*curved arrow*), and calcaneocuboid articulation (*arrowhead*). **D:** Trauma radiograph (technique in *B*) demonstrates a distorted elongated view of the tuberosity. Articulations are not as well demonstrated because of bone overlap.

Distorted projections of the calcaneus may result (see Fig. 2-18D) using this technique.[6,7]

Lateral Calcaneal View. Although the calcaneus is demonstrated on the routine lateral foot view, better definition is obtained when the X-ray beam is centered on the calcaneus (Fig. 2-19).

Weight-Bearing (Coalition View)

Our film series for tarsal coalition includes the following: (1) an AP view of the foot (see Fig. 2-12 for midfoot view); (2) a medial oblique view (see Fig. 2-14); (3) an AP (axial) view of the calcaneus (see Fig. 2-18); (4) a true lateral view of the foot (see Fig. 2-15); and (5) a weight-bearing view.

Talocalcaneal coalition can be evaluated using the weight-bearing view.[33,36] The patient stands with the involved foot on the 8 × 10 inch cassette. The unaffected foot is placed forward to prevent superimposition of the lower leg. The central beam is angled axially 45° and is centered at the posterior ankle joint (Fig. 2-20). The same axial view can also be obtained with patient prone as in Figure 2-18A and B.

Subtalar Views

Many different techniques have been described for evaluation of the subtalar joint.[5,7,8,16,24,33,45] Because of individual patient anatomy, it can difficult to obtain the necessary infor-

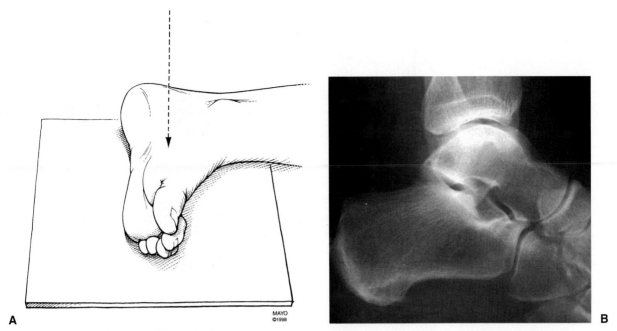

FIG. 2-19. A: Illustration of a patient positioned for the lateral calcaneal view. **B:** Lateral calcaneal view demonstrates the calcaneus and hindfoot more optimally than the standard lateral view of the foot (see Fig. 2-15).

mation on the oblique views (Fig. 2-21). If the area of interest cannot be defined, CT or fluoroscopically positioned films can be performed to delineate specific anatomic areas (see Fig. 2-21E).

Lateral Oblique View. The patient is placed on the affected side with the foot in the lateral position. The limb is externally rotated 60° and rests on a 17° angle board wedge.

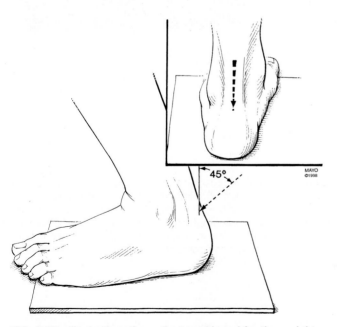

FIG. 2-20. Illustration of a patient positioned for the weight-bearing coalition view. The tube is angled 45°. Weight is forward, forcing the foot into the dorsiflexed position.

The foot should be dorsiflexed with the heel toward the wide end of the sponge. The beam is centered 1 inch below the medial malleolus and is angled 25° to the feet (see Fig. 2-21A). The subtalar joint is usually clearly seen on this view (see Fig. 2-21B). Lateral and axial views of the calcaneus may be indicated to complete the evaluation of the subtalar facets.[6,33]

Medial Oblique View. With the patient in the supine position, the ankle is centered on an 8 × 10 inch cassette. The lower extremity is rotated medially 60° resting on a 30° wedge. Slight dorsiflexion of the foot should be maintained. The beam is centered on the lateral malleolus and is angled 10° to 25° to the head (see Fig. 2-21C). The sinus tarsi region is best demonstrated on this view (see Fig. 2-21D). Because of positioning problems, fluoroscopically positioned spot views may be obtained (see Fig. 2-21E).

Sesamoid Views

Sesamoid fractures, osteonecrosis, and inflammation are not unusual in runners. Routine foot views may not optimally delineate these superimposed, often bipartite structures. The sesamoid view is obtained with the patient supine and the foot dorsiflexed (with gentle traction on the toes using a strip of gauze or tape) (Fig. 2-22A–C). A tangential view of the sesamoids is readily obtained in this manner. The central beam is directed just plantar to the first metatarsal head and perpendicular to the collimated cassette (see Fig. 2-22A–D).[4–6,23,33]

This same view can be taken with the patient seated.[23] The foot is placed with its medial aspect vertical, and the

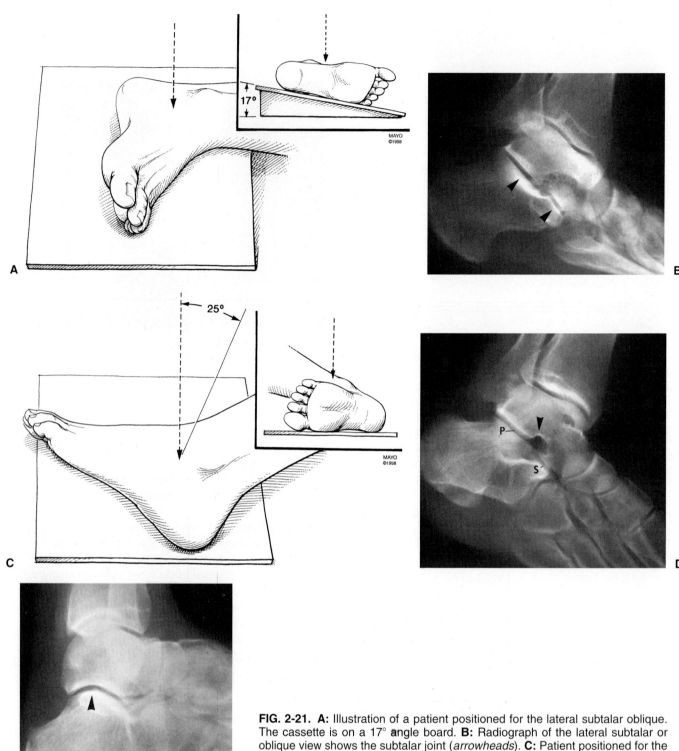

FIG. 2-21. A: Illustration of a patient positioned for the lateral subtalar oblique. The cassette is on a 17° angle board. **B:** Radiograph of the lateral subtalar or oblique view shows the subtalar joint (*arrowheads*). **C:** Patient positioned for the medial subtalar oblique view. **D:** Radiograph of the medial subtalar oblique view demonstrates the posterior facet (*P*), sinus tarsi (*arrowhead*), and sustentacular articulation (*S*). **E:** Fluoroscopically positioned oblique spot film to demonstrate the posterior subtalar joint (*arrowhead*).

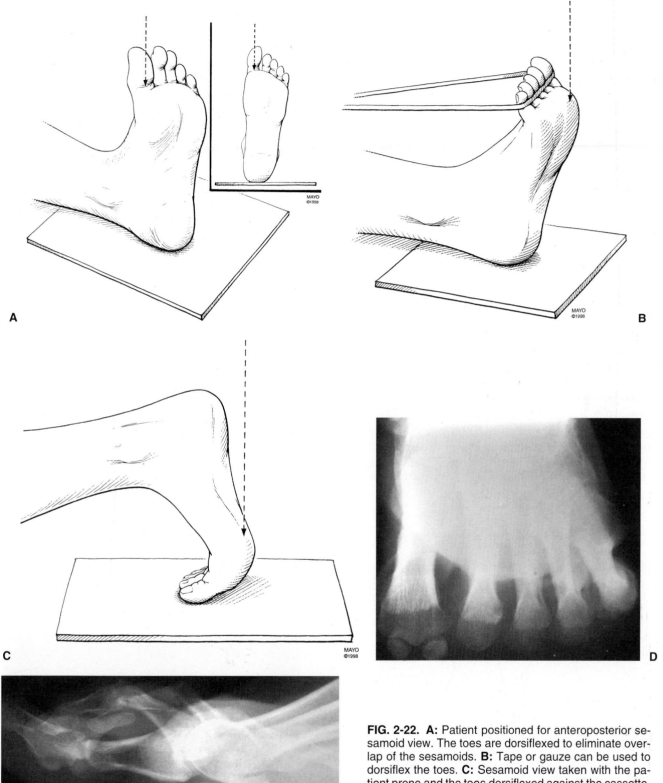

FIG. 2-22. A: Patient positioned for anteroposterior sesamoid view. The toes are dorsiflexed to eliminate overlap of the sesamoids. **B:** Tape or gauze can be used to dorsiflex the toes. **C:** Sesamoid view taken with the patient prone and the toes dorsiflexed against the cassette. **D:** Radiograph of the sesamoids. **E:** Tangential view can separate the sesamoids. Note the bipartite sesamoid (*black arrowhead*).

plantar surface is at an angle of 75° with the cassette. The toes are dorsiflexed as described earlier. The beam is centered on the first metatarsal head. The sesamoids can also be viewed with the patient prone, resting the dorsiflexed great toe on the table so that the metatarsal heads are perpendicular to the cassette (see Fig. 2-22C).

Tangential views of the sesamoids can be obtained with the patient recumbent on the unaffected side and the knees flexed. The cassette is placed under the lower metatarsal heads. The central beam is directed to the first metatarsophalangeal joint and is angled 40° toward the heel. This view can separate the sesamoids of the great toe (see Fig. 2-22E).[6,11,23,33]

Weight-Bearing Views

AP and lateral weight-bearing views are obtained to evaluate the structural changes that may not be detected on the routine, non–weight-bearing views. Articular alignment and important functional measurements can only be obtained with weight-bearing techniques.

Anteroposterior Weight-Bearing View of the Ankle. Standing AP ankle views are useful in evaluating the tibiotalar articulations and alignment. The patient stands on a special wooden holder or sturdy Styrofoam block that supports 10 × 12 inch cassettes. The central beam is centered between both ankle joints (Fig. 2-23). Samuelson and colleagues[50] proposed a double-exposure technique with the patient standing on a Plexiglass support and the malleoli

equidistant from the cassette (Fig. 2-24A). An AP view is obtained using the foregoing standing-ankle technique. A second exposure is made on the same film (the patient must maintain the same position) after angling the tube 20° from horizontal (see Fig. 2-24B). The resulting radiograph shows the hindfoot position (see Fig. 2-24C).[50]

Anteroposterior Weight-Bearing View of Foot. One radiograph of both feet can be made with the patient standing on the cassette. The beam is directed to the center of the 24 × 30 cm cassette and is angled 15° into the metatarsals (Fig. 2-25A). A comparison of the relationships of foot architecture is made using this view (see Fig. 2-24B).[6,7]

Lateral Weight-Bearing View of Ankle and Foot. The patient stands on a low wooden bench and straddles a 24 × 30 cm cassette that fits into the specially constructed bench (Fig. 2-26A). The cassette is centered at the base of the fifth metatarsal. The X-ray beam is centered perpendicular to an area just cephalad to the base of the fifth metatarsal (see Fig. 2-26A). The longitudinal arch of the foot is demonstrated (see Fig. 2-26B). Weight-bearing views of both feet and ankles are usually obtained to allow comparison. For a lateral weight-bearing view of the ankle, the X-ray beam is centered on the hindfoot.[4–6,33]

Axial Weight-Bearing View of Foot. This double-exposure view demonstrates all the bones of the foot. The shadow of the leg is masked.[4] The patient stands on an 8 × 10 inch or 24 × 30 cm cassette on the floor. A mobile unit or a tube is used so that the patient's foot does not change position between exposures. The first view is taken with the opposite foot placed behind the cassette. The X-ray tube is

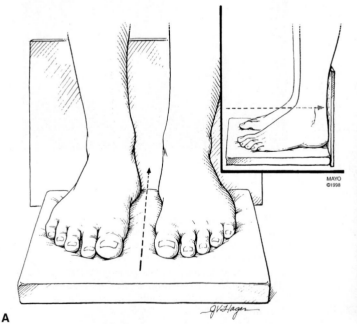

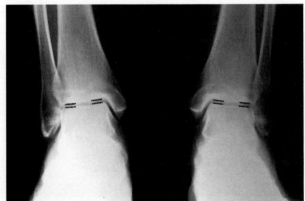

A   **B**

FIG. 2-23. A: Illustration of a patient positioned for AP weight-bearing views of the ankle. **B:** Radiograph of AP weight-bearing view shows symmetry of the tibiotalar joints (*black lines*). The joints are slightly tilted and are not parallel to the floor.

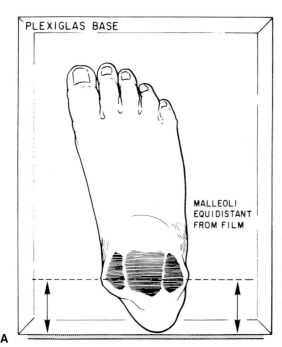

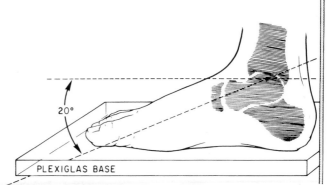

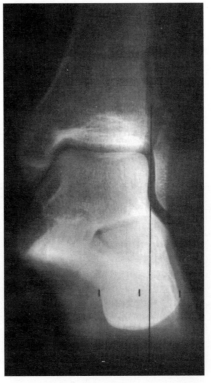

FIG. 2-24. A: Illustration of the malleolar position in relation to film for double-exposure hindfoot view. **B:** Illustration demonstrating the beam angle for second exposure. **C:** Hindfoot anteroposterior view showing the center of the calcaneus in relation to the tibiotalar joint. (From Samuelson et al., ref. 50, with permission.)

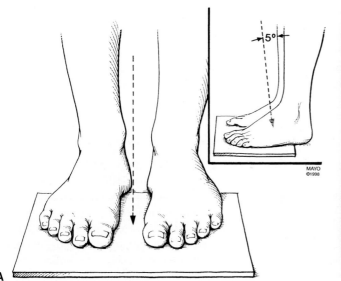

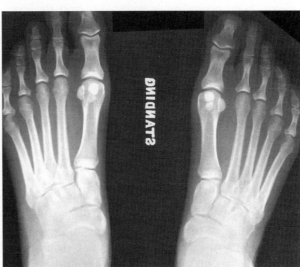

FIG. 2-25. A: Illustration of a patient positioned for the AP weight-bearing view of the feet. **B:** Standing AP radiograph of both feet (see Fig. 2-29 for common measurements).

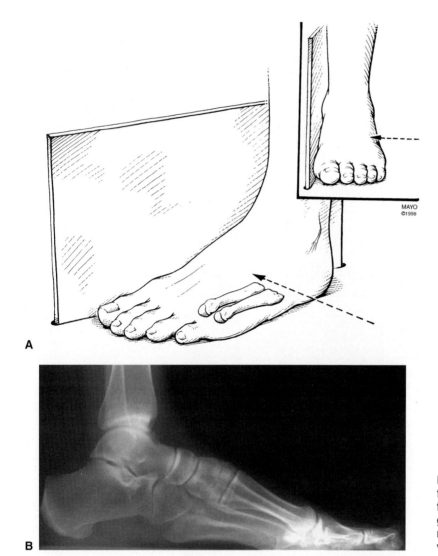

A

B

FIG. 2-26. A: Illustration of a patient positioned for the standing weight-bearing lateral view of the foot and ankle. **B:** Lateral weight-bearing radiograph of the foot and ankle (see Fig. 2-29 for common measurements used on the standing lateral view).

in front of the patient and is angled 15° toward the heel and centered on the navicular bone (similar to AP view of the foot; see Fig. 2-12A). Care must be taken to direct the central ray along the same plane of alignment for both exposures. The patient must not move the affected foot on either exposure. The second exposure is taken with the opposite foot now placed ahead of the cassette. The X-ray tube is placed behind the patient and is angled 25° to the toes (similar to the weight-bearing coalition view; see Fig. 2-16). The central beam is directed to the posterior surface of the ankle (Fig. 2-27).[4-7]

Tangential Anteroposterior Weight-Bearing View of Forefoot. Radiographic evaluation of metatarsalgia is difficult. The non–weight-bearing views of the foot (and sesamoids) do not give the structural status of the forefoot.[12,43]

The patient stands on a low bench or X-ray table.[12] The affected foot is placed in special blocks, and the knee is flexed 30°. Slight toe push is performed, but hyperextension of the metatarsophalangeal joint is avoided. The 8 × 10

inch cassette is placed in front of the toes. The X-ray beam is centered perpendicular to the film and with the plantar surface of the foot.

This projection outlines the metatarsal heads and position of the sesamoids. The height of the arch can also be measured (Fig. 2-28).[8,43]

Radiographic Measurements of the Normal Adult Foot

On the routine AP and lateral weight-bearing views, one sees a wide variety of bony relationships in the normal adult foot.[7,28,29,47,49,51] The techniques for these views were discussed earlier. It is difficult to identify the entire foot on the AP view because of overlap of the hindfoot by the tibia and fibula. Hindfoot evaluation may not be possible in this situation. Only the major relationships are outlined (Fig. 2-29). Comparison of the contralateral foot radiographs is mandatory in the clinical evaluation. The foot is a heterogeneous structure, and abnormal radiographic findings in a

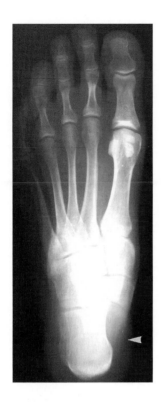

FIG. 2-27. Double-exposure radiograph of the axial weight-bearing foot shows all the bones of the foot. Note overlap and foreshortening of the hindfoot with masking of leg shadows (*white arrowhead*).

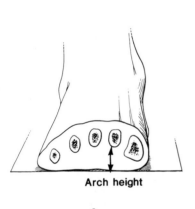

Arch height

A

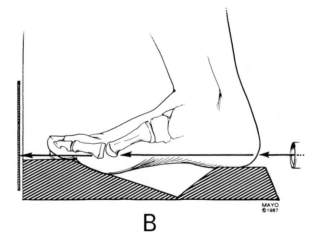

B

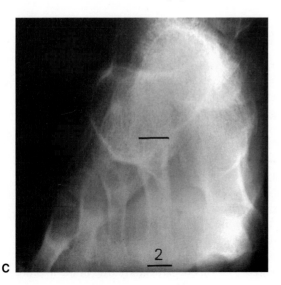

C

2

FIG. 2-28. Illustration of the technique for the anteroposterior weight-bearing view of the forefoot from the front (**A**) and side (**B**). **C:** Radiograph of the tangential weight-bearing view of the forefoot demonstrates the metatarsal heads and sesamoids. The apex is identified as the second metatarsal head (*line*).

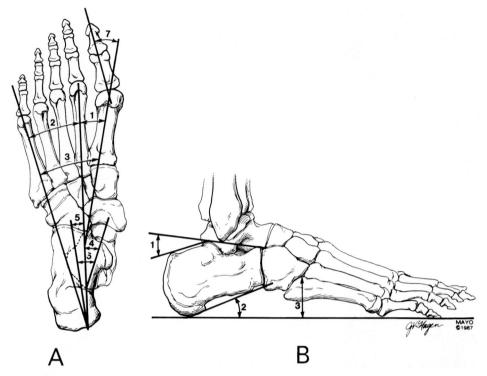

FIG. 2-29. Illustrations of common measurements used for the weight-bearing AP (**A**) and lateral (**B**) views of the foot. **A:** Measurements on the AP view: *1,* intermetatarsal angle (first and second), range 4° to 23°; *2,* intermetatarsal angle (second to fifth), range 8° to 21°; *3,* intermetatarsal angle (first to fifth), range 14° to 35°; *4,* second talometatarsal angle, range 15° to 63°; *5,* second calcaneus-metatarsal angle, range 3° to 35°; *6,* hindfoot angle, range 15° to 63°; *7,* first metatarsophalangeal angle, range 0° to 32°. **B:** Measurements on lateral view: *1,* Böhlers angle, range 22° to 48°; *2,* calcaneal inclination angle, range 11° to 38°; *3,* fifth metatarsal base height, range 2.3 to 3.8 cm.

normal clinical setting should not be aggressively treated.[6,30] Figures 2-30 and 2-31 demonstrate measurements marked on radiographs. The significance of these measurements are discussed in depth in later chapters dealing with adult foot disorders.

The Infant Foot

The two most common indications for radiologic evaluation of the pediatric foot are deformity and trauma.[4,42] Standard views for foot deformity are weight-bearing AP and lateral projections. It is mandatory to evaluate the bones in their functional and structural state. It is important that the films are made of both feet for comparison purposes.

Anteroposterior View of the Foot. The patient stands or lies supine with knees flexed (Fig. 2-32). The foot is placed firmly against the cassette, so the sole is in direct contact with the surface. Care must be taken to align the tibia linearly with the hindfoot. The foot deformity should not be corrected. The central beam is angled 30° toward the head and is centered on the midfoot. Collimation is used on an 8 × 10 inch cassette.[4,33]

Lateral View of Foot. This view is obtained with the patient standing or supine with a board placed under the foot

(see Fig. 2-32C and D). Dorsiflexion is mandatory in either position. The cassette is placed laterally to the foot. The beam is perpendicular to the cassette and is centered on the midfoot. The ankle, not the forefoot, should be placed in the true lateral position to prevent talar dome distortion.[4]

Oblique Views. The oblique views are used in the evaluation of trauma, postsurgical changes, or tarsal coalition.[4,33]

TOMOGRAPHY

Tomography, or body-section radiography, provides a method of blurring out unwanted information to visualize the desired structures better. Laminography, planography, and stratigraphy are terms that have been applied to this technique. Tomography was developed by two Dutch investigators (Ziedes des Plantes and Bart-link) in 1931.[55] During the exposure, the X-ray tube and film move in two parallel planes but in opposite directions. Speeds are maintained at a constant relationship.

Most skeletal structures can be evaluated with routine radiographs or spot films obtained with fluoroscopic monitoring.[63] Thin-section (1- to 3-mm thick) tomography is a useful addition to conventional films when more detailed information is required.[56,61] This is particularly true in the midfoot

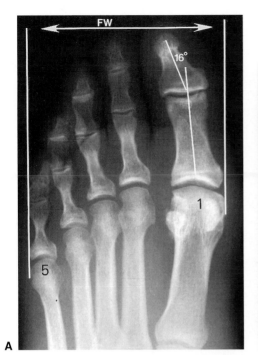

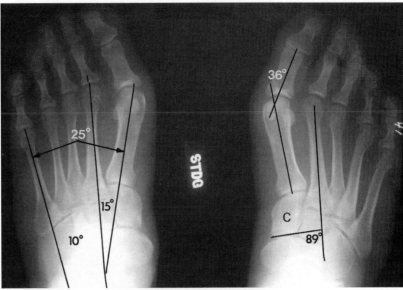

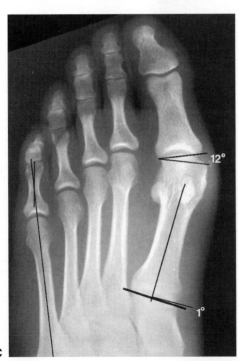

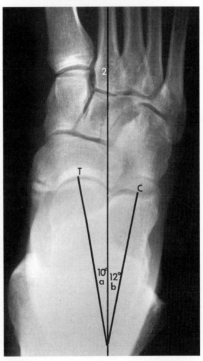

FIG. 2-30. Radiographic measurements on the anteroposterior view.[51] **A:** Forefoot width (*FW*) measured from the first to the fifth metatarsal head margins, range 7.1 to 9 cm. First interphalangeal angle, range 6° to 24°; in this case, the angle is 16°. **B:** First to second intermetatarsal angle, range 4° to 23°; in this case, the left foot is 15°. Second to fifth intermetatarsal angle, range 4° to 21°; in this case, 10°. First to fifth intermetatarsal angle, range 14° to 35°; in this case, the left foot is 25°. First metatarsal phalangeal angle, range 0° to 32°; in this case, 36° in the right foot. Cuneiform proximal articular to the second metatarsal shaft angle, range 84° to 122°; in this case, the right foot angle is 89°. *c,* medial cuneiform. **C:** Fifth metatarsal phalangeal angle, range 1° to 21°; in this case, it is nearly aligned or 0° at the joint. Incongruency angle (measured by lines along articular margins), range −4° to −24°; in this case, −12°. First metatarsal proximal articular angle, range 0° to 15°; in this case, 1°. **D:** Talar-metatarsal 2 shaft angle, range 6° to 42°; in this case, 10°. Calcaneus metatarsal 2 angle, range 3° to 35°; in this case, 12°. Hindfoot or talocalcaneal angle, range 15° to 63°; in this case, the angle formed by the talus (*T*) and calcaneus (*C*) is 22° (10° to 12°).

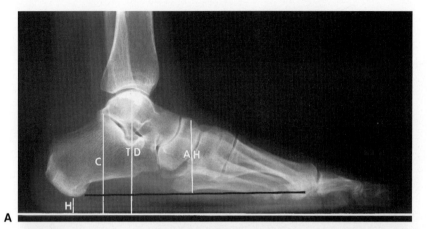

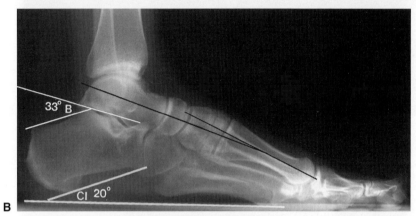

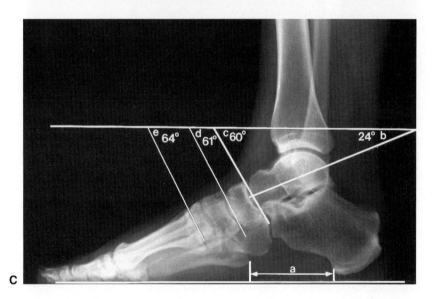

FIG. 2-31. Radiographic measurements on the lateral weight-bearing view.[30,49,51] **A:** *C,* Calcaneal height, range 5.8 to 7.5 cm; *H,* calcaneal soft tissue pad height, range 0.4 to 1.7 cm; *TD,* talar dome height, range 7.3 to 9.5 cm; *AH,* arch height, distance from dorsal navicular to a line from the calcaneal tubercle to the base of the first metatarsal head (*black line*). **B:** *CI,* calcaneal inclination angle, range 11° to 38°; in this case, 20°. *B,* Bohlers angle, range 22° to 48°; in this case, 33°; talar-first metatarsal alignment; in this case, the angle is slightly positive. **C:** *a,* Calcaneal-fifth metatarsal baselength, range 8.1 to 10.7 cm; *b,* talus-base reference angle, range 14° to 36°; in this case, 24°; *c,* proximal navicular articular angle, range 54° to 74°; in this case, 60°; *d,* proximal cuneiform articular angle, range 51° to 78°; in this case, 61°; *e,* proximal first metatarsal articular angle, range 55° to 72°; in this case, 64°.

and hindfoot, where skeletal anatomy and joint alignment are more complex. Conventional tomography provides an image of any selected plane while blurring structures above and below that plane.[59,60] Basic equipment for linear tomography includes (1) an X-ray tube, (2) a connecting rod that moves about a fixed fulcrum, and (3) a cassette and film (Fig. 2-33). As the film moves in one direction, the tube moves in the opposite direction. The plane of interest within the patient (see shaded area in Fig. 2-33) is most commonly selected by adjusting the fulcrum level. Less commonly, the apparatus includes an elevating tabletop to position the plane of interest at a fixed level. Only the plane of interest remains in sharp focus on the tomogram. Planes above and below (see Fig. 2-33) that plane are blurred. Commonly used tomographic motions include simple (linear) and complex (circular, hypocycloidal, elliptic, and trispiral) (Fig. 2-34).[61]

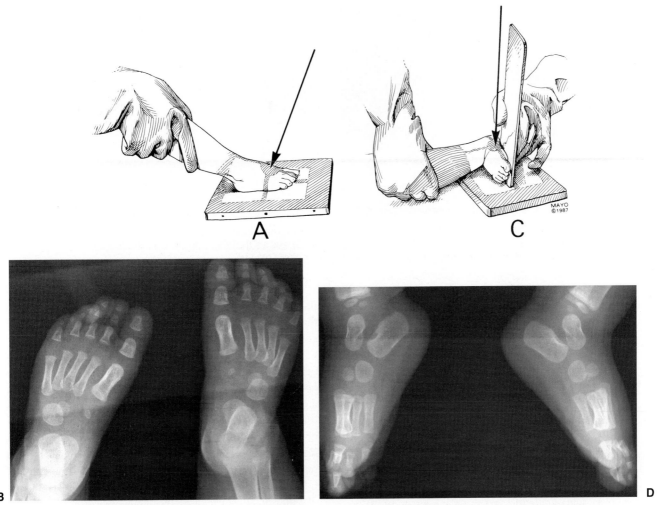

FIG. 2-32. **A:** Illustration of an infant positioned for the AP view of the foot. **B:** AP radiograph of both feet with a compression band in place. **C:** Illustration of an infant positioned for lateral view of the foot. **D:** Lateral radiographs of both feet with a compression band in place.

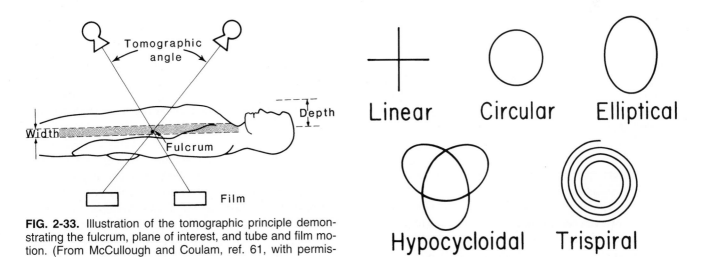

FIG. 2-33. Illustration of the tomographic principle demonstrating the fulcrum, plane of interest, and tube and film motion. (From McCullough and Coulam, ref. 61, with permission.)

FIG. 2-34. Illustration of types of tomographic motion. (From McCullough and Coulam, ref. 61, with permission.)

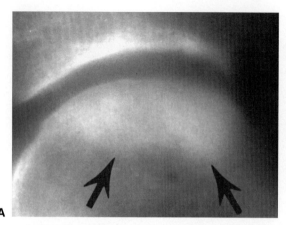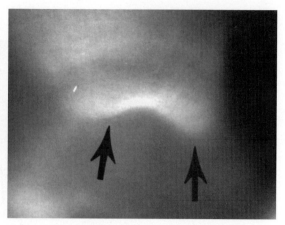

A   B

FIG. 2-35. Trispiral tomograms of the talus: 3-mm thick tomograms of the medial malleolus demonstrate an area of sclerosis (*arrows* in **A**). The adjacent section (**B**) shows that this apparent increased density in **A** was due to partial volume effect of the medial malleolus (*arrows*).

Blurring and Section Thickness

A better understanding of tomography requires a basic understanding of blurring and section thickness. Blurring refers to the effect of the tomographic system on objects outside the focal plane.[58] It depends on (1) the amplitude of tube travel, (2) its orientation, and (3) the distance of the tube from the focal plane. Section thickness refers to the plane that is in sharp focus on the film.[58] It is inversely dependent on (but not proportional to) the amplitude of tube travel. Therefore, the greater the tomographic angle, the thinner is the section.[58,61]

For evaluating skeletal structures (which have high inherent contrast), wide-angle tomography using an arc of 30° to 50° is usually preferred. With the wide angle, maximum blurring of objects outside the focal plane occurs, and therefore phantom images (unwanted images) are less likely to be produced. Despite this, care must be taken to study images in proper sequence to avoid errors caused by partial volume effects. In this setting, portions of structures included in the tomographic plane can mimic pathologic features (Fig. 2-35).

For standard skeletal tomography, we prefer radiographic equipment capable of performing linear (longitudinal, transverse, and diagonal), circular, and trispiral motions. Linear and circular tube travel may be 20°, 30°, or 45°. In trispiral studies, the angle is always 45°. We use 3M XUD film with Lanex regular screens (200 speed system) in special carbon-fiber front cassettes at a 48-inch source-to-film distance. A Bucky grid with a 12 : 1 ratio is used. Exposure factors vary with the body part studied. For foot and ankle imaging, 3-mm thick sections are typically used.

Generally, tomograms are obtained in the AP and lateral planes. However, because of the position of the bones in the foot and off-axis angles of the joints, it is often necessary to position the area of interest fluoroscopically.[54,64] In this situation, two different views are chosen, one in the best image plane and the second, if possible, at a 90° angle to that plane. In certain cases, local pain or the patient's general condition may limit positioning.

In orthopedic practice, tomography is frequently used to evaluate subtle fractures (Fig. 2-36).[56,57,60,62,65] Fracture healing and other clinical problems such as tarsal coalition are also effectively studied with tomography.[62,64] In most orthopedic tomography, the detail is improved with trispiral or complex motion. Occasionally, especially in patients with metallic internal or external fixation devices, linear motion may be more useful than complex motion tomography or CT (Fig. 2-37). Trispiral motion can cause significant loss of bone detail adjacent to the metal. In certain cases, the configuration of the fixation device is such that examination choices are more difficult. Tomography is still often useful in providing increased detail in these situations (see Fig. 2-37).

Summary

The type of tomographic motion used may greatly influence the radiographic findings. There are advantages to simple and complex motion studies. Increased blurring of objects occurs outside the plane in focus because of the greater distance the tube-film moves during the complex motion exposure. This results in elimination of streaking (incomplete blur) in images of structures when their long axis is aligned with the tube-film motion, as seen in linear tomography.[58] Complex motion has decreased tendency to produce phantom images (unreal or unwanted images). The more complex the motion, the less is the likelihood of phantom images. Linear tomography has the advantage of shorter exposure time, which may be useful in uncooperative patients. Linear motion may also be more useful when metal fixation devices are in place. Today, because of the reduced availabil-

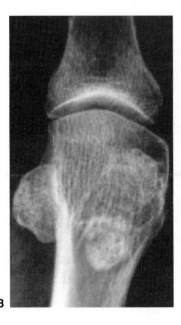 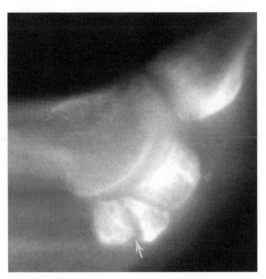

A,B

FIG. 2-36. Jogger with pain under the first metatarsal head. **A:** Routine anteroposterior view of the first metatarsophalangeal joint region is normal. **B:** Lateral tomogram shows a sesamoid fracture (*arrow*).

ity of complex motion equipment, the choice of technique is often limited to linear motion or CT.

MAGNIFICATION RADIOGRAPHY

The technique of magnification radiography was first used in 1940 but did not gain popularity until the last decade.[66] Although initially used for small vessel angiography, magnification is also useful in skeletal radiography. The technique provides accurate and detailed assessment of subtle skeletal abnormalities in articular, metabolic, infectious, neoplastic, and traumatic disorders.[66–71,73]

Equipment and Principles

A thorough understanding of the equipment and principles of magnification is necessary to obtain high-quality magnification radiographs. Proper selection of the X-ray tube is

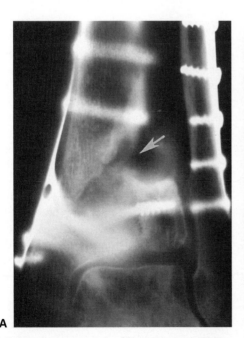 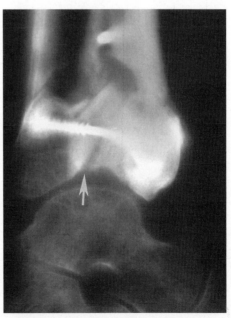

A   B

FIG. 2-37. Anteroposterior (**A**) and lateral (**B**) linear tomograms in a patient with plate-and-screw fixation of the tibia and fibula. The bone loss (*arrow* in **A**) and articular deformity (*arrow* in **B**) are clearly demonstrated.

essential. We use a Machlett DX78E tube with a 0.20-mm focal spot (as specified by the manufacturer). The actual focal spot size (grid-biased) measured 0.10 mm using a star text pattern in accordance with the specifications of the National Electrical Manufacturers Association.[66,72] High-speed rotation of the anode is necessary to prevent X-ray tube damage under heavy exposure conditions. A three-phase generator is also preferred.

For conventional extremity magnification, we use (1) a 44-inch source-film distance, (2) Kodak NMB single emulsion film, (3) Kodak single Min-r intensifying screens (used as a rear screen), and (4) exposure factors of 60 peak kilovolts (kVp), 30 milliamperes/sec (mAs), and 1.25 sec. The part being examined is supported on a Lucite stand (Fig. 2-38) 24 inches above the film. This results in a 2.2 to 1 magnification factor (Fig. 2-39).

Magnification radiography is based on two geometric principles. First, the size of the image is proportional to the distance between the object and the film; and second, the smaller the focal spot of the X-ray tube, the sharper is the image.[66,71] A focal spot size of 0.30 mm or less is required for magnification radiography. Increased image size occurs

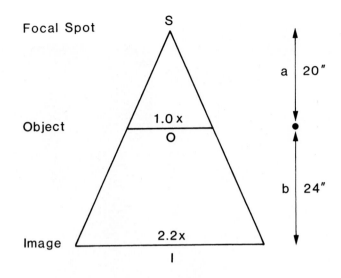

$$Magnification = \frac{a + b}{a} = 2.2$$

FIG. 2-39. Illustration of the principles of magnification. *S,* source; *O,* object; *I,* image. The source-to-image distance (*a–b*) divided by the source-to-object distance results in a magnification factor of 2.2.

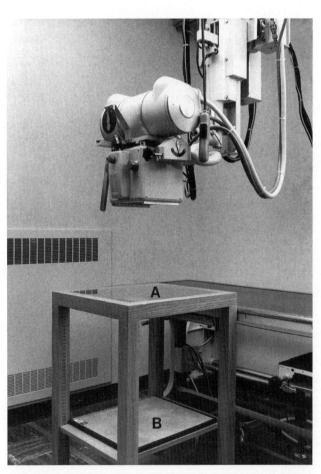

FIG. 2-38. Equipment used for conventional film magnification technique demonstrating the tube, support for the body part (**A**), and film (**B**).

as the distance between the object and film increases (see Fig. 2-39) and as the distance between the focal spot and the object decreases, other factors remaining constant.[66,67] Geometric magnification is defined as the ratio of the source-film distance to the source-object distance for a point-source focal spot (see Fig. 2-39).

Advantages and Limitations

Radiation exposure to the skin is increased in magnification radiography because of the short source-to-skin distance (see Fig. 2-38).[66,72] However, the size of the entrance field (in skull and abdominal magnification) is significantly reduced, thereby lowering total body exposure to nearly the equivalent dose obtained with conventional techniques. Entrance exposure to the skin for the magnified hand or foot using our technique measures 246 milliroentgens (mR) (Webbels W. Unpublished data, St. Mary's Hospital, Rochester, Minnesota, 1983). This exposure is higher than the routine foot films (26 mR) but is accepted, because the magnification technique is used only in selected cases.[68,71] In addition, the foot is among the least radiosensitive body parts. The overall high-quality image is the advantage of this technique. Increased effective sharpness, reduced effective noise, increased subject contrast (the air gap reduces the scattered radiation reaching the film), and improved visual effect of the enlargement contribute to high-quality radiographs (Fig. 2-40).[74]

Limitations of magnification include the following: (1) imaging is limited to small areas; (2) proper positioning of the area of interest may be difficult, especially in the lower

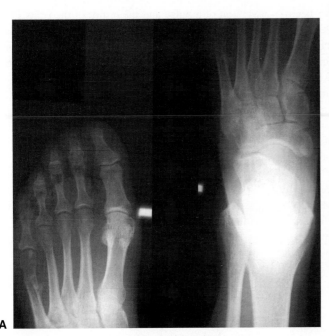
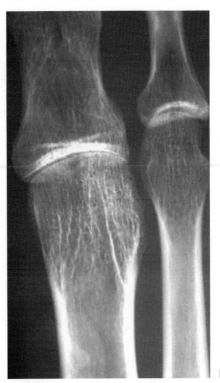

FIG. 2-40. Routine anteroposterior radiographs of the foot (**A**) and magnification view (**B**) of the forefoot. Note the superior trabecular detail using magnification.

extremity; (3) high relative skin exposure and long exposure times may result in limited tube-loading capabilities.[66,74] With the advent of CT and magnetic resonance imaging (MRI), this technique is not frequently used today. In addition, computed radiography allows image magnification on computer monitors.

ULTRASOUND

The term ultrasound refers to mechanical vibrations whose frequencies are above the limit of human audible perception (about 20,000 Hz or cycles/sec). Ultrasound imaging utilizes frequencies in the range of 2 to 10 MHz.[94,97] Doppler ultrasound for peripheral vascular studies is in the 8-MHz range. A central component of any ultrasound instrument is the transducer, which contains a small piezoelectric crystal. It serves as both the transmitter of sound waves into the body and the receiver of the returning echoes. When a brief alternating current is applied to the crystal, it vibrates at a characteristic frequency. By applying this vibrating transducer to the skin surface (through an acoustic coupling medium such as mineral oil or gel), the mechanical energy is transmitted into the body as a brief pulse of high-frequency sound waves. The advancing wave front interacts with tissues and generates small reflected waves that return to the transducer. These cause the crystal to vibrate again, thereby generating an electrical signal that is conducted back to the machine, where it is processed and displayed. With B-mode ultrasound imaging, the returning echoes are displayed as dots of light on an oscilloscope or television screen, with the position of the dot on the screen corresponding to the position in the body where the echo was generated. In this way, the ultrasound image represents a cross-sectional two-dimensional display of the underlying anatomy. Unlike CT, in which the geometric constraints of the scanner itself limit the possible scanning planes obtainable, any conceivable plane or section can be obtained with most ultrasound instruments. Such scanning flexibility can be of great value in demonstrating the continuity or discontinuity of adjacent structures.[94,99]

Static and Real-time Scanners

In ultrasound's early days, static B-mode scanners were utilized in which a two-dimensional static image was created by moving the transducer across the skin surface over the body part being imaged. This technique has been largely replaced by real-time two-dimensional ultrasound scanning that generates rapid sequential B-scan images that permit continuous (real-time) viewing.[75,94,96,97,99,103]

Modern B-mode scanning displays the intensity of returning echoes with at least 256 shades of gray for each pixel. The resulting images therefore demonstrate not only the major boundaries between soft tissue structures, but also their internal structures. This definition permits characterization of diffuse pathologic processes as well as detection of space-occupying lesions. Certainly, the development of gray-scale processing has been a crucial factor in the recent clinical success of ultrasound imaging.[75,87,89,94,96]

High-frequency (7.5 to 10 MHz) transducers have been developed that offer high-resolution images of superficial soft tissue structures.[87,97] It is a fundamental principle of ultrasound that the higher the frequency of the sound, the better the resolution of the images. However, it is also fundamentally true that high-frequency sound waves are attenuated more rapidly in the soft tissues and therefore cannot penetrate deeply. The result of these counterbalancing effects is that the so-called "small-parts" scanner or transducer can obtain submillimeter resolution, but only for structures located within about 5 cm of the skin surface.[84–87,97]

In the future, three-dimensional ultrasound images will be possible as multiple sequential two-dimensional images are stored and then displayed in a three-dimensional format. This advance may have a significant impact on musculoskeletal ultrasound applications.

Doppler Techniques

Doppler ultrasound techniques reflect changes in frequency of moving structures. This technique is commonly used to evaluate blood flow and vascular patency[80,97] (see Chapter 8).

The Doppler effect is based on change in observed frequency from either object motion or observer motion. Changes in frequency indicate that motion or flow is present. When flow is moving toward the ultrasound source, Doppler shift frequency is increased. If flow or motion is in the opposite direction of the emitted wave (away from the source), the frequency decreases (Fig. 2-41).[41,79,89,93]

The simplest Doppler devices utilize continuous-wave rather than pulsed-wave Doppler ultrasound. Continuous-wave systems are inexpensive and can determine the direction of flow. They do not, however, determine the depth of tissue at which the frequency shift is occurring. These devices can be helpful in evaluating patency of superficial vessels.

Because of the continuous-wave limitations, pulsed-wave range-gated Doppler is more widely used for imaging applications. This allows the utilization of the time between transversion of a pulse and the return of the echo 24 as a way of determining depth of where a frequency shift is occurring. Duplex scanners combine a two-dimensional real-time image with the pulsed Doppler data to define precisely where flow is occurring.

Today's modern scanners display Doppler data in a color-coded format known as color-flow Doppler imaging.[92] The use of color saturation to display variations in frequency shift (velocity) allows a semiquantitative estimate of flow from the two-dimensional image.

In recent years, a technique has been developed, termed "power Doppler," which enhances visualization of smaller vessels and slower flow velocities. Power Doppler utilizes color mapping to display the integrated power of the Doppler signal rather than the frequency shift.[98] The image does not display information related to flow direction or velocity.[77,78] This technique improves detection of small vessel perfusion and hyperemia resulting from inflammation or infection.[77,78,82,91]

Musculoskeletal Applications

Until recently, orthopedic applications were limited. However, technical advances and concern for imaging costs have resulted in a new era for musculoskeletal ultrasound (Table 2-2).[82,88,90] Sonographic characteristics of bone-periosteal interfaces and articular cartilage are now better defined, and this knowledge has expanded the clinical utility of this technique for evaluating musculoskeletal disorders.[81,82,85,87,95]

Perhaps the most severe limitation of diagnostic ultrasound imaging is caused by the inability of sound waves to penetrate gas and bone. The strength of an echo generated at the boundary between any two tissues is related to differences in the acoustic impedance of the tissue (a physical property generally dependent on density). Because the acoustic impedances of bone and air are so different from

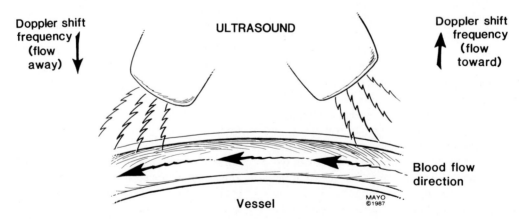

FIG. 2-41. Illustration of Doppler ultrasound showing the relationship of flow direction and the transducer.

TABLE 2-2. *Musculoskeletal ultrasound indications[a]*

Soft tissue masses
Vascular disease
Ligament/tendon tears
Bone
    Osteoporosis
    Fractures
Joint disorders
    Articular cartilage
    Joint fluid
Morton's neuroma
Foreign bodies

[a] Data from references 81 to 85, 88, 91, 95, 100, and 102.

those of human soft tissues, almost all sound energy is reflected off a soft tissue–bone or soft tissue–gas interface, leaving essentially no sound energy left to penetrate and, thus, image deeper structures.[85] The strong echo reflected off such an interface can "overwhelm" the transducer and thus may be displayed as useless noise or artifact in the image.[82,97]

Because this fundamental physical principle prevents ultrasound from passing from soft tissue into bone, the applications of this modality to orthopedics were, until recently, relatively limited. The lower extremity is an exception to the rule. The bones of the lower extremity are deep, except for the subcutaneous portions of the tibia, foot, and ankle, thus allowing easy examination of most soft tissue structures and osseous structures. Recently, evaluation of cortical and trabecular bone has become more feasible and permits ultrasound utilization to evaluate osteoporosis (calcaneus).[85] Muscles, tendons, ligaments, and vessels are generally accessible. Thus, thrombophlebitis, tendon and muscle tears, hematomas, abscesses, and tumors can be evaluated (see Table 2-2). Most structures are within 5 to 6 cm of the skin surface, so high-frequency scans can be performed. Imaging should be performed in both transverse and longitudinal planes of section.[76–78,85,95]

The remarkable sensitivity of ultrasound in distinguishing fluid from solid tissue has made it particularly useful in the characterization of the internal consistency of masses.[76,79] A simple fluid collection, such as an uncomplicated cyst, is represented sonographically as an echo-free area, whereas

solid tissue, or the cells and debris within some fluid masses (such as abscesses), will provide interfaces for sound reflection and will therefore be echogenic.[86] Some masses, of course, demonstrate a complex pattern with both solid and cystic elements. In addition to characterizing a mass by the number of echoes generated within it, it is also important to assess the manner in which sound is transmitted through the mass. Fluid-containing structures cause little attenuation of the sound beam and thereby demonstrate a characteristic ultrasound finding: so-called "enhanced through-transmission." This finding takes the form of stronger or brighter echoes deep to the fluid structure. Solid lesions cause greater attenuation of sound and therefore lack the finding of acoustic enhancement. By evaluating both the internal echogenicity of a mass and the ease of sound propagation through it, one can in virtually all instances characterize the basic contents of the mass as fluid, solid, or mixed. Although such a broad categorization is by no means histologically specific, such information, combined with appropriate clinical data, can often be helpful in patient management.[82,86,90] Power Doppler techniques are capable of defining perfusion changes or hyperemia that may assist in differentiating inflammatory or infected fluid collections from noninflammatory fluid collections.[77,78,91,98]

In addition to defining the internal nature of a soft tissue mass, ultrasound can also play a useful role in defining its size, extent, and relation to adjacent structures. For large or deep-seated lesions, however, the major disadvantage of ultrasound imaging is the inability to demonstrate bony involvement. For this reason, suspected malignant bone or soft tissue tumors are usually better evaluated with CT or MRI. For smaller and more superficially located masses, ultrasound can be a useful diagnostic tool, especially when a high-frequency transducer is used.

More recently, real-time ultrasound has gained acceptance in evaluation of the tendons and other superficial soft tissue structures of the foot and ankle.[75,82–85,87,95] Ultrasound is particularly suited for these structures because of its low cost and ability to study tendon motion (Fig. 2-42). Blei and colleagues[75] studied patients with tendinitis, acute trauma, and previous surgery on the Achilles tendon. Scans were obtained in the transverse and longitudinal planes using a 7.5-MHz transducer (see Fig. 2-36). Tendinitis was par-

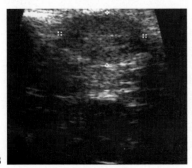
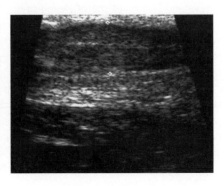

A,B

FIG. 2-42. Transverse (**A**) and longitudinal (**B**) sonograms of the Achilles tendon demonstrate thickening and increased central echogenicity resulting from a partial tear.

ticularly easy to detect because of peritendinous fluid accumulation. Similar success was reported by Fornage and others.[81,82,85,88,94]

Doppler ultrasound is an accurate and simple method for evaluating flow in the lower extremity. This technique is especially useful in evaluating patients with ischemic diseases, but it can also provide a method of accessing the distal vessels after acute trauma.[79,80,82]

Angiography and Doppler techniques can be used to study the arteries in the foot and ankle. Identification of peripheral vessels of the foot can be difficult with routine angiography. Operative angiography and reactive hyperemic angiography are more accurate.

Compared with routine angiography, Campbell and colleagues[80] found Doppler to be more accurate. Doppler ultrasound (pencil probe, 8 MHz) detected 80% (177/220) of patent vessels compared with 58% with routine angiography. Patency of distal arteries is critical in patients with ischemic disease. This has a significant effect on patency of proximal grafts. When comparing Doppler with operative or hyperemic angiography, Roedersheimer and colleagues[97] found that both techniques were equally accurate.

SKELETAL SCINTIGRAPHY

Radionuclide skeletal imaging evolved from the early work with phosphate compounds that had its origins with the introduction of tripolyphosphate by Subramanian and associates.[126,127] Radiopharmaceuticals currently used in bone scanning include compounds with $P==C==P$ bonds (methylenediphosphonate). Diphosphonates are the current agents of choice because of their better stability and soft tissue clearance rates. Phosphate and phosphonate reagents come in sterile, pyrogen-free lyophilized form with stannous ion as a reducing agent. These substances are labeled with technetium-99m (^{99m}Tc) pertechnetate. ^{99m}Tc-pertechnetate is reduced from the $+7$ to the $+4$ state and forms a chelate with the diphosphonate. After compounding, the material is checked for acceptability by quality-control procedures. Generally, thin-layer or paper chromatography is used. The material is injected intravenously. Its localization in bone is dependent on blood flow and osteoblastic activity.[106,109,126,127] The most widely accepted mechanism of localization is believed to be chemiabsorption to the hydroxyapatite crystals of the bone mineral matrix. Approximately 50% of the mineral is cleared by the kidneys and is excreted in the urine. Good hydration and an appropriate interval between administration and scanning are important. Generally, 3 to 4 hours are allowed to elapse between injection and imaging. This allows adequate soft tissue clearance and improved target-to-background ratios. The three-phase bone scan includes a flow study, immediate images (while the tracer is in the extracellular fluid state), and delayed images. This sequence can suggest the acute nature of the problem and is useful to differentiate cellulitis or joint space infections from osteomyelitis.[104,106,115]

Another important radiopharmaceutical, gallium-67 (^{67}Ga) citrate, can be used in patients with suspected infection.[106,111,114,121,130] In the 1950s, gallium isotopes were originally studied as potential bone-scanning agents. Although they do localize in bone, the isotopes of gallium available at that time were not satisfactory for imaging. Later, ^{67}Ga was shown to localize in tumors and sites of infection, its major roles today. The mechanism of localization of gallium in infection sites is not well understood, but it appears to be related to the binding of gallium to lactoferrin at sites of infection, leukocyte labeling, or direct bacterial uptake.[106,111,120] The optimal time from injection to scan is 24 to 48 hr. Because we know that gallium is deposited in bone, care must be taken in the interpretation of gallium uptake when looking for bone or joint infections. A sequence of ^{99m}Tc and gallium scans may be necessary to differentiate reactive bone from inflammatory lesions. Indium-111 (^{111}In) or ^{99m}Tc-labeled white blood cells have replaced gallium for evaluating infections at many institutions.[106,111,118,129,130] The method of cell labeling is beyond the scope of this chapter, but the primary method is based on the work of Thakur and colleagues.[129,130] White blood cells migrate to sites of infection, and localization in the area of bone implies an infectious process. Images may be taken at 4 and 24 hr after the administration of ^{111}In-labeled white cells.[106,130] This time delay is a disadvantage compared with ^{99m}Tc-labeled white blood cells. Technetium images can be obtained 2 to 4 hours after injection, resolution is superior, and the isotope is more readily available.[111] However, technetium also has disadvantages. There is high background activity compared with ^{111}In, and biliary excretion into the bowel occurs at 2 to 4 hr.[111] The latter is not a problem when imaging the foot and ankle.

Instrumentation

Originally, the rectilinear scanner was the most common instrument used for whole-body bone studies. Currently, a gamma camera is the instrument used. The camera allows total-body surveys with a moving table or moving detector. Selected views can also be obtained with this instrument. Radioactivity from the patient passes through a lead collimator and enters a sodium iodide crystal. The photon deposits its energy in the crystal, which, in turn, gives off photons of light that are converted to electrons by the photocathode of the photomultiplier tubes. These electrons are amplified by the photomultiplier tubes and are processed. The resulting data can be placed on film or entered into a computer for further analysis.[105,106]

Collimators are designated according to the resolution and energy levels at which they can be used (i.e., lower energy for ^{99m}Tc agents, medium energy for ^{111}In-labeled white cells or ^{67}Ga studies, and high energy for iodine-131 agents). Collimator holes can be parallel or nonparallel; converging collimators magnify slightly. The pinhole collimator is a single hole that allows for magnification of an area of interest with some geometric distortion.[108] Until recently, this collimator was commonly used to isolate abnormalities in the foot and ankle. Satisfactory evaluation can be obtained by most systems today using coned-down magnification views with parallel hole collimations.[106,108]

Clinical Applications

In general, the most common use of isotope imaging is in oncology, for detection and follow-up of metastatic bone disease primarily from prostatic, breast, and lung cancer.[106, 116] The orthopedic uses of bone scanning primarily include diagnosis of trauma and infection, determination of vascularity, compartmental evaluation of degenerative arthritis of joints, evaluation of patients with painful prosthesis, and evaluation of patients with nonspecific bone pain.[104–107,110, 112,113,115,117,119,124,128,131–133] When evaluating isotope images of the foot and ankle, it is important to remember normal variations in uptake that occur, especially during the growth phases of the skeleton (Fig. 2-43).[106]

Tumors

Bone scanning is perhaps of greatest use in the diagnosis and delineation of metastatic diseases.[106,116] This use is less important in the foot and ankle, in which metastatic disease is not common, although isolated (or solitary) metastasis from lung carcinoma can present in the foot and ankle. Primary tumors in the foot and ankle also occur infrequently.

The bone scan is of limited utility in the evaluation of multiple myeloma, a malignant disease that seems to evoke little reparative response. Conventional radiographs are more sensitive in the evaluation of these patients.[106]

Bone scintigraphy is of little use in the evaluation of benign tumors, except for suspected osteoid osteoma. Plain films are difficult to interpret because of the complex skeletal anatomy, especially in the midfoot and hindfoot. When plain films are negative or atypical, bone scanning is useful to detect the typical focal uptake seen with osteoid osteoma.

The area of abnormal uptake can then be further classified with CT.[123,128]

Trauma

Bone scanning can provide important information in patients with known or suspected trauma. Routine radiographs easily demonstrate the site of fracture in most patients with a clinical history of trauma. In these uncomplicated cases, bone scintigraphy does not add significant additional information. However, when the initial radiographs are normal, as may occur with subtle fractures, the bone scan may play a role in directing the course of management.[106,107,112,119] Fractures are demonstrated as focal areas of increased uptake, with 80% visible in 24 hours and 95% in 72 hours. However, in elderly patients, more time is often required for the onset of activity to occur at the fracture site.[109,111,112,117] Bone scanning is also helpful in patients suspected of having stress fractures. Isotope scans detect stress fractures earlier than radiography. Radiographs may not be positive for several weeks, and if cessation of the stress is instituted, the radiograph may not become positive.[106,109,112,117] A negative scan, with few exceptions, implies that the symptoms are not caused by a stress fracture. Finally, in the battered child syndrome, the bone scan may show the extent of bone trauma, thus allowing for directed radiographic confirmation. The scan may also demonstrate bone contusion not seen radiographically.[106]

Infection

Radionuclide studies play a valuable role in early detection of bone and soft tissue infection (see Chapter 7).[106, 125] Three-phase ^{99m}Tc-pertechnetate studies are sensitive but less specific than newer isotope techniques. More recently, ^{67}Ga- and ^{111}In- or ^{99m}Tc-labeled white blood cells have provided improved specificity.[111,118,122] The latter are particularly useful after trauma or surgery, when detection of subtle infection can be difficult.[122]

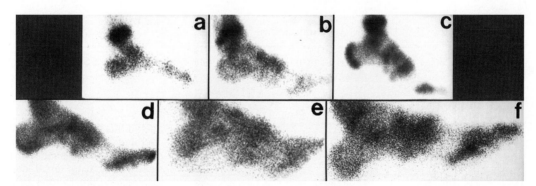

FIG. 2-43. Normal variations in isotope images of the foot with age. *a,* A 22-month-old boy; *b,* a 7-year-old girl; *c,* a 13-year-old boy (note the activity in the calcaneal apophysis); *d,* an 18-year-old man with the apophysis almost completely fused; *e,* an 18-year-old man with a fused apophysis; *f,* a 71-year-old man with increased tarsal uptake because of degenerative arthritis.

Miscellaneous Conditions

Tarsal coalition refers to fusion of two tarsal bones, usually the calcaneus and navicular or the talus and calcaneus.[101] Tarsal coalitions can be difficult to identify radiographically. Reports reveal that ^{99m}Tc methylene diphosphonate scintigraphy is a valuable screening tool in patients with suspected tarsal coalition.[110,113] Confirmation can be obtained using CT or MRI in patients with positive studies (Fig. 2-44). Radionuclide scans are also useful for detection of reflex sympathetic dystrophy. Increased blood flow and intense periarticular uptake are characteristic of this condition.[106]

Other uses for bone scanning are currently being explored. Animal models show that sequential studies can use radionuclide imaging to evaluate fracture healing, although this has not yet been convincingly demonstrated in humans. There does seem to be a role for bone scintigraphy in selecting patients with nonunited fractures for percutaneous electrical stimulation, however, as reported by Desai and colleagues.[109] Their study showed that when diffuse increased activity occurred at the fracture site, 95% of these fractures healed completely with percutaneous electrical stimulation. When a photon-deficient (cold) area was seen at the fracture site, none healed; and only 50% healed when there was low uptake in the fracture site.[109] More specific examples and indications for scintigraphy are discussed in later chapters.

COMPUTED TOMOGRAPHY

CT is a fast and efficacious technique for evaluation of the musculoskeletal system. The basic components of the system are a gantry, which houses a rotating X-ray tube and radiation detectors, and a movable patient table. The output of the radiation detectors is manipulated through a computer to produce the images.[135–138,142,143] The tube and detectors rotate around the patient; the narrowly collimated X-ray

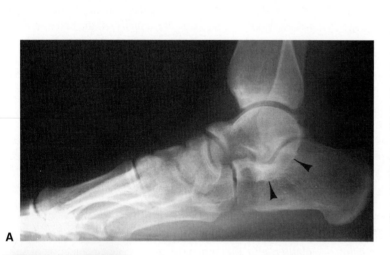

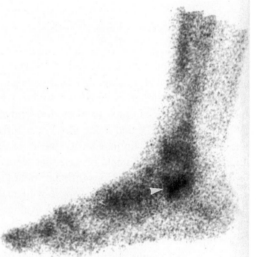

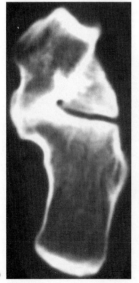

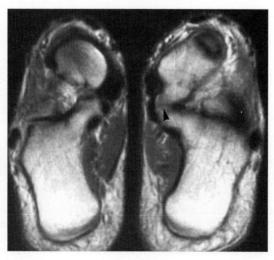

FIG. 2-44. Patient with foot pain and suspected tarsal coalition. **A:** Weight-bearing lateral radiograph of the foot demonstrates a talar beak and C-shaped overlap (*arrowheads*) indicating tarsal coalition. **B:** A technetium-99m isotope scan shows increased tracer in the sustentacular region (*white arrowhead*). **C:** Bony coalition demonstrated on CT. **D:** Bony coalition demonstrated on MRI imaging (*black arrowhead*).

beam produces a cross-sectional image or slice. The table is then moved incrementally, and the next slice is obtained. Spiral (helical) scanners move the patient continuously as the tube and detectors rotate, resulting in a spiral volumetric data set.[134,149,159]

The computer presents the data on a grid or matrix, usually consisting of 512 × 512 picture elements or pixels. The size of each pixel depends on the field of view (FOV) that is reconstructed. Each pixel represents a volume element (voxel) whose depth is the chosen slice thickness. Most commonly, 5-mm slices are used for skeletal work, but thinner slices (1 to 1.5 mm) may be used if reformatting or three-dimensional reconstruction is to be done (Fig. 2-45).[144,147,160] Each picture element is assigned a shade of gray that represents the X-ray attenuation value (CT number) for that voxel. Attenuation values range from air at 1,000, water at 0, and dense bone at 1,000.[127,139–141]

Modern scanners can display a wider range of numbers to allow extremely dense structures to be evaluated. If two tissues of different attenuation are included within one voxel, the resulting CT number will be an average of the two values. This is called partial volume averaging and occurs more often with thicker slices. Therefore, if a fracture line is parallel to and included within a slice, it may not be demonstrated (Fig. 2-46). The viewer manipulates the window width and level to allow tissues of differing attenuation to be evaluated. In this matter, images can be obtained at setting which demonstrate either bone or soft tissues to best advantage. This is critical in musculoskeletal imaging (Fig. 2-47).[137,150,151,154–158]

The use of helical spiral scanners is increasing as earlier generation machines are being replaced. Because the data are acquired as a volume, multiplanar and three-dimensional reconstruction are much improved.[149,159] In addition, patient motion (from pain or inability to maintain a position or hold one's breath) is less of a problem with helical scanners because of decreased scan times. Helical scan times are 20 to 40 sec compared with 4 to 6 min for conventional scan-

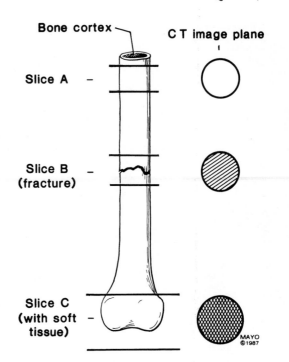

FIG. 2-46. Illustration of partial volume effect. Density is the sum of data in the image slice.

ners.[149,159] Advantages of helical CT include decreased scan time, decreased acquisition time, and more frequent or consistent data sampling. The major disadvantage is that metallic artifact may be increased.

The next generation of CT scanners will employ multiple detector channels, as well as spiral CT technology. This advance will allow faster scanning of larger volumes, as well as retrospective reconstruction of different slice thickness. The utility of these advances for musculoskeletal disease remains to be researched.

Foot and Ankle Techniques

CT examinations of the foot and ankle are particularly useful owing to the complex anatomy. Examination of the hindfoot can be easily accomplished with CT and may demonstrate anatomic changes that may be difficult with special radiographic views or complex motion tomography (see the earlier discussion of routine radiography). The mobility of the foot allows changes in position so that direct image data can be obtained in several planes.

Proper examination of the foot and ankle requires adequate clinical information. Positioning, slice thickness (1 to 1.5 mm may be needed if three-dimensional, sagittal, or coronal reconstruction is contemplated), and need for intravenous contrast medium, for example, must be considered before the examination. All pertinent radiographs and isotope studies should also be reviewed.

Before positioning the patient on the gantry couch, the patient's age, condition, and presence of any orthopedic fixa-

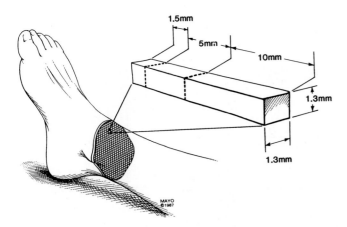

FIG. 2-45. Illustration of CT pixel size and section thickness (1.5-, 5.0-, and 10-mm sections demonstrated).

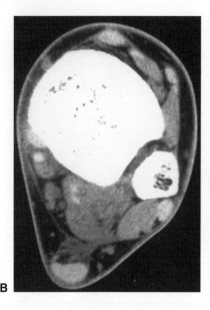 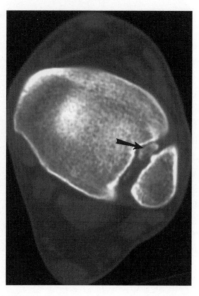

A,B

FIG. 2-47. Axial CT images of the ankle with soft tissue settings (**A**) and bone settings (**B**). Soft tissue anatomy is clearly defined in **A,** and osseous structures including the loose body (*arrow*) are shown in **B.**

tion devices must be considered. Metal fixation devices may degrade the image. Robert Jones dressings and casts should not interfere with image quality, but they restrict positioning. Sedation may be needed for small children, especially those younger than 4 years of age, and pain medication may be needed to allow the patient to maintain the proper position. Examinations, if complex, may take more than 30 min with conventional scanners. Scan time is significantly reduced with helical techniques, which may reduce the need for pain medication or sedation.[149,159]

Ideally, positioning should be comfortable and easily maintained, should provide the proper alignment for the area of interest, and should be reproducible. This may be difficult after acute trauma. Reproducibility can be achieved to some degree with the use of foot boards and angled wedges.[135,139, 145,146,152,153] Donaldson and colleagues[135] advocated using tennis shoes without metal vents (these create image artifacts) to reduce motion and to ensure symmetric positioning in children. The patient's own shoes are preferred, but this group of clinicians keeps multiple pairs of shoes in their department for imaging purposes. This technique has merit, but it may be ineffective after acute trauma or inflammation or in the presence of congenital deformities.

Although positioning and technique vary with individual clinical problems, certain standard techniques can often be applied. A scout view aids with proper positioning and slice selection. Sagittal reformatting and three-dimensional reconstruction are used in selected cases. Axial and coronal images are usually obtained.

Axial images of the foot and ankle are obtained with the patient's feet perpendicular to the gantry table. The knees are extended, and the great toes are together. A foot board can be used to maintain this position and to reduce motion (Fig. 2-48).[137,138,141,149–154]

For coronal images, the patient's knees are flexed with the feet flat against the gantry table (Fig. 2-49). Specific tarsal bones and joints may require the use of a foot wedge

or angling of the gantry, or both, to obtain the alignment desired (see Fig. 2-49).[128,130,131,143] These factors can be determined using the scout view. Positioning is particularly critical in the hindfoot.

Typically examinations are performed using 3- to 5-mm thick slides; 1.0- to 1.5-mm contiguous slides provide superior reconstructed or three-dimensional images. Table 2-3 summarizes the anatomic areas and optical image planes for CT imaging.

Clinical Applications

CT provides excellent bone detail, and assessment of the complex articulations of the foot and ankle is readily accom-

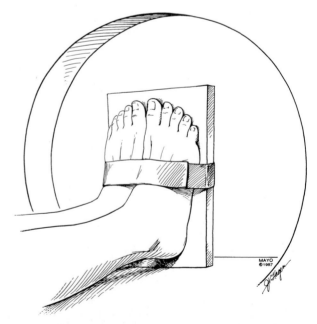

FIG. 2-48. Illustration of feet positioned with a foot board for axial imaging.

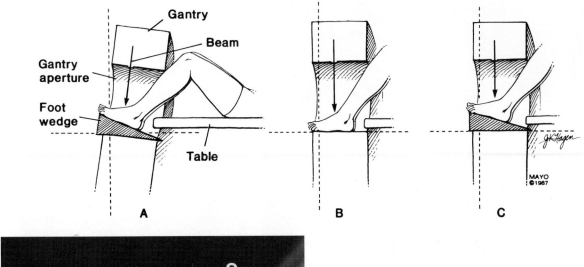

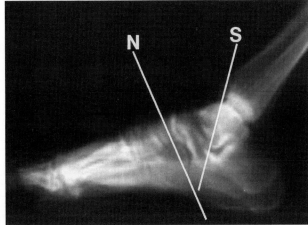

FIG. 2-49. Illustration of positions for coronal images. The gantry can be angled (**A**), or the foot position can be changed (**A–C**) to achieve true coronal images. The scout view (**D**) can be used to confirm positioning and slice selection. Angles required for coronal images of the navicular (*N*) and sustentacular articulation (*S*) are shown. Image planes can be more easily reformatted with new helical scanners.

plished. It may be the technique of choice for the subtalar joint.[136,146,152,155] CT is capable of evaluating the bones and joints to establish diagnoses and to assist in planning conservative or surgical therapy when appropriate.

Foot and ankle neoplasms constitute uncommon indications for CT because of the rarity of these lesions. In addition, MRI, with its superior contrast resolution, lack of beam-hardening artifact, and diminished dependence on fat, is supplanting CT as a method to image foot and ankle neoplasms. However, CT still yields valuable information for defining the extent of a lesion and in planning therapy. Intravenous contrast is often useful to demonstrate tumor vascularity and vascular encasement and to assist in predicting the nature of the lesion (i.e., hemangioma). Coronal and axial imaging are generally adequate for evaluation of neoplasm.

Acute skeletal trauma and posttraumatic arthrosis are also suited to evaluation by CT. This technique is useful in the hindfoot to assess fragmentation, to evaluate the degree of articular involvement, and to check for intraarticular fragments (Fig. 2-50). It is not as helpful for soft tissue injury such as ligamentous tears.[150,158]

When indicated, CT is a valuable addition to radiography in evaluating patients with arthritis, foot deformities, tarsal

TABLE 2-3. *Computed tomography imaging of the foot and ankle*[a]

	Optimal image planes		
	Axial	Coronal	Sagittal (reconstruction)
Posterior subtalar joint	+	+	+
Mid- and anterior talocalcaneal joints		+	
Calcaneus	+		+
Calcaneocuboid joint	+		+
Medial and lateral tendons	+	+	
Tibiofibular syndesmosis	+	+	

[a] Data from references 135, 136, 141, and 156.

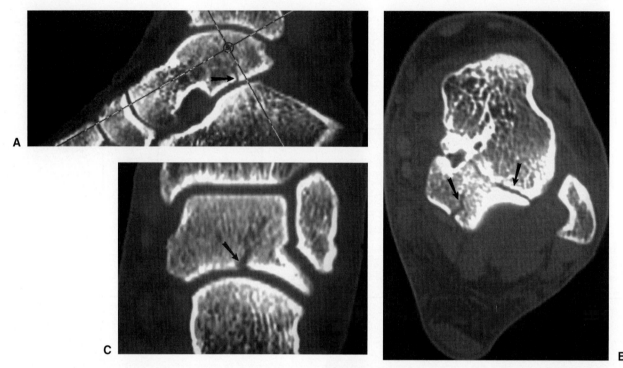

FIG. 2-50. Subtle talar fracture: CT performed for detection and evaluating articular involvement. **A:** Sagittal reformatted image demonstrating angles for optimal axial and coronal planes. Note the fracture entering the posterior joint (*arrow*). **B:** Axial image (*arrows* indicate fractures). **C:** Coronal image (*arrow* indicates fracture).

coalition, and other foot and ankle disorders.[137,146,148,156,157,159] Specific indications and technical variations needed for the examinations are discussed in later chapters.

MAGNETIC RESONANCE IMAGING

Clinical interest in MRI as an imaging modality has increased rapidly in recent years. In 1975, Lauterbur[181] demonstrated the capability of producing axial images using nuclear MRI techniques. Technologic advances have since resulted in significant improvements in MRI.[161–169,172,185,188] Today, MRI is often the second examination selected following routine radiographs.[167]

Principles

An in-depth discussion of the physics of MRI is beyond the scope of this chapter. However, the following paragraphs provide an overview of the factors in MRI that allow image formation.

MRI is based on the principle that nuclei with an odd number of protons or neutrons (^1H, ^{31}P, ^{13}C, ^{23}Na, ^{19}F, ^{17}O) exhibit spin.[171,186] Because of its abundance and favorable magnetic moment, proton imaging (^1H) is most practical at this time. When placed in a strong magnetic field, the normally randomly oriented nuclei tend to produce a net magnetic vector parallel to the magnetic field.[186] Applying a radio frequency (RF) pulse to the spinning nuclei causes

displacement of the nuclei in proportion to the strength of the RF pulse. A pulse resulting in a 90° deflection causes the nuclei to rotate at 90° to the static field. After the RF pulse, the magnetization induces a signal in the receiver coil (the coils around the patient). The nuclei then regress to their original position in the magnetic field. As the nuclei return to their equilibrium position, the signal decreases and two sample-related time constants occur, the spin-lattice (longitudinal) relaxation time (T1), and the spin-spin (transverse) relaxation time (T2).[171,181,186] The relaxation times vary, depending on the tissue being studied. Along with proton density, relaxation times provide the basis for image formation. In general, T1 is always longer than T2, except in liquids, in which the relaxation times are nearly equal.[186]

Clinical Techniques

MRI is particularly suited to evaluation of the complex bone and soft tissue anatomy of the foot and ankle. Examination is facilitated by superior soft tissue contrast and by the ability to image in multiple planes.[165–167,188,195,196] Newer techniques have decreased scan time, improving patient throughput and allowing improved vascular imaging techniques.[162,167,172,178,182,184]

Patient Selection

MRI images are produced using a static magnetic field, magnetic gradients, and RF pulses. There is no ionizing radiation. To date, no biologic hazards have been identified at the currently used field strengths (≤2 Tesla).[167,170,189–191]

Most high-field MRI gantries are more confining than a conventional fluoroscopic unit or CT scanner, although new open and low-field units are less confining. Patients are positioned in the center of the cylindric magnet chamber during the examination. Despite the apparent drawbacks of high-field long-core magnets, we note problems with claustrophobia in only about 5% of patients.[167] Patients with claustrophobic tendencies seem to tolerate MRI examinations more readily if they are in the prone position. The prone position makes positioning of the foot and ankle more difficult. If necessary, mild sedation with oral diazepam (Valium) may be helpful. Obese or significantly claustrophobic patients may more easily tolerate open low-field magnets.

The patient's clinical status must be considered. Patients with significant pain or inability to maintain the necessary positions may not be able to tolerate the potentially lengthy examinations. Premedication with diazepam or meperidine (Demerol) may be useful in these cases. Initially, there was concern that severely ill patients requiring cardiac monitoring and respiratory support could not be examined. Ferromagnetic anesthesia equipment cannot be moved into the magnet room or near the gantry without affecting the images. Our experience shows that these patients can be monitored successfully without interfering with image quality. Initially, we studied 20 patients requiring cardiac and respiratory support. Patients were monitored with a blood pressure cuff with plastic connectors, an Aneuroid Chest Bellows for respiratory rate, and a Hewlett-Packard electrocardiograph (ECG) telemetry system. The respiratory rate and ECG were monitored on a Saturn monitor. Certain problems were encountered during the study. RF pulses caused ECG artifacts, especially when short repetition times were used. This problem was overcome by using a Doppler system to monitor pulse during the imaging sequences. Satisfactory monitoring was achieved in all patients, and the equipment used did not affect image quality.[187]

Magnetic fields may affect certain metal implants and electrical devices. In most situations, the exact chemical structure of the implant cannot be determined.[167,170,180,191] Fortunately, early efforts to determine which implants may be potentially dangerous to the patient or may affect image quality have been successful.[167,168,170,179,191] Synchronous pacemakers convert to the asynchronous mode when placed in MRI scans. The pacemaker power pack may torque in the magnetic field. In addition, significant image degradation may occur if the power pack is in the region examined.[167] Numerous heart valves have been studied at field strengths of 0.35 and 1.5 Tesla. The artifacts created were negligible, and it was concluded that patients with prosthetic valves could safely undergo MRI.[167,191]

Most surgical clips at our institution are nonferromagnetic. However, many aneurysm clips (16/21) are ferromagnetic, and torquing can be demonstrated in a magnetic envi-

ronment.[170,191] Therefore, patients with aneurysm clips or pacemakers are currently not examined by MRI.

Manufacturers of orthopedic appliances (e.g., plates, screws, joint prostheses) generally use high-grade stainless steel, cobalt-chromium, titanium, or multiphase alloys. These materials are usually not ferromagnetic, but they may contain minimal quantities of iron impurities. All the orthopedic appliances at our institution have been tested for magnetic properties (torque in the magnet) and heating. No heating or magnetic response could be detected.[167,168] Davis and colleagues[170] also studied the effects of RF pulses and changing magnetic fields on metal clips and prostheses. No heating could be detected with small amounts of metal. Heating was demonstrated with two adjacent prostheses in a saline medium. However, it was concluded that metal heating in patients should not be a problem even with large prostheses.[180,191]

Metal materials may cause significant artifact on CT images.[168,170] Nonferromagnetic materials cause areas of no signal but less artifact on MRI. The degree of artifact is dependent on the size and configuration of the metal (Fig. 2-51). Screws tend to cause more local image distortion than do smooth tubular or flat metal implants.[168]

External fixation devices may be bulky, but most are not ferromagnetic because the materials are similar to those used in internal fixators. Magnetic properties can be easily checked with a hand-held magnet before the MRI examination. Coil selection may be restricted because of the size of these fixation systems. This can result in a decreased signal-to-noise ratio and may reduce image quality. However, most patients can be examined using head or body coils.

Early experience with metal implants at low and high field strength (0.15 to 1.5 T) shows that artifact is more significant at higher field strengths.[167] Evaluation of patients with casts and bulky dressings (e.g., Robert Jones) is also possible with MRI. We have not detected any reduction in image quality because of these materials.

Patient Positioning and Coil Selection

The patient should be studied with the most closely coupled coil practical and the appropriate FOV to optimize image quality.[165–167,179] It is important to consider the clinical indication when positioning the patient and selecting the coil. For example, if a tendon tear is suspected, enough area must be included to demonstrate the tendon ends, which can be separated by a significant distance.[167]

Conventional surface coils are available in several configurations: flat, partial volume, or circumferential (Fig. 2-52).[165–167,173,175] Different coiled configurations are suited to specific clinical indications and the type of imaging examination required. Generally, flat or coupled flat coils are used for motion studies or when specific position of the foot or ankle is required (see Fig. 2-52). When comparison is indicated, the head or dual coils can be used to reduce examination time (Fig. 2-53).[167]

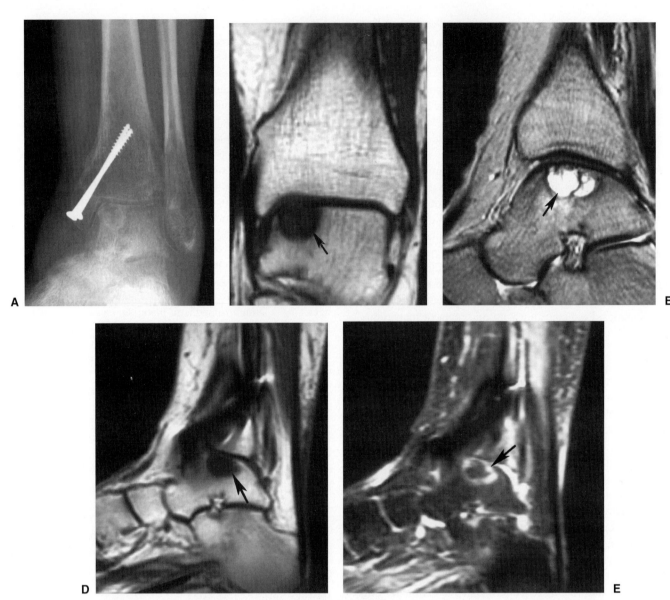

A

B,C

D

E

FIG. 2-51. Patient with ankle pain after appropriate treatment and healing of an ankle fracture. **A:** Mortise view of the ankle demonstrates medial swelling osteopenia and two malleolar screws (partially threaded) for fixation. **B** and **C:** Coronal SE 500/10 (**B**) and sagittal SE 2000/80 (**C**) images demonstrate a large geode (*arrow*) resulting from an old osteochondral fracture. There is no metal artifact. **D** and **E:** Sagittal SE 500/10 (**D**) and fat-suppressed T2-weighted (**E**) images show the defect (*arrows*) with artifacts proximally because of the relationship with the screws in this plane and section.

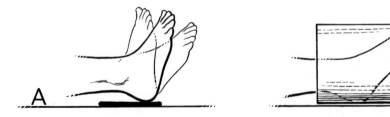

A

B

MAYO
©1985

FIG. 2-52. Patient positioned for examination of the foot and ankle using flat (**A**) and circumferential (**B**) coils. The former allows more flexibility with positioning. The latter provides improved signal uniformity but reduces positioning options. (From Berquist, ref. 167, with permission.)

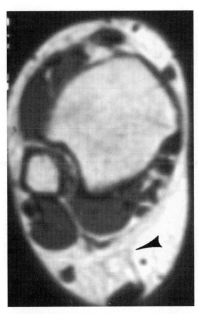 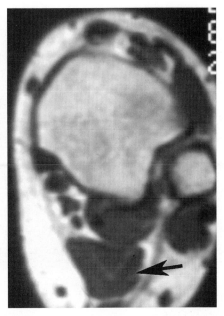

FIG. 2-53. Patient with ankle pain and fullness posteriorly. Examination is performed in the head coil to allow comparison and improved detection of subtle lesions. Axial SE 500/20 images of the ankles demonstrate an accessory soleus muscle on the left (*arrow*), which may have been overlooked if the opposite ankle were not available for comparison. Note the normal pre-Achilles fat on the right (*arrowhead*).

Patients can be examined in the supine or prone position, depending on which anatomic region is being evaluated. The prone position is useful for the midfoot and forefoot and assists in reducing inadvertent motion.[166,167] The prone position is also used when evaluating the posterior soft tissues. This avoids soft tissue compression, which can cause anatomic distortion. The ankle and hindfoot are most often studied in the supine position with the foot neutral to avoid tendon distortion posteriorly, specifically in the Achilles tendon.[167] Motion studies are usually performed using coupled flat coils to allow improved signal and ease of foot movement into the necessary positions to permit a cine loop study.[167]

Image Planes

Coronal, axial, and sagittal image planes are commonly used for foot and ankle examination. In the foot, coronal images are perpendicular to the metatarsals and axial images are along the plane of the metatarsals.[166,188] To achieve patient comfort and to optimize image planes, oblique planes are frequently used in the foot and ankle.[167,188] We generally use a minimum of two image planes at 90° angles to evaluate foot and ankle disorders. Figure 2-54 gives examples of commonly used image planes and patient positions.

Pulse Sequences and Imaging Parameters

Detection and characterization of most lesions in the foot and ankle can be accomplished with conventional spin-echo sequences. We generally perform T1-weighted and T2-weighted spin-echo sequences and use at least two image planes. Conventional spin-echo sequences with one acquisition can be obtained in 3 to 4 min for a T1-weighted sequence and in 8 to 9 min for a T2-weighted sequence.[167] New fast spin-echo sequences are faster, reducing image time. However, in our experience, the contrast is slightly different from that obtained in conventional spin-echo sequences, so subtle lesions, especially in bone marrow, can be overlooked if fat-suppression techniques are not included.[167,183] Short T1 inversion recovery sequences are excellent for subtle marrow and soft tissue abnormalities.

New angiographic sequences provide improved vascular detail with or without intravenous contrast.[167,174,176,178,182,184] Conventional MRI sequences have been replaced with specific fast scan techniques with and without gadolinium injections. These techniques have greatly improved the utility of MRI for arterial and venous studies in the lower extremities.[184,193] Most authors report using two-dimensional time-of-flight or three-dimensional contrast-enhanced MRI for vascular studies of the lower extremity.[162,174,176,178] Bolus chase techniques have become more popular recently. This approach is useful for evaluation of the entire lower extremity (run-off angiogram) and is accomplished by moving the table and patient in steps through the uniform image volume of the magnetic field.[193]

Gadolinium can also be given intravenously to evaluate bone and soft tissue disorders. An arthrographic effect of synovial fluid enhancement occurs 15 to 30 min after intravenous injection.[194] This may be useful for certain arthropa-

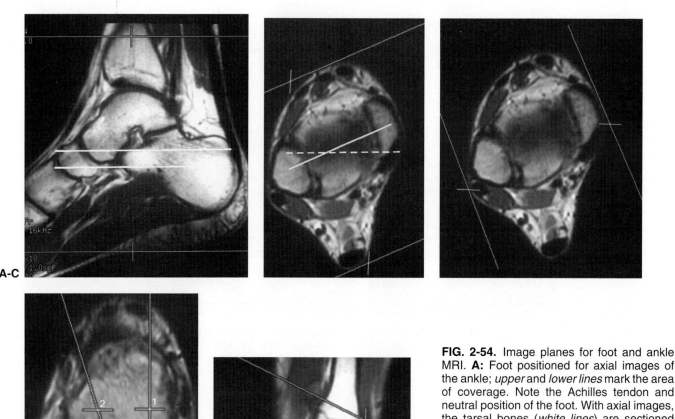

A-C

D,E

FIG. 2-54. Image planes for foot and ankle MRI. **A:** Foot positioned for axial images of the ankle; *upper* and *lower lines* mark the area of coverage. Note the Achilles tendon and neutral position of the foot. With axial images, the tarsal bones (*white lines*) are sectioned out of anatomic alignment. **B:** Image planes obliqued to obtain coronal images through the ankle mortise. The *white line* indicates planes of sections through the mortise. A true coronal plane (*dotted line*) would cut obliquely through the joint and anatomy. **C:** Oblique sagittal image planes to improve anatomic display of the osseous structures in the ankle. **D:** Conventional sagittal image plane (*1*) and obliqued sagittal plane (*2*) to improve evaluation of the Achilles tendon. **E:** Obliqued axial image planes to improve evaluation of the peroneal tendons. *(continued)*

thies (Fig. 2-55). Intraarticular contrast is rarely used in the foot and ankle.[167] Normal saline or iodinated contrast can be used with conventional MRI sequences to provide the necessary fluid to evaluate intraarticular structures. However, most authors prefer gadolinium with fat-suppressed T1-weighted sequences to improve contrast and to reduce image time. The United States Food and Drug Administration has not approved gadolinium for intraarticular use. Therefore, institution review board approval is required.

Intraarticular gadolinium should be injected with fluoroscopic, ultrasonic, or MRI guidance to ensure proper needle position. A small amount of iodinated contrast can be used for this purpose. Gadolinium is diluted with normal saline before intraarticular injection. The mixture is obtained by adding 0.2 ml of gadolinium to 50 ml of normal saline or 1 ml of gadolinium to 250 ml of normal saline.[177] The amount injected varies with the size of the joint being evaluated.[177]

Other image parameters typically include a small FOV (8 to 16 cm), a 256 × 256 or 256 × 192 matrix, and one acquisition. Slice thickness varies depending on the clinical indication. However, 3- to 5-mm thick sections are usually adequate, except for three-dimensional imaging or reformatting. In this case, we use thin (≤1 mm)–section gradient-echo sequences.[167] More specific techniques are provided in later chapters as they apply to specific clinical conditions.

Clinical Applications

Clinical applications of MRI for foot and ankle disorders have expanded. Studies have confirmed its utility as a clinical tool with significant impact on clinical decision making.[167,196] In many cases, MRI is selected as the second technique after screening radiographs.[167]

MRI is most frequently requested to evaluate soft tissue

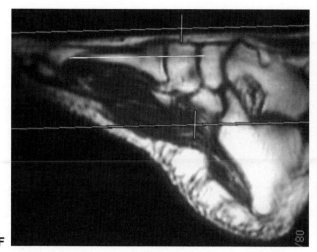

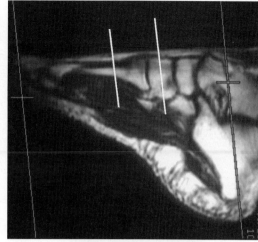

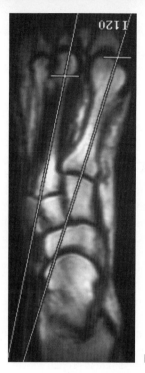

FIG. 2-54. *Continued.* **F:** Scout sagittal image of the mid-foot and forefoot, with the area scanned for images in the planes of the distal tarsal bones and metatarsals (the *white line* indicates the image plane). **G:** Scout sagittal image for imaging perpendicular to the distal tarsal row and metatarsals (*white lines* indicate image sections). **H:** Axial forefoot scout demonstrating oblique planes for sagittal images of the first and second metatarsals.

disorders, specifically tendon and ligament injuries and soft tissue masses.[183,195] Articular and osseous inflammatory and infectious abnormalities can also be detected early with MRI techniques.[167,192] Specific applications are discussed in later chapters, in which MRI is also compared with other imaging techniques.

INTERVENTIONAL ORTHOPEDIC TECHNIQUES

Interventional techniques in the foot and ankle are used for diagnostic and therapeutic purposes. Although MRI has replaced many techniques, arthrography, tenography, sinography, diagnostic and therapeutic injections, and bone and soft tissue biopsy still play a role in evaluating foot and ankle disorders. Proper use of these techniques requires a thorough knowledge of the anatomy and clinical problems. Routine

films, fluoroscopy, CT, ultrasound, and, rarely, MRI may be used to monitor or record the procedures.[198,199,201]

Ankle Arthrography

Arthrography is a safe, valuable method of studying the ligaments, capsule, and articular anatomy of the ankle.[197,198,208,210,227,229–231] Ankle arthrograms are most frequently performed in patients with suspected soft tissue trauma. In the series of Goergen and Resnick,[210] 95% of arthrograms were performed in patients with suspected ligament injury. Arthrograms are less commonly performed to evaluate articular cartilage (talar dome fractures, osteochondritis dissecans) and loose bodies.[198,200,204,219,229,235,236] Evaluation of the joints in children is also useful, because unossified portions of the foot and ankle can be more clearly de-

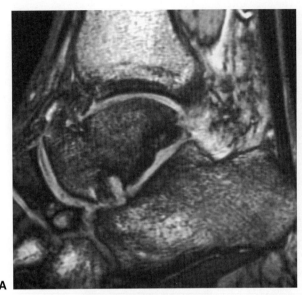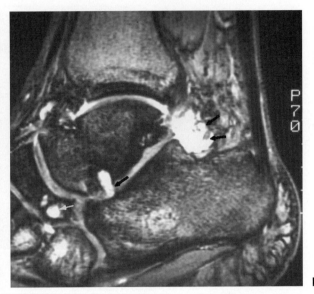

FIG. 2-55. GRE sequences before (**A**) and after (**B**) intravenous gadolinium injection. The joint fluid is enhanced (*arrows* in **B**) 15 min after injection to give an arthrographic effect.

fined.[212,213] Table 2-4 summarizes the indications and technical variations used in ankle arthrography.

Technique

Radiographs (routine and stress views) should be evaluated before obtaining the arthrogram.[205,215] Pertinent clinical information concerning the type of trauma and other indications for the arthrogram are important. Arthrographic technique varies according to clinical indications (see Table 2-4). MRI or CT may be combined with conventional arthrography.[199]

The patient is positioned supine on the fluoroscopic table. The ankle should be examined fluoroscopically to determine whether there is any abnormality (i.e., instability, opaque foreign bodies, or osseous bodies) before injection.[215] The anterior aspect of the ankle is prepared with sterile technique (5-min povidone-iodine [Betadine] scrub). Before needle position, the dorsalis pedis pulse is palpated. The extensor ten-

dons are usually easily located. In most situations, the joint is entered anteriorly and medial to the dorsalis pedis artery (Fig. 2-56).[198,199,208,210] The skin over the injection site is anesthetized with 1% lidocaine (Xylocaine) using a 25-gauge ½-inch needle. A 22-gauge 1½-inch needle is used to perform the arthrogram. Once the needle has penetrated the skin, the ankle can be rotated into the lateral position. This allows one to judge the depth of needle penetration. The joint is entered just inferior to the anterior tibial margin. The needle should be directed slightly inferiorly, to avoid the tibial lip (see Fig. 2-56).[198]

When the needle is within the capsule, any fluid or blood should be aspirated. Appropriate laboratory studies should be obtained in patients with suspected infection or other arthritides. Contrast-material injection depends on the clinical setting (see Table 2-4). For patients with acute trauma, 6 to 8 ml of contrast material (meglumine diatrizoate) is injected. Mixing 2 to 4 ml of lidocaine with the contrast material may facilitate stress views.[198,205,221] If a double-contrast technique is indicated, 1 ml of contrast medium combined with 6 to 8 ml of air is injected.[199,208] Rarely, air alone may be used in patients with significant allergy to iodine. Occasionally, 0.1 to 0.2 ml of 1:1,000 epinephrine is injected with the contrast material. This is helpful if tomography, CT, or MRI is to be used in conjunction with the arthrogram.[199,203,220,232]

Excessive amounts of contrast medium should be avoided, because this can obscure the internal structures of the ankle, especially the articular cartilage. In addition, contrast material may extravasate along the needle tract or may actually leak out of the capsule. The latter is reported in older patients.[199,208,210] These changes should not be confused with ligament injuries.[199]

After the injection, the ankle is stressed and observed fluo-

TABLE 2-4. Ankle arthrography: indications and techniques[a]

Indications	Techniques
Ligament injury	Single contrast, 6 to 8 ml
Articular evaluation	Double contrast
Talar dome fractures	(1 ml contrast and 8 ml air) ± tomography or CT
Osteochondritis dissecans	
Loose bodies	Single contrast ± tomography or CT
Arthritis	Double contrast
Capsulitis	Single contrast and anesthetic distension

[a] Data from references 199, 208, and 210.

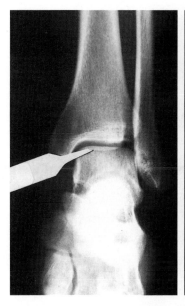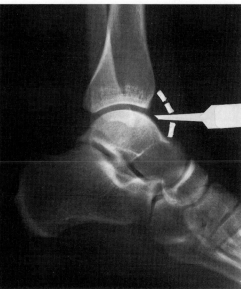

FIG. 2-56. Radiographs demonstrating the typical anteromedial approach for needle entry used for ankle arthrography. (From Berquist, ref. 199, with permission.)

roscopically. Films are obtained in the AP, lateral, and oblique projections. If a ligament injury is suspected, stress views are also obtained.[199,202,214] Vuust and Niedermann[235,236] suggested the oblique axial view to improve detection of calcaneofibular ligament tears.

Normal Arthrographic Anatomy

The anatomy of the ankle is discussed in Chapter 1. Arthrographically, certain anatomic features are easily assessed.

The anterior capsule extends from the neck of the talus to a point 5 mm superior to the distal tibial margin. This anterior recess is best seen on the lateral view (Fig. 2-57). Posteriorly, a second recess is also evident. This recess is more irregular and its size more variable compared with the anterior recess. Medially and laterally, the capsule extends to the tips of the malleoli. The margins should be smooth.[197,199,208,210,216] Superiorly, the capsule extends between the distal tibia and fibula (see Fig. 2-57), forming a syndesmotic recess. Normally, this is smooth and does not extend more than 2.5 cm above the joint space.[199,208,210]

In approximately 10% of patients, the tibiotalar joint communicates with the posterior subtalar joint. Communication with the flexor tendons (posterior tibial and flexor digitorum longus) along the medial aspect of the ankle is noted in approximately 20% of patients (Fig. 2-58).[199,208,210]

Clinical Applications

Considerable controversy exists concerning the management of acute ankle injuries.[199,202,207,225,235,236] Both open and closed methods have been advocated. In young, active persons or in professional athletes, surgical reduction is more commonly performed when both the anterior talofibular and calcaneofibular ligaments are disrupted. Certainly, inadequate management can lead to recurrent injury and instability.[199,202]

Arthrography can provide valuable information regarding the extend of ligament injury.[199,208,210] In the acute postinjury period, arthrography is easily performed and is more accurate than stress views.[199,214,227] Accuracy in assessing ligament injury decreases if the arthrogram is performed more than 72 hours after the injury. Ideally, the test should be performed within 48 hours.[199,208,227]

The ligaments of the ankle are not directly visible arthrographically. The medial complex (deltoid ligament) is broad and triangular. The fibers pass from the medial malleolus to insert on the talus and calcaneus.[199,208,210] Laterally, there are three major ligaments. The anterior talofibular ligament extends from the lateral malleolus to the talus and blends with the anterior capsule. The calcaneofibular ligament is not intimately associated with the capsule. The posterior talofibular ligament extends posteriorly from the fibula to the talus.[199,208,210,217]

The anterior talofibular ligament is most frequently disrupted. This is usually the result of an inversion injury. The capsule is also torn, allowing contrast material to extravasate laterally and anterior to the distal fibula.[199,229] The abnormality is best localized on the external oblique view. The contrast material is projected lateral to the fibula if extravasation has occurred anteriorly. The lateral view is also useful (Fig. 2-59). Contrast medium may reach the tip of the lateral malleolus and may extend superiorly. Anterior talofibular ligament tears may seal within 48 hr. Thus, arthrograms performed more than 2 days after injury may appear negative if they are not properly performed by an experienced examiner.[199,208]

More significant ankle injuries may involve both the anterior talofibular and calcaneofibular ligaments. This injury

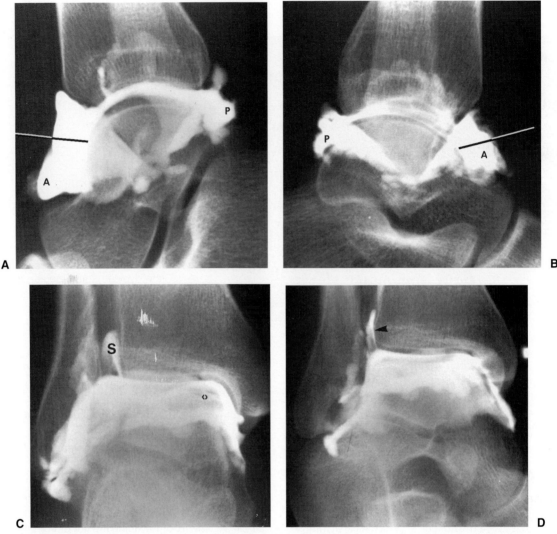

FIG. 2-57. Normal ankle arthrogram. **A** and **B:** Normal lateral views demonstrating the anterior (*A*) and posterior (*P*) recesses. *Black and white lines* indicate the needle entry site and angle. **C:** Anteroposterior view from an ankle arthrogram demonstrating the syndesmotic recess (*S*) and needle entry site (*< >*). **D:** Mortise view after contrast injection demonstrates articular cartilage thickness and the syndesmotic recess (*arrowhead*).

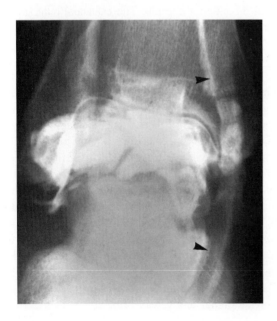

FIG. 2-58. Anteroposterior radiograph from an ankle arthrogram demonstrates normal filling of the medial tendon sheaths (*arrowheads*).

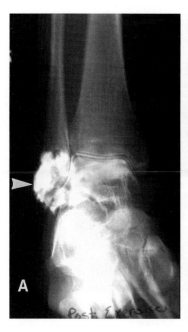 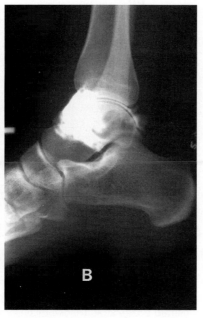

FIG. 2-59. Anteroposterior (**A**) and lateral (**B**) views of an ankle arthrogram demonstrating an anterior talofibular ligament tear with contrast extravasation (*arrowhead*) but no filling of the peroneal tendon sheaths.

classically results in filling of the peroneal tendon sheaths as well as capsular extravasation (Fig. 2-60).

Diagnosis of calcaneofibular ligament tears may be difficult. Spiegel and Staples[231] reported 8 false-negative arthrograms in 26 patients with surgically proven calcaneofibular ligament tears. Difficulty in diagnosis of calcaneofibular tears may be caused by decompression of the capsule by the associated anterior talofibular ligament and capsular tear. The contrast material takes the path of least resistance.[199, 208,231] Olson[224] suggested that lack of resistance in filling the joint with massive extravasation indicates disruption of both ligaments. Prearthrographic injection of the joint with lidocaine, followed by exercise and stress, or repeated exercise views after the arthrogram may be helpful in more accurate assessment of the calcaneofibular ligament.[199]

Extravasation of contrast material posterior and lateral to the malleolus may also indicate a tear, even though the peroneal tendon sheaths are not filled. This finding is best seen on the internal oblique or axial oblique view.[235,236] Direct injection of the peroneal tendon sheath probably provides the most accurate method of diagnosing calcaneofibular ligament tears.[200,206,209] Isolated tears of the calcaneofibular ligament are rare. If peroneal tendon sheath filling occurs without an associated anterior talofibular ligament tear, one can assume that the injury is not acute.[199,200,208,210,241] Occasionally, incomplete, old, or partially healed tears are noted.

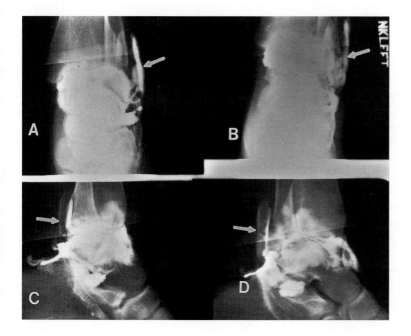

FIG. 2-60. Anteroposterior (**A and B**), lateral (**C**), and oblique (**D**) radiographs of an ankle arthrogram demonstrating peroneal tendon sheath filling (*arrows*) owing to calcaneofibular and anterior talofibular ligament disruption.

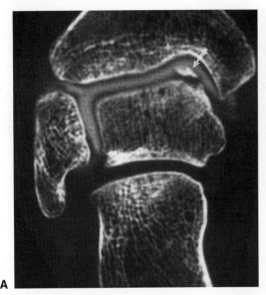 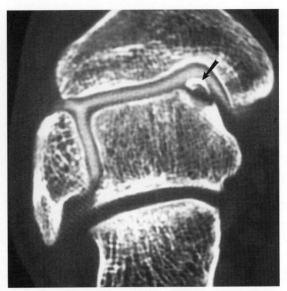

FIG. 2-61. Patient with ankle pain after inversion injury. Coronal CT images obtained after contrast with bone (**A**) and soft tissue (**B**) settings demonstrate a displaced medial talar dome fracture (*arrow*).

These injuries present with subtle irregularity of the capsule or ulcer-like projections.[199]

Tears of the posterior talofibular ligament are unusual and do not occur as isolated injuries. In this setting, gross instability is usually evident clinically, obviating the need for arthrography.[199,202]

Medial ligament injuries are less common and usually involve both the deltoid ligament and distal tibiofibular syndesmosis. The arthrogram demonstrates extravasation around the tip of the medial malleolus and extension, disruption, or irregularity of the syndesmotic recess.[199,204] The lateral view demonstrates loss of the normal lucent zone anterior to the distal tibia. (Isolated complete tears of the anterior tibiofibular ligament are uncommon.)

After treatment of ankle injuries, arthrography with or without CT may be useful in evaluating patients with persistent pain or instability.[199,203,232] Persistent instability, adhesive capsulitis, and other complications are clearly demonstrated.[199]

Arthrography is less commonly performed to evaluate subtle articular or synovial changes. Articular cartilage is best studied using double-contrast technique (see Table 2-4). The combination of reduced contrast medium and air provides better detail of the articular surface. This is particularly useful in evaluating osteochondral defects such as talar dome fractures and osteochondritis dissecans (Fig. 2-61).[199,203,232] Additional information is provided by using tomography or CT in conjunction with the double-contrast technique. Subtle synovial changes and loose bodies can also be evaluated with arthrotomography.[199,232]

After trauma, persistent pain and decreased range of motion may indicate adhesive capsulitis. In this clinical setting, single-contrast technique is most useful. Injection may be more difficult because of the constricted capsule.[199]

Goergen and Resnick[210] described the use of ankle arthrography in patients with arthritis, ganglia, and total joint replacement, but these are uncommon indications. Subtraction arthrography is less effective for the evaluation of arthroplasty in the ankle than in the hip. The surface area of the components is smaller, and overlying contrast material may obscure the bone-cement interface.[199]

Arthrography of the Subtalar and Other Joints

Arthrograms of the tarsal joints, subtalar joints, and foot are infrequently performed. Diagnostic and therapeutic injections are usually performed in conjunction with these arthrograms to localize the source of pain.[198,218,220] The sub-

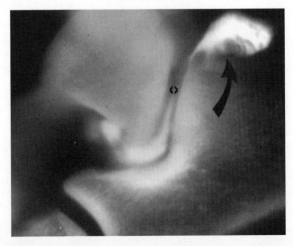

FIG. 2-62. Subtalar arthrogram showing the injection site (< >), normal articular cartilage, and slight synovial irregularity posteriorly (*curved arrow*).

talar joint can be easily entered medially or laterally, depending on the anatomy and on whether any joint or posttraumatic deformity exists.[198,218,226] The patient should be on his or her side and the posterior talocalcaneal facet positioned fluoroscopically. The same sterile preparation and needles are used as in ankle arthrography. Fluoroscopic guidance allows a straight vertical approach into the joint. Fluoroscopic spot films are useful, but conventional tomography and CT are often used to improve anatomic detail after the injection of 2 to 4 ml of contrast medium (Fig. 2-62).[198,199]

The normal subtalar joint should be clearly outlined, with equal thickness of the articular surfaces and a smooth synovial lining.[199,226] The examination is most often performed in patients with persistent posttraumatic pain or to ensure proper needle position for aspiration or therapeutic injections. If the articular cartilage is abnormal, one will see irregularity, hazy enhancement (degenerative changes), or thin-

ning. Synovitis causes irregularity of the synovial lining with small filling defects.[199,226]

Injection of other tarsal, metatarsophalangeal, and interphalangeal joints can be accomplished easily with a fluoroscopically guided dorsal approach (Fig. 2-63). Usually, the 25-gauge anesthetic needle has adequate length to penetrate the more superficial joints. When this is inadequate, as in the case of soft tissue swelling, a 22-gauge 1½-inch needle can be used. Because the joint capacity is small, single-contrast technique is almost always used. AP, lateral, and oblique spot films are taken. In certain situations, CT or conventional tomography may provide additional information.[198,218]

Indications for these arthrograms are more limited. Tarsal coalition and clubfoot deformities (especially in children with unossified osseous structures), needle position for diagnostic or therapeutic injections or biopsy, and determination

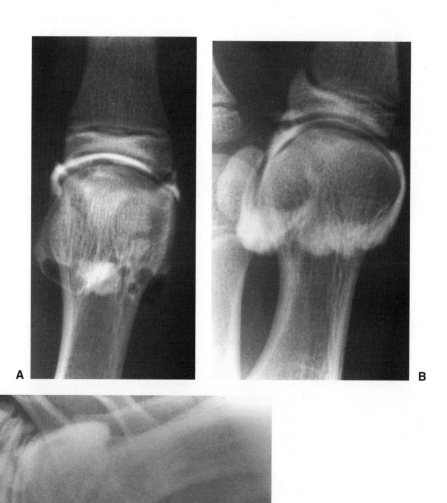

FIG. 2-63. Anteroposterior (**A**), oblique (**B**), and lateral (**C**) single-contrast arthrogram of the first metatarsophalangeal joint demonstrating the normal capsule and articular cartilage.

of articular or capsular abnormalities are the primary indications.[199,212,218]

Tenography

Injection of contrast medium into the tendon sheaths is generally used to diagnose inflammatory or posttraumatic conditions.[199,207,209,228,233] The technique is slightly more difficult than arthrography, and experience is required to perform and interpret the studies. Studies may be performed on the lateral group (peroneus longus and brevis), medial tendons (tibialis posterior, flexor digitorum longus, and flexor hallucis longus), or the anterior tendons (tibialis anterior, extensor hallucis longus, extensor digitorum longus). The Achilles tendon does not have a tendon sheath.[199,209]

Technique and Normal Anatomy

Clinical history and all pertinent imaging studies should be reviewed. Fluoroscopic examination of the foot and ankle should be performed before the injection. This technique allows palpation and localization of the tendons to be injected, evaluation of range of motion, snapping, and detection of osseous abnormalities. The skin is prepared using the same sterile technique described earlier for arthrography. Before injection, the vascular structures should be localized and the foot dorsiflexed and plantar flexed to localize the tendon (Fig. 2-64).

Lateral Tendons

The peroneal tendon sheaths are injected by entering the sheaths posterior and just cephalad to the lateral malleolus

(Fig. 2-65). The injection site may vary slightly, depending on the site of suspected injury (i.e., slightly higher for suspected peroneal tendon subluxation). After sterile preparation, the skin is anesthetized with 1% lidocaine using a 25-gauge ¾-inch needle. In certain cases, this needle is adequate for the study, but generally a 22-gauge 1½-inch needle is required. This needle is directed from above and enters the tendon sheath obliquely so the bevel will be entirely within the sheath. When the needle enters the tendon, a slight resistance is felt. The needle is then withdrawn slightly, and a small test injection is made using fluoroscopic observation. If the needle is properly positioned, the contrast will outline the tendon and will flow away from the needle tip. The injection is monitored fluoroscopically to ensure that the proper amount of contrast is used, to prevent overdistension and to detect sites of obstruction, extravasation, or filling of the ankle joint. In general, 10 to 12 ml of contrast (Hypaque-M, 60) is required.[199,209,233]

The peroneus longus and brevis tendons share a common tendon sheath to the distal third of the calcaneus.[199,209,233] The sheath divides at this point, and the peroneus brevis inserts in the base of the fifth metatarsal. The peroneus longus takes an oblique course via the sole of the foot to insert in the inferior aspects of the medial cuneiform and first metatarsal base (see Fig. 2-65).[209,233] After the injection, the foot is exercised during fluoroscopic monitoring to be certain that the sheaths are completely filled and to allow spot films of any abnormal findings.

Medial Tendons

The same preparation and examination technique described for the peroneal tendons is used for the medial tendons. The main difference is the injection sites. The tibialis posterior tendon is the most anterior and is entered just poste-

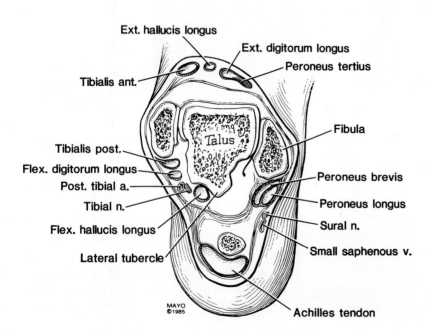

FIG. 2-64. Axial illustration of the ankle demonstrating the tendons and neurovascular structures.

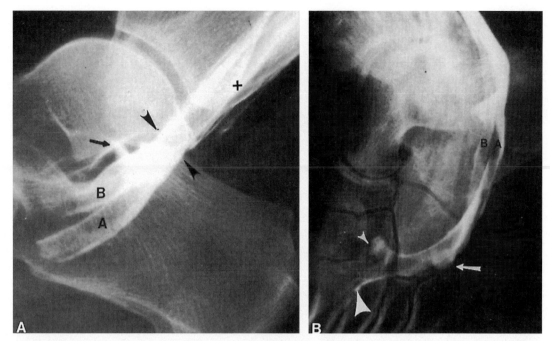

FIG. 2-65. Lateral (**A**) and oblique (**B**) views of the peroneal tendon sheaths after contrast injection. **A:** The peroneus brevis (labeled *B*) and peroneus longus (labeled *A*) have a common tendon sheath (*large black arrowheads*) to the midcalcaneal level. The *small arrow* shows a normal outpouching, and the *plus sign* (+) marks the needle entry site. **B:** Oblique view with the *small white arrow* indicating the peroneus brevis insertion on the fifth metatarsal. *Double arrowheads* indicate the peroneus longus insertion on the first metatarsal base and medial cuneiform. (From Teng et al., ref. 233, with permission.)

rior to the metaphysis of the medial malleolus (see Fig. 2-64). The flexor digitorum longus and flexor hallucis longus are more posterior (see Fig. 2-64).[199,233] The posterior tibial tendon sheath begins 3 to 4 cm above the tibiotalar joint space and extends to the level of the navicular. Here the tendon spreads its expanded insertions on the navicular, cuneiforms, and metatarsal (second through fourth) bases.[209]

The flexor digitorum longus and flexor hallucis longus lie posterior to the tibialis posterior (see Fig. 2-64). In up to 25% of patients, these tendons share a common sheath.[209] The flexor digitorum longus can be injected initially because it is more easily located. These tendon sheaths also begin 3 to 4 cm above the tibiotalar joint and extend distally crossing inferior to the talonavicular junction. The flexor digitorum longus divides and inserts in the bases of the distal phalanges of the lateral four toes. The flexor hallucis longus inserts in the base of the distal phalanx of the great toe.[209]

Anterior Tendons

The anterior tendons (tibialis anterior, extensor hallucis longus, and extensor digitorum longus) are less often studied than the medial and lateral groups. These tendons can be entered 2 to 3 cm above the tibiotalar joint or can be injected inferiorly using the dorsalis pedis artery as a landmark. The injection is made in the proximal dorsal foot. The tibialis anterior is most medial, the extensor hallucis longus just

medial to the dorsalis pedis artery, and the extensor digitorum longus is lateral to the artery (Fig. 2-66).[209,233]

The tibialis anterior tendon sheath begins approximately 5 cm above the tibiotalar joint and extends to the level of the first cuneiform.[209] The extensor hallucis longus is just lateral to the tibialis anterior and begins about the same level, extending a variable distance, usually to the distal shaft of the first metatarsal. The combined tendon sheaths of the extensor digitorum longus begin just above the tibiotalar joint and end at the level of the tarsometatarsal joints.[209,233]

Clinical Indications

Tenography is most commonly used to evaluate posttraumatic or overuse syndromes. The lateral tendons are most commonly studied. Black and colleagues[200] found tenography more accurate than arthrography in detection of calcaneofibular ligament tears. If a ligament tear has occurred, injection of the tendon sheath will result in communication with the ankle joint. This does not occur normally.[199,200] Extravasation can be normal and does not indicate a ligament tear (Fig. 2-67).[198,199] Other traumatic conditions such as subluxation, dislocation, or stenosis of the tendon sheath after calcaneal fractures can also be evaluated with tenography.[199,207,228]

MRI provides excellent image detail of the tendon and fluid in the tendon sheath. This technique is more commonly

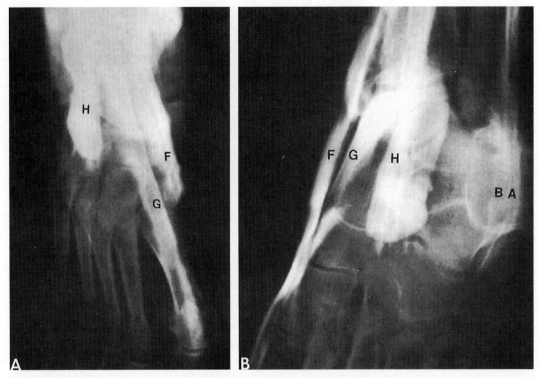

FIG. 2-66. Anteroposterior (**A**) and oblique (**B**) views of the anterior tendon sheaths. *F,* tibialis anterior tendon; *G,* extensor hallucis longus tendon; *H,* extensor digitorum longus tendon; *A,* peroneus longus tendon; *B,* peroneus brevis tendon. (From Teng et al., ref. 233, with permission.)

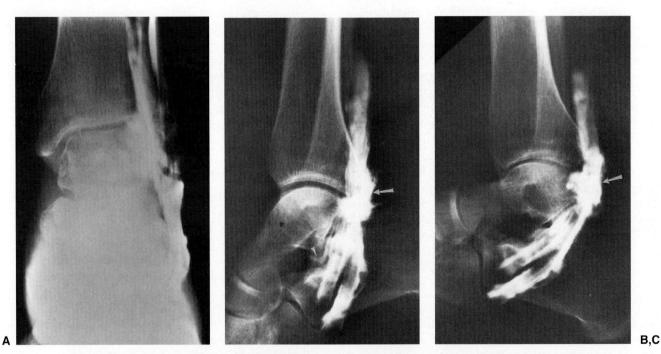

FIG. 2-67. Anteroposterior (**A**) and lateral (**B**) views after peroneal tenogram just after injection. Some extravasation is present at the injection site (*arrow*). The lateral views are obtained with the foot plantar flexed (**B**) and dorsiflexed (**C**). Note the filling of the subtalar joint with the foot plantar flexed (*small arrowheads*) (**C**) indicating calcaneofibular ligament injury.

used today than tenography. However, tenography offers the advantage of including an anesthetic agent to confirm the site of symptoms.[198]

Diagnostic Injection, Aspirations, and Biopsy

Fluoroscopy, CT, MRI and ultrasound can all be used to assist joint or tendon sheath injections.[199,201,220,222] Bone and soft tissue biopsy, contrast injection, and diagnostic and therapeutic injections (anesthetic with or without steroid) can all be monitored in this fashion. In most cases, fluoroscopy is adequate and readily available at most centers.[198,199] Diagnostic and therapeutic injections are commonly performed in the foot and ankle. Injections can localize the site of abnormality so that surgery can be planned or to allow steroid and anesthetic injection for therapeutic purposes.[198,218,220]

These techniques are used in the same manner and using the same sterile precautions described earlier. For injection, we generally use bupivacaine hydrochloride 25% (Marcaine Hydrochloride) because it is longer acting than lidocaine. This agent is used alone if surgery is contemplated or if a total joint arthroplasty is in place. Diagnostic anesthetic injections are commonly used along with CT to plan joint fusions in the foot.[198,218,220,221] We also do not inject steroid if aspirated fluid is abnormal or if infection is suspected. When steroid is used, we combine 1 ml of betamethasone (Celestone) with 2 to 3 ml of bupivacaine hydrochloride or use this ratio, depending on the volume of the joint or sheath to be injected (Figs. 2-68 and 2-69).[198]

If a biopsy is being performed, an 18- or 15-gauge sure-cut needle is used in most cases. If intact cortical bone is present, a larger Jamshidi needle may be required. Biopsy

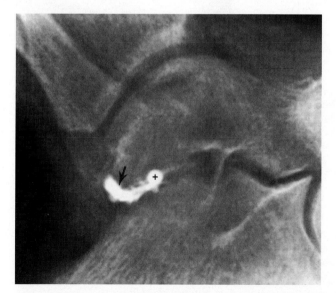

FIG. 2-68. Fluoroscopic spot view obtained during subtalar joint injection. Contrast (*arrow*) flows away from the needle tip (+) confirming position in the joint before injecting anesthetic and steroid.

procedures can be monitored most easily with fluoroscopy, but occasionally CT or even MRI may be used.[199,222]

In patients with open wounds or sinus tracts, it may be useful to inject these tracts with contrast material to determine the extent of bone or soft tissue involvement.[199,211] This can be easily accomplished using fluoroscopy, small pediatric feeding tubes to cannulate the sinus tract, and the same contrast medium used for arthrography. The extent of the sinus tract can be clearly defined and documented with spot films.[199,211]

Complications

Complications secondary to arthrography, tenography, and other diagnostic injections using contrast medium are rare. Newberg[223] reviewed 126,058 arthrogram cases. There were no deaths, 61 patients developed hives related to contrast medium, 83 patients experienced vasovagal episodes, and 5 patients noted severe joint pain after the arthrogram. The total number of complications was 150 in 126,058 cases or 0.1%. Similar results have been reported by others authors.[207,210]

We have not observed any significant complications associated with the interventional techniques described earlier. Neural injury may potentially occur if the injection site is improperly selected. The only neurologic problem we have noted is transient deficit resulting from the anesthetic injection that may affect an adjacent nerve. This clears as the local anesthetic loses its effect.[199]

VASCULAR TECHNIQUES

Until recently, arterial and venous invasive techniques were relied on heavily both for the diagnosis of vascular disease entities and anomalies and for the performance of any subsequent therapeutic vascular interventions. However, the emergence of vastly improved noninvasive diagnostic imaging techniques, such as magnetic resonance angiography, CT angiography, and ultrasound, has greatly reduced reliance on these invasive techniques simply for vascular diagnosis. Increasingly, invasive vascular procedures are being reserved for the performance of specific therapeutic interventions on entities identified noninvasively or to confirm a diagnosis when noninvasive techniques are not possible or are not definitive. Venography of the lower leg is reserved for instances in which ultrasound is inconclusive or when venous malformations are suspected. Lymphangiography is seldom of much value for diagnosis of entities below the knee.[237,241,250,267,268]

Although these techniques are used sparingly in the foot and ankle, the appropriate use of invasive vascular procedures demands careful attention to technique and a thorough knowledge of the relevant indications for each examination if proper diagnosis is to result and therapies are to be performed with minimal complications.

Arterial invasive procedures of the foot and ankle are most

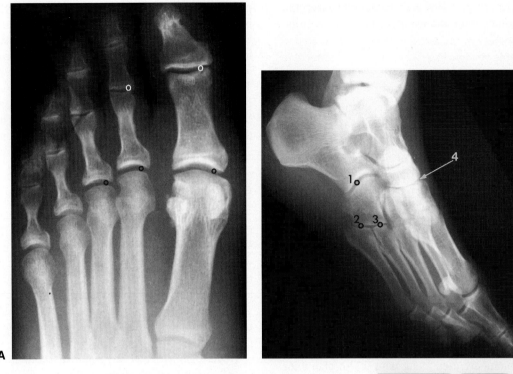

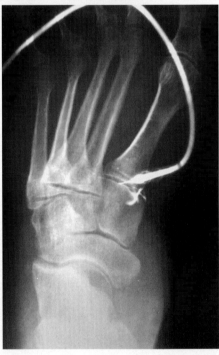

FIG. 2-69. A: Anteroposterior view of the forefoot demonstrating needle entry sites (*0*) for the metatarsophalangeal and phalangeal joints. An off-center dorsal approach is used to avoid the extensor tendon and neurovascular structures. **B:** Oblique view of the foot demonstrating entry sites (*0*) for the calcaneocuboid (*1*), (*2* and *3*) cuboid fourth to fifth metatarsal, and (*4*) navicular cuneiform (*white arrow*) articulations. **C:** Fluoroscopic spot view of test injection with contrast before anesthetic injection of the medial cuneiform first metatarsal joint.

often performed utilizing a percutaneous transfemoral approach, a technique first described by Seldinger.[270] Diagnostic arteriograms are most commonly performed following retrograde placement of a catheter into the lower abdominal aorta, whereas therapeutic interventions in the foot and ankle are most effectively performed using an antegrade puncture with catheter placement into the ipsilateral common femoral artery. In certain instances in which a transfemoral approach is not feasible, an axillary approach can be employed.[237]

An axillary or high brachial approach, using small-caliber catheters, is also becoming more popular in the outpatient population, to hasten ambulation and discharge. The translumbar approach to lower extremity angiography is rarely employed, and there is no effective means of performing therapeutic interventions via this route.

Several technologic advances in the design and manufacture of angiographic equipment and contrast agents have particularly served to encourage development and refinement of transluminal therapeutic interventional techniques involving the vasculature of the foot and ankle. The proliferation of a wide variety of miniaturized catheters and guidewires from multiple vendors has made possible the effective cannulation of even the small vessels of the foot and ankle, thereby allowing these interventions.[242,245,249]

Paralleling the development of new catheters and guidewire systems has been the evolution of newer intravascular contrast agents. These have been developed primarily in an attempt to decrease the occurrence of adverse systemic events associated with their use. Although life-threatening idiosyncratic reactions are of the greatest concern, they occur infrequently. More commonly, nonidiosyncratic reactions such as nausea, vomiting, nephrotoxicity, and cardiac arrhythmia occur. These reactions are more commonly associated with the use of older (ionic) high-osmolality contrast materials (HOCM) than with the newer (nonionic) low-osmolality contrast materials (LOCM).[249] Because renal vascular disease and peripheral vascular disease frequently occur together, nephrotoxicity related to the use of contrast material during lower extremity diagnostic and therapeutic interventions is of particular concern. For this reason, there has been a significant shift from use of HOCM to LOCM for use in invasive vascular diagnosis and intervention.[237,249,258,260,263,267]

In distinction to the adverse systemic effects of contrast material, such as nausea and vomiting, that are more commonly experienced from the venous route of agent administration, local effects are also associated with intraarterial injection of contrast material. These local effects consist of pain and a burning sensation and are most prevalent with injection of contrast material into the arteries of the extremities. Although these local effects are less severe with LOCM compared with HOCM, the sensations of heat and pain are still frequent.[257] An isotonic, nonionic contrast material (Visipaque, Nycomed Imaging AS, Oslo, Norway) has become commercially available. Early clinical investigations have found this agent to cause significantly reduced local effects during intraarterial administration. Use of this agent can make peripheral arteriography, especially selective studies of the foot and ankle, more acceptable to patients.[257]

Occasionally, patients with compromised renal function or a documented serious allergic reaction to iodinated contrast material must undergo angiography, either before radiologic intervention or for presurgical diagnosis. Although the risk of contrast-induced nephrotoxicity is reduced when LOCM is chosen over HOCM, there is still a significant risk of renal damage with the low-osmolar agents, particularly in azotemic patients.[249,277] Alternative contrast agents are available and have been used increasingly in patients with azotemia. Gadolinium is a commonly used MRI contrast agent that has not shown nephrotoxicity even with doses as high as 0.4 mml/kg of body weight.[258,263] Allergic reaction to gadolinium preparations are also rare. This agent has been

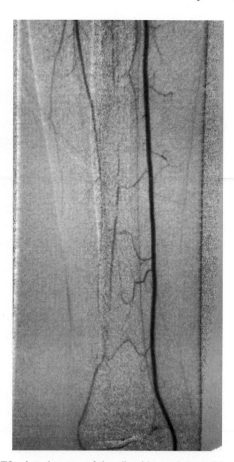

FIG. 2-70. Arteriogram of the distal lower leg performed with gadolinium instead of iodinated contrast material in a patient with severe renal insufficiency.

successfully utilized in diagnostic (Fig. 2-70) and interventional angiographic procedures in patients with azotemia [258,263] and contrast allergy.[260] Because of the increased cost of gadolinium preparations compared with iodinated contrast materials, its use is most appropriately reserved for subselective injections in which low volumes of gadolinium can be administered. This agent is, therefore, particularly well suited to angiography of the foot and ankle, in which these smaller injections of contrast material are utilized. Arteriography performed with intraarterial injection of carbon dioxide has also been shown this gas to be an effective contrast material in patients with iodine allergy or azotemia.[253,254] Because carbon dioxide is rapidly dissolved in the blood, study of the foot and ankle must be performed with the catheter subselectively placed in the lower superficial femoral or popliteal artery. No known toxicity is associated with the peripheral use of carbon dioxide.[253]

All peripheral vascular procedures, regardless of their location, require recording images of the findings. Several different imaging methods may be utilized. At a minimum, a high-resolution image intensifier and television chain with standard arteriographic filming capabilities, including at least a 14 serial film changer, are required. Long-leg film

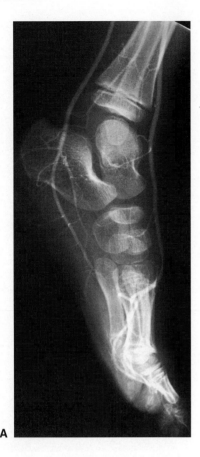

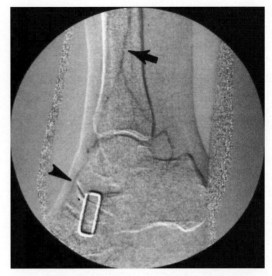

FIG. 2-71. A: Lateral view of a normal arteriogram of the left foot in a child. **B:** Digital subtraction angiogram performed with venous injection demonstrates peroneal (*upper arrow*) and refilled anterior tibial artery (*lower arrowhead*) in an elderly patient with atherosclerotic disease.

changers are sufficient for arteriography of the lower extremities if serial film changers or digital subtraction systems are available for acquiring localized supplemental views. Large FOV, totally digital, angiographic acquisition systems with high spatial resolution have become available and are becoming increasingly better accepted within the angiographic community. These newer systems offer an acceptable alternative to conventional film systems in all aspects of angiography. Because of an unacceptably high patient and operation radiation dose, the use of cineradiography or small-field mobile image intensifiers is inappropriate for peripheral angiography and intervention.[237,277]

Digital subtraction angiography (DSA) has proven a valuable adjunct to angiography, especially in procedures involving the smaller vessels of the ankle and foot. The newer digital angiographic equipment is capable of a 2k × 2k image matrix that permits outstanding small vessel resolution. In addition, acquisition rates of up to 30 frames/sec are valuable in eliminating motion effects, which are a particular problem with foot and ankle imaging. Magnification views of selected anatomic regions are also easily obtained using DSA.

Additionally, DSA is sensitive to low concentrations of contrast materials. This is especially important in distal extremity studies because lower concentrations of iodinated contrast material may be used, thus decreasing the local symptoms of pain and burning (Fig. 2-71). Use of alternative contrast materials such as carbon dioxide and gadopentate is also possible with DSA.[253,254,258,260]

Arterial Interventions

The indications for diagnostic and therapeutic arterial interventions of the foot and ankle are many. They include occlusive arterial disease, trauma, tumors, vascular malformations, vasculitis, and the preoperative delineation of arterial vascular anatomy.[244,255,256,264,272–274,282] The relative frequency of these indications varies depending on regional practice differences; however, occlusive arterial disease is generally the most common. Occlusive arterial disease may be the result of atherosclerosis, thrombosis, embolism, or a combination thereof. Atherosclerotic narrowing of arteries is most common and primarily affects older patients, particularly men older than 50 years and postmenopausal women. Various predisposing factors include smoking, hypertension, hyperlipidemia, hypercholesterolemia, obesity, family history, diabetes, and genetic factors. Diabetes is particularly implicated in the accelerated narrowing of the small arteries of the foot and ankle.[237,277] Most patients with arterial insufficiency of the lower extremities present with intermittent claudication; few cases are initially heralded by a threatened limb.[237,247] Intermittent claudication is characterized by muscle pain that is induced by exercise and relieved with rest. The level of exercise necessary to induce claudication is typically constant.[247] The pain usually develops in the muscles of the calf in patients harboring disease in the superficial femoral arteries and in the thigh and buttocks in patients with involvement in the aortoiliac artery segments.[247] Whereas claudication implicates arterial insufficiency in the thigh, buttocks, and calf regions, it is an unusual indicator of foot and ankle vascular disease, although foot claudication can be a presenting feature in Buerger's disease.[279]

Ischemic rest pain, ulceration, and gangrene are common indicators of severe lower extremity vascular insufficiency, and they typically occur in the region of the foot and ankle.[248,277] In these patients with critical limb ischemia, multilevel vascular disease is common. Advanced atherosclerotic disease tends to involve the pelvic, infrainguinal, and infrageniculate arteries concurrently, with a predisposition to the more proximal vessels. Diabetes, on the other hand, disproportionately affects the infrageniculate and submalleolar vessels to a greater degree than the proximal vessels.[277,280]

Treatment of arterial insufficiency in the foot and ankle may be a complex undertaking. Because atherosclerosis tends to be a diffuse disease, the potential exists for multiple sequential sites of vascular constriction proximal to the foot and ankle that need to be addressed to optimize therapeutic outcome.[280] In addition, the status of the coronary arteries must be assessed because of the increased risk of myocardial infarction during surgical intervention.[243] Currently, various percutaneous endoluminal interventions are available as treatment options below the knee. These are discussed in more detail in Chapter 8. Briefly, these percutaneous interventions include angioplasty[242,281] and thrombolysis using chemical infusion[256,264,269] or mechanical[244,273,274,281] techniques.

Trauma represents the second most common reason for arteriography of the foot and ankle (Fig. 2-72). There is divergent opinion in the literature about the use of arteriography in blunt or penetrating trauma of the lower extremity, much depending on the nature of the individual practices. Generally, patients with definite clinical findings, such as absent pulses, pulsatile hemorrhage, large expanding hematoma, and distal ischemia, proceed directly to emergency surgery.[255,277] Although emergency arteriography may be employed in these patients if the area of injury is not readily amenable to exploration, this technique is frequently reserved for patients with softer clinical findings such as neurologic deficit, stable hematoma, or a history of arterial bleeding.[255] Elective arteriography is indicated when the likelihood of finding significant occult arterial injury is low and the patient has no pulse deficit.[255,267,277] This topic is addressed more thoroughly in Chapter 8.

Complications related to arteriography happen infrequently, but when they occur, they usually present at the arterial puncture site or involve the circulation distal to the puncture.[265,277] Serious puncture site complications occur in 0.4% of studies,[278] depending on evaluation criteria and include hematoma formation, pseudoaneurysm formation,

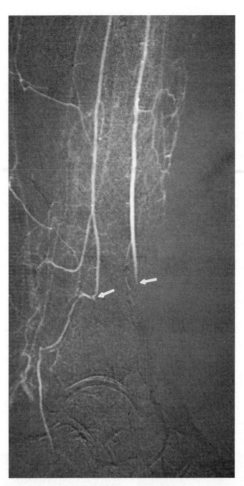

FIG. 2-72. Arteriogram after a distal tibial fracture demonstrates occlusion of the anterior tibial and peroneal arteries (*arrows*).

thrombosis, and arteriovenous fistula.[237,239,259,261,275–277] Puncture site complications are less frequent with the transfemoral approach and are most common with the transaxillary approach.[278] The risk factor most commonly associated with hematoma formation, the most frequently encountered complication, is obesity.[246] Interestingly, catheter size, advanced age, hypertension, and coagulation deficits do not appear to increase the risk of hematoma.[246] During femoral artery access, punctures distal to the common femoral artery significantly increase the risk of creating a pseudoaneurysm or arteriovenous fistula.[239] Two-thirds of these abnormalities may close spontaneously, without necessitating surgical repair.[259] Patients receiving concomitant continuous anticoagulation present with a greater chance of requiring surgical repair of pseudoaneurysms and arteriovenous fistulae.[259]

The second major groups of complications related to arteriography are caused by the catheter, with thromboembolism representing the most common complication within this particular group.[275] Embolization of thrombus in the catheter can most effectively be prevented by frequent and vigorous flushing of the catheter with heparinized saline. Atheroembolization is caused by dislodgement of vessel plaque by catheter manipulations and may occur in up to 30% of arteriograms in which the catheter traverses the aorta.[265] Fortunately, most of these occurrences are subclinical events.

Venous Interventions

Ultrasound techniques have largely replaced lower extremity venograms in the evaluation of potential deep venous thrombosis. B-mode compression combined with color duplex flow imaging of the lower extremity deep veins is accurate in excluding or including the diagnosis of deep vein thrombosis.[268] However, venography remains a low-risk, albeit invasive, technique that is highly available and quite useful for the evaluation of the lower extremity deep veins when ultrasound studies are indeterminate or when clinical suspicion persists in the face of a negative venous ultrasound study (Fig. 2-73).[240,241]

Whenever possible, lower extremity venography should be performed with the patient in a 30° to 45° upright position, to facilitate pooling of the contrast material in the lower leg veins.[251] Proximal leg and pelvic veins can be filled by lowering the examination table so that the patient is in the supine position. Elevation of the involved extremity enhances visualization of the pelvic vessels. Dilute ionic

(HOCM) contrast material and, most commonly, nonionic (LOCM) contrast material is used for venous opacification.

The most commonly encountered local complications of peripheral venography are postvenographic syndrome, postvenographic venous thrombosis, and contrast extravasation resulting in tissue necrosis and gangrene.[276] The postvenographic syndrome consists of pain, tenderness, swelling, and erythema of the ankle or calf. These symptoms and signs typically appear 2 to 12 hr after venography and then resolve within 5 days.[276] The incidence of this syndrome appears to increase proportionately with the concentration of ionic contrast material utilized.[240,241] Its occurrence is unusual with nonionic contrast material.[238]

Postvenographic thrombosis of the deep venous system occurs in fewer than 3% of patients.[238,240] This rate has diminished markedly from previous studies as a result of more universal use of nonionic contrast material. The occurrence of postvenographic syndrome and thrombosis can also be reduced or prevented by early ambulation, leg elevation, and flushing of the extremity with 200 to 300 ml of heparinized saline following venography. All these maneuvers enhance the clearing of contrast material from the venous system.[276,277]

Perivenous extravasation of contrast material during venography is usually of a small degree and has no consequence. However, extravasation of greater than 10 ml may result in skin necrosis and gangrene.[262] With extravasation, the contrast injection should be halted and the site massaged, the leg elevated, and warm compresses applied.[276] These maneuvers are intended to facilitate dissipation of contrast material from the site of injection. The suggestion exists that extravasation of nonionic contrast material leads to fewer instances of necrosis and gangrene; however, further study is needed.[245]

Catheter-directed treatment of lower extremity deep venous thrombosis using urokinase has been advocated to facilitate rapid thrombus resolution in symptomatic patients and to avoid future postphlebitic complications. The procedure works best for patients with acute iliofemoral deep vein thrombosis isolated to the iliac and femoral veins.[271] The procedure involves placement of a thrombolysis catheter into the popliteal vein and using ultrasound guidance.[271]

REFERENCES

Routine Radiography

1. American College of Radiology (ACR). Appropriateness Criteria for 1996. Reston, VA, ACR, 1996.
2. Anis AH, Stiell IG, Stewart DG, Laupacis A. Cost-effective analysis of the Ottawa ankle rules. Ann. Emerg. Med. 1995; 26(4):422–428.
3. Arimoto HK, Forrester DM. Classification of ankle fractures. An algorithm. AJR Am. J. Roentgenol 1980; 135:1057–1063.
4. Ballinger WP. Merrill's Atlas of Roentgenographic Positive and Standard Radiologic Procedures. 8th Ed. St. Louis, C.V. Mosby, 1995.
5. Barks RT, Morgan J. Anatomy of the lateral ankle ligaments. Am. J. Sports Med. 1994; 22:72–77.
6. Bernau A, Berquist TH. Orthopedic Positioning in Diagnostic Radiology. Baltimore, Urban & Schwarzenberg, 1983.

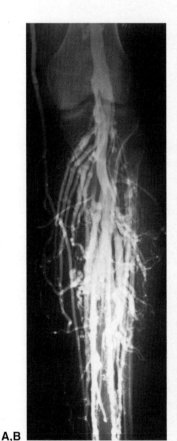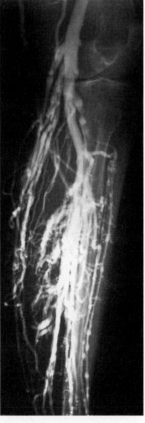

A,B

FIG. 2-73. Anteroposterior (**A**) and oblique (**B**) views of a negative left calf venogram.

7. Berquist TH. Imaging of Orthopedic Trauma. 2nd Ed. New York, Raven Press, 1992; pp. 1–7.

8. Brage ME, Holmes JR, Sangeorzan BJ. The influence of x-ray orientation on the first metatarsocuneiform joint angle. Foot Ankle Int. 1994; 15:495–497.

9. Brantigan JW, Pedegana LR, Lippert, FG. Instability of the subtalar joint. J. Bone Joint Surg. Am. 1977;59:321–324.

10. Brostrom L. Sprained ankles. III. Clinical observations in recent ligament ruptures. Acta Chir. Scand. 165;130:560–569.

11. Causton J. Projection of sesamoid bones in the region of the first metatarsophalangeal joint. Radiology 1943; 9:39–40.

12. Chang JW, Griffiths H, Chan DPK. A new radiological technique for the forefoot. Foot Ankle 1984; 5:77–83.

13. Clark TWI, Janzen DL, Logan PM, Ho K, Connell DG. Improving the detection of radiographically occult ankle fractures. Positive predictive value of an ankle joint effusion. Clin. Radiol. 1996; 51: 632–636.

14. Ebraheim NA, Wong FY. External rotation views in the diagnosis of posterior colliculus fracture of the medial malleolus. Am. J. Orthop. 1996; 25(5):380–382.

15. Evans GA, Frenyo SD. The stress-tenogram in the diagnosis of ruptures of the lateral ligament of the ankle. J. Bone Joint Surg. Br. 1979; 61:347–351.

16. Feist JH, Mankin HJ. The tarsus. I. Basic relationships and motions in the adult and definition of optimal recumbent oblique projection. Radiology 1962; 79:250–263.

17. Foster SC, Foster RR. Lisfranc's tarsometatarsal fracture dislocation. Radiology 1976; 120:79–83.

18. Fox IM, Collier D. Imaging of injuries to the tarsometatarsal joint complex. Clin. Podiatr. Med. Surg. 1997; 14(2):357–368.

19. Frolich H, Gotzen L, Adam D. Evaluation of stress roentgenograms of the upper ankle joint. Unfallheikunde 1980; 83:457–461.

20. Hasegawa A, Kimura M, Tomizawa S, Shirakura K. Separated ossicles of the lateral malleolus. Clin. Orthop. 1996; 330:157–165.

21. Ho K, Clark TWI, Janzen DL, Connell DG, Blachut P. Occult ankle fracture detected by ankle effusion on plain radiography. A case report. J. Emerg. Med. 1996; 14(4):455–459.

22. Höcker K. The skeletal radiology of the distal tibiofibular joint. Arch. Orthop. Trauma Surg. 1994; 133:345–346.

23. Holly EW. Radiography of the tarsal sesamoid bones. Med. Radiogr. Photogr. 1955; 31:73–80.

24. Isherwood I. A radiological approach to the subtalar joint. J. Bone Joint Surg. Br. 1961; 43:566–574.

25. Ishii T, Miyagawa S, Fukubayashi T, Hayashi K. Subtalar stress radiography using forced dorsiflexion and supination. J. Bone Joint Surg. Br. 1996;78:56–60.

26. Johannsen A. Radiologic diagnosis of lateral ligament lesion of the ankle. A comparison between talar tilt and anterior drawer sign. Acta Orthop. Scand. 1978; 49:259–301.

27. Jonsson K, Fredin HO, Cederlund CG. Width of the normal ankle joint. Acta Radiol. Diagn. 1984; 25:147–149.

28. Karasick D, Schweitzer ME. Tear of the posterior tibial tendon causing asymmetric flat foot. Radiographic findings. AJR Am. J. Roentgenol. 1993; 161:1237–1240.

29. Kell PM. A comparative radiologic examination for unresponsive plantar fasciitis. J. Manipulative Physiol. Ther. 1994; 17(5):329–334.

30. Kitaoka HB, Lundberg A, Luo ZP, An K-N. Kinematics of the normal arch of the foot and ankle under physiologic loading. Foot Ankle Int. 1995; 16(8):492–499

31. Lewis RW. Non-routine views in roentgen examination of the extremities. Surg. Gynecol. Obstet. 1938; 69:38–45.

32. Lilienfeld L. Anordnung der normalisierten Routgenaufnahmen des menschlichen Korpers. 4th Ed. Berlin, Urban & Schwarzenberg, 1927; p. 36.

33. Long BW, Rafert JA. Orthopaedic Radiology. Philadelphia, W.B. Saunders, 1995.

34. Louwerens JWK, Ginai AZ, Van Linge B, Siiders CJ. Stress radiography of the talocrural and subtalar joints. Foot Ankle Int. 1995; 16(3): 148–155.

35. Martin DE, Kaplan PA, Kahler DM, Dussault R, Randolph BJ. Retrospective evaluation of graded stress examination of the ankle. Clin. Orthop. 1996; 328:165–170.

36. Newmark H III, Olken SM, Mellon WS Jr. A new finding in the radiographic diagnosis of Achilles tendon rupture. Skeletal Radiol. 1982; 8:223–224.

37. Norfray JF, Gelins RA, Steinberg RI, Galinski AW, Gilula LA. Subtleties of Lisfranc fracture-dislocations. AJR Am. J. Roentgenol. 1981; 137:1151–1156.

38. O'Keefe D, Nicholson DA, Driscoll PA, Marsh D. The ankle. BMJ 1994; 308:331–336.

39. O'Mary RA, Kaplan PA, Dussault RG, Hornsby PP, Carter CT, Kahler DM, Hullman BJ. The impact of ankle radiographs on diagnosis and management of acute ankle injuries. Acad. Radiol. 1996; 3:758–765.

40. Olson RW. Ankle arthrography. Radiol. Clin. North Am. 1981; 19: 255–268.

41. Ostrum RF, De Meo P, Subramanian R. A critical analysis of the antero-posterior radiographic anatomy of the ankle syndesmoses. Foot Ankle Int. 1995; 16(3):128–131.

42. Ozonoff MB. Pediatric Orthopedic Radiology. Philadelphia, W.B. Saunders, 1995.

43. Pritsch M, Heim M, Horoszowski H, Farine I. The significance of the axial foot projection in diagnosis of metatarsal pathology. Arch. Orthop. Trauma Surg. 1981; 98:139–141.

44. Ray RG, Christensen JC, Gusman PN. Critical evaluation of anterior drawer measurement methods in the ankle. Clin. Orthop. 1997; 334: 215–224.

45. Rhea JT, Salvatore AD, Sheehan J. Radiographic anatomy of the tarsal bones. Med. Radiogr. Photogr. 1983; 59(1):28.

46. Rogers LF, Campbell RE. Fractures and dislocations of the foot. Semin. Roentgenol. 1978; 13:157–166.

47. Saltzman CL, Brandser EA, Berbaum KS, DeGnore L, Holmes JR, Katcherian DA, Teasdall RD, Alexander IJ. Reliability of standard foot radiographic measurements. Foot Ankle Int. 1994; 15(12): 661–665.

48. Saltzman CL, El-Khoury GY. The hindfoot alignment view. Foot Ankle Int. 1995; 16(9):572–576.

49. Saltzman CL, Nawoczenski DA, Talbot KD. Measurement of the medial longitudinal arch. Arch. Phys. Med. Rehabil. 1995; 76:45–49.

50. Samuelson KM, Harrison R, Freeman MAR. A roentgenographic technique to evaluate and document hindfoot position. Foot Ankle 1981; 1:286–289.

51. Steel MW III, Johnson KA, DeWitz MA. Radiographic measurements of the normal adult foot. Foot Ankle 1980; 1:151–158.

52. Towbin R, Dunbar JS, Towbin J. Teardrop sign. Plain film recognition of ankle effusion. AJR Am. J. Roentgenol. 1980; 134:985–990.

53. Vangsness CT, Carter V, Hunter T, Kerr R, Newton E. Radiographic diagnosis of ankle fractures. Are three views necessary? Foot Ankle Int. 1994; 15(4):172–174.

Tomography

54. Bailey DS, Perillo JT, Forman M. Subtalar joint neutral. A study using tomography. J. Am. Podiatr. Assoc. 1984; 74(2):59–64.

55. Berrett A, Brunner S, Valvassori GE. Modern Thin Section Tomography. Springfield, IL, Charles C Thomas, 1973.

56. Bokstrom, I. Principles of vertebral tomography. Acta Radiol. Suppl. 1955:103:5–109.

57. Burkus JK, Sella EJ, Southwick WO. Occult injuries of the talus diagnosed by bone scan and tomography. Foot Ankle 1984; 4: 316–324.

58. Curry TS, Dowdey JE, Murray RC. Christensen's Physics of Diagnostic Radiology. 4th Ed. Philadelphia, Lea & Febiger, 1990; pp. 242–256.

59. Eastman Kodak Co. Fundamentals of Radiology. 12th Ed. Rochester, NY, Eastman Kodak Co., 1980.

60. Ho K, Connell DG, Jansen DJ, Grunfeld A, Clark TWI. Using tomography to diagnose occult ankle fractures. Ann. Emerg. Med. 1996; 27:600–605.

61. McCullough EC, Coulam CM. Physical and dosimetric aspects of diagnostic geometrical and computer assisted tomographic procedures. Radiol. Clin. North Am. 1976; 14:3–13.

62. Norman A. The value of tomography in the diagnosis of skeletal disorders. Radiol. Clin. North Am. 1970; 8:251.

63. Pavlov H, Torg JS, Freiberger RH. Tarsal navicular stress fractures. Radiographic evaluation. Radiology 1983; 148:641–645.

64. Resnick D, Niwayama G. Diagnosis of Bone and Joint Disorders. Philadelphia, W.B. Saunders, 1995.

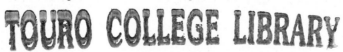

Magnification Radiography

66. Curry TS, Dowdey JE, Murray RC. Christensen's Physics of Diagnostic Radiology. 4th Ed. Philadelphia, Lea & Febiger, 1990; pp. 219–241.
67. Eastman Kodak Co. The Fundamentals of Radiology. 12th Ed. Rochester, NY, Eastman Kodak Co., 1980.
68. Fletcher DE, Rowley KA. Radiographic enlargements in diagnostic radiology. Br. J. Radiol. 1951; 24:598–604.
69. Genant HK, Kunlo D, Mall JC, Sickles EA. Direct magnification for skeletal radiography. Radiology 1977; 123:47–55.
70. Gordon SL, Greer RB, Wiedner WA. Magnification roentgenographic technique in orthopedics. Clin. Orthop. 1973; 91:169–173.
71. Lee SM, Lee RGL, Wilinsky J, Balogh K, Clouse ME. Magnification radiography in osteomyelitis. Skeletal Radiol. 1986; 15(8):625–627.
72. Nemet A, Cox WF. The improvement of definition of x-ray image magnification. Br. J. Radiol. 1956; 29:335–337.
73. Wagner LK, Cohen G, Wong W, Amtey SR. Dose efficiency and the effects of resolution and noise detail perceptibility in radiographic magnification. Med. Phys. 1981; 8:24–32.
74. Weiss A. A technique for demonstrating fine detail in the bones of the hand. Clin. Radiol. 1972; 23:185–187.

Ultrasound

75. Blei CL, Nirschl RP, Grant EG. Achilles tendon. US diagnosis of pathologic conditions. Radiology 1986; 159:765–767.
76. Bluth EI, Merritt CR, Sullivan MA. Gray scale ultrasound evaluation of the lower extremities. JAMA 1982; 247:3127–3129.
77. Braumstein EM, Silver TM, Martel W, Jaffe M. Ultrasonographic diagnosis of extremity masses. Skeletal Radiol. 1981; 6:157–163.
78. Breidahl WH, Adler RS. Ultrasound guided injection of ganglia with corticosteroids. Skeletal Radiol. 1996; 25:635–638.
79. Breidahl WH, Newman JS, Taljanovic MS, Adler RS. Power Doppler sonography in the assessment of musculoskeletal fluid collections. AJR Am. J. Roentgenol. 1996; 166:1443–1446.
80. Campbell WB, Fletcher EL, Hands LJ. Assessment of distal lower limb arteries. A comparison of arteriography and Doppler ultrasound. Ann. R. Coll. Surg. Engl. 1986; 8:37–39.
81. Carpenter JR, Hattery RR, Hunder GG, Bryan RS, McLeod RA. Ultrasound evaluation of the popliteal space. Comparison of arthrography and physical examination. Mayo Clin. Proc. 1976; 51:498–503.
82. Fornage BD. Achilles tendon. US examination. Radiology 1986; 159:759–764.
83. Frankel DA, Bargiela JA, Craig JG, Shirazi KK, van Holsbeck MT. Synovial joints. Evaluation of intra-articular bodies with US. Radiology 1998; 206:41–44.
84. Harcke HT, Grissom LE, Farkelstein MS. Evaluation of the musculoskeletal system with sonography. AJR Am. J. Roentgenol. 1988; 150:1253–1261.
85. Jacobson JA, Van Holsbeck MT. Musculoskeletal ultrasonography. Orthop. Clin. North Am. 1998; 29(1):135–167.
86. Kaufman RA, Tarskins RB, Babcock DS, Crawford AH. Arthrosonography in the diagnosis of pigmented villonodular synovitis. AJR Am. J. Roentgenol. 1982; 139:396–398.
87. Koski JM. Detection of plantar tenosynovitis of the forefoot by ultrasound in patients with early arthritis. Scand. J. Rheumatol. 1995; 24:312–313.
88. Lawson IL, Mittler S. Ultrasonic evaluation of extremity soft tissue lesions with arthrographic correlation. J. Can. Assoc. Radiol. 1978; 29:58–61.
89. Leopold GR. Ultrasonography of superficially located structures. Radiol. Clin. North Am. 1980; 18:161–173.
90. Lund PJ, Nisbet JK, Valencia FG, Ruth JT. Current sonographic applications in orthopedics. AJR Am. J. Roentgenol. 1996; 166:889–895.
91. Marinoli C, Derchi LE, Pastoreno C, Bertolotto M, Silvestri E. Analysis of echo texture of tendons with US. Radiology 1993; 186:839–843.
92. Merritt CRB. Doppler colorflow imaging. J. Clin. Ultrasound 1987; 15:591–597.

93. McDicken WN. Diagnostic Ultrasonics. Principles and Use of Instruments. New York, John Wiley and Sons, 1981.
94. McDonald DG, Leopold GR. Ultrasound B-scanning in the differentiation of Baker's cyst and thrombophlebitis. Br. J. Radiol. 1972; 45:729–732.
95. Nazarean LN, Rawool NM, Morten CE, Schweitzer ME. Synovial fluid in the hindfoot and ankle. Detection of amount and distribution with US. Radiology 1995; 197:275–278.
96. Newman JS, Adler RS, Bude RO, Rubin JM. Detection of soft-tissue hyperemia. Value of power Doppler sonography. AJR Am. J. Roentgenol. 1994; 163:385–389.
97. Roedersheimer LR, Feins R, Green RM. Doppler evaluation of the pedal arch. Am. J. Surg. 1981; 142:601–604.
98. Rubin JM, Bude RO, Carson PL, Bree RL, Adler RS. Power Doppler US. A potentially useful alternative to mean frequency-based color Doppler US. Radiology 1994; 190:853–856.
99. Sarti DA, Sample WF. Diagnostic Ultrasound. Text and Cases. Boston, G.K. Hall, 1980.
100. Shapiro PP, Shapiro SL. Sonographic evaluation of interdigital neuromas. Foot Ankle 1995; 16(10):604–606.
101. Silber TM, Washburn RL, Stanley JC, Gross WS. Gray scale ultrasound evaluation of popliteal artery aneurysms. AJR Am. J. Roentgenol. 1977; 129:1003–1006.
102. Van Holsbeeck M, Introcaso JH. Musculoskeletal Ultrasound. St. Louis, C.V. Mosby, 1991.
103. Winsberg F, Cooperberg PL. Real Time Ultrasonography. New York, Churchill Livingstone, 1982.

Skeletal Scintigraphy

104. Berggren A, Weiland AJ, Ostrup LT. Bone scintigraphy in evaluating the viability of composite bone grafts revascularized by microvascular anastomosis, conventional autologous bone grafts, and free non-revascularized periosteal grafts. J. Bone Joint Surg. Am. 1982; 64:799–809.
105. Brown ML. Skeletal scintigraphy. In Berquist TH, ed. Imaging of Orthopedic Trauma and Surgery. Philadelphia, W.B. Saunders, 1986; pp. 16–21.
106. Brown ML, Swee RG, Johnson KA. Bone scintigraphy of the calcaneus. Clin. Nucl. Med. 1986; 11(7):530–536.
107. Burkus JK, Sella EJ, Southwick WO. Occult injuries of the talus diagnosed by bone scan and tomography. Foot Ankle 1984; 4:316–324.
108. Connolly LP, Treves ST, Connally SA, Zimmerman RE, Bar-Sever Z, Itrato D, Davis RT. Pediatric skeletal scintigraphy. Applications of pinhole magnification. Radiographics 1998; 18:341–351.
109. Desai A, Alvi A, Dalinka M, Brighton C, Esterhai J. Role of bone scintigraphy in the evaluation and treatment of non-united fractures. Concise communication. J. Nucl. Med. 1980; 21:931–934.
110. Deutsch AL, Resnick D, Campbell G. Computed tomography and bone scintigraphy in evaluation of tarsal coalition. Radiology 1982; 144:137–140.
111. Donohoe KH. Skeletal topics in orthopedic nuclear medicine. Orthop. Clin. North Am. 1998; 29(1):85–102.
112. Geslien JE, Thrall JH, Espinosa JL, Older RA. Early detection of stress fractures using Tc-99m polyphosphate. Radiology 1976; 121:683–687.
113. Goldman AB, Pavlov H, Schneider R. Radionuclide bone scanning in subtalar coalition. Differential considerations. AJR Am. J. Roentgenol. 1982; 138:427–432.
114. Hoffer P. Gallium. Mechanisms. J. Nucl. Med. 1980; 21:282–285.
115. Intenzo C, Kim S, Millin J, Park C. Scintigraphic patterns of the reflex sympathetic dystrophy syndrome of the lower extremities. Clin. Nucl. Med. 1989; 14:657–661.
116. Jacobson AF, Stouper PC, Cronin EB, Stomper PC, Kaplan WD. Bone scans with one or two new abnormalities in cancer patients with known metastasis. Frequency and serial scintigraphic behavior of benign and malignant lesions. Radiology 1990; 175:229–232.
117. Matin P. The appearance of bone scans following fractures, including immediate and long-term studies. J. Nucl. Med. 1979; 20:1227–1231.
118. Mauer AH, Millmond SH, Knight LC, Mesgazadeh M, Siegel JA, Shuman CR, Adler LP, Greene GS, Malmud LS. Infection in diabetic osteoarthropathy. Use of indium-labeled leukocytes for diagnosis. Radiology 1986; 161:221–225.

119. Pavlov H, Torg JS, Freiberger RH. Tarsal-navicular stress fractures. Radiographic evaluations. Radiology 1983; 148:641–645.

120. Rosenthal L, Kloiber R, Damten B, Al-Majed H. Sequential use of radiophosphate and radiogallium imaging in the differential diagnosis of bone, joint, and soft tissue infection. Quantitative analysis. Diagn. Imaging 1982; 51:249–258.

121. Rosenthal L, Lisbona R, Hernandez M, Hadjipavlou A. Tc-99m-pp and Ga-67 imaging following insertion of orthopedic devices. Radiology 1979; 133;717–721.

122. Schauwecker DS. Scintigraphic diagnosis of osteomyelitis. AJR Am. J. Roentgenol. 1992; 182:849–854.

123. Smith FW, Gilday DL. Scintigraphic appearance of osteoid osteoma. Radiology 1980; 137:191–195.

124. Spencer RB, Levinson ED, Baldwin RD, Sziktas JJ, Witek JT, Rosenberg R. Diverse bone scan abnormalities in "shin splints." J. Nucl. Med. 1979; 20:1271–1272.

125. Stadalnik RC. "Cold spot" bone imaging: gamet. Semin. Nucl. Med. 1979; 9:2–3.

126. Subramanian G, Mcafee JG. A new complex for skeletal imaging. Radiology 1971; 99:192–196.

127. Subramanian G, McAfee JG, Bell EG, Blair RJ, Omara RE, Ralston PH. Tc-99m–labeled polyphosphate as a skeletal imaging agent. Radiology 1972; 102:701–704.

128. Swee RG, McLeod RA, Beabout JW. Osteoid osteoma. Detection, diagnosis and localization. Radiology 1979; 130:117–123.

129. Thakur ML, Coleman RE, Mayhall CG, Welch MJ. Preparation and evaluation of III In-labeled leukocytes as an abscess imaging agent in dogs. Radiology 1976; 119:731–732.

130. Thakur ML, Coleman RE, Welch MJ. Indium lll-labeled leukocytes for the localization of abscesses. Preparation, analysis, tissue distribution in comparison with gallium-67 citrate in dogs. J. Lab. Clin. Med. 1977; 89:217–228.

131. Urman M, Ammann W, Sisler J, Leuthe BC, Lloyd-Smith R, Loomer R, Fisher C. The role of bone scintigraphy in evaluation of talar dome fractures. J. Nucl. Med. 1991; 32:2241–2244.

132. Weissberg DL, Resnick D, Taylor AK, Becker M, Alazraki N. Rheumatoid arthritis and its variants. Analysis of scintiphotographic, radiographic and clinical examination. AJR Am. J. Roentgenol. 1978; 131: 665–673.

133. Wilcox JR, Miniot AL, Green JP. Bone scanning and the evaluation of exercise-related injuries. Radiology, 1997; 123:699–703.

Computed Tomography

134. Berland LL, Smith KL. Multidetector array CT. Once again technology creates new opportunities. Radiology 1998; 209:327–329.

135. Donaldson JS, Poznanski AK, Kieves A. CT of children's feet. An immobilization technique. AJR Am. J. Roentgenol. 1987; 148: 169–170.

136. Floyd EJ, Ransom RA, Dailey JM. Computed tomography scanning of the subtalar joint. J. Am. Podiatr. Assoc. 1984; 74(11):533–537.

137. Genant HK, Heller M. CT improves evaluation of musculoskeletal trauma. Diagn. Imaging 1984; 11:116–119.

138. Genant HK, Helms CA. Computed tomography of the appendicular musculoskeletal system. In Moss AA, Gamsu G, Genant HK, eds. Computed Tomography of the Body. Philadelphia, W.B. Saunders, 1983; pp. 475–533.

139. Guyer BH, Levinsohn EM, Fredrickson BE, Bailey GL, Formikell M. Computed tomography of calcaneal fractures. Anatomy, pathology, dosimetry and clinical relevance. AJR Am. J. Roentgenol. 1985; 145. 911–919.

140. Heger L, Wulff K. Computed tomography of the calcaneus. Normal anatomy. AJR Am. J. Roentgenol. 1985; 75:123–129.

141. Heger L, Wulff K, Seddigi MSA. Computed tomography of calcaneal fractures. AJR Am. J. Roentgenol. 1985; 145:131–137.

142. Herto BR, Perl J II, Sevey C, Lieber ML, Davros WJ, Baker ME. Comparison of examination times between CT scanners. Are the newer scanners faster? AJR Am. J. Roentgenol. 1998; 170:13–18.

143. Hillman BJ. New imaging technology cost and containment. AJR Am. J. Roentgenol. 1994; 162:503–506.

144. Kuszyk BS, Heath DG, Bliss DF, Fishman EK. Skeletal 3-D CT. Advantages of volume rendering over surface rendering. Skeletal Radiol. 1996; 25:207–214.

145. Lee TH, Wapner KL, Moyer DP, Hecht PJ. Computed tomographic demonstration of the vacuum phenomenon in the subtalar and tibiotalar joints. Foot Ankle 1994; 15(7):382–385.

146. Martinez S, Herzenberg JE, Apple JS. Computed tomography of the hindfoot. Orthop. Clin. North Am. 1985; 16:481–496.

147. Morrison R, McCarty J, Cushing FR. Three-dimensional computerized tomography. A quantum leap in diagnostic imaging. J. Foot Ankle Surg. 1994; 33(1):72–76.

148. Nyska M, Pomerany S, Porat S. The advantage of computed tomography in locating a foreign body in the foot. J. Trauma 1986; 26(1): 93–95.

149. Pretorius ES, Fishman EK. Helical (spiral) CT of the musculoskeletal system. Radiol. Clin. North Am. 1995; 33(5):949–979.

150. Rosenberg ZS, Feldman F, Singson RD. Peroneal tendon injuries. CT analysis. Radiology 1986; 161:743–748.

151. Rosenthal DF, Mankin HJ, Bauman RA. Musculoskeletal applications for computed tomography. Bull. Rheum. Dis. 1983; 33(3):1–4.

152. Sarno RC, Carter BL, Bankoff MS, Semine MC. Computed tomography of tarsal coalition. J. Comput. Assist. Tomogr. 1984; 8(6): 1155–1160.

153. Seeram E. Computed Tomography: Physical Principles Clinical Applications and Quality Control. Philadelphia, W.B. Saunders, 1994.

154. Seltzer SE, Weissman BN, Braunstein EM, Adams DF, Thomas WH. Computed tomography of the hind foot. J. Comput. Assist. Tomogr. 1984; 8(3):488–497.

155. Smith RW, Staple TW. Computerized tomography (CT) scanning technique for the hindfoot. Clin. Orthop. 1983; 177:34–38.

156. Solomon MA, Gilula LA, Oloff LM, Oloff J. CT scanning of the foot and ankle. II. Clinical applications and a review of the literature. AJR Am. J. Roentgenol. 1986; 146:1204–1214.

157. Solomon MA, Gilula LA, Oloff LM, Oloff J, Compton T. CT scanning of the foot and ankle. I. Normal anatomy. AJR Am. J. Roentgenol. 1986; 146:1192–1203.

158. Szczukowski M, St. Pierre RK, Fleming LL, Somogyi J. Computerized tomography in evaluation of peroneal tendon dislocation. A report of 2 cases. Am. J. Sports Med. 1983; 11(6):444–447.

159. Wexler RJ, Schweitzer ME, Karasick D, Deely DM, Morrison W. Helical CT of calcaneal fractures. Technique and imaging fractures. Skeletal Radiol. 1998; 27:1–6.

160. Woolson ST, Porvati D, Fillingham LL, Vassiliadis A. Three-dimensional imaging of the ankle joint from computerized tomography. Foot Ankle 1985; 6(1):2–6.

Magnetic Resonance Imaging

161. Aerts P, Disler DG. Abnormalities of the foot and ankle. MR image findings. AJR Am. J. Roentgenol. 1995; 165:119–124.

162. Alley MT, Shifrin RY, Pele NJ, Herfkens RJ. Ultrafast contrast enhanced three-dimensional MR angiography. State of the art. Radiographics 1998; 18:273–285.

163. Anzilotti K, Schweitzer ME, Hecht P, Wapner K, Kahn M, Ross M. Effect of foot and ankle MR imaging on clinical decisions making. Radiology 1996; 201:515–517.

164. Arakawa M, Crooks LE, McCarten B, Hoenninger JC, Watts JC, Kaufman L. A comparison of saddle-shaped and solenoidal coils for magnetic resonance imaging. Radiology 1985; 154:227–228.

165. Beltran J. MRI techniques and practical applications. Magnetic resonance imaging of the ankle and foot. Orthopedics 1994; 17(11): 1075–1082.

166. Beltran J, Nato AM, Mosure JC, Shaman, OM, Weiss KL, Zuelger WA. Ankle. Surface coil MR imaging at 1.5 T. Radiology 1986; 161: 203–209.

167. Berquist TH. MRI of the Musculoskeletal System. 3rd Ed. New York, Lippincott–Raven, 1996.

168. Berquist TH. Preliminary experience in orthopedic radiology. Magn. Reson. Imaging 1984; 2:41–52.

169. Daffner RH, Reimer BL, Lupetin AR, Dash N. Magnetic resonance imaging of acute tendon ruptures. Skeletal Radiol. 1986; 15(8): 619–621.

170. Davis PL, Crooks L, Arakawa M, McRee R, Kaufman L, Margulis AR. Potential hazards of MR imaging. Heating and effects of changing magnetic fields and RF fields on small metallic implants. AJR Am. J. Roentgenol. 1981; 137:857–860.

171. des Plantes BGZ, Falke THM, den Boer JA. Pulse sequences and

contrast in magnetic resonance imaging. Radiographics 1984; 4: 869–883.

172. Deutsch AL, Mink JH, Kear R. MRI of the Foot and Ankle. New York, Raven Press, 1992.

173. Fisher MR, Barker B, Amparo EG, Brandt G, Brant-Zawadzki M, Hricak H, Higgens CB. MR imaging using special coils. Radiology 1985; 157:443–447.

174. Forster BB, Houston G, Machan LS, Doyle L. Comparison of two-dimensional time-of-flight dynamic magnetic resonance angiography with digital subtraction angiography in popliteal artery entrapment syndrome. Can. Assoc. Radiol. J. 1997; 48(1):11–18.

175. Hajek PC, Baker LL, Bjorkingren A, Sartoris DJ, Neuman CH, Resnick D. High resolution MRI of the ankle. Normal anatomy. Skeletal Radiol. 1986; 15(7):536–540.

176. Hany F, Schmidt M, Davis CP, Göhde SC, Debatin JF. Diagnostic impact of four post processing techniques in evaluating contrast-enhanced three-dimensional MR angiography. AJR Am. J. Roentgenol. 1998; 170:907–912.

177. Helgason JW, Chandnani VP, Yu JS. MR arthrography. A review of current techniques and applications. AJR Am. J. Roentgenol. 1997; 168:1473–1480.

178. Kaufman JA, McCarter D, Geller SC, Waltman AC. Two-dimensional time-of-flight MR angiography of the lower extremities. Artifacts and pitfalls. AJR Am. J. Roentgenol. 1998; 171:129–135.

179. Kneeland JB; Knowles RJR; Cahill PT. Magnetic resonance imaging systems. Optimization in clinical use. Radiology 1984; 153:473–478.

180. Lackman RW, Kaufman B, Han JS, Nelson DA, Clampitt M, O'Block AM, Haaga JR, Alfidi RJ. MR imaging in-patients with metallic implants. Radiology 1985; 157:711–714.

181. Lauterbur P. Magnetic resonance zugimatography. Pure Appl. Chem. 1975; 40(2):149–157.

182. Lee JM, Wang Y, Sostman HD, Schwartz LH, Khilani NM, Trost DW, de Arellans ER, Teeger S, Bush HL Jr. Digital lower extremity arteries. Evaluation with two-dimensional MR digital subtraction angiography. Radiology 1998; 207:505–512.

183. Mitchell MJ, Sartoris DJ, Resnick D. The foot and ankle. Top. Magn. Reson. Imaging 1989; 1:57–73.

184. Moody Ar, Pollock JG, O'Connor AR, Bagnail M. Lower-limb deep venous thrombosis. Direct MR imaging of the thrombus. Radiology 1998; 209:349–355.

185. Moon KL, Genant HK, Helms CA, Chafetz NI, Crooks LE, Kaufman L. Musculoskeletal applications of nuclear magnetic resonance. Radiology 1983; 147:161–171.

186. Pykett I. Principles of nuclear magnetic resonance imaging. Radiology 1982; 143:157–168.

187. Roth JL, Nugent M, Gray JE, Julsrud PR, Berquist TH, Sill JC, Kispert DB, Hayes DL. Patient monitoring during magnetic resonance imaging. Anesthesiology 1985; 62:80–83.

188. Rubin DA, Towers JD, Britton CA. MR imaging of the foot. Utility of complex oblique imaging planes. AJR Am. J. Roentgenol. 1996; 166:1079–1084.

189. Saunders RD. Biological effects of NMR clinical imaging. Appl. Radiol. 1982; 11:43–46.

190. Schwartz JL, Crooks LE. NMR imaging produces no observable mutations or cytotoxicity in mammalian cells. AJR Am. J. Roentgenol. 1982; 139:583–585.

191. Shellock FG, Kanal E. MRI report. Policies, guidelines and recommendations for MR imaging safety and patient management. J. Magn. Reson. Imaging 1991; 1:97–101.

192. Sierra A, Potchen EJ, Moore J, Smith HG. High field magnetic resonance imaging of aseptic necrosis of the talus. J. Bone Joint Surg. Am. 1986; 68:927–928.

193. Wang Y, Lee HM, Khilani NM, Trost Dw, Jagust MB, Winchester PA, Bush HL, Sos TA, Sostman HD. Bolus-chase MR digital subtraction angiography in the lower extremity. Radiology 1998; 207:263–269.

194. Winalski S, Aliabadi P, Wright RJ, Shortkroff S, Sledge CB, Weissman BW. Enhancement of joint fluid with intravenously administered gadopentate dimeglumine. Techniques, rationale and implications. Radiology 1993; 187:179–181.

195. Yu JS, Vitellas KM. The calcaneus. Applications of magnetic resonance imaging. Foot Ankle Int. 1996; 17(12):771–780

196. Zanetti M, DeSimoni C, Wetz HH, Zollinger H, Hodler J. Magnetic resonance imaging of injuries to the ankle joint. Can it predict the outcome? Skeletal Radiol. 1997; 26:82–88.

Interventional Orthopedic Techniques

197. Ala-Ketola L, Puronen J, Koivisto E, Purepera M. Arthrography in the diagnosis of ligament injuries and classification of ankle injuries. Radiology 1977; 125:63–68.

198. Berquist TH. Diagnostic and therapeutic injections as an aid to musculoskeletal diagnosis. Semin. Intervent. Radiol. 1993; 10(4):326–343.

199. Berquist TH. Imaging of Orthopedic Trauma. 2nd Ed. New York, Raven Press, 1992; pp. 26–33.

200. Black HM, Brand RL, Eichelberger MR. An improved technique for the evaluation of ligamentous injury in severe ankle sprains. Am. J. Sports Med. 1978; 6(5):276–282.

201. Breidahl WH, Adler RS. Ultrasound-guided injection of ganglia with corticosteroids. Skeletal Radiol. 1996; 25:635–638.

202. Cass JR, Morrey BF. Ankle instability. Current concepts, diagnosis and treatment. Mayo Clin. Proc. 1984; 59:165–170.

203. Dihlman W. Computed tomography of the ankle joint. Chirug 1982; 53:123–126.

204. Dory MA. Arthrography of the ankle joint in chronic instability. Skeletal Radiol. 1986; 15(4):291–294.

205. Edeiken J, Colter JM. Ankle injury. The need for stress films. JAMA 1978; 240(11):1182–1184.

206. Evans GA, Frenyo SD. The stress tenogram in diagnosis of ruptures of the lateral ligament of the ankle. J. Bone Joint Surg. Br. 1979; 61: 347–351.

207. Fitzgerald RH, Coventry,B. Post-traumatic peroneal tendinitis. In Bateman JE, Trolt AW, eds. The Foot and Ankle. New York, Thieme–Stratton, 1980; pp. 102–1009.

208. Freiberger RH, Kaye J. Arthrography. New York, Appleton-Century-Crofts, 1979.

209. Gilula LA, Oloff L, Caputi R, Destouet JM, Jacobs A, Solomon MA. Ankle tenography. A key to unexplained symptomatology. Radiology 1984; 151:581–587.

210. Goergen TG, Resnick D. Arthrography of the ankle. In Dalinka M, ed. Arthrography. New York, Springer-Verlag, 1981.

211. Goldman F, Manzi J, Carver A, Torre R, Rechter R. Sinography in diagnosis of foot infection. Am. J. Podiatry 1981; 71(9):497–502.

212. Hjelmstedt EA, Sahlstedt B. Arthrography as a guide in the treatment of congenital clubfoot. Acta Orthop. Scand. 1980; 51:321–334.

213. Ho AMW, Blane CE, Klung TF Jr. The role of arthrography in management of dysplasia epiphysealis hemimelia. Skeletal Radiol. 1986; 15(3):224–227.

214. Horsfield D, Murphy G. Stress views of the ankle joint in lateral ligament injury. Radiography 1985; 51:7–11.

215. Hudson TM. Joint fluoroscopy before arthrography. Detection and evaluation of loose bodies. Skeletal Radiol. 1984; 12:199–203.

216. Johannsen A. Radiologic diagnosis of lateral ligament lesion of the ankle. Acta Orthop. Scand. 1978; 49:295–301.

217. Kaye JJ, Bohne WHO. A radiographic study of the ligamentous anatomy of the ankle. Radiology 1977; 125:659–667.

218. Khoury NJ, El-Khoury GY, Saltzman CL, Brandser EA. Intra-articular foot and ankle injections to identify source of pain before arthrodesis. AJR Am. J. Roentgenol. 1996; 167:669–673.

219. Lindholmer E, Andersen A, Andersen SB, Funder V, Jorgensen JF Nudermann B, Vuust M. Arthrography of the ankle. Acta Radiol. 1983; 24(3):217–223.

220. Lucas PE, Hurwitz SR, Kaplan PA, Dussault RG, Maurer EJ. Fluoroscopically guided injections into the foot and ankle. Localization of the source of pain as a guide to treatment prospective study. Radiology 1997; 204:411–415.

221. Mitchell MJ, Bielecki D, Bergman AG, Kursunogli-Brahine S, Sartoris DJ, Resnick D. Localization of specific joint causing hindfoot pain. Value of injecting local anesthetics into individual joints during arthrography. AJR Am. J. Roentgenol. 1995; 164:1473–1476.

222. Mueller PR, Stark DD, Simeone JF, Saini S, Butch RJ, Edelman RR, Wittenberg J, Ferrucci JT. MR guided aspiration biopsy. Needle design and clinical trials. Radiology 1986; 161:605–609.

223. Newberg AH. Presentation. Contrast reactions in arthrography. In ACR categorical course in diagnostic techniques in the musculoskeletal system, Sept. 13–14, Baltimore, 1986.

224. Olson RW. Ankle arthrography. Radiol. Clin. North Am. 1981; 19(2): 255–268.
225. Parisien JS, Vangsness T. Operative arthroscopy of the ankle. Three year experience. Clin. Orthop. 1985; 199:46–53.
226. Pavlov H. Ankle and subtalar arthrography. Clin. Sports Med. 1982; 1(1):47–69.
227. Raatikainen T, Puronen J. Arthrography for diagnosis of acute lateral ligament injuries of the ankle. Am. J. Sports Med. 1993; 21(3): 343–347.
228. Resnick D, Goergen TG. Peroneal tenography in patients with previous calcaneal fractures. Radiology 1975; 115:211–213.
229. Sauser DD, Nelson RC, Lavine MH, Wa CW. Acute injuries of the lateral ligaments of the ankle. Comparison of stress radiography and arthrography. Radiology 1983; 148:653–657.
230. Schweigel JF, Knickerbocher WJ, Cooperberg P. A study of ankle instability utilizing ankle arthrography. J. Trauma 1977; 17(11): 878–881.
231. Spiegel PK, Staples, OS. Arthrography of the ankle joint. Problems in diagnosis of acute lateral ligament injuries. Diagn. Radiol. 1975; 114:587–590.
232. Tehranzedek J, Galrieli OF. Intra-articular calcified bodies. Detection by computed arthrotomography. South Med. J. 1984; 77(6):703–710.
233. Teng MMH, Desfouet JM, Gilula, LA, Resnick D, Hembree JL, Oloff LM. Ankle tenography. A key to unexplained symptomatology. I. Normal tenographic anatomy. Radiology 1984; 151:575–580.
234. Termansen NB, Hansen H, Damholt. Radiological and muscular status following injury to the lateral ligaments of the ankle. Acta Orthop. Scand. 1979; 50:705–708.
235. Vuust M. Arthrographic diagnosis of ruptured calcaneofibular ligament. I. A new projection tested on experimental post mortem. Acta Radiol. Diagn. 1980; 21:123–128.
236. Vuust M, Niedermann B. Arthrographic diagnosis of ruptured calcaneofibular ligament. II. Clinical evaluation of a new method. Acta Radiol. Diagn. 1980; 21:231–234.

Vascular Techniques

237. Abrams HL. Abrams Angiography. Boston, Little, Brown, 1983.
238. Albrechtsson U, Olsson CG. Thrombosis after phlebography. A comparison of two contrast media. Cardiovasc. Radiol. 1979; 2:9–18.
239. Altin RS, Flicker S, Naidech HJ. Pseudoaneurysm and arteriovenous fistula after femoral catheterization. Association with low femoral punctures. AJR Am. J. Roentgenol. 1989; 152:629–631.
240. Bettman MA, Paulson S. Leg phlebography. The incidence, nature and modification of undesirable side effects. Radiology 1977; 122: 102–104.
241. Bettman MA, Robbins A, Braun SD, Wetzner S, Dunnick NR, Finkelstein J. Contrast venography of the leg: diagnostic efficacy, tolerance and complication rates with ionic and non-ionic contrast media. Radiology 1987; 165:113–116.
242. Bull PG, Mendel H, Hold M, Schlegl A, Denck H. Distal popliteal and tibioperoneal transluminal angioplasty. Long-term follow-up. J. Vasc. Intervent. Radiol. 1992; 3:45–53.
243. Bunt JJ. The role of defined protocol for cardiac risk assessment in decreasing peri-operative myocardial infarction in vascular surgery. J. Vasc. Surg. 1992; 15:626.
244. Cleveland TJ, Amberland DC, Gaires PA. Percutaneous aspiration thromboembolectomy to manage the embolic complications of angioplasty and as an adjunct to thrombolysis. Clin. Radiol. 1994; 49: 549–552.
245. Cohan RH, Dunnick NR, Leder RA, Baker ME. Extravasation of non-ionic radiologic contrast media. Efficacy of conservative treatment. Radiology 1990; 176:65–67.
246. Cragg AH, Nakagawa N, Smith TP, Berbaum KS. Hematoma formation after diagnostic arteriography. Effect of catheter size. J. Vasc. Intervent. Radiol. 1991; 2:231–233.
247. Craids E, Ramadan F, Keagy B. Intermittent claudication. Surg. Gynecol. Obstet. 1991; 173:163.
248. Edmonds ME. The diabetic foot. Pathophysiology and treatment. Endocrinol. Metab. 1986; 15:889–916.
249. Ellis JH, Cohan RH, Sonnad SS, Cohan NS. Selective use of radiographic low-osmolality contrast media in the 1990s. Radiology 1996; 200:297–311.
250. Freidman SA. Diagnosis and medical management of vascular ulcers. Clin. Dermatol. 1990; 8:30–39.
251. Greitz T. Technique of ascending phlebography of the lower extremity. Acta Radiol. 1954; 42:421–441.
252. Harmovec H. Patterns of arteriosclerotic lesions of the lower extremity. Arch. Surg. 1967; 95:918 933.
253. Hashimoto S, Hiramatsu K, Sato M. CO_2 as an intra-arterial digital subtraction angiography (IADSA) agent in the management of trauma. Semin. Intervent. Radiol. 1997; 14:163–173.
254. Hawkins IF. Carbondioxide digital subtraction angiography. AJR Am. J. Roentgenol. 1982; 139:19–24.
255. Hawks SE, Pentecost MJ. Angiography and transcatheter treatment of extremity trauma. Semin. Intervent. Radiol. 1992; 9:19–27.
256. Holden RW. Plasminogen activators. Pharmacology and therapy. Radiology 1990; 174:993–1001.
257. Justesen P, Downes M, Grynne BH, Lang H, Rasch W, Seim E. Injection-associated pain in femoral arteriography. A European multicenter study comparing tolerability and efficacy of Iodoxonal and Iopromide. Cardiovasc. Intervent. Radiol. 1997; 20(4):251–256.
258. Kaufman JA, Geller SC, Waltman AC. Renal insufficiency. Gadotetate dimeglumine as a contrast agent during peripheral vascular interventional procedures. Radiology 1996; 198:579–581.
259. Kent KC, McArdle CR, Kennedy B, Baim DS, Anninos E, Skillman JJ. A prospective study of the clinical outcome of femoral pseudoaneurysms and arteriovenous fistulas induced by femoral punctures. J. Vasc. Surg. 1993; 17:125–131.
260. Kinno Y, Odagiri K, Andoh K, Itoh Y, Tarao K. Gadopentetate dimeglumine as an alternate contrast material for use in angiography. AJR Am. J. Roentgenol. 1993; 160(6):1293–1294.
261. Lang E. A server of the complications of percutaneous retrograde arteriography. Radiology 1971; 81:257–263.
262. Lea TM, MacDonald LM. Complications of ascending phlebography of the leg. BMJ 1989; 2:317–318.
263. Matchett WJ, McFarland DR, Russell DK, Sailors DM, Moursi MM. Azotemia. Gadopentetate dimeglumine as a contrast agent at digital subtraction angiography. Radiology 1996; 201(2):569–571.
264. Motarjeme A. Thrombolytic therapy of arterial occlusion and graft thrombosis. Semin. Vasc. Surg. 1989; 2(3):155–178.
265. Ramirez G, O'Neill WM Jr, Lambert R, Bloomer HA. Cholesterol embolism as a complication of angiography. Arch. Intern. Med. 1978; 138(9):1430–1432.
266. Ritz G, Friedman S, Osbourne A. Diabetes and peripheral vascular disease. Clin. Podiatr. Med. Surg. 1992; 9:125–137.
267. Roberts AC, Kaugman JA, Geller SC. Angiographic assessment of peripheral vascular disease. In Straudness DE, van Breda A, eds. Vascular Diseases. Surgical and Interventional Therapy. New York, Churchill Livingstone, 1994; pp. 201–235..
268. Rose SC. Venous duplex ultrasound. In RSNA Categorical Course in Vascular Imaging. Chicago, 1997.
269. Sasalara AA. Fundamentals of fibrinolytic therapy. Cardiovasc. Intervent. Radiol. 1998; 11:53–55.
270. Seldinger SI. Catheter replacement of needle in percutaneous arteriography. New technique. Acta Radiol. 1953; 39:368–376.
271. Semba CP, Dake MD. Thrombolysis in venous and pulmonary occlusive disease. In RSNA Categorical Course in Vascular Imaging, Chicago, 1997.
272. Sharfuddin JHA, Hicks ME. Current status of mechanical thrombectomy. III. Present and future applications. J. Vasc. Intervent. Radiol. 1998; 9:209–224.
273. Sharafuddin MJA, Hicks ME. Current status of percutaneous mechanical thrombectomy. II. Devices and mechanisms of action. J. Vasc. Intervent. Radiol. 1998; 9:15–31.
274. Sharafuddin MJA, Hicks ME. Current status of percutaneous mechanical thrombectomy. I. General principles. J. Vasc. Intervent. Radiol. 1997; 8:911–921.
275. Spies JB, Complications of diagnostic arteriography. Semin. Intervent. Radiol. 1994; 2:93–101.
276. Stokes KR. Complications of diagnostic venography. Semin. Intervent. Radiol. 1994; 2:102–106.
277. Strandness DE, van Breda A. Vascular Diseases. Surgical and Interventional Therapy. New York, Churchill Livingstone, 1994.
278. Suh JS, Skin KH, Na JB, Won JY, Hahn SB. Venous malformations. Sclerotherapy with a mixture of ethanol and lipiodol. Cardiovasc. Intervent. Radiol. 1997; 20(4):268–273.

279. Treiman RL. Peripheral vascular disease in diabetic patients. Evaluation and treatment. Mt. Sinai J. Med. 1987; 54:241.

280. Veith FJ, Gupta SK, Wengester KR, Goldsmith J, Rivers SP, Bakal CW, Dietzek AM, Cynamon J, Sprayregen S, Gliedman ML. Changing arteriosclerotic disease patterns and management strategies in lower limb threatening ischemia. Ann Surg. 1990; 212(4):402–412.

281. Wagner JH, Starck EE, McDermio HJL. Infra-popliteal percutaneous transluminal re-vascularization. Results of a prospective study on 148 patients. J. Intervent. Radiol. 1993; 8:81–90.

282. Wagner HJ, Starck EE, Reuter D. Long-term results of percutaneous aspiration embolectomy. Cardiovasc. Intervent. Radiol. 1994; 17: 241–246.

Radiology of the Foot and Ankle, Second Edition,
edited by Thomas H. Berquist.
© 2000 by Mayo Foundation.
Published by Lippincott Williams & Wilkins, Philadelphia.

CHAPTER 3

Soft Tissue Trauma and Overuse Syndromes

Thomas H. Berquist

Numerous soft tissue injuries and overuse syndromes affect the foot and ankle. Up to 10% of emergency room visits are due to ankle sprains.[12,27] Proper utilization of imaging techniques is essential for detection and treatment of acute and chronic disorders of the foot and ankle.

LIGAMENT INJURIES

The anatomy of the ligaments and supporting structures of the ankle is discussed in Chapter 1. However, certain aspects of ankle anatomy bear repeating in order to understand ligament injuries fully.

The distal tibia and fibula are supported by a system of anterior, posterior, and interosseous ligaments (Fig. 3-1).[12,16,64,128] The anterior inferior tibiofibular ligament is about 2 cm wide and extends from the anterior tibial tubercle to insert on the roughened anterior surface of the lateral malleolus. Posteriorly, the posterior inferior tibiofibular ligament extends from the posterior tibial tubercle to the lateral malleolus. The inferior transverse tibiofibular ligament lies just below and deep to the former structure (see Fig. 3-1B).[12,64,128] The interosseous membrane extends from the posterior tibial border (see Fig. 3-1A) obliquely to insert on the fibular margin. More inferiorly, the membrane thickens, forming

the interosseous ligament (see Fig. 3-1A).[12,64,128] The anterior inferior tibiofibular ligament is about 2 cm wide and extends from the anterior tibial tubercle to insert on the roughened anterior surface of the lateral malleolus. Posteriorly, the posterior inferior tibiofibular ligament extends from the posterior tibial tubercle to the lateral malleolus and the inferior transverse tibiofibular ligament lies just below and deep to the former structure (see Fig. 3-1B).[12,64,128] The interosseous membrane extends from the posterior tibial border (see Fig. 3-1A) obliquely to insert on the fibular margin. More inferiorly, the membrane thickens, forming the interosseous ligament (see Fig. 3-1A).[12,64,128] Other ligament structures maintain the ankle joint (Fig. 3-2). Medially, the deltoid ligament is triangular and broadens as it extends from the medial malleolus to its talar and calcaneal insertions. The deltoid ligament (see Fig. 3-2B) is composed of anterior and posterior superficial and an intermediate deep or tibiotalar ligament.[12,64] The ligament is essentially a triangular thickening with medial capsule. There are three ligaments laterally (see Fig. 3-2C). The anterior talofibular ligament extends from the anterior fibula to insert in the lateral talus just below the articular surface. With the ankle in a neutral position, this ligament is horizontally oriented and resists internal rotation. Studies also indicate that it is significant in resisting varus tilt, particularly with the ankle in plantar flexion.[60] The posterior tibiofibular ligament extends from the posterior fibula to the posterior talus. The calcaneofibu-

T. H. Berquist: Mayo Medical School, Mayo Clinic Jacksonville, Jacksonville, Florida 32224; Mayo Foundation, Mayo Clinic, Rochester, Minnesota 55905.

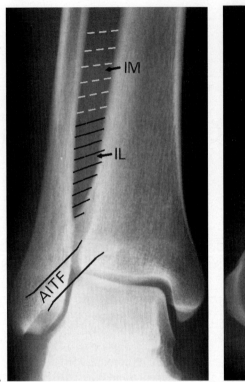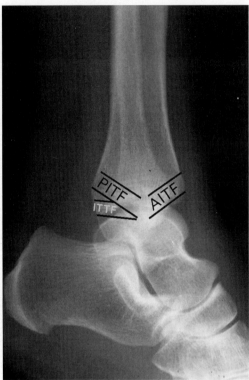

FIG. 3-1. Mortise (**A**) and lateral (**B**) radiographs of the ankle demonstrating the interosseous and distal tibiofibular ligament complex. *AITF,* anterior inferior tibiofibular ligament; *IL,* interosseous ligament; *IM,* interosseous membrane; *ITTF,* inferior transverse tibiofibular ligament; *PITF,* posterior inferior tibiofibular ligament.

lar ligament originates at the lateral malleolar tip and inserts on the calcaneus, restricting inversion. The calcaneofibular ligament supports both the ankle and subtalar joints and is intimately associated with the peroneal tendon sheaths.[12,27,60]

Ankle sprains are most commonly caused by inversion with internal rotation of the foot. The injury commonly occurs during sporting events or falls on uneven surfaces.[22,27,96] The lateral ligaments are most frequently involved. Combination injuries can occur with more severe injuries. Isolated rupture of the deltoid ligament (an eversion injury) is rare. Syndesmotic sprains can occur with the same mechanisms that result in medial or deltoid ligament tears. These mechanisms include eversion, pronation, or pronation and external rotation.[21,120,128] Boyim and colleagues[121] suggested that syndesmotic sprains may account for up to 10% of ankle injuries. Clinically, ankle sprains present with varying degrees of pain, swelling, and ecchymosis. Pain and tenderness are usually evident on ankle examination. There is tenderness to palpation over the involved ligaments. Patients with syndesmotic sprains usually have tenderness to palpation over the anterior and posterior inferior tibiofibular ligaments.[21,27,128] In assessing ankle sprains, it is important to classify the degree of injury so proper treatment can be instituted and chronic instability can be avoided.[96] Typically,

ankle sprains (inversion injuries) are divided into three grades.[12,39] Patients with grade 1 sprains present with mild stretching of the ligaments but no disruption or instability. These patients can still ambulate and generally have mild swelling with pain and tenderness over the anterior talofibular ligament or involved structure. Grade 2 sprains are incomplete ligament tears. There is generally significant pain, marked swelling, and ecchymosis. Patients are difficult to evaluate on physical examination. Discomfort on palpation over the calcaneal fibular ligament is not uncommon. Grade 3 sprains are complete ligament tears. Both the anterior talofibular and calcaneofibular may be involved, resulting in ankle instability.[27,96] The degree of swelling is variable, but the patient usually has tenderness over both the anterior talofibular and calcaneofibular ligaments.[12,27]

Diagnosis

Diagnosis of ligament disruption usually requires special studies. Routine ankle views (anteroposterior [AP], lateral, and mortise views) are not usually effective in differentiating the types of ankle sprains. However, secondary signs are important in determining which additional techniques may be most useful.[12,27,42,112] Patients with grade 1 sprains generally present with mild soft tissue swelling over the lateral

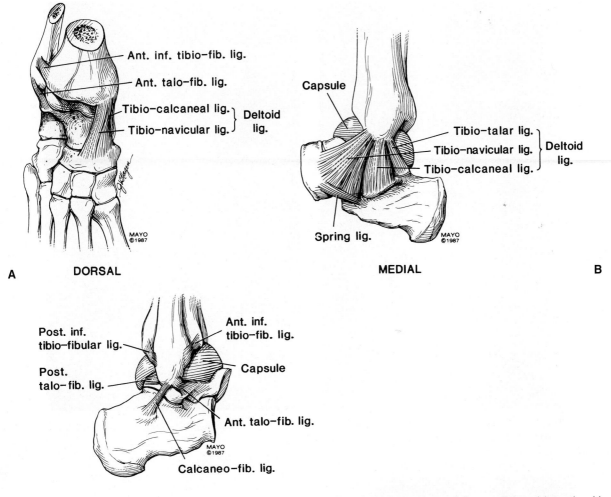

A   DORSAL

B   MEDIAL

C   LATERAL

FIG. 3-2. Illustrations of the medial and lateral ankle ligaments seen dorsally (**A**), medially (**B**), and laterally (**C**).

malleolus. This can be identified on the AP and mortise views. A bright light is frequently needed to evaluate the soft tissues on conventional films. Window level-width or gray-scale reversal can be used with computed radiography. No fracture or effusion is evident on the lateral view. Grade 2 and 3 sprains have more significant swelling that can be identified clinically and on both AP and lateral radiographs. However, this finding has little value. Attempts at correlating ligament injury with the degree of swelling seen radiographically have been unsuccessful. The presence of an effusion in the joint is somewhat useful in that it generally indicates the capsule is intact (Fig. 3-3). Effusions are best seen on the lateral view. Small avulsion fractures (grade 4 sprain) can also be seen on plain films (Fig. 3-4). Measuring the tibiotalar joint to differentiate second and third degree sprains is not usually helpful.[86,114] However, if the talus is shifted, resulting in asymmetry of the ankle mortise, a ligament injury is generally present.

Specific imaging techniques for ligament injury include stress views, arthrography, tenography, and magnetic resonance imaging (MRI).[2,12,24,26,29,97,108] Stress views of the ankle are useful in diagnosing ligament disruption.[12,57] However, this technique requires adequate joint anesthesia and is highly dependent on the experience of the examiner. Comparison with the normal ankle is also necessary. The ankles should be stressed in varus and valgus positions with the foot in neutral and plantar-flexed positions. AP stress views (drawer sign) should also be performed.[12]

For best results, the examination should be fluoroscopically guided to ensure proper positioning and monitoring. When performing varus and valgus stress tests, it is important to remember normal variations in ankle motion. Normal talar tilt ranges from 5° to 23°.[27,35,59] This problem is overcome by comparing the injured and uninjured sides. Measuring varus and valgus stress views can be accomplished using angles or distance measurements. When using the angle technique, a line is drawn along the talar dome and tibial plafond (Fig. 3-5). The change in the angle with stress is measured,

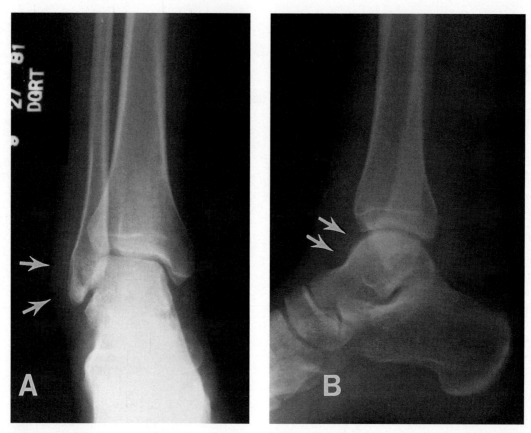

FIG. 3-3. AP (**A**) and lateral (**B**) radiographs demonstrate soft tissue swelling over the lateral malleolus (*arrows* in **A**) and an effusion (*arrows* in **B**) on the lateral view.

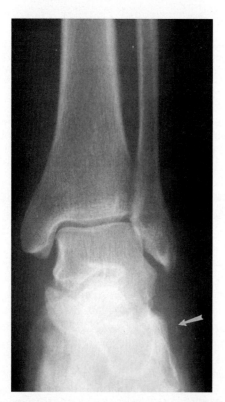

FIG. 3-4. AP radiograph of the ankle demonstrating a small fragment (*arrow*) from a calcaneofibular ligament avulsion.

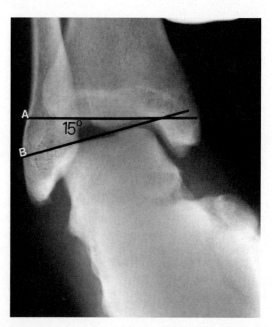

FIG. 3-5. AP varus stress view using the angle technique with lines drawn along the tibial (**A**) and talar (**B**) articular surface. The angle with stress measures 15°.

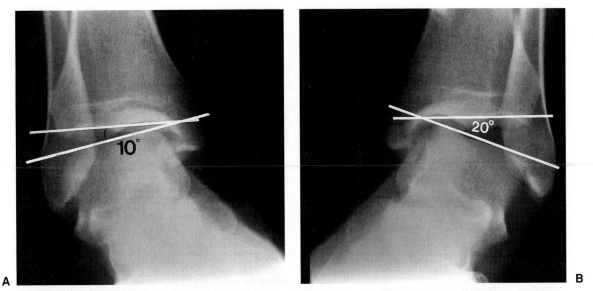

FIG. 3-6. Varus stress views of the normal (**A**) and injured (**B**) ankle. The normal ankle measures 10°, and the injured side is 20°. The 10° difference indicates tears of both the anterior talofibular and calcaneofibular ligaments.

and both ankles are compared (Fig. 3-6). If the angle (talar tilt) of the injured ankle is approximately 10° greater than the normal side, it generally indicates both the anterior talofibular and calcaneofibular ligaments are torn.[27,52] These changes should be noted with the foot in both plantar-flexed and neutral positions during stress. In neutral, if the angle is 6° greater than the normal side, both ligaments are probably torn. If this only occurs in plantar-flexed stress, it is likely that only the anterior talofibular ligament is torn.[52] It has been demonstrated experimentally that accuracy is best with 10° of plantar flexion and the leg internally rotated 25°.[77] The change in height from the talar dome to the plafond can also be measured. A difference of 3 mm between the normal and injured ankle indicates ligament disruption (Fig. 3-7).[12] AP stress can be applied using several techniques. For consistency, I prefer the double-exposure technique with the foot neutral or slightly plantar flexed (Fig. 3-8).[12,77] This allows the change in talar or tibial position to be easily measured on one film. Both ankles are studied for comparison purposes. Sauser and colleagues[107] studied 55 patients with stress views and arthrography within 72 hours of injury. This study noted stress views were accurate if talar tilt increased by 10° or more, but the test was only positive in 38% of patients with positive arthrograms.

Blanchard and associates,[16] Black and colleagues,[15] and Schweigel and associates[109] reported significantly improved accuracy, approaching 96%, using stress tenography to evaluate the calcaneofibular ligament. False-negative studies using conventional arthrography approached 21%.[15,114] As noted in Chapter 2, the ankle tenogram is positive when contrast injected into the peroneal tendon sheath enters the joint space (Fig. 3-9). However, this maneuver decompresses the sheath and can make it more difficult to demonstrate

anterior talofibular ligament tears. The latter and deltoid ligaments are intimately associated with the capsule, and, therefore, ankle arthrography is more useful in demonstrating these ligament injuries (Fig. 3-10). Because stress views are most accurate after anesthetic injection, it would seem wise to combine arthrograms or tenograms with stress views to allow the most accurate assessment of the injury. Therefore,

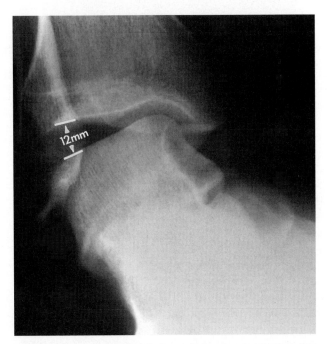

FIG. 3-7. Varus stress view of the ankle demonstrates opening of the lateral joint space to 12 mm. The normal side measured 7 mm.

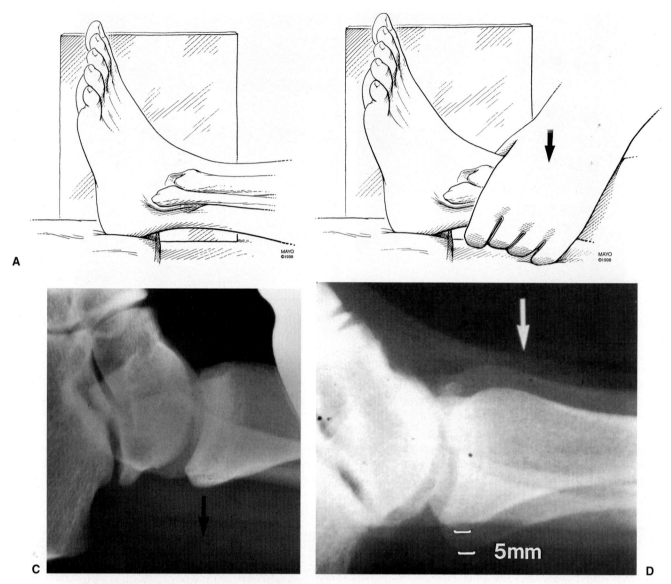

FIG. 3-8. AP stress view technique. **A:** Illustration of ankle positioned with heel on a block and film positioned for the cross-table lateral technique. **B:** The same film is exposed before and after stress. **C:** Cross-table lateral view of the normal ankle. **D:** Double-exposed view of the injured ankle shows a 5-mm shift, which is easily measured using the double-exposure technique.

I recommend using one of these combinations in assessing acute ankle injury. This decision should be based on clinical findings and whether surgery or treatment modifications will be made based on the degree of ligament injury. Surgical intervention is a more important consideration in professional athletes or young active persons. Generally, assessment of the calcaneofibular ligament is most critical because conservative treatment is most often used if only the anterior talofibular ligament is torn. Therefore, a stress tenogram is the invasive technique of choice.[16,43]

Contrast extravasates medially when there is deltoid ligament disruption and may extend beyond the normal 2.5-cm syndesmotic recess when the patient has a syndesmotic sprain.[12,128] Contrast extending between the tibia and the

fibula on the mortise view or seen anterior to the tibiofibular ligament on the lateral view is also indicative of a syndesmotic tear.[128] However, care must be taken not to mistake extravasation along the anterior needle tract for a ligament tear.[2,12]

In recent years, MRI has been used in place of stress studies and arthrotenography to evaluate the ankle ligaments and syndesmotic region.[10,24,26,29,108] Both conventional MRI (no intraarticular contrast) and MR arthrography can be used to evaluate the ligaments of the ankle. The complexity of ligament anatomy (see Figs. 3-1 and 3-2) makes it difficult to demonstrate all potential ligament injuries without special positioning, specific image planes, or three-dimensional gradient-echo techniques.[12,74,108] Using conventional image

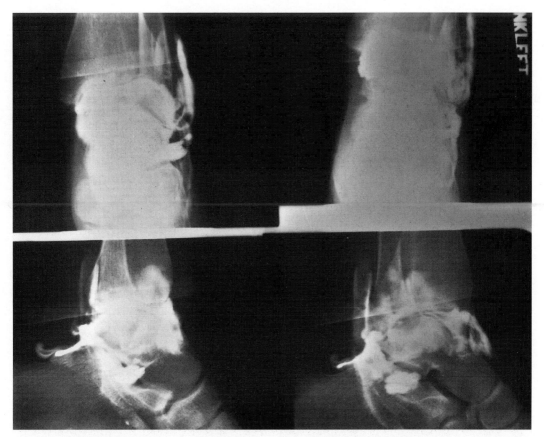

FIG. 3-9. Peroneal tenogram. Contrast injected into the peroneal tendon sheath enters the joint space, thus indicating a calcaneofibular ligament tear.

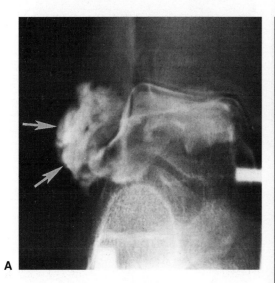

A

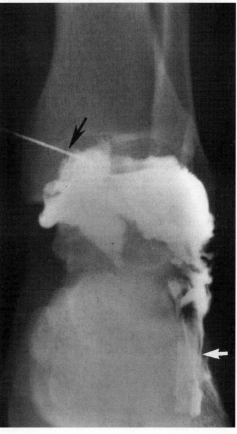

B

FIG. 3-10. Ankle arthrograms. **A:** AP view after ankle injection demonstrates extravasation laterally (*arrows*) resulting from an anterior talofibular ligament tear. There is no filling of the peroneal tendon sheath. **B:** AP radiograph taken during ankle injection (*black arrow* shows medial entry of the needle). There is filling of the peroneal tendon sheaths (*white arrow*) resulting from calcaneofibular ligament disruption.

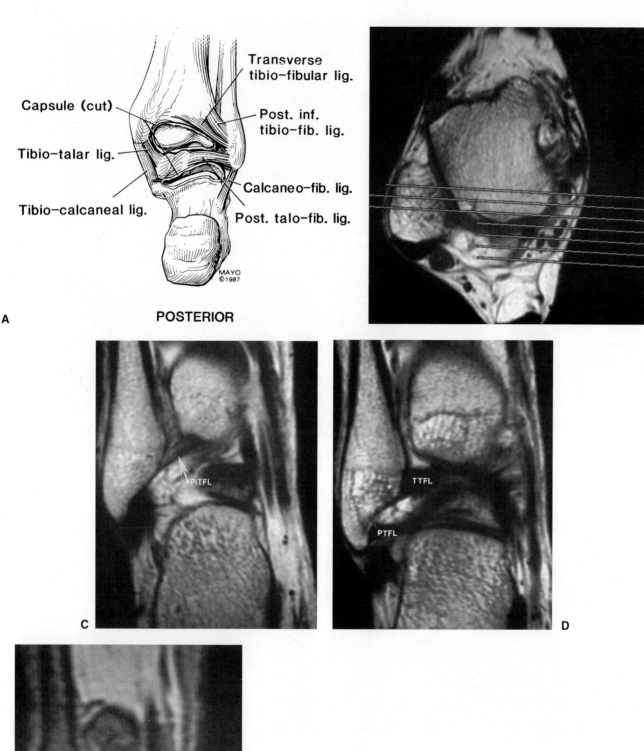

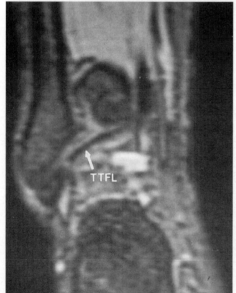

FIG. 3-11. MRI of the posterior tibiofibular ligament complex. **A:** Illustration of ligaments of the ankle seen posteriorly. **B:** Axial scout image with planes selected for oblique coronal sections in the plane of the posterior ligaments. **C** and **D:** Coronal SE 500/11 images demonstrating the posterior ligaments. *PITFL,* posterior inferior tibiofibular ligament; *PTFL,* posterior talofibular ligament; *TTFL,* transverse tibiofibular ligament. **E:** GRE echo image demonstrating the transverse tibiofibular ligament (*TTFL*).

112

planes, Kier and associates[70] identified the anterior talofibular ligament on 20% of sagittal images and on 75% of axial images and failed to identify this structure on any coronal images. The posterior tibiofibular ligament was seen on 7% of sagittal images and on all axial images and was not demonstrated on coronal images.[70]

Special positions or obliqued image planes are necessary to demonstrate the ligaments using conventional MRI.[12,29,108] Schneck and colleagues[108] demonstrated that the distal anterior and posterior tibiofibular ligaments were most easily appreciated on axial images with the foot dorsiflexed 10° to 20° (Fig. 3-11). Coronal images were optimal for evaluating the talocalcaneal interosseous ligament (Fig. 3-12). Axial images with the foot plantar flexed 40° to 50° were optimal for demonstrating the calcaneofibular ligament.[108] These foot positions may be difficult to maintain following acute injury or if there is persistent ankle pain.

Selected image planes (Figs. 3-13 and 3-14) or three-dimensional gradient-echo sequences (T2*) improve the likelihood of defining ligament anatomy and tears with greater accuracy.[12,73,74] Gradient-echo three-dimensional images can be obtained (see Fig. 3-11E) using 30/10 (TR/TE), 70% flip angle, a 14-cm field of view, 256 × 256 or 256 × 192 matrix, and effective section thicknesses of 0.7 to 1 mm.[73] This sequence should be added to screening examinations of patients with suspected ligament injuries.[10]

MR arthrography can be performed using saline, conventional arthrographic contrast agents, or gadolinium. Using standard iodinated contrast agents has advantages. Needle

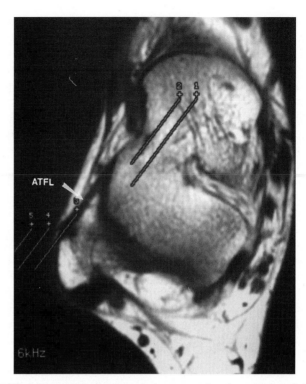

FIG. 3-13. Axial scout image demonstrating the anterior talofibular ligament (*ATFL; arrow*) with image planes selected for oblique sagittal images of the structure.

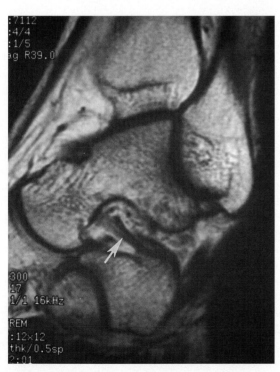

FIG. 3-12. Oblique coronal SE 500/11 image demonstrating the normal talocalcaneal interosseous ligament (*arrow*).

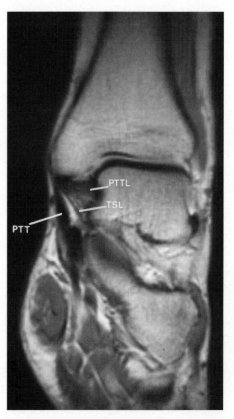

FIG. 3-14. Oblique coronal SE 400/10 image demonstrating the medial ligaments. *PTT,* posterior tibial tendon; *PTTL,* posterior tibiotalar ligament; *TSL,* tibiospring ligament.

position can be documented so extravasation or improper injections can be avoided. Local anesthetics can be injected with contrast so stress views and symptomatic relief can be evaluated. This adds additional information to MRI images and, in some cases, may solve the problem so that the MRI examination can be avoided, thereby reducing patient costs. Most institutions use gadolinium for MR arthrography after confirming needle position with a small test injection of iodinated contrast. Small amounts of iodinated contrast are used because T1 and T2 relaxation times are dose dependent.[55] Gadolinium is diluted with normal saline (0.2 ml of gadopentetate dimeglumine with 50 ml of normal saline or 1 ml of gadopentetate dimeglumine with 250 ml of saline), and about 12 to 15 ml is injected, using the technique discussed in Chapter 2. The joint is exercised, and T1-weighted MRI images are obtained using appropriate image planes to study the suspected injury. Imaging can be performed immediately after injection or any time during the next few hours.[55] The accuracy, especially for subtle injuries, is much greater with MR arthrography than with conventional MRI. Sensitivities and specificities in the 90% to 100% range have been reported.[29,55]

Ligament tears in the foot and ankle resemble ligament injuries in other anatomic regions. Grade 1 injuries present as subtle areas of increased signal intensity and slight thickening. Overlying subcutaneous edema is usually present. Grade 2 ligament tears involve about half the fibers, so signal intensity changes are more dramatic and ligament thickening is more obvious. Grade 3 ligament tears (Fig. 3-15) are complete, with separation of the ligament fragments and high-intensity signal between the torn fragments. On conventional

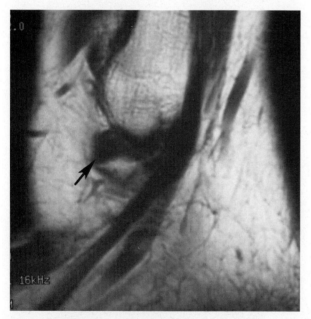

FIG. 3-15. Sagittal T1-weighted MRI shows a focal area of low signal intensity (*arrow*) resulting from a thickened remnant of a completely torn calcaneofibular ligament.

MRI, these changes are most easily appreciated on T2 or T2* sequences.[12,29,108]

Treatment

Imaging of ankle sprains should be based on philosophy of treatment, on clinical findings, and on whether surgery may be indicated. Treatment of ligament injuries of the ankle is controversial.[27,96,122,128] Accurate assessment of the degree of injury (anterior talofibular alone or with calcaneofibular ligament), the history of recurrent sprains, chronic instability, patient's age and activity, and the presence of systemic disease or steroid therapy all play a part in the decision to treat surgically or conservatively. Many authors believe that conservative treatment is superior to early operative intervention.[96] Brand and Collins[22] reported that only 12% of ankle sprains were surgically repaired. Cass and Morrey[27] also recommended conservative therapy. Grade 1 and 2 sprains are treated with taping, air splints, or casting if the patient is unable to ambulate with taping alone. Patients with grade 3 sprains are treated with walking casts for 3 to 6 weeks. Patients are generally allowed to return to normal activity as symptoms dictate. This treatment approach is based on their data, which indicates repair after acute injury does not provide any advantage to delayed repair if chronic instability occurs.[27] Chronic instability can develop in 15 to 25% of patients after ligament injury.[55,62,128] However, surgery is not required in all cases.

Imaging of ankle sprains, as with treatment, can be controversial. Routine radiographs should be obtained to exclude fracture when physical findings are significant (pain, ecchymosis, pain with weight bearing or inability to bear weight). Some authors do not believe that additional studies are indicated unless surgery will be performed or the patient is young or a professional athlete.[12,24,27] Brestenseher and associates[24] suggested that MRI be reserved for patients on whom surgery is contemplated or with talar tilt on stress views of 6 to 14°. An additional advantage of MRI is the ability to detect talar dome and peroneal tendon injury that may mimic ankle sprains. Our current approach still includes use of stress views and arthrotenography or MRI, depending on the acute or chronic nature of the injury. The algorithm demonstrated below suggests imaging approaches to acute and chronic ankle sprains.

Patients treated conservatively or surgically may require radiographic follow-up when symptoms persist. Early degenerative changes and certain signs of chronic instability may be evident on standing AP and lateral views (Figs. 3-16 and 3-17).[54] Usually, changes are more subtle, and stress testing is required. These tests are generally believed to be most accurate within 72 hours of acute injury; however, chronic changes can be documented. When stress tests yield a talar tilt greater than or equal to 6° or when symptoms cannot be effectively explained, based on existing radiographs, arthrotenography or MRI should be performed.

Ankle Sprain
Imaging Techniques

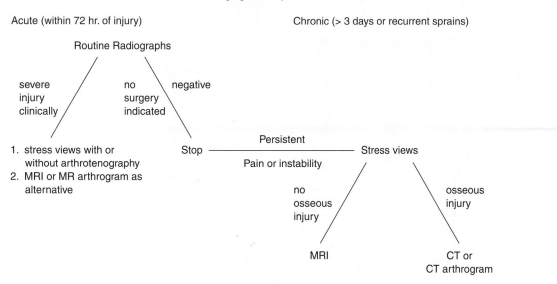

Acute (within 72 hr. of injury)   Chronic (> 3 days or recurrent sprains)

Routine Radiographs

severe   no   negative
injury   surgery
clinically   indicated

1. stress views with or   Stop ——— Persistent ——— Stress views
   without arthrotenography   Pain or instability
2. MRI or MR arthrogram as   no   osseous
   alternative   osseous   injury
                                                   injury
                                                     MRI   CT or
                                                                  CT arthrogram

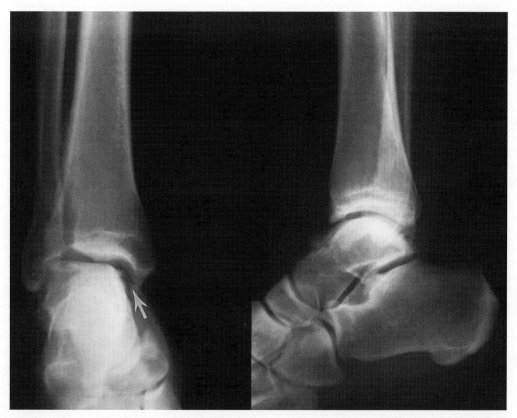

FIG. 3-16. AP and lateral views of the ankle in a patient with chronic instability after ankle sprain. There is degenerative arthritis with talar shift, widening of the medial ankle mortise (*arrow*), and intraarticular fragments.

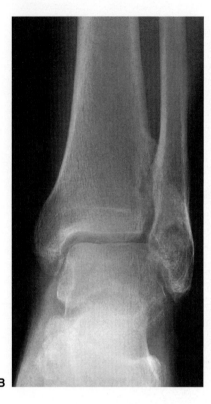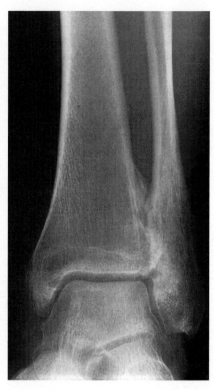

A,B

FIG. 3-17. AP (**A**) and mortise (**B**) views of the ankle in a patient with previous syndesmotic sprain resulting in ossification of the interosseous ligament and membrane.

These studies can demonstrate partially healed tears, chronic tears in the calcaneofibular ligament (see Fig. 3-15), adhesive capsulitis, and residual instability.[16,41,108] Axial images provided by MRI are particularly useful in evaluating the tibiofibular syndesmosis.[128] Table 3-1 summarizes the late complications of ligament injuries.

TENDON INJURIES

Thirteen tendons cross the ankle.[10,64] These tendons include the following: the peroneus brevis and longus laterally; the Achilles tendon posteriorly, the tibialis posterior, flexor digitorum longus, and flexor hallucis longus medially; and anteriorly, the tibialis anterior, extensor hallucis longus, tendons of the extensor digitorum longus, and peroneus tertius. All tendons are enclosed in sheaths, with the exception of the Achilles tendon. Tendon injury may occur as an isolated event, in association with a fracture, or because of a previous fracture with degenerative joint disease. Tendons may also rupture in patients receiving steroid therapy (systemic or direct injection) or in those with chronic inflammatory diseases.[51,81,87,101–103]

Peroneal Tendons

The peroneal muscles assist in pronation and eversion of the foot (Fig. 3-18).[64,102] The peroneus brevis tendon is anterior to the peroneus longus as they pass posterior to the lateral malleolus (Fig. 3-19). Approximately 80% of patients have a notch (varies in size) in the fibula that accommodates the peroneus brevis. In 20% of patients, this notch is shallow or absent, a feature that may lead to subluxation or dislocation (Fig. 3-20).[12,102] The tendons also pass deep to the superior and inferior peroneal retinacula (see Fig. 3-19). It is between these two structures that the tendons are immediately adjacent to the calcaneofibular ligament.[12,27] The peroneal tendons share a common sheath to the inferior margin of the superior retinaculum. At this point, the peroneus longus separates from the peroneus brevis (see Fig. 3-19; Fig. 3-21). The peroneus longus progresses inferior to the peroneal tubercle of the calcaneus to the plantar aspect of the foot, where it inserts on the base of the first metatarsal and medial cuneiform (see Fig. 3-19B). The peroneus brevis passes inferiorly, inserting on the base of the fifth metatarsal (see Fig. 3-19A). Evaluation of the tendons and normal sulci is easily accomplished using tenography, MRI, or computed tomography (CT) (see Figs. 3-20 and 3-21).[8,10,80,119]

Diagnosis of peroneal tendon injury first requires that the problem be considered. Many patients present with sprained

---

TABLE 3-1. *Sequelae of ankle ligament injuries*[a]

Recurrent instability (15–25%)
Recurrent sprains
Peroneal nerve palsy
Peroneal tendon dislocation/subluxation
Degenerative arthritis
Sural nerve injury (usually following surgical repair)

[a] Data from references 12, 27, 54, and 55.

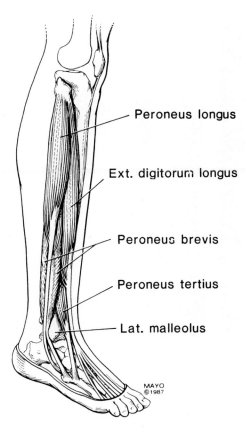

FIG. 3-18. Illustration of the leg demonstrating the peroneal muscles and tendons, the evertors of the foot.

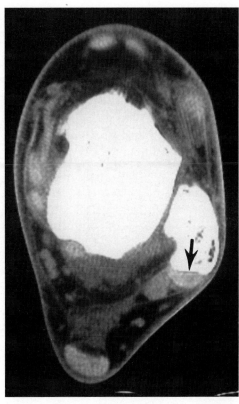

FIG. 3-20. Axial CT image at the level of the fibular notch showing the peroneal tendons and a shallow fibular notch (*arrow*).

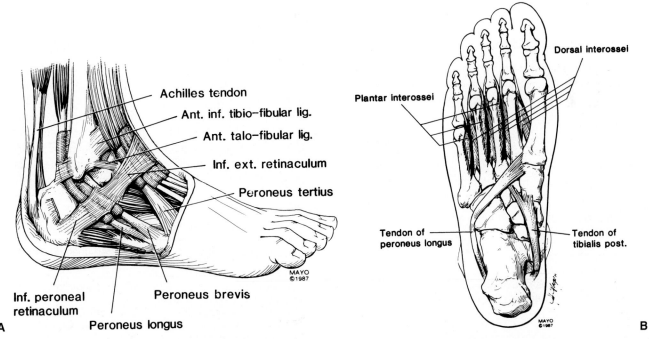

FIG. 3-19. A: Illustration of the peroneal tendons and retinacula. **B:** Plantar illustration of the foot demonstrating the insertions of the peroneus longus and tibialis posterior tendons.

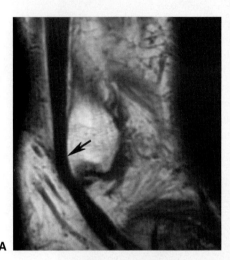
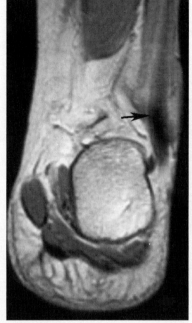
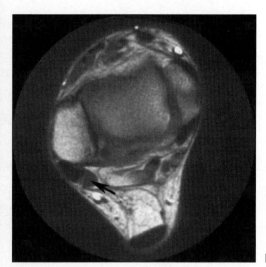

A   B

FIG. 3-21. MRI images of the peroneal tendons in the sagittal (**A**), coronal (**B**), and axial (**C**) planes (*arrow*).

ankle or repeated giving-way, and disorders of the peroneal tendon are not considered (Tables 3-2 and 3-3).[1,27,29,87]

Recognition of peroneal tendon disorders and their image features has been reemphasized with the evolving role of MRI.[6,12,69,101,124] Table 3-3 summarizes peroneal tendon injuries and our preferred imaging approach to detection and classification of injuries.

Peroneal Tendon Subluxation/Dislocation

Peroneal tendon dislocations and subluxations are not common. Subluxations have been reported with ski injuries and in patients with chronic ankle sprains with retinacular laxity and shallow or convex fibular grooves.[38,69,124] The mechanism of injury is not clear, but dislocation is most likely caused by an inversion-dorsiflexion or abduction-dorsiflexion injury. Patients present with pain and swelling over the posterior superior aspect of the lateral malleolus. Certain patients can voluntarily dislocate the peroneal tendons.[87]

Swelling may make actual palpation of the tendon difficult, and pain with motion can limit the detection of subluxation on physical examination. Routine radiographs demonstrate soft tissue swelling laterally, but the distribution is not characteristic or different from an inversion sprain (see Table 3-2). A characteristic longitudinal flake fracture along the distal fibular metaphysis is useful when present.[87] This is best seen on the internal oblique view.[12,119] Murr[88] reported this finding in 15 to 50% of peroneal tendon dislocations (Fig. 3-22). Usually, other imaging procedures are more useful. CT, MRI, or tenography should be considered to confirm the diagnosis. CT provides excellent bone detail and is useful

TABLE 3-2. *Ankle sprains: differential diagnosis[a]*

Fractures
Talus
Neck
Dome
Lateral process
Posterior process
Calcaneus
Anterior process
Cuboid
Malleolar fractures or avulsions
Fifth metatarsal base
Soft tissue injuries
Peroneal tendon
Subtalar subluxation/dislocation
Deltoid ligament
Talonavicular subluxation/dislocation

[a] Data from references 27, 33, 39, and 69.

TABLE 3-3. *Peroneal tendon injuries[a]*

Type of injury	Preferred imaging technique
Peroneal subluxation or dislocation	MRI > tenogram
Tenosynovitis	MRI
Stenosing tenosynovitis	Tenogram ≥ MRI with motion study
Peroneal tendon tears	MRI
Peroneus tendon split syndrome	MRI

[a] Data from references 12, 69, 101, and 110.

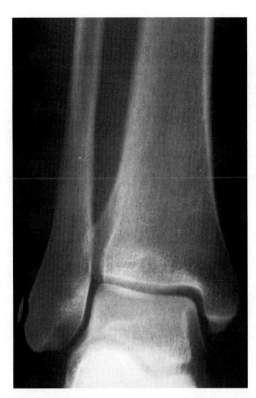

FIG. 3-22. Internal oblique view of the ankle demonstrating a fibular flake fracture associated with peroneal tendon dislocation.

in assessing the peroneal notch in the fibula (see Fig. 3-20).[102,103] The tendons are less clearly demonstrated with CT than MRI.[12] Subtle tears or complete disruptions are more easily seen on MRI, in which the tendons are normally of low signal intensity (black) compared with the high intensity seen in the tendon that has torn. These noninvasive techniques do have disadvantages. For example, if the tendons have returned to normal position or are only slightly displaced, fluoroscopic observation after tenography may be more useful in demonstrating subluxation (see Table 3-3). This situation may also be possible to demonstrate with newer fast-scan (gradient-echo) MRI techniques. Today, MRI is preferred because it is easily performed and does not require the technical skill of tenography (see Table 3-3).[12,122]

Rupture of the Peroneal Tendon

Rupture of the peroneal tendons is not common. However, the lesion may be overlooked as a cause of ankle instability, and therefore the true incidence is not known.[1] Patients may present acutely with an ankle sprain or may have symptoms of chronic instability. The latter is more common in patients with chronic inflammatory arthritis or patients receiving systemic steroids. Cavovarus foot and compartment syndromes have also been reported with peroneal tendon

rupture.[19,37,39] When the tendons are torn, the patient is unable to evert the foot effectively.[1,12,33]

Peroneal tendon tears have been classified as degenerative, partial, and complete (Fig. 3-23). Most tears are partial with a longitudinal configuration.[69] The mechanism of injury and clinical features for the peroneus longus and peroneus brevis may vary. Peroneus longus injury may be acute or chronic. Acute injuries are uncommon and are most often seen in patients with an os peroneum (Fig. 3-24) who have inversion injuries with the foot supinated.[6,69,110] When the os peroneum is present, the sesamoid may be displaced or avulsed. Chronic peroneus longus injuries are usually due to degeneration, resulting in a longitudinal split that usually begins at the lateral malleolar margin and extends proximally and distally. The tear may also occur at the level of the peroneal process on the calcaneus.[69,110] Systemic diseases such as diabetes mellitus may also lead to degeneration and peroneus longus tears.[69]

Peroneus brevis tendon tears are usually longitudinal and are associated with subluxation-dislocation. Other causes include a lax superior retinaculum, bone irregularity in the fibular groove, compression between bone and the peroneus longus tendon, and an anomalous peroneus quadratus muscle or low-lying peroneus brevis muscle belly.[6,32,64,101,110,133]

Imaging of the peroneal tendons is important because clinical features and physical findings may be subtle or confusing. Routine radiographs are usually not useful. However, displacement of the os peroneum (see Fig. 3-24) may indicate peroneal rupture.[121] A fibula flake fracture may also be evident (see Fig. 3-22).[88] Tenography may demonstrate the site of the tear, but because this technique outlines the tendon and does not provide direct assessment, it is less useful than MRI. Both CT and MRI have been described as useful techniques for evaluating the peroneal tendons.[8,12,102,103] CT is useful for demonstrating abnormalities in the peroneal groove fibular abnormalities (see Fig. 3-20) and prominence of the peroneal tubercle of the calcaneus and for demonstrating peroneal tendon changes related to calcaneal fractures.[18,102,103]

MRI is useful for defining osseous and soft tissue changes. Axial and sagittal images using T2-weighted sequences are most useful to detect and classify injuries. Some authors use oblique axial images to more accurately follow the course of the tendons (Fig. 3-25). T2-weighted images reduce confusion that may be caused by magic angle effect (Fig. 3-26). Magic angle effect is seen as increased signal in tendons angled approximately 55° to the bore of the magnet on short TE/TR sequences.[12,110]

Positioning of the foot is also important. If the foot is dorsiflexed, the peroneus brevis muscle moves distally and can be confused with an anomalous muscle or low-lying muscle belly (Fig. 3-27).[98] Magic angle effect is also more likely with the foot in neutral position. Some authors suggest plantar flexion to correct this problem.[69]

MRI can clearly define peroneal tendon tears. Complete tears are seen as an area of bright signal intensity on T2-

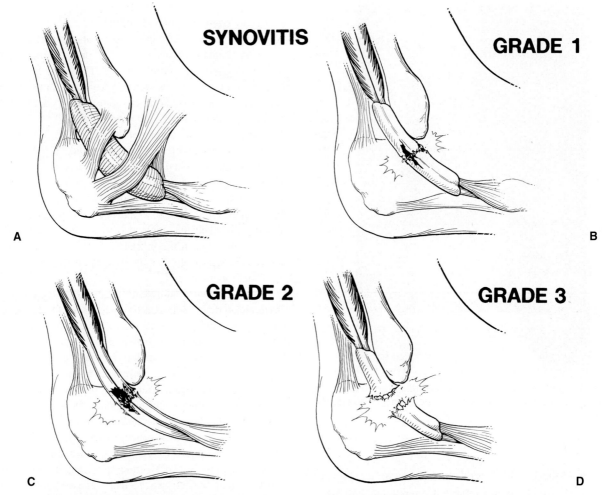

FIG. 3-23. Classification of tendon tears. **A:** Tendons intact with synovitis-tenosynovitis. **B:** Grade 1 tear: minimal fiber disruption. **C:** Grade 2 tear: approximately 50% of fibers are disrupted. **D:** Grade 3 tear: complete disruption of the tendon.

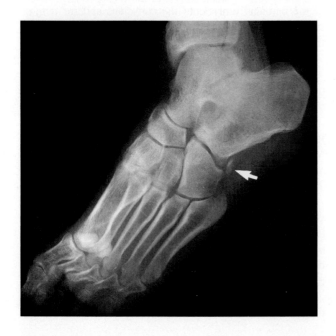

FIG. 3-24. Oblique radiograph of the foot demonstrating the os peroneum (*arrow*).

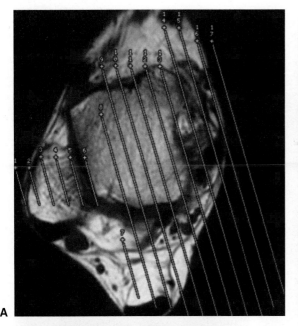

A

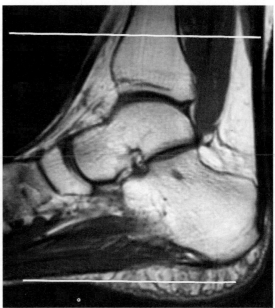

B

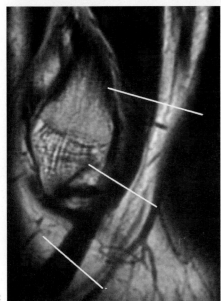

C

FIG. 3-25. MRI planes for evaluating peroneal tendon injuries. **A:** Axial scout image with 3- to 4-mm thick sagittal images selected. **B:** Sagittal image with conventional axial images to include the peroneus longus insertion on the plantar aspect of the foot (see Fig. 3-19B). **C:** Sagittal scout image with image planes selected for oblique axial images. Variations in foot position and anatomy can result in the need to use different angles of obliquity. I do not use oblique axial images.

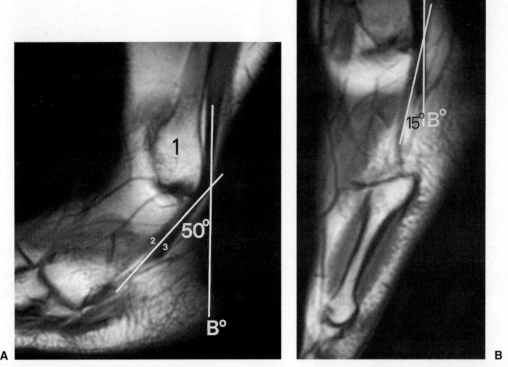

FIG. 3-26. A: Sagittal SE 500/20 image demonstrating the tendon angle in relation to the magnet (B°). In this case, the angle is 50°. The magic angle effect can be particularly difficult to differentiate from tendinosis on short TE/TR sequences. *1,* fibula; *2,* peroneus brevis; *3,* peroneus longus. **B:** Sagittal image with foot plantar flexed straightens the peroneal tendons reducing the likelihood of magic angle effects.

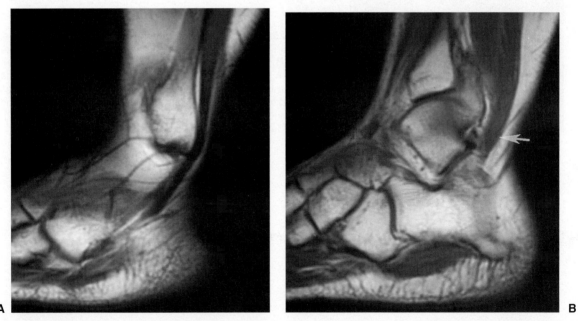

FIG. 3-27. Position of the peroneus brevis muscle may vary with foot position. **A:** Normal-appearing tendons with foot slightly plantar flexed. **B:** The muscle extends distally (*arrow*) when the foot is dorsiflexed.

TABLE 3-4. *Magnetic resonance imaging features of tendon injuries*

Injury category	MRI features
Acute complete tear (grade 3)	Tendon ends separated completely with ↑ signal intensity on T2-weighted sequence; fluid in tendon sheaths
Acute partial tear (grade 1–2)	Tendon thickening with increased signal intensity ≤ 50% of tendon thickness on T2-weighted sequence
Chronic partial tear or tendinosis	Tendon thickened with intermediate signal on proton density image that does not ↑ significantly on T2-weighted image
Synovitis	Tendon normal to slightly thickened; fluid in tendon sheath with ↑ signal surrounding tendon on T2-weighted sequence

weighted images with separation of the torn tendon segments (Table 3-4). In this setting, a larger field of view (16 to 24 cm) may be necessary to demonstrate the proximal retracted portion of the tendon. Demonstrating the tendon margins is essential for operative planning (Fig. 3-28). Acute injuries (Fig. 3-29) usually have significant soft tissue changes that can make image interpretation more confusing.[12]

Peroneus brevis tendon tears are usually seen as longitudinal splits that may extend for 2.5 to 5.0 cm.[69,101,110,124] Multiple splits may be identified at surgery.[69] Axial images are most useful for evaluating peroneus brevis tendon splits (Fig. 3-30). However, both sagittal and axial images should be reviewed (see Fig. 3-30B and C). Partial tears of the peroneus longus (Fig. 3-31) are also most easily demonstrated on axial images. The tendon is usually thickened, with increased signal intensity involving a portion of the tendon (see Table 3-4).[10]

Tenosynovitis and stenosing tendonitis may also develop because of chronic microtrauma, recurrent subluxation, or previous fracture.[10,18] Stenosing tendinitis is associated with calcaneal fractures and prominence of the peroneal process of the calcaneus.[18] MRI is preferred to evaluate synovitis (Fig. 3-32). Stenosing tenosynovitis requires motion studies and sufficient fluid in the tendon sheath to evaluate entrapment. Therefore, in this setting, tenography (Fig. 3-33) may be more useful (see Table 3-3).[10,12]

Treatment

Treatment of peroneal tendon injury depends on the degree of injury. In patients with dislocation, considerations include deepening the fibular groove and reinforcing the superior retinaculum. The latter can be accomplished using a pedical fascial flap, a strip of Achilles tendon, or a portion of the distal plantaris. The tendons can also be rerouted medial to the calcaneofibular ligament.[64]

Incomplete tendon tears can be treated conservatively. In patients with complete disruption, operative intervention

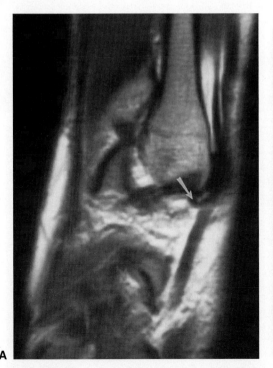
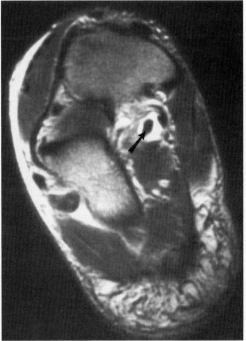

A   **B**

FIG. 3-28. Acute peroneus longus tendon tear. **A:** Sagittal SE 2000/20 image demonstrates the proximal end of the torn peroneus longus (*arrow*) at the malleolar margin. **B:** Axial SE 2000/60 image demonstrates the distal segment (*arrow*) with fluid in the sheath.

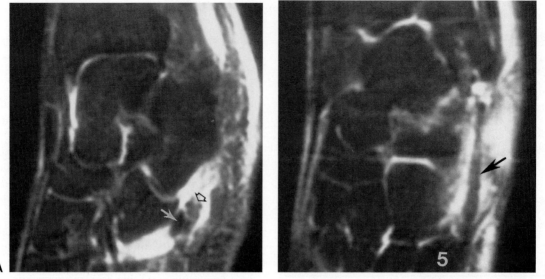

FIG. 3-29. A: Oblique coronal STIR image demonstrates extensive soft tissue injury with a torn peroneus longus (*open arrow*) near the os peroneum (*white arrow*). **B:** Oblique STIR image in a different plane demonstrates the intact peroneus brevis (*arrow*) inserting on the base of the fifth metatarsal (*5*).

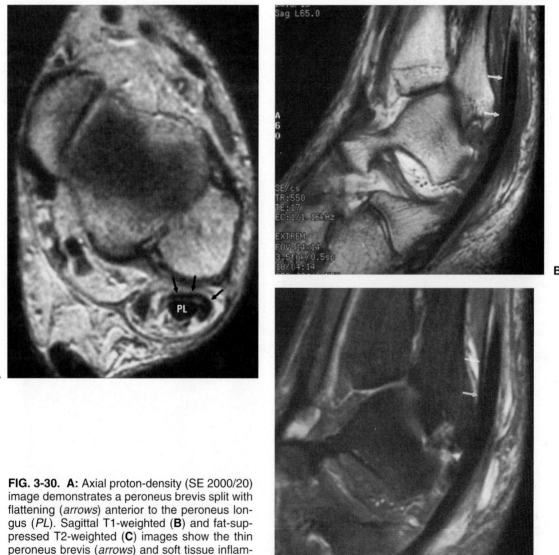

FIG. 3-30. A: Axial proton-density (SE 2000/20) image demonstrates a peroneus brevis split with flattening (*arrows*) anterior to the peroneus longus (*PL*). Sagittal T1-weighted (**B**) and fat-suppressed T2-weighted (**C**) images show the thin peroneus brevis (*arrows*) and soft tissue inflammation.

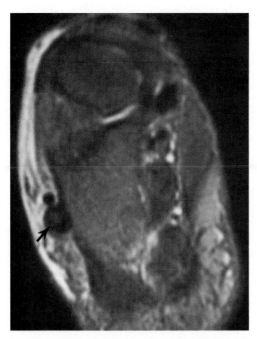

FIG. 3-31. Axial SE 2000/80 image demonstrates thickening with increased signal intensity in the peroneus longus tendon (*arrow*).

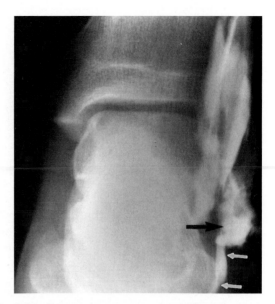

FIG. 3-33. Peroneal tenogram shows fluid in the tendon sheath to the calcaneal level with distal narrowing (*white arrows*). There is proximal extravasation (*black arrow*).

provides the best results. This can be accomplished by repairing the torn ends or using soft tissue grafts. Follow-up evaluation is most easily accomplished using MRI. MRI can determine whether the tendon is intact and provides valuable baseline data should postoperative infection or recurrent rupture take place.[12,64]

Achilles Tendon

The Achilles tendon is the largest and strongest tendon in the foot and ankle. The tendon originates as the gastrocnemius and soleus tendons join and inserts on the posterior calcaneus. In its axial presentation, the tendon thickens distally, becoming elliptic with concave anterior and convex posterior surfaces (Fig. 3-34). Approximately 2 to 6 cm above its calcaneal insertion, the fibers in the tendon cross.

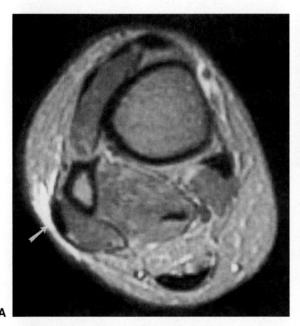

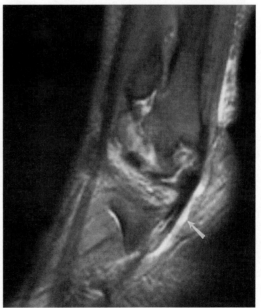

FIG. 3-32. Axial (**A**) and sagittal (**B**) T2-weighted images demonstrate fluid in the tendon sheaths (*arrow*) and local edema (*arrow*) resulting from synovitis secondary to recurrent subluxation.

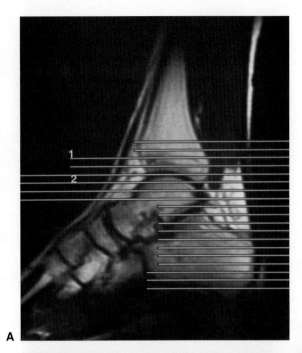

A

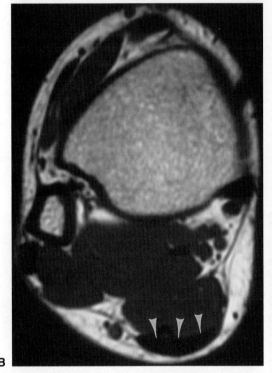

B

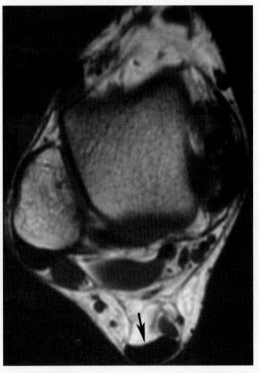

C

FIG. 3-34. Normal MRI anatomy of the Achilles tendon. **A:** Sagittal MRI demonstrating levels for axial images of the Achilles tendon. **B:** Axial image at level 1 shows a concave anterior border (*white arrowheads*). The soleus muscle is still evident. **C:** Axial image at level 2 shows the tendon (*arrow*) contrasted against the high-intensity pre-Achilles fat.

The posterior fibers course medial to lateral, and anterior fibers lateral to medial before inserting in the calcaneus. Most tendon tears occur just above this, perhaps partially owing to the reduced blood supply in this region. The Achilles tendon does not have a true tendon sheath.[10,64]

The Achilles tendon, although strong, is commonly torn. Ruptures are usually the result of indirect trauma. The injury can occur during athletic activity at any age. Injuries usually occur during strenuous activities, with frequent plantar flex-

ion during raising up on the toes or with pushing off or jumping with the knee extended. Falling or landing on the forefoot, which leads to abrupt dorsiflexion of the foot, can also cause Achilles rupture. In nonathletes, the injury is most common from 30 to 50 years of age.[64] Certain systemic and local conditions predispose to tendon disruption. Gout, systemic lupus erythematosus, rheumatoid arthritis, hyperparathyroidism, chronic renal failure, steroids, and diabetes have all been implicated.[10,90] Patients receiving systemic steroids or with other systemic diseases noted earlier may rupture both Achilles tendons simultaneously. Local steroid injections may also lead to partial or complete disruption.[76]

Diagnosis

Clinically, patients present with pain, local swelling, and inability to raise up on their toes on the affected side.[64] If completely torn, a defect may be palpable on physical examination. However, clinical examination is not always accurate. The exact nature of the injury can be misdiagnosed in over 25% of patients. This is because a gap in the tendon may not be palpable (especially in incomplete tears) and the patient may be able to plantar flex the foot with the toe flexors. Differentiation of Achilles tears from gastrocnemius or plantaris tears may also be difficult.[94] Thompson's test may be useful. This test is performed by squeezing the gastrocnemius muscle belly. If the Achilles tendon is intact, the foot will plantar flex during the maneuver (positive response). If the tendon is torn, the foot will not respond (negative response).[123] O'Brien[91] described a similar test using a needle placed in the Achilles tendon 10 inches above the calcaneus. The motion of the needle hub is observed while the foot is in the dorsiflexed and plantar-flexed positions. When the hub moves in the opposite direction of foot motion, the tendon is intact.[91]

Imaging of Achilles tendon disorders can be accomplished using several modalities. Routine radiographs are usually nonspecific. However, Newmark and associates[90] described fracture of a calcaneal osteophyte in association with Achilles tendon avulsion. Low kVp X-ray studies (soft tissue technique) may demonstrate swelling, thickening of the tendon, and irregularity of the pre-Achilles fat or Kager's triangle.[12, 28] These findings are best seen on the lateral view (Fig. 3-35). Patients with chronic trauma or previous surgery may develop ossification in the Achilles tendon (Fig. 3-36).[132]

Ultrasound can also be effective for evaluating the architecture of the tendon.[4,17,46] Ultrasound is less expensive and can detect tendinosis (degeneration) and Achilles tears with accuracy that approaches that of MRI. Aström and colleagues[4] reported an accuracy of 81% for ultrasound compared with 96% for MRI when studying tendinosis and tears of the Achilles tendon (Figs. 3-37 to 3-39). Tendon thickness and tears can be assessed. Tendinosis may be seen as areas of hypoechoic texture in the tendon. Tendon ruptures show increased thickness and abnormal echo texture (see Figs. 3-37 to 3-39).[4,17,46]

CT and MRI, although more expensive than the foregoing techniques, provide more information about the tendon and surrounding structures. MRI is particularly useful because of its superior soft tissue contrast and ability to obtain images in the axial, sagittal, coronal, and off-axis oblique planes.[7, 9,36] Axial and sagittal T2-weighted images are usually adequate for detection and classification of injuries. I prefer dual-echo spin-echo (SE) sequences, although fast SE sequences may also be used.[10] The proton-density images (SE

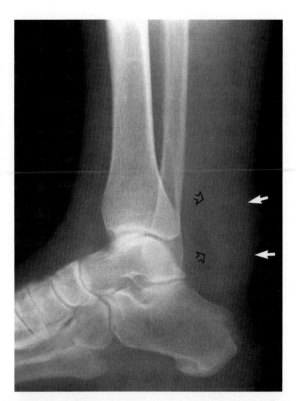

FIG. 3-35. Lateral view of the ankle demonstrates distortion of the pre-Achilles fat with marked thickening of the Achilles tendon (*black open arrows,* anterior margin; *white arrows,* posterior margin).

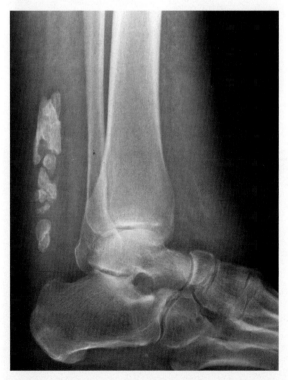

FIG. 3-36. Lateral view of the ankle demonstrates areas of ossification in the Achilles tendon resulting from recurring injuries.

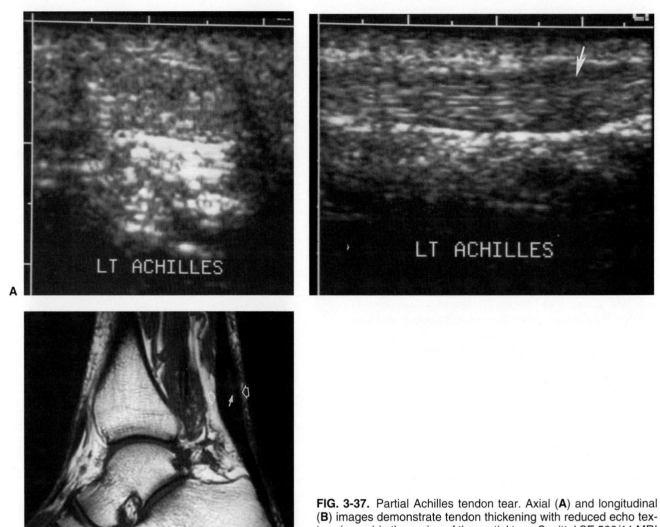

FIG. 3-37. Partial Achilles tendon tear. Axial (**A**) and longitudinal (**B**) images demonstrate tendon thickening with reduced echo texture (*arrow*) in the region of the partial tear. Sagittal SE 500/11 MRI images show the tendon thickening (*open arrows*) with a subtle area (*arrow*) of increased signal intensity in the region of the partial tear. (Courtesy of J. W. Charboneau, Mayo Clinic, Rochester, MN.)

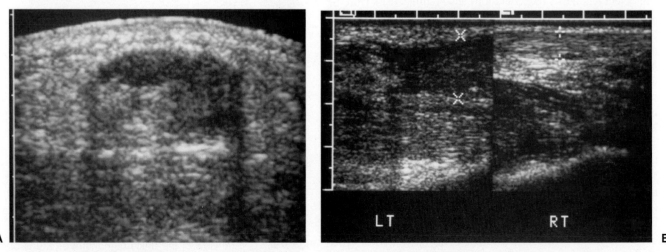

FIG. 3-38. Transaxial (**A**) and longitudinal (**B**) ultrasound images of a left Achilles rupture. Normal right longitudinal image presented in **B.** (Courtesy of J. W. Charboneau, Mayo Clinic, Rochester, MN.)

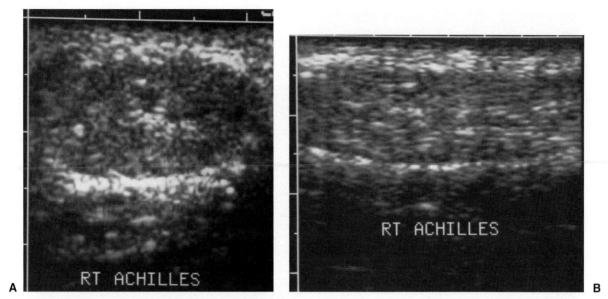

FIG. 3-39. Transaxial (**A**) and longitudinal (**B**) ultrasound images demonstrate thickening (22 mm) and abnormal echo texture resulting from a partial tear in the Achilles tendon. (Courtesy of J. W. Charboneau, Mayo Clinic, Rochester, MN.)

2000/20) provide excellent anatomic display. Increases in signal intensity between the first echo (proton density) and T2-weighted second echo (SE 2000/80) are useful for differentiating acute (increased signal intensity on second echo) from chronic (no change or minimal increase in signal intensity on second echo) injuries or tendinosis.[10] I find MRI useful for detecting complete, incomplete, and old Achilles injuries (see Table 3-4; Figs. 3-40 to 3-44), as well as for evaluating bursitis and other causes of Achilles tendon disorders.[10] The extent of involvement can be accurately assessed with MRI. In addition, patients can be followed to determine whether healing is progressing normally or whether operative intervention is necessary.[10] Another uncommon problem may mimic an Achilles injury or soft tissue tumor. This

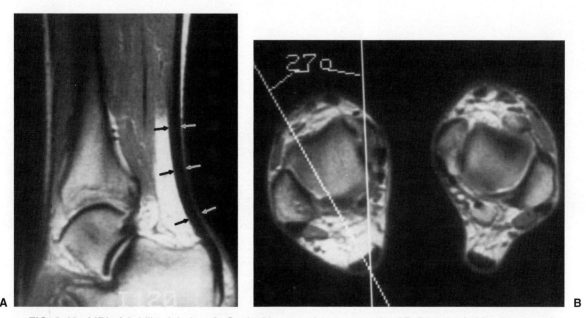

FIG. 3-40. MRI of Achilles injuries. **A:** Sagittal images demonstrate the AP diameter (*white arrows* and *black arrow*) and pre-Achilles fat triangle. Normal tendons are uniform in AP dimensions and have low signal intensity. The foot should be in neutral position to avoid tendon buckling, seen when the foot is plantar flexed. **B:** Axial image of the Achilles tendon showing selection of an oblique sagittal plane to optimize sagittal images. The tendon is angled 27° in this position.

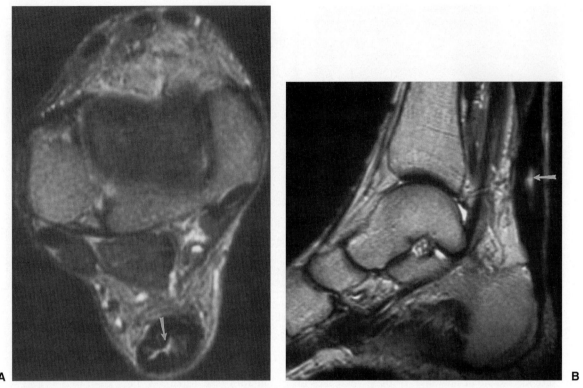

FIG. 3-41. Axial (**A**) and sagittal (**B**) SE 2000/80 images demonstrate a grade 1 tear (*arrow*). The tendon is significantly thickened and has lost the normally concave anterior margin seen on axial images (compare with Fig. 3-40B).

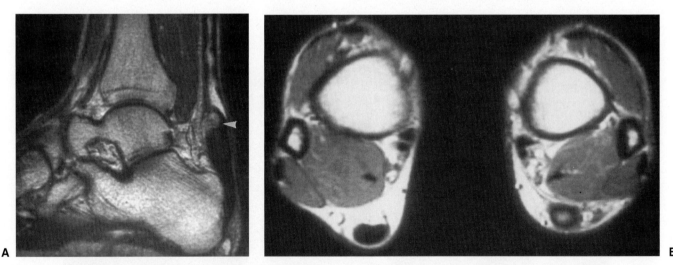

FIG. 3-42. Sagittal (**A**) and axial (**B**) images of a near-complete tear of the Achilles tendon. The fat has herniated into the tendon defect (*arrowhead* in **A**).

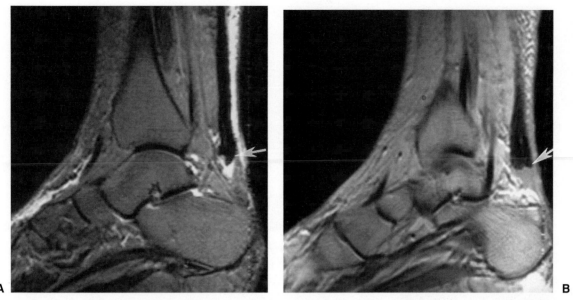

FIG. 3-43. Complete Achilles tears in both ankles. Sagittal SE 2000/80 image of the right (**A**) and SE 2000/20 image (**B**) of the left ankle demonstrate complete tears of the Achilles tendon with thickening (*arrow*) and retraction of the tendons.

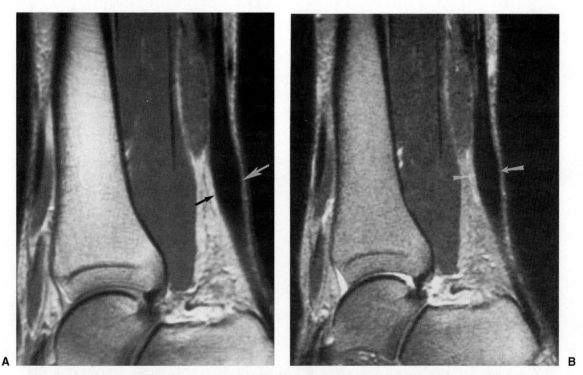

FIG. 3-44. Sagittal SE 2000/20 (**A**) and SE 2000/80 (**B**) image of an old low-grade tear that has filled in with scar tissue. There is tendon thickening (*arrows*) but no increased signal intensity.

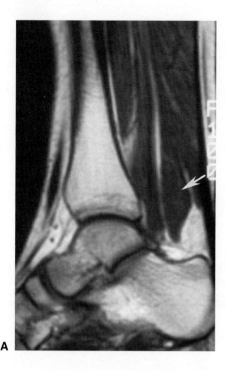

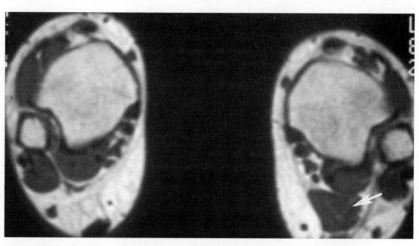

FIG. 3-45. Sagittal (**A**) and axial (**B**) SE 500/20 images demonstrating an accessory soleus muscle (*arrow*).

situation is created by the presence of an accessory soleus muscle (Figs. 3-45 and 3-46).[100,131] It is not uncommon for patients with this anomaly to experience pain after exercise.[40] Either CT or MRI can easily diagnose the condition, but MRI can more easily distinguish the accessory soleus from a soft tissue tumor or hematoma (see normal fat triangle, Fig. 3-40A). Gastrocnemius tears, plantaris tears, and deep vein thromboses can also be confused with Achilles tendon injuries (Fig. 3-47). Another pitfall must also be considered when evaluating the Achilles tendon. The soleus tendon may incorporate into the distal Achilles tendon, thereby giving the appearance of thickening or a partial tear.[84]

Treatment

Decisions regarding treatment of Achilles tendon tears depend on the age and activity status of the patient, on the degree of tear (partial or complete), and on whether the pa-

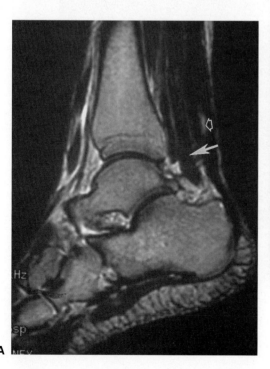

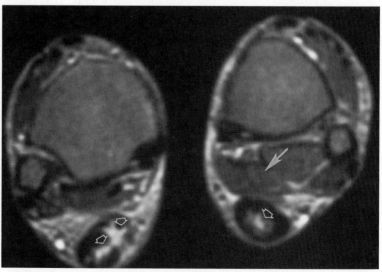

FIG. 3-46. Sagittal (**A**) and axial (**B**) SE 2000/80 images demonstrate an accessory soleus (*arrow*) on the left and bilateral partial Achilles tendon tears (*open arrows*).

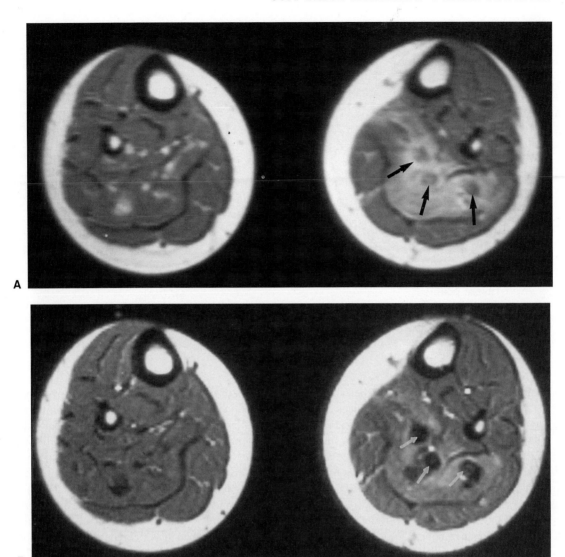

FIG. 3-47. Axial SE 2000/20 (**A**) and SE 2000/80 (**B**) images of the calf in a patient with suspected Achilles injury. The patient has thrombus in the deep veins (*arrows*) and soleus inflammation.

tient has predisposing factors such as systemic disease or steroids. As with many soft tissue injuries, treatment can be controversial.

Generally speaking, minor tears (less than 50%, grade 2) can be treated conservatively. This may be accomplished using a below-the-knee cast with the foot plantar flexed for 8 weeks. After cast removal, a shoe with an elevated heel (2.5 cm) for an additional 4 weeks is commonly used.[64] It is essential to follow the healing process to be certain that recurrent injury does not occur or the incomplete tear may become complete. This can be easily accomplished using MRI (see Figs. 3-41 to 3-44).

Percy and Conochie[94] reported excellent surgical results in 64 patients with complete Achilles ruptures. In their series, 4 incomplete tears eventually ruptured after conservative management. Inglis and colleagues[58] treated 48 patients surgically and 31 conservatively. The surgically treated patients

were more satisfied with the end result. Cybex testing demonstrated that patients treated conservatively only achieved 72% of normal strength. Therefore, it may be best to consider conservative therapy for older, inactive persons or for patients with underlying systemic disease. Surgical repair should be considered in more active patients.[58,64] Surgical treatment consists of repairing the torn tendon ends and reestablishing continuity. Plantaris or other fascial or tendon grafts may be needed to approximate the torn ends of the tendon.[64]

Medial Tendons

The posterior tibial, flexor digitorum longus, and flexor hallucis longus tendons make up the medial tendon group and are located anterior to posterior in the foregoing order (Fig. 3-48). The posterior tibial tendon (most anterior) with

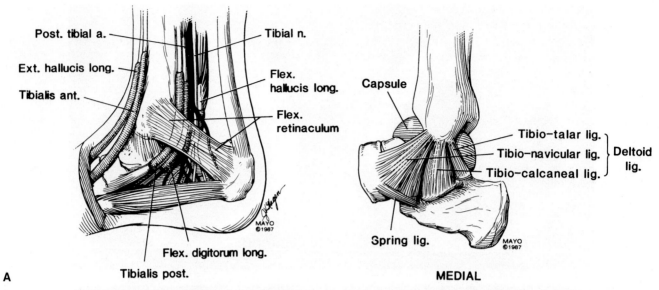

FIG. 3-48. A: Medial tendon anatomy demonstrating the flexor retinaculum and relationships of the three tendons and neurovascular structures. **B:** Medial ligament structures. The plantar calcaneonavicular or spring ligament is a stabilizer of the longitudinal arch of the foot.

its tendon sheath passes just posterior to the medial malleolus, lateral to the flexor retinaculum, and broadens at its insertion in the navicular tuberosity and base of the medial cuneiform. The flexor digitorum longus takes a similar course proximally lying between the posterior tibial tendon and posterior tibial artery (see Fig. 3-48). As it turns toward the plantar aspect of the foot, it passes superficially to the flexor hallucis longus before dividing into tendon slips that insert in the bases of the second through fifth distal phalanges. The flexor hallucis longus tendon is located more posteriorly and laterally. It passes through a fibroosseous tunnel beneath the sustentaculum tali and along the medial plantar aspect of the foot to insert in the base of the distal phalanx of the great toe.[48,51,64]

The calcaneonavicular or spring ligament (see Fig. 3-48B) is an important stabilizer of the longitudinal arch. This ligament is important to evaluate in patients with posterior tibial tendon dysfunction. Unfortunately, the spring ligament can be difficult to demonstrate with MRI or other imaging techniques.[10,30,105]

Abnormalities of the medial tendons include degeneration, inflammation, partial or complete tears, and dislocation or subluxation (see Table 3-4).[7,10,35]. The posterior tibial tendon is most commonly involved. However, classification systems used for this tendon can also be applied to the flexor digitorum longus, flexor hallucis longus, and other tendons about the ankle.[5,10,30,34,50,67]

Diagnosis

Posterior tibial tendon dysfunction occurs in patients with multiple risk factors. These include mechanical foot abnormalities, inflammatory osteopathies, previous trauma, con-

genital disorders, and obesity.[48,50,67,85] Patients with this condition present with ankle pain, instability, and foot deformities.[67] Clinical examination may demonstrate loss of the longitudinal arch and inability to perform a heel-rise maneuver, and the tendon may not be palpable on physical examination.[48,85]

Imaging of posterior tibial dysfunction begins with careful evaluation of routine standing radiographs of the foot and ankle. Acute trauma rupture of the posterior tibial tendon has been described in association with medial malleolar fractures.[39] The fracture is a mirror image of the flake fracture seen with peroneal tendon dislocation (see Fig. 3-22). It occurs longitudinally along the distal medial tibial metaphysis.[116]

Numerous plain film features of posterior tibial tendon dysfunction, specifically complete tears, have been described. The AP view may demonstrate an accessory navicular. This finding is commonly associated with posterior tibial tendon tears.[48,67] Karasick and Schweitzer[61] described radiographic foot deformities in 50% of patients with complete

TABLE 3-5. *Radiographic features: complete posterior tibial tendon tears[a]*

Fracture	Incidence
↓ Calcaneal inclination angle	50%
↑ Lateral talometatarsal angle	47%
↑ Anterior talocalcaneal angle	43%
Osteopenia	37%
Medial soft tissue swelling	27%
Accessory navicular	17%
↑ Lateral talocalcaneal angle	13%

[a] Data from references 61 and 67.

posterior tibial tendon tears. Flatfoot deformity is common. Radiographic features associated with complete tears are summarized in Table 3-5 (Figs. 3-49 and 3-50).[49,61]

Stress tenograms may also be useful for evaluating the posterior tibial tendon.[51,52] However, the technique is more difficult compared with peroneal tenography.[12] Ultrasound and CT are also useful, but I prefer MRI to evaluate the tendon, synovial sheath, and surrounding ligamentous anatomy.[10,61]

MRI of the posterior tibial tendon is easily performed using axial and sagittal T2-weighted sequences.[10,34] It is important to define the distal insertion (see Fig. 3-50) and to

include enough of the ankle and lower leg to define the proximal segment of the tendon when complete tears are detected. This may require a larger field of view. We generally prefer to position the foot in neutral or mild plantar flexion. It is important to evaluate the spring ligament.[30,50] This ligament may be difficult to demonstrate on conventional axial and sagittal images. Rule and colleagues[105] suggested that the plantar aspect of the ligament is most easily seen on oblique sagittal images (45° to the long axis of the calcaneus). The medial position of the ligament may be most easily demonstrated on oblique axial images through the talonavicular joint (Fig. 3-51).[105]

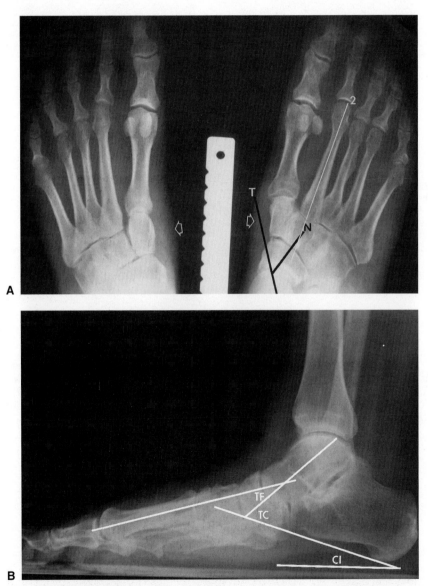

FIG. 3-49. Standing AP (**A**) and lateral (**B**) radiographs of an elderly female with bilateral posterior tibial tendon tears. **A:** There is medial soft tissue swelling (*open arrows*) bilaterally. The foot is pronated with the talar axis (*T*) projecting medially and the navicular (*N*) is rotated laterally. The second metatarsal axis (*2*) is medial to the talocalcaneal angle. **B:** The calcaneal inclination angle (*CI*) is reduced to 11°. The talus is plantar flexed increasing the talocalcaneal angle (*TC*) to 60°. The talar first metatarsal angle (*TF*) should be zero, but in this case it is −28°.

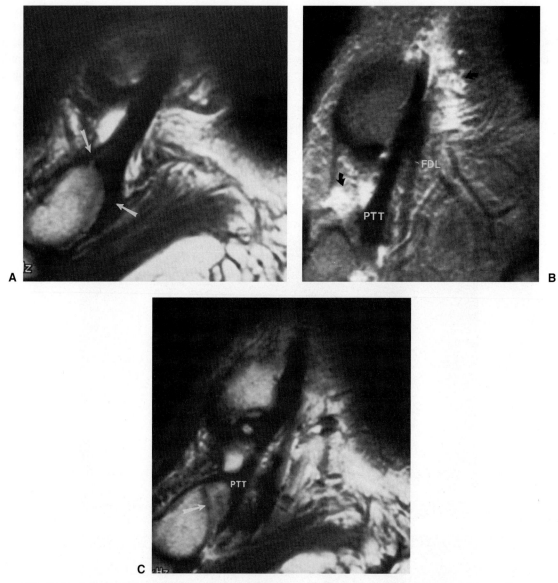

FIG. 3-50. Insertion of the posterior tibial tendon on the navicular. **A:** Sagittal SE 500/11 image demonstrates the normal fanning of the tendon at its insertion (*arrows*). The foot is slightly plantar flexed. **B:** Sagittal SE 2000/80 image with foot plantar flexed shows the posterior tibial tendon (*PTT*) and flexor digitorum longus tendon (*FDL*). *Arrows* indicate edema. **C:** Sagittal SE 500/11 image shows the posterior tibial tendon (*PTT*) insertion on an accessory navicular (*arrow*).

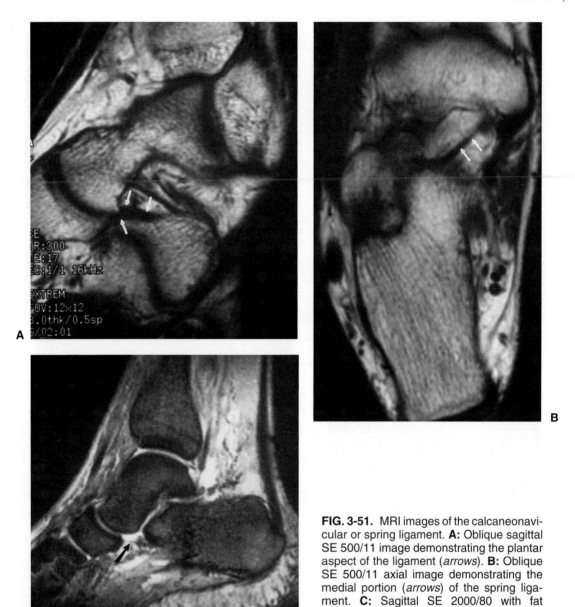

FIG. 3-51. MRI images of the calcaneonavicular or spring ligament. **A:** Oblique sagittal SE 500/11 image demonstrating the plantar aspect of the ligament (*arrows*). **B:** Oblique SE 500/11 axial image demonstrating the medial portion (*arrows*) of the spring ligament. **C:** Sagittal SE 2000/80 with fat suppression shows complete disruption of the spring ligament (*arrow*).

MRI features of tendon injuries are summarized in Table 3-4. Normal tendons are of low intensity, and there is little fluid in the tendon sheath. Fluid surrounding the tendon is usually termed tendonitis, peritendinitis, or tenosynovitis (Fig. 3-52). These terms are frequently used loosely to describe inflammation of the sheath, tendon, or both. Tenosynovitis is most often applied to fluid in the tendon sheath with a normal tendon. Peritendinitis may involve both.[31] A thickened tendon with no increased signal intensity but surrounded by fluid in the tendon sheath may be tendinosis (degeneration) or an old tear.[31,67] Thickened tendons with increased signal involving only a portion of the fibers are partial tears (Fig. 3-53). Complete tears have high-signal-intensity fluid separating the torn ends of the tendons (Figs.

3-54 and 3-55). In some cases, evaluating both ankles separately or using the head coil is useful for comparison purposes (Fig. 3-56).[10,67]

Disorders of the flexor digitorum longus and flexor hallucis longus occur less frequently than posterior tibial tendon dysfunction. However, clinical and image features may be similar.[10,31,49] Garth[49] reported rupture of the flexor hallucis longus tendon in ballet dancers (Fig. 3-57). Patients present with posterior ankle pain that is exaggerated by flexion and extension of the great toe.

Routine radiographs may be useful. Soft tissue changes in the posterior capsular recess with irregularity of the adjacent fat may be seen with flexor hallucis tendinitis, disruption, and os trigonum syndrome.[10,49,62,115]

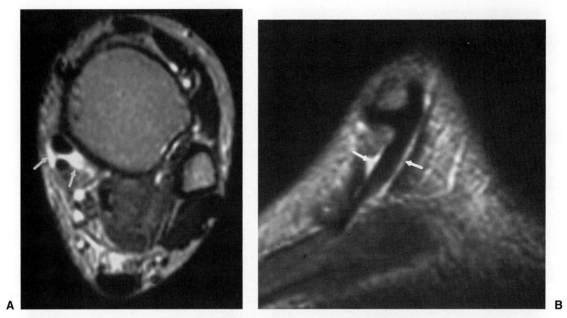

FIG. 3-52. A middle-aged woman with medial ankle pain. Axial (**A**) and sagittal (**B**) SE 2000/80 images demonstrate fluid in the tendon sheaths (*arrows*) of the posterior tibial and flexor digitorum longus tendon sheaths resulting from synovitis. The tendon size and signal intensity are normal.

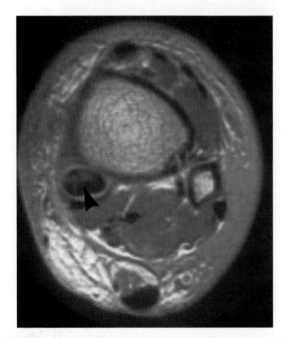

FIG. 3-53. Axial SE 2000/80 image demonstrates thickening with fluid in the tendon sheath and increased signal in the tendon substance (*arrowhead*) resulting from a partial tear.

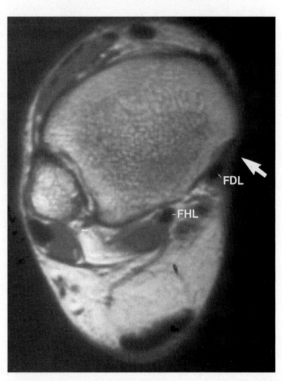

FIG. 3-54. Axial SE 2000/20 image demonstrates the flexor hallucis longus (*FHL*), flexor digitorum longus (*FDL*), and complete absence (*arrow*) of the posterior tibial tendon resulting from an old complete tear. There is no swelling or edema.

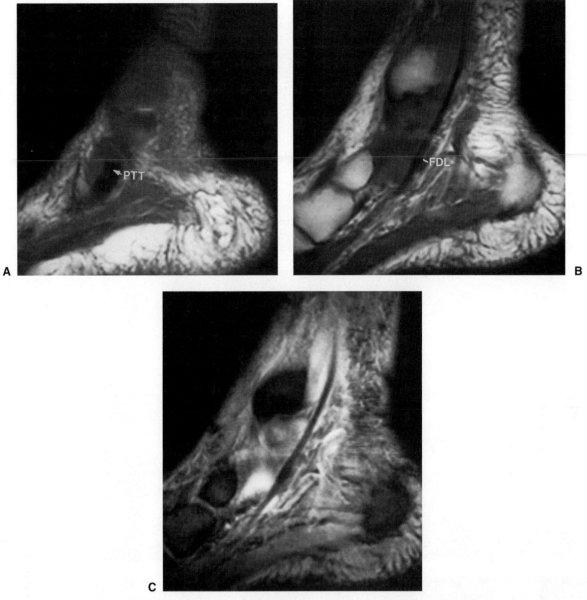

FIG. 3-55. Proton-density sagittal images at different levels (**A** and **B**) demonstrate the distal segment of the posterior tibial tendon (*PTT*) and the flexor digitorum longus tendon (*FDL*). Sagittal SE 2000/80 image with fat suppression shows a long segment of absent PTT resulting from retraction of the proximal segment. The flexor digitorum longus tendon is intact.

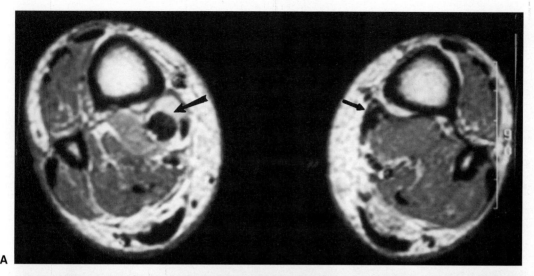

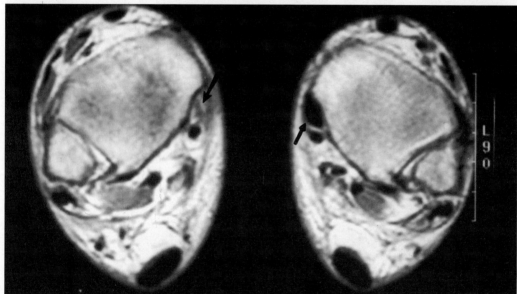

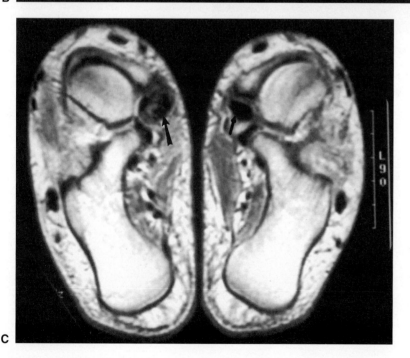

FIG. 3-56. Axial proton density images of both ankles for comparison. **A:** Axial image above the ankle shows a thickened posterior tibial tendon on the right (*arrow*) and normal tendon on the left (*small arrow*). **B:** Axial image at the level of the syndesmosis shows a normal tendon on the left and nearly complete tear on the right (*arrow*) **C:** Axial image just below the sustentaculum shows the thickened distal segment with increased signal on the right (*arrow*) and normal left tendon (*small arrow*).

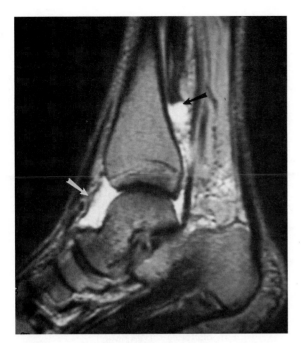

FIG. 3-57. Sagittal SE 2000/80 image demonstrating a complete tear in the flexor hallucis longus tendon (*black arrow*). Note the large effusion anteriorly (*white arrow*). (From Berquist, ref. 10, with permission.)

MRI is the technique of choice for evaluating the flexor digitorum longus (Fig. 3-58) and flexor hallucis longus (see Fig. 3-57) tendons. Axial and sagittal T2-weighted images (conventional SE or fast SE with fat suppression) are generally adequate for detection and classification or these disorders.[10]

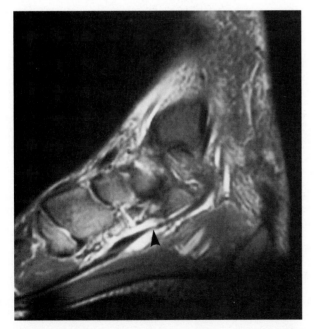

FIG. 3-58. Sagittal SE 2000/80 fat suppressed image shows thinning of the flexor digitorum longus (*arrowhead*) with fluid in the tendon sheath.

Treatment

Most older patients or patients with systemic disease are treated conservatively. However, more active persons usually prefer surgical repair. Funk and associates[48] described the operative findings of posterior tibial tendon disorders. Group 1 tears were avulsions of the tendon insertion, group II midsubstance tears, group patients with no tear but synovitis. Mann and Thompson[81] reported results of posterior tibial tendon repair using the flexor digitorum longus tendon in 17 patients. Results were excellent in 13 of 17, fair in 3 of 17, and poor in 1 patient. In this patient, an alternative procedure, arthrodesis, was performed. Using their grading system, Funk and colleagues[48] found that surgical repair of group I (avulsion at insertion) was not successful. Patients with midsubstance (group II) tears had good results. Patients with incomplete tears had even better resolution of symptoms after surgery.

Anterior Tendons

Anteriorly, the anterior tibial, extensor hallucis longus, and extensor digitorum longus tendons are all enclosed in tendon sheaths (Fig. 3-59). Acute tears are unusual, but in patients with previous fractures, degenerative arthritis, or other predisposing factors, tendon rupture can occur.[51,64] Most patients with anterior tibial tendon ruptures are men in the 50- to 70-year age range.[68] Injury to the anterior tibial tendon may also occur in runners. Rupture of the anterior tibial tendon usually occurs as it exits the superior retinaculum. The distal segment retracts and can be palpated between the superior and inferior retinaculum. Clinically, pain and swelling occur over the ankle anteriorly. There may also be decreased dorsiflexion of the foot on physical examination.[64]

Radiographically, patients demonstrate minimal to prominent soft tissue swelling anteriorly. This is most easily identified on the lateral and oblique views (Fig. 3-60).[61] Tenography demonstrates abnormalities in the tendon sheaths, but more specific information can be obtained with ultrasound or MRI (Fig. 3-61).[10,11,14,68] MRI examinations should be performed in the axial and sagittal planes. T2-weighted sequences are generally best for the high intensity of fluid, and blood provides excellent contrast with the black tendon (Figs. 3-62 and 3-63).[10] Conservative treatment is adequate in older, less active patients. Surgical repair is indicated in active patients.[64]

MISCELLANEOUS DISORDERS AND OVERUSE SYNDROMES

Numerous other traumatic conditions involve the ankle, hindfoot, midfoot, and forefoot. Certain other related syndromes are also reviewed in this section. Disorders are reviewed by location because symptoms related to anatomic regions may be caused by multiple conditions that can be

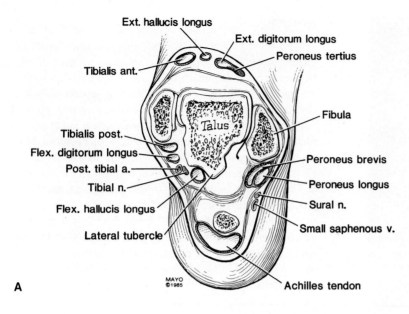

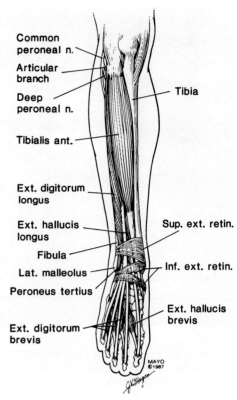

FIG. 3-59. A: Illustration of the tendons and neurovascular structures about the ankle. **B:** Frontal illustration of the anterior muscles and tendons and the superior and inferior retinacula.

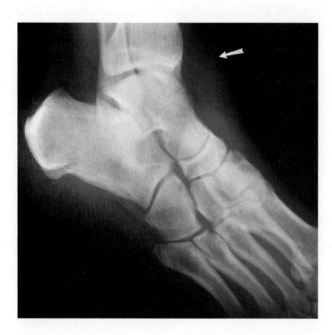

FIG. 3-60. Oblique radiographs in a patient with anterior tibial tendon rupture. There is focal anterior soft tissue swelling (*arrow*).

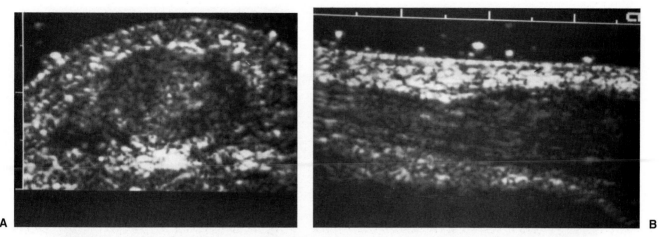

FIG. 3-61. Transaxial (**A**) and longitudinal (**B**) sonograms of the anterior tibial tendon demonstrating thickening and hyperechoic changes resulting from an anterior tibial tendon tear. (Courtesy of J. W. Charboneau, Mayo Clinic, Rochester, MN.)

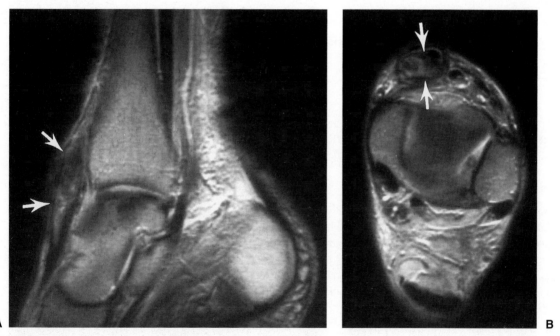

FIG. 3-62. Sagittal (**A**) and axial (**B**) SE 2000/80 images demonstrate focal thickening (*arrows*) between the retinacula (see Fig. 3-59B) with increased signal intensity resulting from a partial tear in the anterior tibial tendon.

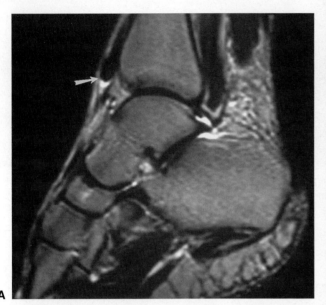
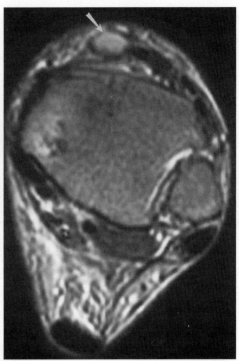

FIG. 3-63. Sagittal (**A**) and axial (**B**) SE 2000/80 images demonstrate a complete tear in the anterior tibial tendon (*arrow*).

confused clinically. Imaging plays a significant role in sorting out the origin of these foot and ankle conditions.

Heel Pain

The causes of heel pain are numerous. Karr[63] listed a differential diagnosis of 43 causes of subcalcaneal heel pain that included multiple categories (e.g., inflammation, neoplastic, metabolic, degenerative) of local and systemic conditions. This discussion focuses on common overuse syndromes that result in heel or posterior ankle pain (Table 3-6).[9,63,117]

Subcalcaneal Heel Pain

Subcalcaneal heel pain may be related to the fat pad, plantar fascia, or numerous other conditions noted in Table 3-6. This common orthopedic problem can be perplexing clinically. Determination of the origin and treatment are challenging.

The heel pad (Fig. 3-64) absorbs 20 to 25% of contact force during heel strike. There are free nerve endings in the heel fat, so pain could arise from this region without other associated abnormalities.[63]

The plantar fascia or aponeurosis consists of medial, central, and lateral components. The lateral and medial segments are thinner and cover the abductor digiti minimi and abductor

TABLE 3-6. *Heel pain: differential diagnoses[a]*

Local osseous causes
  Calcaneal stress fracture
  Calcaneal periostitis
  Calcaneal spurs
  Sever's disease
  Arthropathies
  Os trigonum syndrome
  Tarsal coalition
  Haglund's deformity
Local soft tissue causes
  Subcalcaneal pain syndrome
  Painful heel pad
  Nerve entrapment
  Plantar fasciitis
  Retrocalcaneal bursitis
  Retro-Achilles bursitis
  Tarsal tunnel syndrome
  Achilles tendon injury
  Flexor hallucis longus tendon injury
  Peroneal tendon injury
Systemic causes[b]
  Ankylosing spondylitis
  Reiter's syndrome
  Psoriatic arthritis
  Rheumatoid arthritis
  Gout

[a] Data from references 9, 63, 117, and 127.
[b] 16% of patients with heel pain.

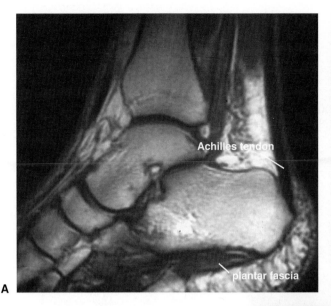

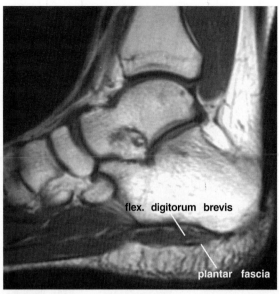

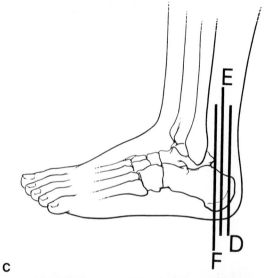

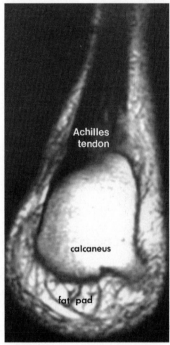

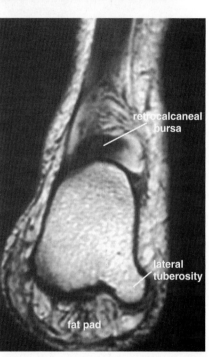

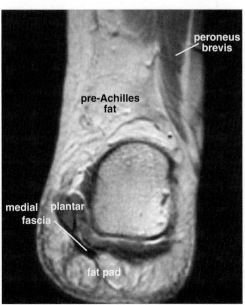

FIG. 3-64. Normal MRI images of the heel. **A** and **B:** Sagittal MRI images demonstrating the heel pad plantar fascia and Achilles tendon insertion. **C:** Coronal illustration localizing coronal images. **D:** Coronal image at the Achilles insertion. **E:** Coronal image just anterior to the Achilles tendon. **F:** Coronal image through the calcaneus.

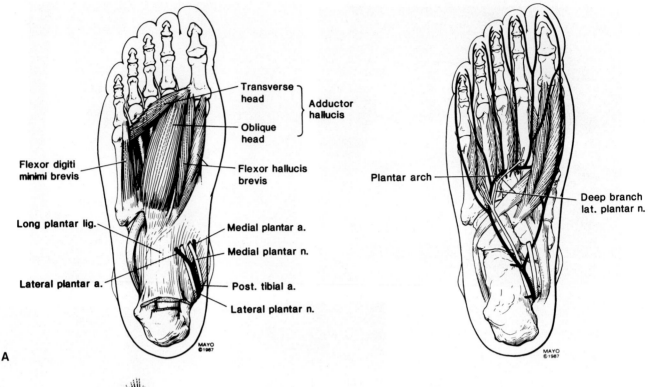

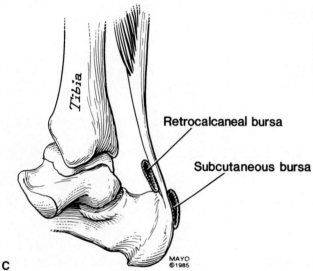

FIG. 3-65. Anatomic illustrations of the plantar aspect of the foot and calcaneus. **A:** Plantar fascia and nerves. **B:** Deep plantar nerves. **C:** Relationship of retrocalcaneal and subcutaneous (retro-Achilles) bursae with the calcaneus and Achilles tendon.

hallucis muscles (Fig. 3-65).[10,63,64] The thickest portion of the plantar fascia extends distally from the medial calcaneal tuberosity. Distally, the fascia splits into five bands that insert on proximal phalanges. Near the calcaneal attachment, the plantar fascia is 3 to 4 mm thick on sagittal and coronal MRI (see Fig. 3-64).[9]

The posterior tibial nerve and its branches (see Figs. 3-48A and 3-65) pass posteriorly to the posterior tibial and flexor digitorum longus tendons deep to the flexor retinaculum. Branches of the medial calcaneal nerve exit the main trunk at the medial malleolus to innervate the fat pad.[63] The plantar nerves (medial and lateral) enter the plantar aspect of the foot under the sustentaculum tali (Fig. 3-65).[9,10,63]

Plantar Fasciitis

Plantar fasciitis is a painful condition with debilitating results. Pain may be associated with exercise (mild) or constant with walking or standing.[9] Physical examination reveals tenderness to palpation over the medial and proximal plantar aspects of the foot. Pain is exaggerated by dorsiflexion of the great toe. Fascia rupture and flexor hallucis longus tendinitis are included in the differential diagnosis along with conditions summarized in Table 3-6.[9,63,65]

Imaging of this condition may be accomplished with radionuclide scans and routine radiographs (Fig. 3-66). Other conditions, such as stress fractures (Fig. 3-67), can also be excluded.

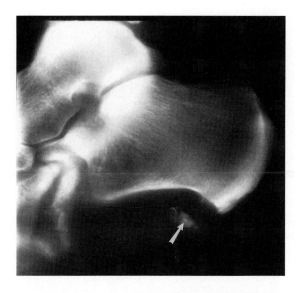

FIG. 3-66. Lateral radiograph of the calcaneus demonstrates an avulsed osteophyte (*arrow*) in a patient with chronic heel pain with a recent acute exacerbation.

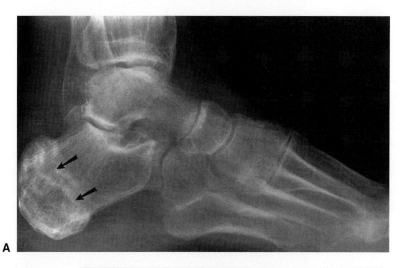

A

FIG. 3-67. Lateral radiograph (**A**) and isotope bone scan (**B**) in a patient with heel pain resulting from calcaneal stress fracture (*arrow*).

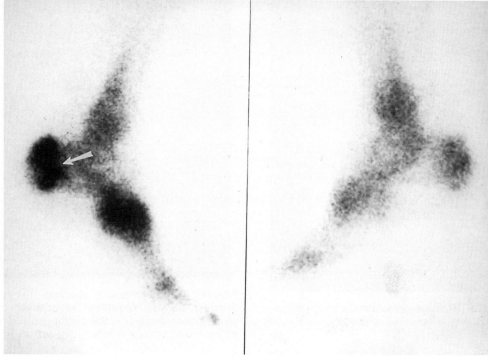

B

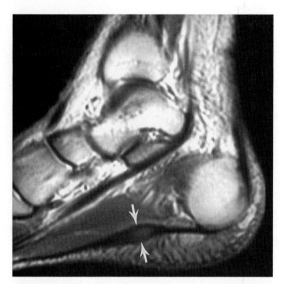

FIG. 3-68. Sagittal SE 2000/20 image demonstrates thickened fascia with a partial tear (*arrows*) distal to the calcaneal attachment.

MRI is more specific for diagnosis of fascial inflammation and partial or complete rupture. MRI if more specific for diagnosis of fascial inflammation and partial or complete rupture. MRI can also exclude other causes of heel pain.[10] T2-weighted sequences in the sagittal and axial and coronal planes are most useful to measure the fascia and to detect inflammatory changes or tears. These changes are seen as areas of increased signal intensity contrasted with the normal low-intensity plantar fascia. The plantar fascia is normally 3 to 4 mm thick (Figs. 3-68 to 3-72).[9]

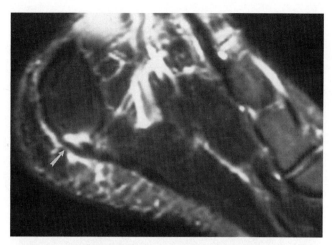

FIG. 3-70. Sagittal fat-suppressed T2-weighted image demonstrates fasciitis with fascial irregularity and edema (*arrow*).

Treatment is almost always conservative. Rest, ice, antiinflammatory medications, and heel pads or orthotics.[9] Patients who do not respond to conservative treatment may be injected with steroids. Surgery is reserved for refractory cases or when nerve entrapment is suspected.[9,63,64]

Bursitis/Haglund's Deformity

The heel has two bursae (see Fig. 3-65C). One is located between the calcaneus and Achilles tendon, and the other is superficial to the tendon.[10,64,117] Bursal prominence or projection was originally described by Haglund in

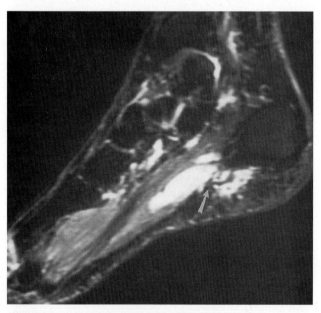

FIG. 3-69. Sagittal STIR image demonstrates a tear (*arrow*) in the plantar fascia with edema and inflammation in the fat and muscles deep to the fascia.

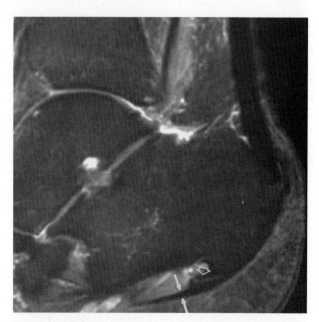

FIG. 3-71. Chronic fascial changes. Fat-suppressed T2-weighted fast SE sequence demonstrates an osteophyte (*open arrow*) and fascial thickening (*small arrows*). There is no increased signal intensity to suggest active inflammation.

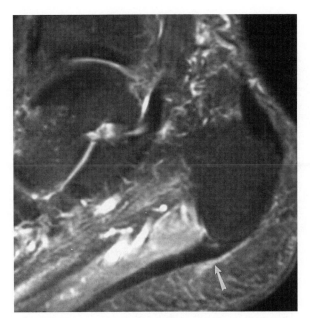

FIG. 3-72. Chronic fasciitis. Sagittal fat-suppressed fast SE image demonstrates marked thickening with proximal inflammation.

1928.[117] This condition is commonly seen in adolescent and younger women, when footwear change to higher heels is common. Bursal inflammation has also been reported in patients with arthropathy (rheumatoid arthritis) and in ice skaters.[47,118,125]

Patients present with retrocalcaneal prominence located anterior to the distal Achilles tendon. The superficial bursa may also be prominent. The tendon may be inflamed and tender to palpation.[47,117] Heel varus is often seen in association with this condition. Differential diagnostic considerations are primarily arthropathies such as Reiter's syndrome, gout, and rheumatoid arthritis.[117,118]

Radiographs may demonstrate bony erosive changes (Fig. 3-73), prominence of the superior calcaneus, inflammatory changes in the pre-Achilles fat, and thickening of the Achilles tendon.[10,12,117] Measurements made on standing lateral radiographs of the ankle or calcaneus can be used to determine approaches to therapy. The Phillips and Fowler angle is measured by a line drawn tangent to the anterior calcaneal tubercle and medial tuberosity. A second line is drawn along the posterior calcaneal projection and posterior tuberosity. The angle formed by these two lines should not exceed 75° (Fig. 3-74).[47,125] Parallel pitch lines can also be used to evaluate the posterior calcaneal projection. The lower line is constructed along the plantar calcaneal surface. A perpendicular line (Fig. 3-75) is drawn from this line to the posterior margin of the subtalar joint. A second parallel line is drawn at this level. If the bursal projection is below or just touching the superior line, it is considered normal. If the calcaneal projection extends above this line, it is abnormal (see Fig. 3-75).[47,125] Ultrasound may be used to evaluate the tendon

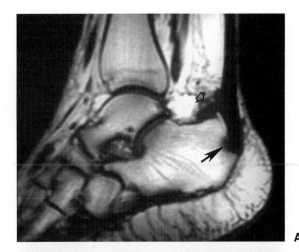

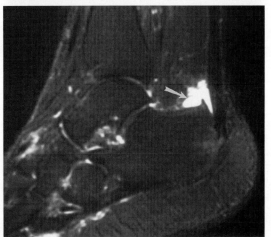

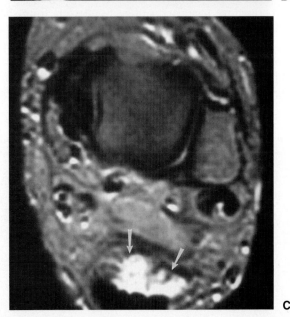

FIG. 3-73. Retrocalcaneal bursitis with bone erosion and prominence of the posterior superior calcaneus. (**A**) sagittal SE 500/11 MRI shows bone erosion (*arrow*) and an enlarged bursa extending into the pre-Achilles fat (*open arrow*). Sagittal (**B**) and axial (**C**) T2-weighted images using fat suppression demonstrate the high-signal-intensity distended retrocalcaneal bursa (*arrow*).

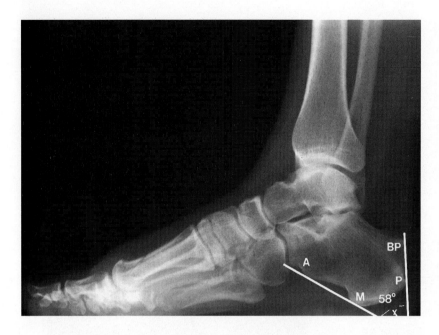

FIG. 3-74. Lateral view of the foot demonstrating the Fowler and Phillips angle. Normal is less than or equal to 75°. The angle is formed by a line drawn tangent to the anterior tubercle (*A*) and midtuberosity (*M*). A second line is drawn along the bursal projection (*BP*) and posterior tuberosity (*P*). In this case, the angle is 58°. (Data from refs. 47 and 125.)

and bursae.[17,89] Bursography (Fig. 3-76) is invasive and is generally reserved for therapeutic or diagnostic injections in our practice.[12]

MRI is preferred to evaluate the bursae, Achilles tendon, and adjacent bony changes. Early changes with only small amounts of fluid in the bursa are most easily detected with the foot slightly plantar flexed (Fig. 3-77).[10,20] Sagittal and axial T2-weighted images are optimal for evaluating bursitis and Achilles tendon changes (see Fig. 3-73; Fig. 3-78).[10,20]

Conservative treatment with heel protection from shoes or footwear changes is used initially. Bursal injections (see Fig. 3-76) may be useful in some cases. Direct injection of the Achilles tendon should be avoided because it can lead to further structural weakening and rupture. When conservative measures fail, surgical correction may be necessary. Tech-

niques include calcaneal osteotomy and resection of the posterior superior calcaneal prominence. In the latter procedure, the bursal tissue is also resected (Fig. 3-79 and 3-80).[117]

Os Trigonum Syndrome

The os trigonum is analogous to a secondary ossification center. It is formed in a cartilaginous posterior extension of the talus (Fig. 3-81).[53] The os trigonum is connected to the talus by a cartilaginous synchondrosis. Ossification of this process occurs between the ages of 7 and 13 years. Fusion usually occurs within a year of ossification forming Stieda's process (see Fig. 3-81B). A separate ossicle remains in 7 to 14% of patients. This condition is frequently bilateral.[53,62]

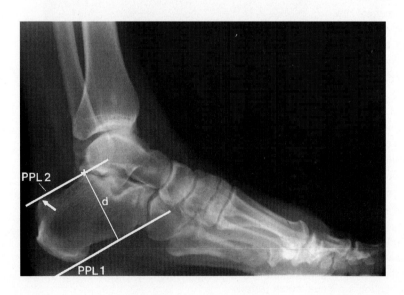

FIG. 3-75. Two parallel pitch lines can also be used. The lower line (*PPL1*) is drawn along the inferior margin, similar to Figure 3-74. A perpendicular line (*d*) is drawn to the margin of the posterior facet (+). If the bursal projection (*arrow*) touches or lies below line 2, it is normal. (Data from refs. 47 and 125.)

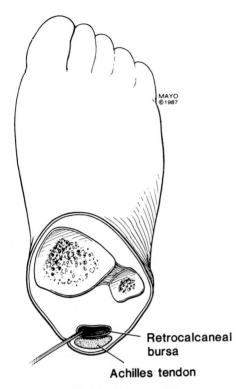

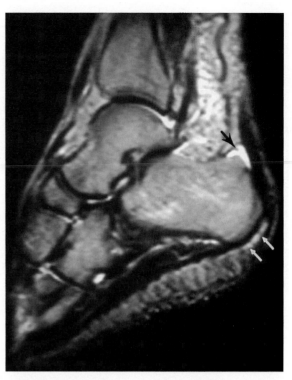

FIG. 3-76. Illustration of needle approach for retrocalcaneal bursal injection or aspiration. The bursa normally has a volume of about 1.5 cc. (From Stephens, ref. 117, with permission.)

FIG. 3-77. Sagittal T2-weighted (SE 2000/80) image with the foot slightly plantar flexed. The retro-Achilles bursa contains fluid (*arrow*). There is also slight inflammation in the deep heel pad (*small arrows*).

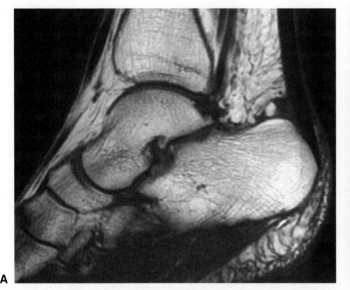

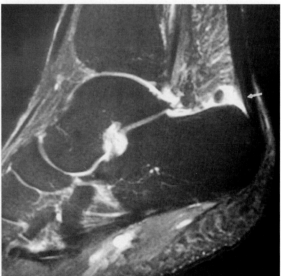

FIG. 3-78. Sagittal SE 500/11 (**A**) and fat-suppressed fast SE (**B**) images demonstrate bursitis and inflammation in the adjacent Achilles tendon (*small arrow* in **B**).

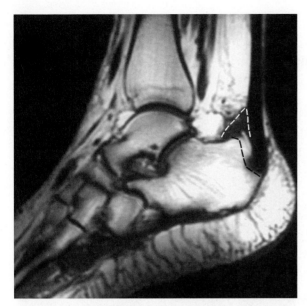

FIG. 3-79. Sagittal SE 500/11 image (same patient as Fig. 3-73) demonstrating the area of resection used for surgical treatment (*broken lines*).

In the adult, the ununited ossification center may be difficult to differentiate from an old fracture.[78]

Os trigonum syndrome may be due to acute trauma or overuse (repetitive microtrauma). The syndrome includes process fracture, flexor hallucis longus tendinitis, and posterior tibiotalar impingement.[62, 93,127] Patients present with posterior ankle pain and swelling. Physical examination reveals posterior ankle tenderness anterior to the Achilles tendon. Pain is often exaggerated by plantar flexion of the foot.[62,127]

Os trigonum syndrome is difficult to diagnose clinically. Therefore, the role of imaging to suggest or confirm the diagnoses is important.[127] The identification of an os trigonum radiographically is not sufficient to make the diagnosis. However, irregularity at the margins or associated distortion of the pre-Achilles fat may suggest acute fracture or inflammation (Fig. 3-82).[127] Stress views or plantar flexion studies may demonstrate posterior impingement and may recreate the patient's symptoms (Fig. 3-83).[11,13,127] Bone scanning may be useful because increased tracer in the region of the os trigonum should at least indicate further study. A normal bone scan excludes the diagnosis of os trigonum syndrome.[62,78,127]

CT may be useful for detection of acute fractures or defining the osseous margins more clearly (see Fig. 3-81). However, MRI is most useful to detect soft tissue changes (edema, flexor hallucis longus tendinitis) and subtle bone changes resulting from impingement.[12,62,127] MRI should be performed using a small (10 to 14 cm) field of view. T2-weighted images are most useful (Fig. 3-84).[12] I use axial and sagittal image planes (Fig. 3-85). However, specifically for os trigonum syndrome, images with the foot plantar flexed or sagittal gradient-recalled echo motion studies are more useful. Impingement and motion of the os trigonum are more clearly demonstrated using the latter approach.[12,127]

Treatment of os trigonum syndrome is conservative in most cases. Direct injection of the synchondrosis or space between the talus and os trigonum is useful to confirm the source of pain and to provide therapy by injection a mixture of bupivacaine (Marcaine) and celestone.[11,62] Immobilization with a short leg cast for 4 to 6 weeks may also be selected for initial treatment. When conservative measures

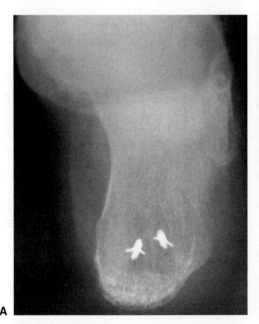

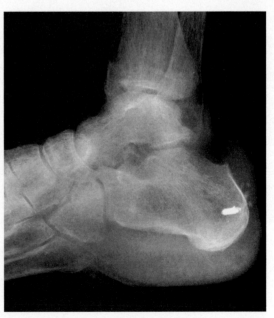

FIG. 3-80. Axial (**A**) and lateral (**B**) radiographs after surgical repair with two Mytek soft tissue anchors in the calcaneus. There are residual areas of ossification in the soft tissues.

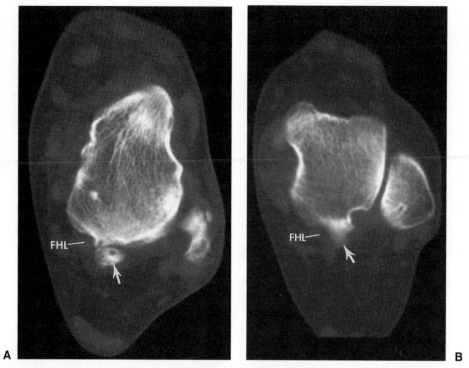

A   **B**

FIG. 3-81. CT images of the ankle demonstrating the os trigonum (*arrow*) (**A**) and a fused Stieda's process (*arrow*) (**B**). Note the relationship of the flexor hallucis longus tendon (*FHL*). There are degenerative changes along the synchondrosis of the os trigonum in (**A**).

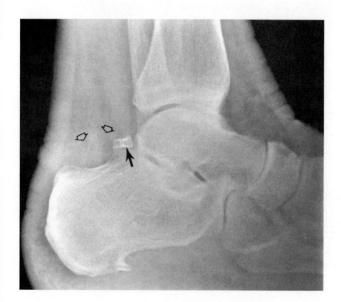

FIG. 3-82. Lateral computed radiographic image (*CR*) of the calcaneus shows an os trigonum (*black arrow*) and edema (*open arrows*) in the pre-Achilles fat resulting from os trigonum syndrome.

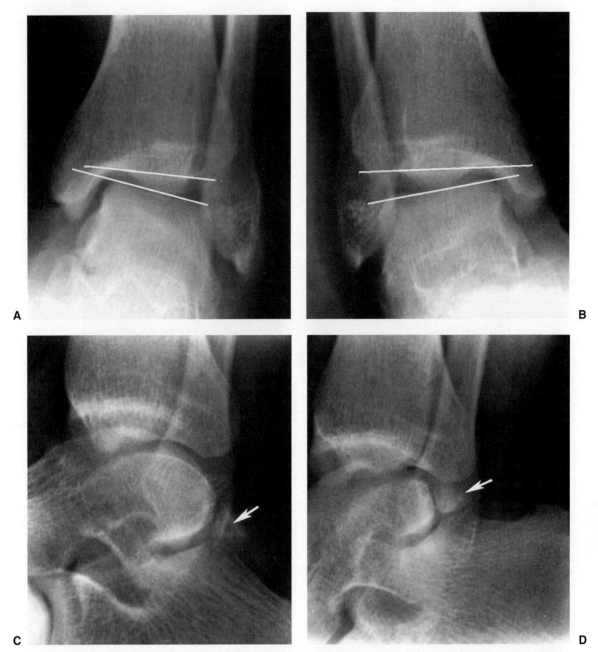

FIG. 3-83. A 23-year-old man with ankle pain referred for stress views to assess the ligaments. Varus stress views (**A** and **B**) of both ankles failed to demonstrate lateral ligament injury. There is no significant difference in the angles (abnormal greater than or equal to 6° compared with the normal side). Lateral spot views in the dorsiflexed (**C**) and plantar flexed (**D**) positions show posterior impingement (**D**) and motion of the os trigonum (*arrow*).

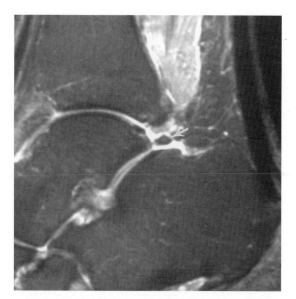

FIG. 3-84. Sagittal fat-suppressed fast SE T2-weighted image demonstrating fluid and inflammation around the os trigonum (*arrow*). The foot is plantar flexed.

fail, resection of the os trigonum is indicated. Results of resection are excellent in most patients. When there is associated flexor hallucis longus tendinitis (see Fig. 3-85), some surgeons also perform a tendon release.[92,129]

Tarsal Tunnel Syndrome

Tarsal tunnel syndrome is caused by neuropathy of the posterior tibial nerve in the tarsal tunnel. The tarsal tunnel

TABLE 3-7. *Tarsal tunnel syndrome etiology*[a]

Trauma
    Fractures
    Posttraumatic fibrosis
Talocalcaneal coalition
Soft tissue masses
    Ganglion cysts
    Lipomas
Varicosities
Synovial hypertrophy
Hypertrophy of abductor hallucis
Muscle anomalies

[a] Data from references 56, 66, 95, and 106.

is located in the posteromedial ankle and extends from just above the medial malleolus to the abductor hallucis muscle in the foot (see Fig. 3-49).[10,56,68] The boundaries of the tarsal tunnel are summarized as follows:

Medial: Flexor retinaculum.
Lateral: Calcaneus, talus.
Superior: Upper margin of flexor retinaculum.
Inferior: Abductor hallucis muscle.

Unlike the carpal tunnel in the wrist, the tarsal tunnel has numerous transverse septa that segment the tarsal tunnel so that small lesions may have more significant impact on the nerve.[66] Space-occupying lesions such as ganglion cysts, fracture fragments, osseous projections, and postsurgical or posttraumatic scarring are the most common causes of tarsal tunnel syndrome.[56,95,106] Table 3-7 provides a more in-depth summary of causes.

Clinical findings and nerve conduction studies may lead

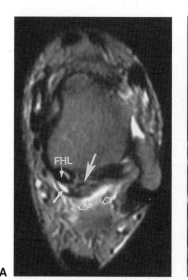 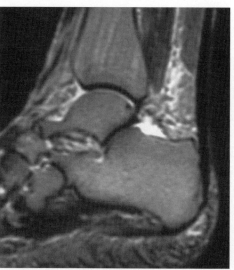 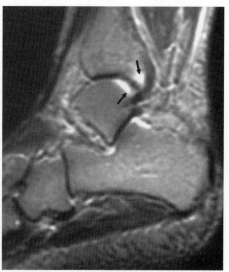

A   B,C

FIG. 3-85. Os trigonum syndrome. **A:** Axial fat-suppressed SE 2000/80 image demonstrates edema (*open arrows*) and fluid (*small white arrow*) around the flexor hallucis longus tendon (*FHL*). The irregularly appearing os trigonum (*large white arrow*) is not clearly demonstrated on this section. Sagittal SE 2000/80 (**B**) and SE 2000/20 (**C**) images demonstrate fluid posteriorly and marginal tibiotalar edema (*arrows*) resulting from associated impingement.

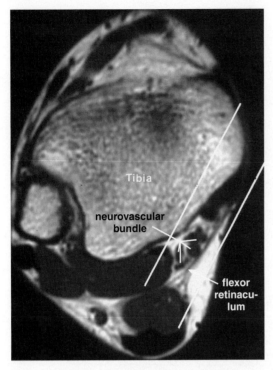

FIG. 3-86. Axial SE 500/10 image demonstrating structures in the tarsal tunnel. In addition to axial images, oblique sagittal images (*white lines*) can be obtained.

to the diagnosis. Patients usually present with subtle symptoms of intermittent paresthesias, burning in the foot, or plantar anesthesia.[106] Pressure on the nerve, percussion of the nerve, or sustained inversion and eversion of the foot may produce the symptoms.[56,95]

Imaging of the tarsal tunnel can be accomplished with routine radiographs, CT, ultrasound and MRI. Osseous abnormalities (see Table 3-7) such as fracture deformity or tarsal coalition can be demonstrated with radiographs and CT.[10,12] Ultrasound may also assist with ganglion cysts and soft tissue abnormalities in this superficial compartment.[89] MRI is superior for identifying soft tissue and neural abnormalities. Axial and sagittal or oblique sagittal images (Fig. 3-86) are most useful. Conventional SE sequences are usually sufficient to detect and characterize the abnormalities (Fig. 3-87).[10,66] Rarely, additional image planes and pulse sequences are required. Gadolinium may be useful to clarify certain soft tissue lesions further (Fig. 3-88).[10]

Treatment of tarsal tunnel syndrome is usually surgical decompression. Some authors report good to excellent results in 79 to 95% of patients. However, results may be difficult to evaluate because the only parameter to evaluate may be pain relief.[95] Pfeiffer and colleagues[95] followed 32 procedures on 30 patients for an average of 31 months. Excellent results were obtained in only 44%. Demonstrating a mass or space-occupying lesion is the best indication for operative intervention, and excellent results are more likely. Therefore, optimal imaging approaches are essential to select patients most likely to achieve positive results with surgery.

Sinus Tarsi Syndrome

Sinus tarsi syndrome is due to a pathologic process in the tarsal canal and sinus. Most patients present with a history of ankle sprain or inversion injury. Characteristically, the patient has lateral ankle or hindfoot pain with point tenderness to palpation or pressure over the tarsal sinus.[71,75] Most patients also describe a sense of ankle or hindfoot instability.[72] Up to 70% of patients have a history of inversion injury. Therefore, there is a high incidence of ligament injury in the tarsal sinus and associated lateral ligament tears in the ankle. Seventy-nine percent of patients with sinus tarsi syndrome had associated calcaneofibular ligament tears.[75]

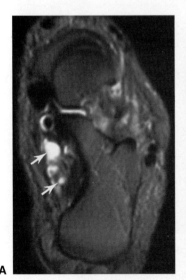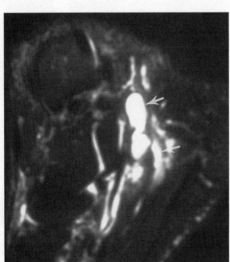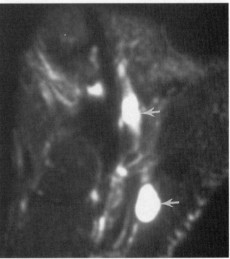

A
B,C

FIG. 3-87. Axial (**A**) and sagittal (**B** and **C**) SE 2000/80 images with fat suppression demonstrate multiple high-signal-intensity varicose veins (*arrows*) causing tarsal tunnel syndrome.

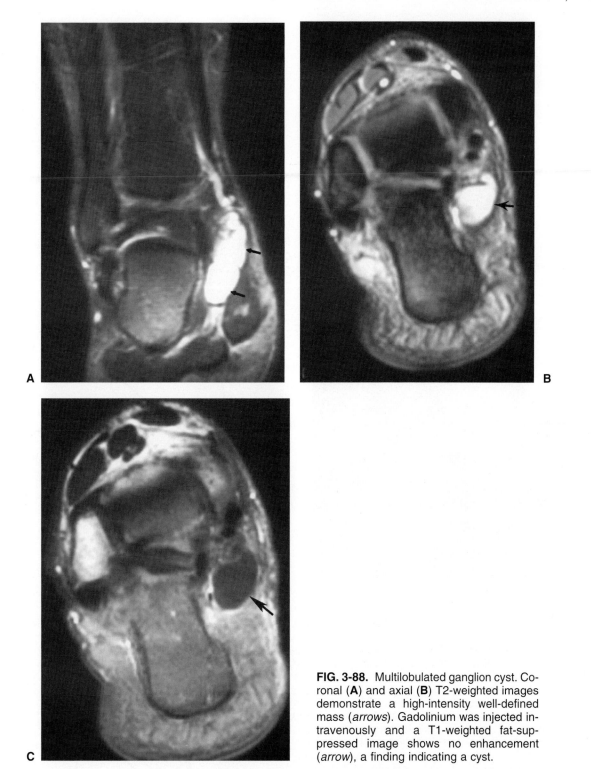

FIG. 3-88. Multilobulated ganglion cyst. Coronal (**A**) and axial (**B**) T2-weighted images demonstrate a high-intensity well-defined mass (*arrows*). Gadolinium was injected intravenously and a T1-weighted fat-suppressed image shows no enhancement (*arrow*), a finding indicating a cyst.

Other conditions such as arthropathy, subtalar capsular hypertrophy, and space-occupying lesions may also cause sinus tarsi symptoms.[71,72,75]

The anatomy of the tarsal canal and sinus is important to understand in order to select proper imaging techniques. Klein and Spreitzer[75] provided an excellent summary of osseous, neurovascular, and ligamentous anatomy of this region. The tarsal canal and sinus extend in a posteromedial to anterolateral course at an angle of approximately 45° to the calcaneal axis (Fig. 3-89).[25] The tarsal canal is the narrow posteromedial portion between the posterior and middle facets (Fig. 3-90). The sinus is cone shaped and widens progressively as it extends lateral and anterior to the posterior facet (Fig. 3-91).[25,75]

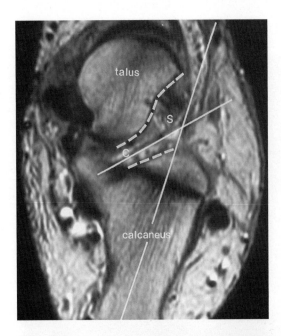

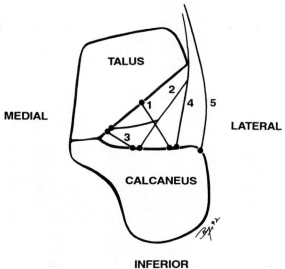

FIG. 3-89. Axial SE 500/11 MRI demonstrating the configuration (*broken lines*) of the tarsal canal and sinus. The relationship to the calcaneal axis (*white lines*) is about 45°. *C,* canal; *S,* sinus.

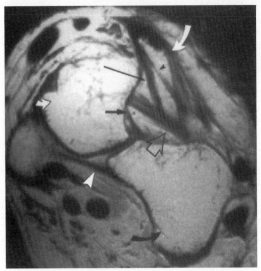

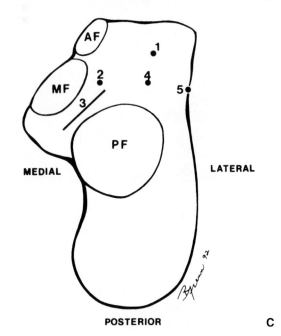

FIG. 3-90. A: Coronal SE 600/15 image of the normal tarsal canal and sinus. The ligament of the tarsal canal (*short black arrow*), the cervical ligament (*open arrow*), and the medial (*long black arrow*), intermediate (*small black arrowhead*), and lateral (*long curved arrow*) roots of the inferior extensor retinaculum are seen as low-intensity structures coursing through the high-intensity fat in the tarsal canal and sinus. The talus (*short curved white arrow*) and calcaneus (*long curved black arrow*) are evident along with the plantar calcaneonavicular ligament (*white arrowhead*) on the medial aspect of the foot. **B:** Coronal anatomic illustration demonstrating the attachment sites of the cervical ligament (*1*), the ligament of the tarsal canal (*3*), the medial (*2*), intermediate (*4*), and lateral (*5*) roots of the inferior extensor retinaculum. **C:** Overhead anatomic illustration of the calcaneus demonstrates the attachment sites of the cervical ligament (*1*), ligament of the tarsal canal (*3*), and medial (*2*), intermediate (*4*), and lateral (*5*) roots of the inferior extensor retinaculum. *AF,* anterior facet; *MF,* middle facet; *PF,* posterior facet. (From Klein and Spreitzer, ref. 55, with permission.)

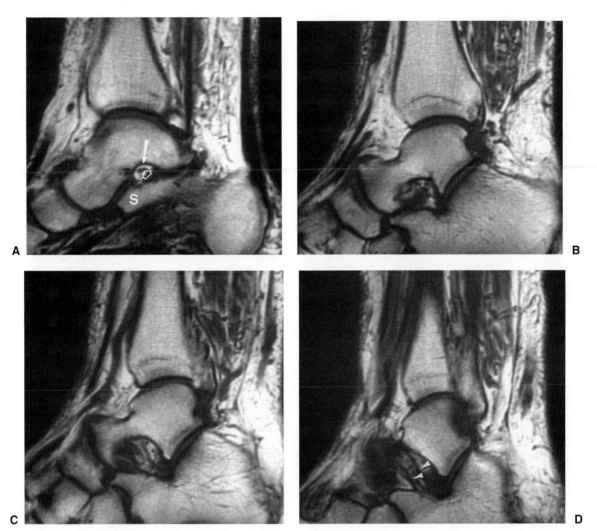

FIG. 3-91. Sagittal SE 500/11 MRI images demonstrating the increase in size of the sinus as it extends from medial to lateral (see also Fig. 3-89). **A:** Sagittal image at the level of the sustentaculum (*S*) shows the small tarsal canal (*arrow*) with fat and the ligament of the tarsal canal (*open arrow*) seen on end. **B:** Sagittal image at the level of the posterior and anterior facets shows widening of the sinus with low-intensity neurovascular and ligament structures seen in the high-intensity fat. **C:** Sagittal image at the lateral margin of the posterior and anterior facets. **D:** Sagittal image at the lateral margin of the sinus demonstrating the lateral and intermediate roots (*white arrowheads*) of the inferior extensor retinaculum.

The tarsal canal and sinus contains fat, neurovascular structures, and is bordered by the synovial capsules of the subtalar facets. There are five distinct ligaments (see Fig. 3-90).[75] These ligaments are the medial, intermediate, and lateral roots of the inferior extensor retinaculum, the ligament of the tarsal canal, and the cervical ligament (see Figs. 3-90 and 3-91).[25] The cervical ligament (see Fig. 3-90) extends from the anterior calcaneus laterally to the neck of the talus. The ligament of the tarsal canal is the most posteromedial of the five ligaments and extends from the calcaneus to the talus in an oblique plane (see Fig. 3-90). The three roots of the inferior extensor retinaculum (medial, intermediate, and lateral) divide on the lateral margins of the tarsal sinus and extend for variable depths into the sinus to attach in sequence to the upper anterior calcaneus (see Figs. 3-90 and 3-91).[25,75]

Imaging of the tarsal canal and sinus can be accomplished with routine radiographs, subtalar arthrography, CT, and MRI. Lateral and oblique radiographs may demonstrate subtalar arthrosis, osseous fragments, or fractures involving the margins of the tarsal canal and sinus. Stress views of the ankle and subtalar joint may be useful to confirm ligament injury and instability.[12,23] Subtalar arthrography and diagnostic injections are useful in selected cases. However, I reserve these invasive techniques for treatment planning or to confirm the source of pain.[11,12,82]

Both CT and MRI provide advantages over the foregoing techniques. In our practice, we prefer MRI because of image plane flexibility and the ability to evaluate the structures in and around the tarsal canal and sinus more thoroughly. MRI can be accomplished using convention axial and sagittal T1- and T2-weighted SE sequences (Fig. 3-92). Off-axis oblique

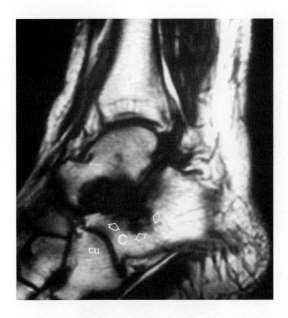

FIG. 3-92. Sagittal SE 500/11 image at the lateral margin of the tarsal sinus near the calcaneocuboid articulation. *C,* calcaneus; *cu,* cuboid. The normal high-intensity fat is replaced by low-signal-intensity inflammatory tissue (*arrow*), and there are erosions (*open arrows*) in the calcaneus.

planes designed to provide views aligned with the tarsal canal and sinus can also be used when the indication is for specific evaluation of this region (Fig. 3-93). However, because most patients are referred for generalized lateral pain or instability, orthogonal sagittal, axial. and coronal images are usually sufficient. T1-weighted SE, fast SE with fat suppression and short T1 inversion recovery (STIR) sequences are also useful (Figs. 3-94 and 3-95). Gadolinium is rarely indicated and reserved for selected situations such as neuromas or soft tissue masses in the tarsal sinus.[10,12,75]

Klein and Spreitzer[75] report MRI findings in 33 patients with abnormal findings in the tarsal canal and sinus. There was a calcaneofibular ligament tear in about 80% of patients with associated infiltrative changes in the sinus tarsi on T1- and T2-weighted sequences. Abnormal fluid collections in the tarsal sinus were noted in 15% of patients.[75]

Treatment of sinus tarsi syndrome may be dictated by associated ligament and tendon injury. Conservative treatment with cast immobilization or direct injection may be warranted initially.[11,75] Surgical repair, when indicated,

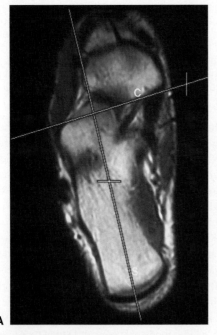
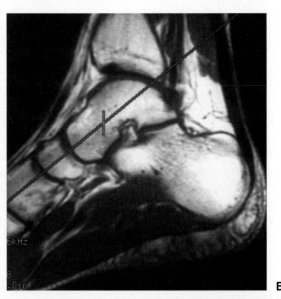

FIG. 3-93. MRI approaches to the tarsal canal and sinus. **A:** Axial image demonstrating oblique sagittal (*S*) and oblique coronal (**C**) image planes selected. **B:** Sagittal scout demonstrating the plane for oblique axial images.

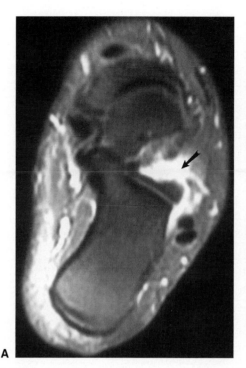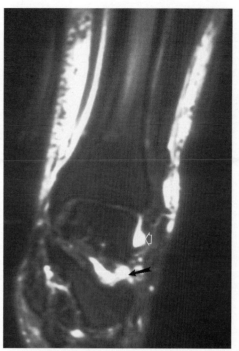

FIG. 3-94. Axial fat-suppressed fast SE (**A**) and coronal STIR (**B**) sequences demonstrating diffuse edema in the lower leg with areas of increased signal (*arrow*) in the tarsal sinus and fluid (*open white arrow*) in the anterior talofibular ligament region resulting from inversion injury with sinus tarsi syndrome.

should include the lateral ligament complex and any disrupted ligament (see Fig. 3-95) in the tarsal canal and sinus. For this reason, imaging of ligament injuries in the ankle should always include evaluation of the ligamentous structures of the tarsal canal and sinus. If left unexplored, chronic instability may result.[23,75]

Impingement Syndromes

Impingement syndromes in the ankle may be related to bone or soft tissue abnormalities. Posterior impingement has been discussed in relation to os trigonum syndrome (see Fig. 3-85). Anterior impingement may be related to osseous changes in the tibia, talus, or soft tissue abnormalities.[44,104,126] The former is usually related to osseous changes in the tibia, talus, or both articular margins.[126] Soft tissue impingement is related to abnormal soft tissue proliferation in the anterior aspect of the tibiotalar joint. This most commonly occurs in the anterolateral ankle. The syndrome is commonly associated with ankle sprain with scarring or synovitis in the anterolateral gutter.[44] Patients typically present with deep anterior ankle pain swelling and limited dorsiflexion of the foot.[104] The origin may be related to hypertrophy of synovial tissue, fibroses, or osseous changes.[5,130] Diagnosis is based on clinical and image features. Differential diagnostic considerations include anterolateral ligament injury, peroneal tendon disorders, sinus tarsi syndrome, and osteoarthritis.[44,104]

Imaging of anterior impingement syndrome may be ac-

complished with routine radiographs or lateral stress views with dorsiflexion and plantar flexion of the foot.[12] Bone changes at the anterior articular margin of the ankle may be obvious. When diagnosis is in doubt or when other clinical syndromes described earlier are considered, additional techniques may be indicated. CT may be preferred when subtle osseous changes are evident (Fig. 3-96). When radiographs are normal, MRI should be considered. MRI is more useful for excluding other conditions and for detecting subtle anterior soft tissue changes (Fig. 3-97).[104]

Treatment of this disorder may be initiated with conservative approaches such as rest, cast immobilization, and antiinflammatory medications. When conservative therapy fails, arthroscopic or open surgery is indicated.[126,130]

Midfoot and Forefoot Syndromes

Osseous and soft tissue overuse syndromes in the midfoot and forefoot are not uncommon. Stress fractures in the tarsal and metatarsal regions are common (Fig. 3-98).[3,13,125] These injuries are discussed in Chapter 4. Midfoot injuries may be due to ligament injury or in association with fractures, especially Lisfranc's injuries.[19,111] Compartment syndrome in adults and children is most often associated with acute injury and is not discussed in this section.[111]

Many forefoot syndromes are diagnosed clinically and do not require imaging when they respond to conservative therapy. Imaging plays a more significant role when conservative measures fail. In this setting, properly selected imaging

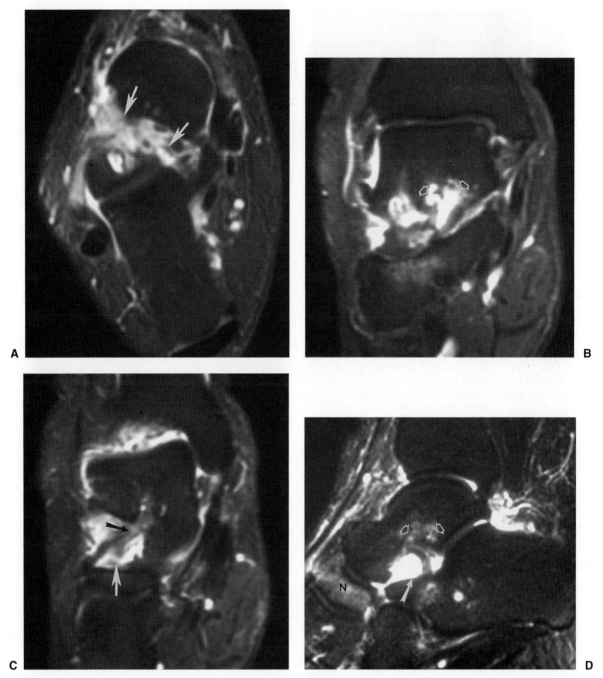

FIG. 3-95. Axial (**A**), coronal (**B** and **C**), and sagittal (**D**) fat-suppressed fast SE T2-weighted images in a patient with chronic instability and subtalar arthrosis. Note the high signal intensity (*arrows*) in the tarsal canal and sinus with articular erosions (*open arrows*). There is also a bone bruise in the navicular (*N*) on the sagittal image (**D**). The cervical ligament is partially torn near the talar attachment on image **C** (*black arrow*).

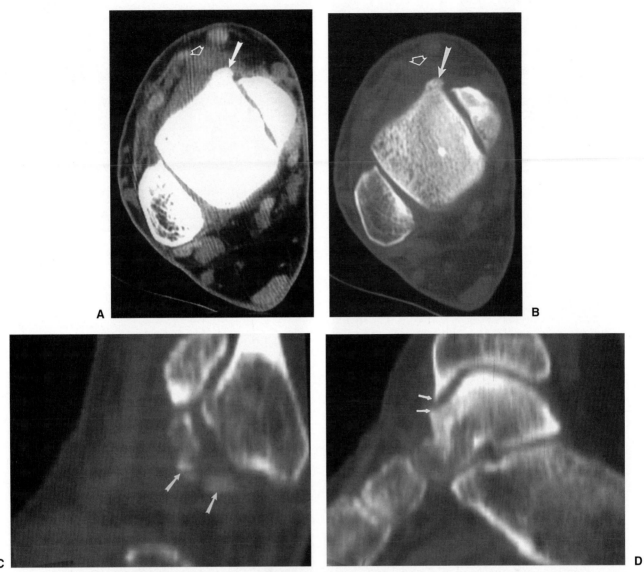

FIG. 3-96. Anterolateral impingement syndrome. Axial CT images with soft tissue (**A**) and bone (**B**) settings demonstrate marginal osteophytes anterolaterally (*arrow*) and soft tissue hypertrophy (*open arrows*). Reformatted sagittal images demonstrate osseous fragments (**C**) and tibiotalar osteophytes (**D**).

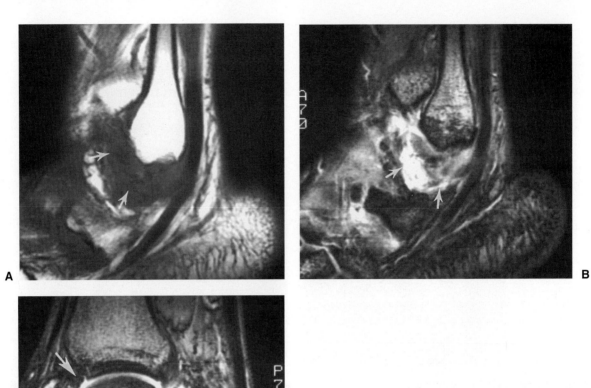

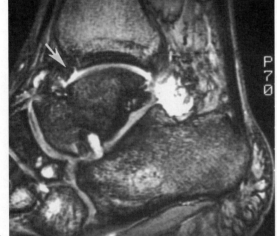

FIG. 3-97. Arterolateral impingement. **A:** Sagittal SE 500/11 image shows low intensity soft tissue thickening (*arrows*) around and anterior to the lateral malleolus. Sagittal GRE postgadolinium images demonstrate soft tissue enhancement (*arrows* in **B**) and anterior tibial osteophytes (*arrow* in **C**).

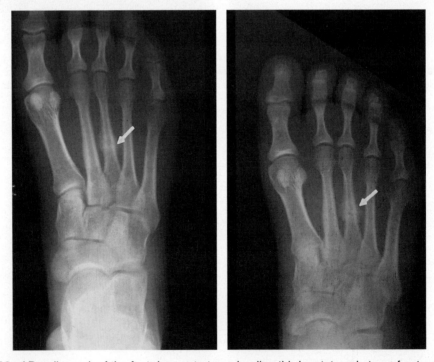

FIG. 3-98. AP radiograph of the foot demonstrates a healing third metatarsal stress fracture (*arrow*).

TABLE 3-8. *Forefoot pain syndromes*[a]

Metatarsalgia
Sesamoiditis
Osteochondritis
Metatarsophalangeal subluxation/synovitis
Hallux rigidus
Neuromas
Turf toe
Stress fractures

[a] Data from references 13, 79, 83, and 113.

techniques are necessary to define conditions not responding to common conservative approaches. Table 3-8 summarizes common forefoot syndromes.[13,45,79,83,113]

Forefoot pain is a common problem in athletes and patients with occupational activity that involves weight bearing for long periods of time.[3,13,115] Metatarsalgia may be related to a long second metatarsal or hypermobile first metatarsal.[79] More generalized metatarsal pain may be evident in athletes with a tight Achilles tendon or anterior ankle impingement.[13] Routine radiographs are usually adequate for identifying metatarsal length. In certain cases, MRI may be required to detect plantar bursae or other abnormalities causing forefoot pain.[10]

Sesamoid pain syndromes are common in runners.[4,45,92] The medial and lateral sesamoids lie in the medial and lateral slips of the flexor hallucis brevis.[68] The sesamoids function to elevate the (Fig. 3-99) first metatarsal head, disperse impact forces, to protect the flexor hallucis tendon, and to increase the mechanical advantage of the flexor hallucis brevis.[10,13,45] Sesamoids may become inflamed, fracture, or undergo osteonecrosis. In addition to pain, physical examination may cause discomfort with dorsiflexion of the great toe.[45]

Routine radiographs including AP, oblique, lateral, and sesamoid views (Fig. 3-100) may be diagnostic.[13,45] The sesamoid may be fragmented, sclerotic, or fractured (see Figs. 3-101 and 3-102). Soft tissue swelling over the in-

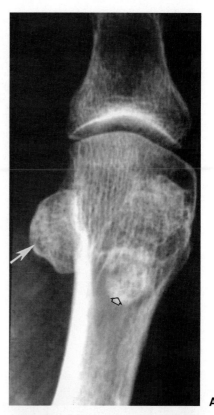

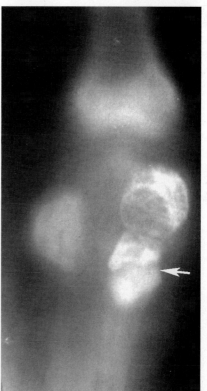

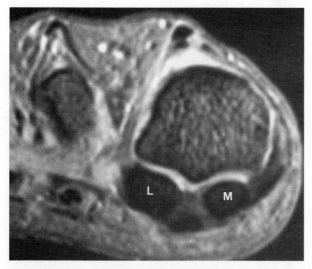

FIG. 3-99. Axial fat-suppressed fast SE image demonstrating the medial (*M*) and lateral (*L*) sesamoids seated in the metatarsal grooves.

FIG. 3-100. A long-distance runner with pain in the plantar aspect of the great toe. **A:** AP radiograph shows rotation of the lateral sesamoid (*arrow*). The medial sesamoid appears bipartate and the proximal portion (*open arrow*) looks sclerotic. **B:** AP tomogram shows a sclerotic fractured sesamoid (*arrow*).

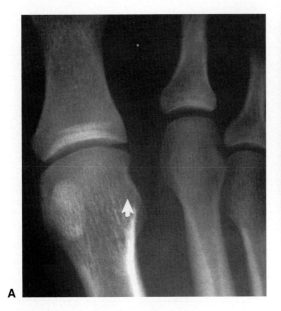

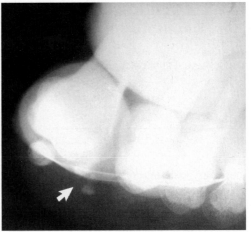

FIG. 3-101. A long-distance runner with chronic pain under the first metatarsal head. AP (**A**) radiograph shows an absent lateral sesamoid (*arrow*). Sesamoid view (**B**) shows only a small remnant (*arrow*) of the lateral sesamoid resulting from avascular necrosis and bone resorption.

volved sesamoid is usually present as well. In subtle cases, radionuclide bone scans are useful (Fig. 3-103). Increased tracer occurs in the presence of sesamoid disorders. A normal scan excludes the diagnosis. In some cases MRI is required for evaluating unresponsive sesamoid pain.[10,13]

Treatment of sesamoid disorders is usually conservative initially. Footwear changes, a sesamoid pad, and antiinflammatory medications may be sufficient. When conservative measures fail, surgical resection is recommended.[45]

Osteochondritis may also lead to forefoot pain. Osteonecrosis of the second metatarsal head occurs most frequently. Women are affected more often than men.[99] Routine radiographs are usually diagnostic. However, when indicated, MRI is useful to confirm the diagnosis and exclude other conditions such as synovitis.[113] In the latter, intravenous gadolinium may be useful to detect early synovial changes.[10] Synovitis, like osteonecrosis, also more commonly involves the second metatarsophalangeal joint.[113]

Hallux rigidus usually results from chronic trauma. Athletes involved in track and football are commonly affected.[78] Joint space narrowing without hallux valgus deformity may be the only radiographic finding initially. If the condition is left untreated, marked narrowing (Fig. 3-104) and prominent osteophytes may develop. Surgical resection may be indicated in advanced cases.

Morton's neuromas may also result from chronic trauma to the interdigital nerve. Symptoms are classically described between the third and fourth metatarsal heads. Paresthesia and numbness of the sensory distribution of the nerve are common. Clinical history and physical examination are usually diagnostic. MRI (Fig. 3-105) is useful in selected cases. Neuromas are also reviewed in Chapter 6.

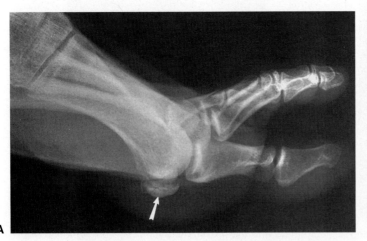

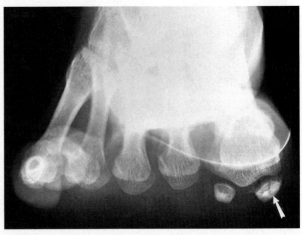

FIG. 3-102. Lateral (**A**) and sesamoid (**B**) views demonstrating sclerosis and fragmentation of the medial sesamoid (*arrow*) resulting from avascular necrosis.

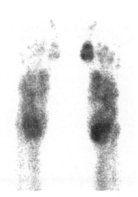

FIG. 3-103. A: Technetium-99m methylene diphosphonate bone scan shows increased tracer in the sesamoids and first metatarsophalangeal joint resulting from degenerative joint disease and early avascular necrosis of the sesamoids.

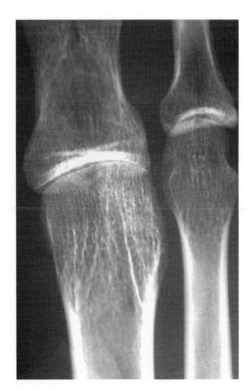

FIG. 3-104. Coned-down AP radiograph of the great toe demonstrates marked joint space narrowing with no angular deformity. The second MTP joint is also narrowed and slightly subluxed.

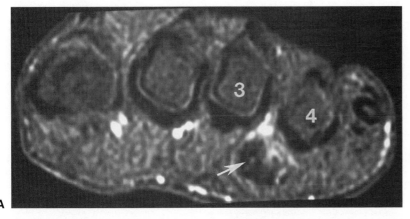

A

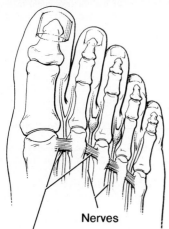

B Intermetatarsal ligaments

Nerves

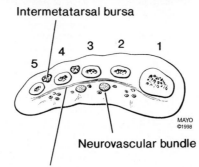

Intermetatarsal bursa

Neurovascular bundle

Transverse metatarsal ligament

MAYO
©1998

FIG. 3-105. A: Axial fat-suppressed postgadolinium image demonstrates a large Morton's neuroma (*arrow*) between the third (*3*) and fourth (*4*) metatarsal heads. **B:** Illustration of the location of Morton's neuromas and bursae with relation to the transverse metatarsal ligament.

167

REFERENCES

1. Abraham E, Sternaman JE. Neglected rupture of the peroneal tendon causing recurrent sprains of the ankle. J. Bone Joint Surg. Am. 1979; 61:1247–1248.
2. Ala-Ketola L, Peranen J, Kosivisto E, Puupera M. Arthrography in the diagnosis of ligament injuries and classification of ankle injuries. Radiology 1977; 125:63–68.
3. Andrews JR. Overuse syndromes of the lower extremity. Clin. Sports Med. 1983; 2:137–148.
4. Aström M, Gentz C-F, Nilsson P, Rausing A, Sjöberg S, Westlin N. Imaging in chronic Achilles tendinopathy. A comparison of ultrasonography, magnetic resonance imaging and surgical findings in 27 histologically verified cases. Skeletal Radiol. 1996; 25:615–620.
5. Bassett FH, Gates HS, Billys JB, Morris HB, Nikolaou PK. Talar impingement by the anteroinferior tibiofibular ligament. J. Bone Joint Surg. Am. 1990; 72:55–59.
6. Bassett FH, Speer KP. Longitudinal rupture of the peroneal tendons. Am. J. Sports Med. 1993; 21:354–357.
7. Bencardino J, Rosenberg ZS, Beltran J, Booker M, Cheung Y, Rosenberg LA, Schweitzer M, Hamilton W. MR imaging of dislocation of the posterior tibial tendon. AJR Am. J. Roentgenol. 1997; 169: 1209–1112.
8. Beltran J, Noto AM, Mosure JC, Shamain OM, Weiss KL, Zueler WA. Ankle. Surface coil MR imaging at 1.5 T. Radiology 1986; 161: 203–209.
9. Berkowitz JF, Kier R, Rudicel S. Plantar fasciitis: MR imaging. Radiology 1991; 179:665–667.
10. Berquist TH. MRI of the Musculoskeletal System. 3rd Ed. New York, Lippincott–Raven, 1996.
11. Berquist TH. Diagnostic and therapeutic injections as an aid to musculoskeletal diagnosis. Semin. Intervent. Radiol. 1993; 10(4):326–343.
12. Berquist TH. Imaging of Orthopedic Trauma. 2nd Ed. New York, Raven Press, 1992.
13. Berquist TH. Imaging of Sports Injuries. Gaithersburg, MD, Aspen Press, 1992.
14. Bianchi S, Zwass A, Abdelwahab IF, Zoccola C. Evaluation of tibialis anterior tendon rupture by ultrasonography. J. Clin. Ultrasound 1994; 22:564–566.
15. Black HM, Brand RL, Eichelberger MR. An improved technique for the evaluation of ligamentous injury in severe ankle sprains. Am J. Sports Med. 1978; 6(5):276–282.
16. Blanchard KS, Finlay DBL, Scott DJA, Ley CC, Suggins D, Allen MJ. A radiological analysis of lateral ligament injuries of the ankle. Clin. Radiol. 1986; 37:247–251.
17. Blei CL, Nirschl RP, Grant EG. Achilles tendon. US diagnosis of pathologic conditions. Radiology 1986; 159:765–767.
18. Boles MA, Lomasney LM, Demos TC, Sage RA. Enlarged peroneal process with peroneus longus tendon entrapment. Skeletal Radiol. 1997; 26:313–315.
19. Bonutti PM, Bell GR. Compartment syndrome of the foot. J. Bone Joint Surg. Am. 1986; 68:1449–1450.
20. Bottger BA, Schweitzer ME, El-Noueam KI, Desai M. MR imaging of the normal and abnormal retrocalcaneal bursae. AJR Am. J. Roentgenol. 1998; 170:1239–1241.
21. Boyim MJ, Fischer DA, Neumann L. Syndesmotic ankle sprains. Am J. Sports Med. 1991; 19:294–298.
22. Brand RL, Collins MDF. Operative management of ligamentous injuries of the ankle. Clin. Sports Med. 1982; 1(1):117–130.
23. Brantigan JW, Pedegana LR, Lippert FG. Instability of the subtalar joint. Diagnosis with stress radiography in 3 cases. J. Bone Joint Surg. Am. 1977; 59:321–324.
24. Brestenseher MJ, Trattnig S, Kukla C, Gaebler C, Kaider A, Baldt MM, Haller J, Imhof H. MRI vs. lateral stress radiography in acute lateral ankle ligament injuries. J. Comput. Assist. Tomogr. 1997; 21(2):280–285.
25. Cahill DR. Anatomy and function of the contents of the human tarsal sinus and canal. Anat. Rec. 1965; 153:1–18.
26. Cardone BW, Erickson SJ, Den Hartog BD, Carrera GF. MRI of injury to the lateral collateral ligamentous complex of the ankle. J. Comput. Assist Tomogr. 1993; 17(1):102–107.
27. Cass JR, Morrey BF. Ankle instability. Current concepts diagnosis, and treatment. Mayo Clin. Proc. 1984; 59:165–170.
28. Cetti R, Andersen I. Roentgenographic diagnosis of ruptured Achilles tendons. Clin. Orthop. 1993; 286:215–221.
29. Chandnani VP, Harper MT, Ficke JR, Gagliardi JA, Rolling L, Christensen KP, Hansen MF. Chronic ankle instability. Evaluation with MR arthrography MR imaging, and stress radiography. Radiology 1994; 192:189–194.
30. Chen JP, Allen AM. MR diagnosis of traumatic tear of the spring ligament in a pole vaulter. Skeletal Radiol. 1997; 26:310–312.
31. Cheung Y, Rosenberg ZS, Magee T, Chinitz L. Normal anatomy and pathologic conditions of ankle tendons. Current imaging techniques. Radiographics 1992; 12:429–444.
32. Cheung YY, Rosenberg ZS, Ramsinghani R, Beltran J, Jahss MH. Peroneus quartus muscle. MR imaging features. Radiology 1997; 202: 745–750.
33. Church CC. Radiographic diagnosis of acute peroneal tendon dislocation. AJR Am. J. Roentgenol. 1977; 129:1065–1068.
34. Clark HD, Kitaoka HB, Berquist TH. Imaging of tendon injuries about the ankle. Orthopedics 1997; 20(7):639–643.
35. Cox JS, Hewes TF. Normal talar tilt angle. Clin. Orthop. 1979; 140: 37–41.
36. Daffner RH, Riemer BL, Lupetin AR, Dash N. Magnetic resonance imaging in acute tendon ruptures. Skeletal Radiol. 1980; 15(8): 619–621.
37. Davies JAK. Peroneal compartment syndrome secondary to rupture of the peroneus longus. J. Bone Joint Surg. Am. 1979; 61:783–784.
38. DeLuca PA, Bauta JV. Pes cavovarus as a late consequence of peroneus longus tendon rupture. J. Pediatr. Orthop. 1985; 5:582–583.
39. Dezwart DF, Davidson JSA. Rupture of the posterior tibial tendon associated with ankle fractures. J. Bone Joint Surg. Am. 1983; 65: 260–261.
40. Dokter G, Lundaw LA. The accessory soleus muscle. Symptomatic soft tissue tumor or accidental finding. Neth. J. Surg. 1981; 33(3): 146–149.
41. Dory MA. Arthrography of the ankle joint in chronic instability. Skeletal Radiol. 1986; 15(9):291–294.
42. Edwards GS, DeLee JC. Ankle diastasis without fracture. Foot Ankle 1984; 4(6):305–312.
43. Evans GA, Frenyo SD. The stress-tenogram in diagnosis of rupture of the lateral ligament of the ankle. J. Bone Joint Surg. Br. 1979; 61: 347–351.
44. Farooki S, Yao H, Seeger LL. Anterolateral impingement of the ankle. Effectiveness of MR imaging. Radiology 1998; 207:357–360.
45. Fleischli J, Cheleuitte E. Avascular necrosis of the hallucial sesamoids. J. Foot Ankle Surg. 1995; 34(4):358–365.
46. Fornage BD. Achilles tendon. US examination. Radiology 1986; 159: 759–764.
47. Fowler A, Phillip JF. Abnormality of the calcaneus as a cause of painful heel. Br. J. Surg. 1945; 32:494–498.
48. Funk DA, Cass JA, Johnson KA. Acquired adult flat foot secondary to posterior tibial tendon pathology. J. Bone Joint Surg. Am. 1986; 68:95–102.
49. Garth WP. Flexor hallucis tendinitis in ballet dancers. J. Bone Joint Surg. Am. 1981; 63:1489.
50. Gazdag AR, Cracchiolo A. Rupture of the posterior tibial tendon. Evaluation of injury of the spring ligament and clinical assessment of tendon transfer and ligament repair. J. Bone Joint. Surg. Am. 1997; 79:675–681.
51. Gilula LA, Oloff L, Caputi R, Destouet JM, Jacobs A, Solomon MA. Ankle tenography. A key to unexplained symptomatology. II. Diagnosis of chronic tendon disabilities. Radiology 1984; 151:581–587.
52. Goergen TG, Resnick D. Arthrography of the ankle and hindfoot. In Dalinka MK, ed. Arthrography. New York, Springer-Verlag, 1980; pp. 137–153.
53. Grogan DP, Walling AK, Ogden JA. Anatomy of the os trigonum. J. Pediatr. Orthop. 1990; 10:618–622.
54. Harrington KD. Degenerative arthritis of the ankle secondary to long standing ligament instability. J. Bone Joint Surg. Am. 1979; 61: 354–361.
55. Hilgason JW, Chandnani VP, Yu JS. MR arthrography. A review of current technique and applications. AJR Am. J. Roentgenol. 1997; 168:1473–1480.
56. Ho VW, Peterfly C, Helms CA. Tarsal tunnel syndrome caused by strain of an anomalous muscle. An MRI-specific diagnosis. J. Comput. Assist. Tomogr. 1993; 17(5):822–823.

57. Horsfield D, Murphy G. Stress views of the ankle joint in lateral ligament injury. Radiography 1985; 51:7–11.

58. Inglis AE, Scott N, Sculo TP, Patterson AH. Rupture of the tendon Achilles. An objective assessment of surgical and non-surgical treatment. J. Bone Joint Surg. Am. 1976; 58:990–993.

59. Johannsen A. Radiologic diagnosis of lateral ligament lesion of the ankle. Acta Orthop. Scand. 1978; 49:295–301.

60. Johnson EE, Morkolf KL. The contribution of the anterior talofibular ligament to ankle laxity. J. Bone Joint Surg. Am. 1983; 65:81–88.

61. Karasick D, Schweitzer ME. Tear of the posterior tibial tendon causing asymmetric flatfoot. Radiologic findings. AJR Am. J. Roentgenol. 1993; 161:1237–1240.

62. Karasick D, Schweitzer ME. The os trigonum syndrome. Imaging features. AJR Am. J. Roentgenol. 1996; 166:125–129.

63. Karr SD. Subcalcaneal heel pain. Orthop. Clin. North Am. 1994; 25(1):161–175.

64. Kelikian H, Kelikian AS. Disorders of the Ankle. Philadelphia, W.B. Saunders, 1985.

65. Kell PM. A comparative radiologic examination for unresponsive plantar fasciitis. J. Manipulative Physiol. Ther. 1994; 17(5):329–334.

66. Kerr R, Frey C. MR imaging in tarsal tunnel syndromes. J. Comput. Assist. Tomogr. 1991; 15:280–286.

67. Khoury, NJ, El-Khoury GY, Saltzman CL, Brandser EA. MR imaging of posterior tibial tendon dysfunction. AJR Am. J. Roentgenol. 1996; 167:675–682.

68. Khoury NJ, El-Khoury GY, Saltzman CL, Brandser EA. Rupture of the anterior tibial tendon. Diagnosis with MR imaging. AJR Am. J. Roentgenol. 1996; 167:351–354.

69. Khoury NJ, El-Khoury GY, Saltzman CL, Kathol MH. Peroneus longus and brevis tendon tears. MR imaging evaluation. Radiology 1996; 200:833–841.

70. Kier R, Dietz MJ, McCarthy SM, Rudicel SA. MR imaging of the normal ligaments and tendons of the ankle. J. Comput. Assist. Tomogr. 1991; 15:477–482.

71. Kjaerguard-Anderson P, Anderson K, Soballe K, Pilgaard S. Sinus tarsi syndrome. Presentation of 7 cases and review of the literature. J. Foot Surg. 1989; 28:3–6.

72. Kjaerguard-Anderson P, Wethslund JD, Helmig P, Soballe K. The stabilizing effect of the ligamentous structures in the sinus and canalus tarsi on movement in the hindfoot. An experimental study. Am. J. Sports Med. 1988; 16:512–516.

73. Klein MA. MR imaging of the ankle. Normal and abnormal findings in the medial collateral ligament. AJR Am. J. Roentgenol. 1994; 162: 377–383.

74. Klein MA. Reformatted three-dimensional fourier transform gradient-recalled echo MR imaging of the ankle. Spectrum of normal and abnormal findings. AJR Am. J. Roentgenol. 1993; 161:831–836.

75. Klein MA, Spreitzer AM. MR imaging of the tarsal sinus and canal. Normal anatomy, pathologic findings, and features of sinus tarsi syndrome. Radiology 1993; 186:233–240.

76. Kleinman M, Gross AE. Achilles tendon rupture following steroid injection. J. Bone Joint Surg. Am. 1983; 65:1345–1347.

77. Larson E. Experimental instability of the ankle. A radiographic investigation. Clin. Orthop. 1986; 204:193–200.

78. Lawson JP. Clinically significant radiologic anatomic variants of the skeleton. AJR Am. J. Roentgenol. 1994; 163:249–255.

79. Lillich JS, Baxter DE. Common forefoot problems in runners. Foot Ankle 1986; 7:145–151.

80. Lurk SC, Erickson SJ, Timins ME. MR imaging of the ankle and foot. Normal structures and anatomic variants that may simulate disease. AJR Am. J. Roentengol. 1993; 161:607–612.

81. Mann RA, Thompson FM. Rupture of the posterior tibial tendon causing flat foot. J. Bone Joint Surg. Am. 1985; 67:556–561.

82. Meyer JM, Garcia J, Hoffmeier P, Fritschy D. Subtalar sprain. A roentgenographic study. Clin. Orthop. 1988; 226:169–173.

83. Marshall P. The rehabilitation of overuse foot injuries in athletes and dancers. Clin. Podiatr. Med. Surg. 1989; 6:639–655.

84. Mellado J, Rosenberg ZS, Beltran J. Low incorporation of soleus tendon. A potential diagnostic pitfall of MR imaging. Skeletal Radiol. 1998; 27:222–224.

85. Michelson J, Easley M, Wigley FM, Hellmann D. Posterior tibial tendon dysfunction in rheumatoid arthritis. Foot Ankle Sut. 1995; 16(3):156–161.

86. Montague AP, McQuillan RF. Clinical assessment of the apparently sprained ankle and detection of fracture. Injury 1985; 16:545–546.

87. Morti R. Dislocation of the peroneal tendon. Am J. Sports Med. 1977; 5(1):19–22

88. Murr S. Dislocation of the peroneal tendon with marginal fracture of the lateral malleolus. J. Bone Joint Surg. Br. 1961; 43:563–565.

89. Nazarian LN, Rawool NM, Martin CE, Schweitzer ME. Synovial fluid in the hindfoot and ankle. Detection of amount and distribution with US. Radiology 1995; 197:275–278.

90. Newmark H, Olken SM, Mellon WS, Malhotra AK, Halls J. A new finding in radiographic diagnosis of Achilles tendon rupture. Skeletal Radiol. 1982; 8:223–224.

91. O'Brien T. The needle test for complete rupture of the Achilles tendon. J. Bone Joint Surg. Am. 1984; 66:1099–1101.

92. Paty JG. Diagnosis and treatment of musculoskeletal running injuries. Semin. Arthritis Rheum. 1988; 18:48–60.

93. Paulos LE, Johnson CL, Noyes FR. Posterior compartment fractures of the ankle. Am J. Sports Med. 1983; 11:439–443.

94. Percy EC, Conochie LB. Surgical treatment of ruptured tendo Achilles. J. Bone Joint Surg. Br. 1975; 57:535.

95. Pfeiffer WH, Cracchiolo A. Clinical results after tarsal tunnel decompression. J. Bone Joint Surg. Am. 1994; 76:1222–1230.

96. Povacz P, Unger F, Miller K, Tockner R, Resch H. A randomized prospective study of operative and non-operative treatment of injuries of the fibular collateral ligaments of the ankle. J. Bone Joint Surg. Am. 1998; 80:345–349.

97. Raatikainen T, Puronen J. Arthrography for diagnosis of acute lateral ligament injuries of the ankle. Am. J. Sports Med. 1993; 21(3): 343–347.

98. Rademaker J, Rosenberg ZS, Beltran J, Colon E. Alterations of the distal extension of the musculus peroneus brevis with foot movement. AJR Am. J. Roentgenol. 1997; 168:787–789.

99. Rettig AC, Shelbournek D, Beltz HF, Robertson DW, Afken P. Radiographic evaluation of foot and ankle injuries in athletes. Clin. Sports Med. 1987; 6:905–919.

100. Romanus B, Landahl S, Stener B. Accessory soleus muscle. A clinical and radiographic presentation of 11 cases. J. Bone Joint Surg. Am. 1986; 68:731–734.

101. Rosenberg ZS, Beltran J, Cheung YY, Colon E, Herraiz F. MR features of longitudinal tears of the peroneus brevis tendon. AJR Am. J. Roentgenol. 1997; 168:141–147.

102. Rosenberg ZS, Feldman F, Singson RD. Peroneal tendon injuries: CT analysis. Radiology 1986; 161:743–748.

103. Rosenberg ZS, Feldman F, Singson RD, Price GJ. Peroneal tendon injury associated with calcaneal fractures. CT findings. AJR Am. J. Roentgenol. 1987; 149:125–129.

104. Rubin DA, Tishkoff NW, Britton CA, Conti SF, Towers JD. Anterolateral soft tissue impingement in the ankle. Diagnosis using MR imaging. AJR Am. J. Roentgenol. 1997; 169:829–835.

105. Rule J, Yao L, Seeger LL. Spring ligament of the ankle. Normal MR anatomy. AJR Am. J. Roentgenol. 1993; 161:1241–1244.

106. Sammarco GJ, Conti SF. Tarsal tunnel syndrome caused by an anomalous muscle. J. Bone Joint Surg. Am. 1994; 76:1308–1314.

107. Sauser DD, Nelson RC, Lavine MH, Wu CW. Acute injuries of the lateral ligaments of the ankle. Comparison of stress radiography and arthrography. Radiology 1983; 148:653–657.

108. Schneck CD, Mesgarzadeh M, Bonakdarpour A, Ross GJ. MR imaging of the most commonly injured ankle ligaments. I. Normal anatomy. Radiology 1992; 184: 499–506.

109. Schweigel JF, Knickerbacher WJ, Cooperberg P. A study of ankle instability utilizing ankle arthrography. J. Trauma 1977; 17(11): 878–881.

110. Schweitzer ME, Eid ME, Deely D, Wapner K, Hecht P. Using MR imaging to differentiate peroneal splits from other peroneal disorders. AJR (Am. J. Roent) 1997; 168:129–133.

111. Silas SI, Herzenberg JE, Myerson MS, Sponseller PD. Compartment syndrome of the foot in children. J. Bone Joint Surg. Am. 1995; 77: 356–361.

112. Simon RR, Hoffman JR, Smith M. Radiographic comparison of plain films on second and third degree ankle sprains. Am. J. Emerg. Med. 1986; 4(5):387–389.

113. Smith RW, Reischl SF. Metatarsophalangeal joint synovitis in athletes. Clin. Sports Med. 1988; 7:75–88.

114. Spiegel PK, Staples OS. Arthrography of the ankle joint. Problems in diagnosis of acute leg injuries. Radiology 1975; 114:587–590.

115. Stanish WD. Lower leg, foot and ankle injuries in athletes. Clin. Sports Med. 1995; 14(3):651–668.
116. Stein RE. Rupture of the posterior tibial tendon in closed ankle fractures. J. Bone Joint Surg. Am. 1985; 67:493–494.
117. Stephens MM. Haglund's deformity and retrocalcaneal bursitis. Orthop Clin. North Am. 1994; 25(1):41–46.
118. Sturgill BC, Allen JH. Rheumatoid like nodules presenting as pump bumps in a patient without rheumatoid arthritis. Arthritis Rheum. 1970; 13:175–180
119. Szczukowski M, St. Pierre RK, Fleming LL, Somogyi J. Computerized tomography in the evaluation of peroneal tendon dislocation. A report of 2 cases. Am. J. Sports Med. 1983; 11(6):444–447.
120. Taylor DE, Englehardt DL, Bassett FH. Syndesmotic sprains of the ankle. The influence of heterotopic ossification. Am. J. Sports Med. 1992; 20:146–150.
121. Tehranzadeh J, Stoll DA, Gabriele OM. Posterior migration of the os peroneum of the left foot indicating a tear of the peroneal tendon. Skeletal Radiol. 1984; 12:44–47.
122. Termansen NB, Hansen H, Damvolt V. Radiologic and muscular status following injury to the lateral ligaments of the ankle. Acta Orthop. Scand. 1979; 50:705–708.
123. Thompson TC. A test for rupture of the tendo Achilles Acta Orthop. Scand. 1962; 32:461–465.
124. Ton ERT, Schweitzer ME, Karasick D. MR imaging of peroneal tendon disorders. AJR Am. J. Roentgenol. 1997; 168:135–140.
125. Torg JS, Pavlov H, Torg E. Overuse injuries in sport. The foot. Clin. Sports Med. 1987; 6:291–320.
126. Vogler HW, Stienstra JJ, Montgomery F, Kipp L. Anterior ankle impingement arthropathy. Clin. Podiatr. Med. Surg. 1994; 11(3):425–447.
127. Wakely CJ, Johnson DP, Watt I. The value of MR imaging in the diagnosis of os trigonum syndrome. Skeletal Radiol. 1996; 25:133–136.
128. Ward DW. Syndesmotic ankle sprain in a recreational hockey player. J. Manipulative Physiol. Ther. 1994; 17(6):385–394.
129. Wredmark T, Carlstedt CA, Bauer H, Saertok T. Os trigonum syndrome. A clinical entity in ballet dancers. Foot Ankle 1991; 11:404–406.
130. Wokin I, Glassman F, Siderman S, Leventhal DH. Internal derangement of the talofibular component of the ankle. Surg. Gynecol. Obstet. 1950; 91:193–200.
131. Yu JS, Resnick D. MR imaging of the accessory soleus muscle appearance in six patients and review of the literature. Skeletal Radiol. 1994; 23:525–528.
132. Yu JS, Witte D, Resnick D, Pogue W. Ossification of the Achilles tendon. Imaging abnormalities in 12 patients. Skeletal Radiol. 1994; 23:127–131.
133. Zanetti M, DeSimoni C, Wetz HH, Zollinger H, Hodler J. Magnetic resonance imaging of injuries to the ankle joint. Can it predict clinical outcome? Skeletal Radiol. 1997; 26:82–88.

Radiology of the Foot and Ankle, Second Edition,
edited by Thomas H. Berquist.
© 2000 by Mayo Foundation.
Published by Lippincott Williams & Wilkins, Philadelphia.

CHAPTER 4

Fractures/Dislocations

Thomas H. Berquist

INTRODUCTION TO FRACTURES

Management of foot and ankle fractures is a common problem for orthopedic surgeons, emergency room physicians, family practice physicians, and radiologists. Appropriate use of imaging techniques is important in today's cost-conscious environment. Clinical algorithms have been developed in an attempt to reduce unnecessary imaging of foot and ankle injuries.[2,3,9,10,11,24] For example, the Ottawa ankle rules were instituted to reduce costs of ankle radiographs. Ninety percent of ankle injuries are radiographed, but the fracture detection yield is less than 15%.[24] Application of the Ottawa ankle rules (pain over one or both malleoli and one or more of the following: (1) patient 55 years old or older; (2) inability to bear weight; and (3) bone tenderness at malleolar tip) before ordering radiographs may reduce costs in treating ankle injuries by 16 to 22%.[11,24]

Identification of most fractures radiographically is not complex. However, detection of subtle fractures and evaluating the extent of soft tissue injury may be more difficult. Thus, it is essential for those interpreting images to be aware of the manner in which various fractures and soft tissue injuries present so the images can be correctly and thoroughly evaluated. Soft tissue changes may be the only clue to a

subtle fracture or ligament rupture. Soft tissue swelling, obliteration of the fat planes or pre-Achilles fat triangle, and the presence of an effusion can be useful in identifying the location of subtle fractures (Fig. 4-1).[18,23]

It is also important to understand the clinical significance of certain fracture patterns. Fractures may be complete (involve both cortices) or incomplete (one cortex fractured). The latter are more common in children. Fractures may be comminuted (multiple fragments) or compound (open).[1,9,18]

Terms other than complete or incomplete are also used in describing fractures. Avulsion fractures occur at the insertion of ligaments or tendons. Compression is a term usually reserved for vertebral fractures, but it can also be used to describe talar or calcaneal fractures.[18] Pathologic fractures involve bone with underlying abnormality such as osteoporosis or neoplasm. Stress fractures occur in normal bone that is exposed to unusual stress. The metatarsals in military recruits and the tibia and fibula in long-distance runners are commonly involved.[1,12,18] An insufficiency fracture is a category of stress fracture that occurs in abnormal bone under normal stress. This may occur in a patient with rheumatoid arthritis who becomes active too soon after joint arthroplasty.[15,18] Certain eponyms have been applied to many injuries about the foot and ankle.[3–6,13,14,16,20,22] These terms are frequently used, especially by orthopedists, and it is important to understand what they imply. However,

T. H. Berquist: Mayo Medical School, Mayo Clinic Jacksonville, Jacksonville, Florida 32224; Mayo Foundation, Mayo Clinic, Rochester, Minnesota 55905.

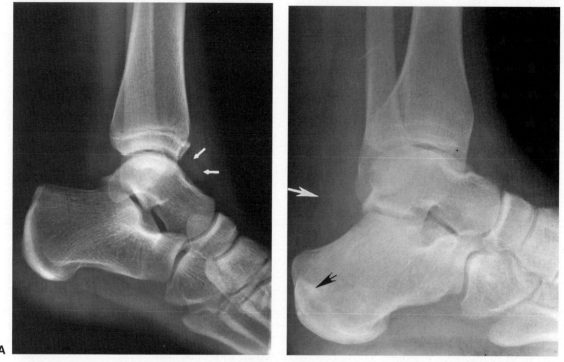

FIG. 4-1. Soft tissue findings with subtle injuries. **A:** Lateral radiograph demonstrates an effusion anteriorly with the tear drop sign (*white arrows*). **B:** Lateral radiograph demonstrating edema (*white arrow*) in the pre-Achilles fat resulting from a subtle calcaneal fracture (*black arrow*).

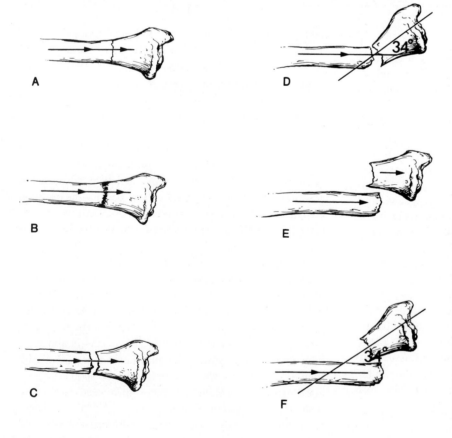

FIG. 4-2. Illustration of fractures and descriptive terms. **A:** Undisplaced complete fracture with normal alignment. No angulation or shortening. **B:** Impacted fracture with trabecular compression. Minimal shortening, no angulation. **C:** Distracted fracture with separation of fragments but normal alignment and no angulation. **D:** Complete fracture with dorsal displacement of the distal fragment or 34° volar angulation. **E:** Complete fracture with dorsal displacement and no angulation. **F:** Complete fracture with no apposition. One sees shortening and 34° of angulation.

TABLE 4-1. *Fractures of the foot and ankle*

Eponym or descriptive term	Definition
Aviator's astragalus	Fractures and fracture dislocations of the talus (Fig. 4-4) (20)
Bosworth's fracture	Fracture of the distal fibula with locking of the proximal fibular fragment behind the tibia (1,2,11,16)
Chopart's fracture dislocation	Injury involving the midtarsal (talonavicular and calcaneocuboid) joints (Fig. 4-5) (20)
Cotton's fracture	Trimalleolar fracture with the posterior tibial fragment posteriorly and superiorly displaced; medial malleolar fracture line continuing posteriorly and separating the posterior tibia; usually fibular fracture above the joint level; certain physicians refer to the posterior tibial fracture as Cotton's fracture (Fig. 4-6) (1,4–8,20)
Dupuytren's fracture	
High	Fracture of the fibular shaft above the ankle with rupture of the interosseous membrane and distal tibiofibular ligaments; lateral talar shift with medial malleolar fracture or deltoid ligament tear (Fig. 4-7A) (1,20)
Low	Fracture of the fibula near the ankle joint with rupture of the anterior tibiofibular ligament or anterior tibial avulsion and medial malleolar fracture or deltoid ligament rupture (Fig. 4-7B) (20)
Gosselin's fracture	"V"-shaped fracture of the distal tibia that may enter the tibial plafond (Fig. 4-8) (20)
Green-stick fracture	Incomplete fracture involving one cortex with angulation and bowing (20)
Jones fracture	Fracture of the fifth metatarsal approximately ¾ inch distal to the tuberosity (Fig. 4-3) (9–11,21)
LeFort's fracture	Vertical fracture of the anteromedial distal fibula owing to anterior tibiofibular ligament avulsion (Fig. 4-9) (20)
Lisfranc's fracture dislocation	Any of a variety of fracture dislocations of the tarsometatarsal joints (Fig. 4-10) (20)
Maisonneuve's fracture	Fracture of the proximal fibula near the head with rupture of the interosseous membrane and distal tibiofibular syndesmosis; there is usually an associated deltoid ligament tear or medial malleolar fracture (Fig. 4-11) (1,23)
March fracture	Stress fracture of the metatarsal commonly seen in military recruits (Fig. 4-12) (1,20)
Pilon fracture	Comminuted fracture of the tibial plafond (8,15)
Pott's fracture	Fracture of the fibula 2 to 3 inches above the ankle with rupture of the deltoid ligament (or avulsion of the medial malleolus) and tibiofibular syndesmosis (Fig. 4-13) (1,20)
Shepherd's fracture	Fracture of the lateral tubercle of the posterior talar process; may be confused with os trigonum (Fig. 4-14) (1,20)
Tillaux's fracture	Fracture of the distal tibial articular surface; may involve anterior or posterior tubercle; usually triad of (a) deltoid rupture or medial malleolar avulsion, (b) fibular fracture 5 to 6 cm above the ankle joint; and (c) avulsion of tibial tubercles with diastasis of syndesmosis (1,20)
Juvenile Tillaux's fracture	Salter-Harris III fracture of the lateral epiphysis; medial physis is closed; may separate because of distal tibiofibular ligament (Fig. 4-15)
Torus fracture	Incomplete fracture with buckling of the cortex (Fig. 4-16) (1,20)
Triplane fracture	Three fragment fracture with (a) tibial shaft, (b) anterolateral epiphyseal fragment, and (c) remaining epiphysis and posterior metaphyseal fragment with attached fibula (Fig. 4-17) (13,14,16)

eponyms can be confusing and inaccurately used (Figs. 4-3 to 4-17).[1,19,112] For example, the Jones fracture (Table 4-1) was originally described as a fracture of the proximal fifth metatarsal. However, radiographs were so poor at that time that the fracture site was not clear. Today, the term Jones fracture (see Fig. 4-3) is commonly used to describe a fracture distal to the tuberosity, a condition that is more difficult to treat than a tuberosity fracture.[1,7,8,19,21,23] The most commonly used eponyms are summarized in Table 4-1 (Figs. 4-3 to 4-17).

A systematic approach should be used when describing the imaging features of a fracture or fracture dislocation so the injury is completely assessed.[17,18] Eponyms can be confusing and should not be used without describing the associated fractures and soft tissue injury. The time, date, and views or imaging technique should be described first. This method makes it easier to keep examinations in chronologic

order. This is followed by a general description of the fracture location, orientation (transverse, oblique, spiral), degree of displacement, angulation, and alignment (see Fig. 4-18). Angulation can be described using the direction of the distal fragment or the apex of the fragments.[1,11] I prefer the latter method of describing angulation (Fig. 4-2).[1] Articular involvement, including the degree of separation or articular irregularity and the percentage of the articular surface involved, should be described. Soft tissue injury should also be carefully described (see Fig. 4-2).[1,17]

After the interpretation of available images, one should suggest further techniques that may assist in more clearly defining the injury. Postreduction (closed or open) images should be clearly labeled chronologically because more than one film may be taken during manipulation (Fig. 4-18). Position of fragments should be carefully assessed using the

(Text continues on page 180)

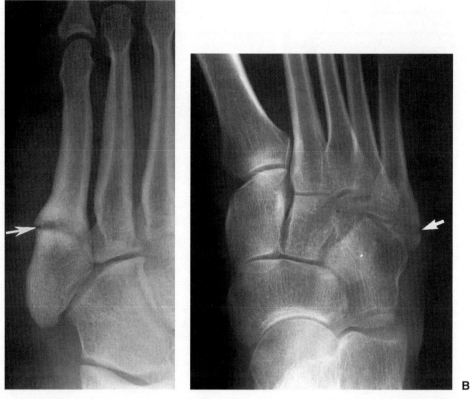

A   B

FIG. 4-3. **A:** United Jones fracture (*arrow*). **B:** Typical proximal avulsion fracture (*arrow*) for comparison.

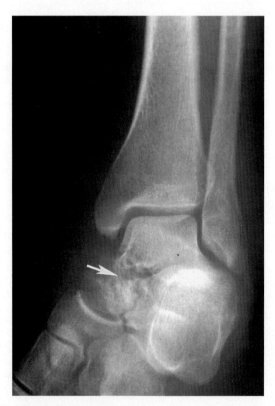

FIG. 4-4. Mortise view of the ankle demonstrating a comminuted talar neck fracture (*arrow*).

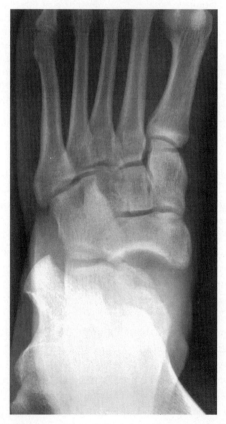

FIG. 4-5. AP view of the midfoot demonstrating a talonavicular fracture dislocation.

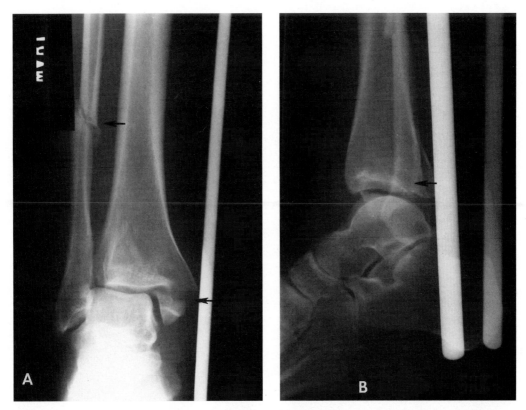

FIG. 4-6. Cotton's fracture. AP (**A**) and lateral (**B**) radiographs demonstrate a medial malleolar fracture (*arrow*) and displaced posterior tibial fracture (*arrow,* lateral view, **B**). Note the high fibular fracture (*upper arrow*) in **A**.

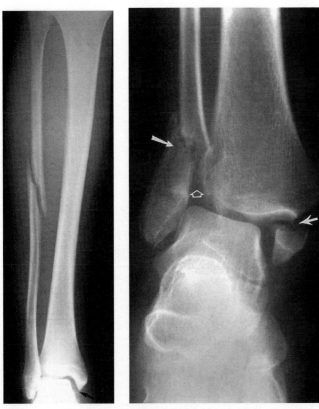

FIG. 4-7. Dupuytren's fracture. **A:** High fibular fracture with deltoid ligament rupture (*black arrow*). **B:** Low fibular fracture (*arrow*) with rupture of the tibiofibular ligaments (*open arrow*) and a medial malleolar fracture (*arrow*).

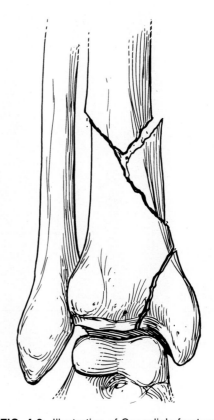

FIG. 4-8. Illustration of Gosselin's fracture.

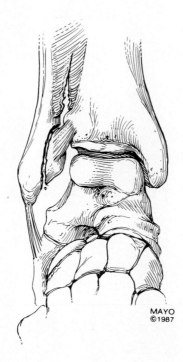

FIG. 4-9. Illustration of LeFort's fracture.

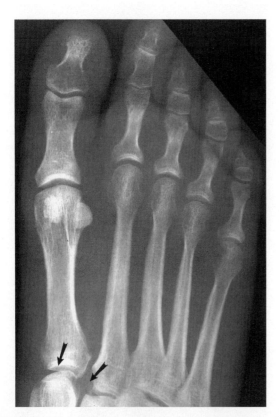

FIG. 4-10. AP radiograph of the foot demonstrating a fracture dislocation at the first to second tarsometatarsal joints (*arrows*).

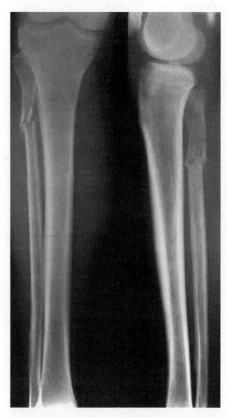

FIG. 4-11. Maisonneuve's fracture. High fibular fracture just below the proximal tibiofibular articulation. The ankle must also be imaged to detect the medial ligament disruption.

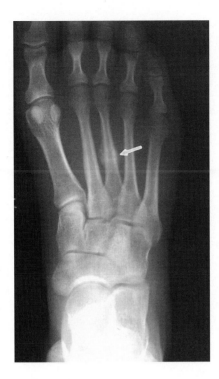
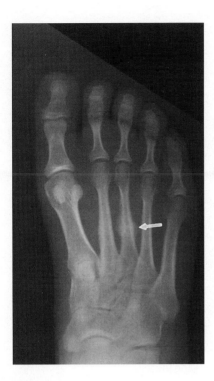

FIG. 4-12. March fracture. Metatarsal stress fracture (*arrow*).

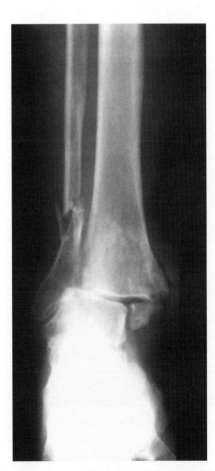

FIG. 4-13. Pott's fracture. Fracture of the fibula 2 to 3 inches above the joint with talar shift and medial malleolar avulsion.

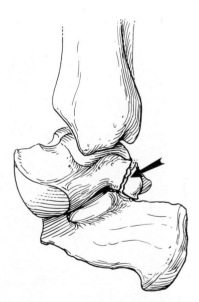

FIG. 4-14. Illustration of Shepherd's fracture (*arrow*). This can be difficult to distinguish from an os trigonum.

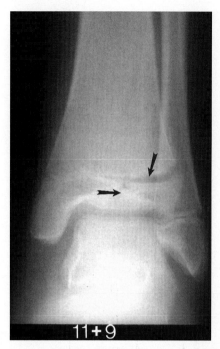

FIG. 4-15. AP radiograph of the ankle demonstrating juvenile Tillaux's fracture (*arrows*).

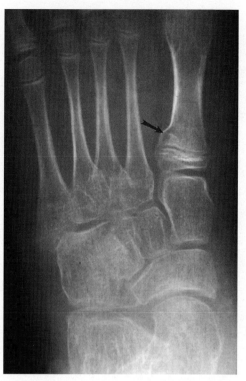

FIG. 4-16. AP radiograph of the foot demonstrating a torus fracture at the first metatarsal base (*arrow*).

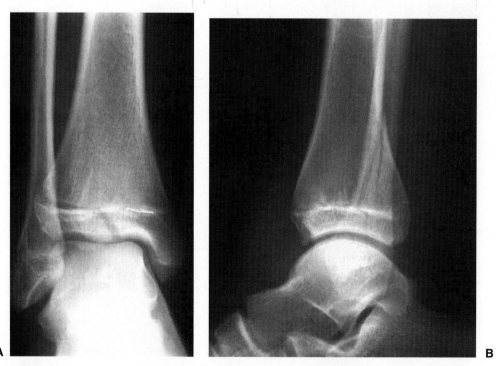

FIG. 4-17. AP (**A**) and lateral (**B**) radiographs demonstrate a triplane fracture. The fracture looks like a Salter-Harris III fracture on the AP view and a type II on the lateral view.

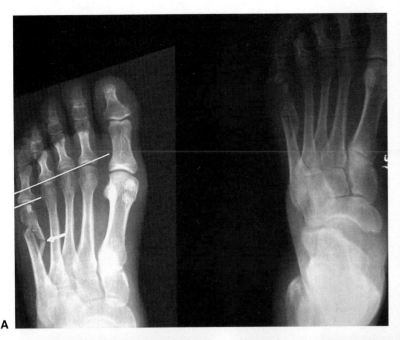
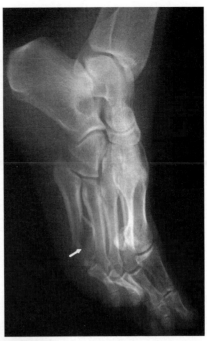
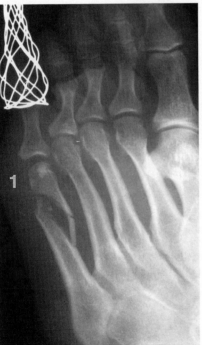
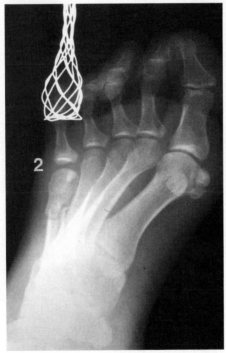

FIG. 4-18. Radiographs from initial diagnosis through treatment and healing of a metatarsal fracture. Initial interpretation: AP (**A**) and lateral (**B**) views of the left foot demonstrate a comminuted oblique fracture of the distal fifth metatarsal diaphysis (*arrow*). There is dorsomedial displacement of the major distal fragment and slight shortening (note the *line* on metatarsal heads). Films taken with traction show improvement in length with the change in traction between image *1* (**C**) and *2* (**D**). *(continued)*

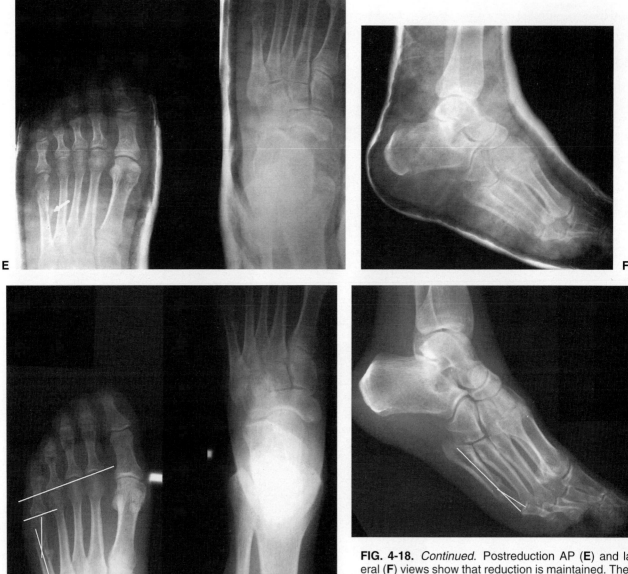

FIG. 4-18. *Continued.* Postreduction AP (**E**) and lateral (**F**) views show that reduction is maintained. There is a small medial fragment (*arrow*). Cast immobilization. AP (**G**) and lateral (**H**) views 5 months after injury show that the fracture has healed with slight angular deformity. Shortening of the fifth metatarsal (*lines* on metatarsal leads) persists.

same process applied to the original diagnostic studies. Joint space evaluation or failure to reduce a fracture with usual methods may indicate soft tissue interposition or osteochondral fragments, which prevent good position and alignment of fragments. Generally, these changes are evident to the physician reducing the fracture. If noted, after reduction one should suggest the best technique to demonstrate the problem.[17,18]

Discussion of specific foot and ankle fractures and fracture dislocations is most easily accomplished by using anatomic regions. Therefore, ankle, hindfoot, midfoot, and forefoot injuries are discussed separately. Both adult and pediatric disorders are included.

ANKLE FRACTURES

Ankle fractures may be simple or complex with associated ligament rupture[81,124]. The latter is more common in adults. Generally, fractures in patients oolder than 15 to 16 years of age are classified and treated using adult criteria. For discussion purposes, it is more effective to review adult and pediatric ankle injuries separately.

Pediatric Fractures

The appearance of ankle fractures in children depends on the age (growth plate development), relationship of the lig-

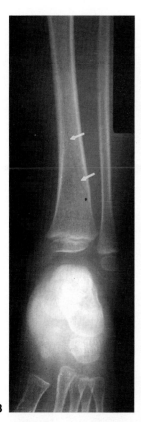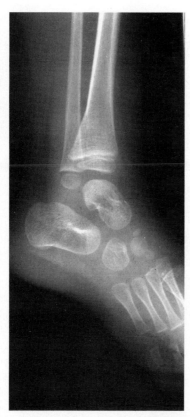

,B

FIG. 4-19. AP (**A**) and lateral (**B**) views of the ankle demonstrate a subtle undisplaced spiral fracture (*arrows*) that is only visible on the AP (**A**) view.

aments with the epiphysis, and mechanism of injury.[26,35,46] Distal diaphyseal and metaphyseal fractures are frequently incomplete. In most cases, there is a posterior cortical break with buckling (torus fracture) of the anterior cortex above the growth plate (Figs. 4-19 and 4-20).[33] Fractures of the distal tibia and fibula frequently involve the growth plates (Fig. 4-21). The distal tibia epiphysis is the second most common site for growth plate fracture.[47] In Rogers series,[52] 25% of 188 physeal injuries involved the distal tibia or fibula. Physeal fractures can result in growth or articular deformity if proper diagnosis and treatment are not implemented.[33,52]

There are two types of epiphysis. Pressure epiphyses are located in the ends of long bones and are subject to weight-bearing forces and forces acting on the joint. Traction epiphyses occur at sites of muscle or tendon insertions (i.e., greater and lesser trochanter). The latter are not directly associated with weight bearing.[52,53] The pressure epiphyses of the distal tibia and fibula contribute 45% and 40%, respectively, of the growth of the tibia and fibula. The proximal epiphysis of the tibia contributes 55%, and the proximal epiphysis of the fibula, 60%.[53] The distal tibial and fibular epiphyses appear at the age of 2 years. The tibial epiphysis fuses by age 15 in girls and by age 17 in boys. The fibular epiphysis remains open longer and fuses at age 20.[35]

Histologically, the growth plate is divided into four zones.

Progressing distally from the metaphysis, these zones include (1) the zone of provisional calcification, (2) the hypertrophic cartilage zone, (3) the proliferating zone, and (4) the resting zone (Fig. 4-22).[52,53] The cartilage cells are surrounded by longitudinally oriented collagen fibers and a chondroitin sulfate matrix. This substance is less abundant in the hypertrophic zone, a feature that at least partially explains why this zone is the most susceptible to fracture (see Fig. 4-22).[52,53] The blood supply to the epiphysis and metaphysis of the long bones is separate, with the exception of the proximal radial and femoral epiphysis. Therefore, when fracture of the growth plate occurs, the blood supply is generally not disrupted. This spares the proliferating zone, so normal growth can occur after healing.[57]

Fracture Classification and Mechanism of Injury

The same forces that cause fracture and ligament disruption in adults also cause fractures in children. In children, the growth plates are two to five times weaker than the ligaments, so fractures of the physis occur more commonly than ligament injuries.[38] The fracture patterns that evolve are thus related to age, the ligamentous attachments, and the type of force applied. All ligament structures about the ankle attach to the epiphyses, except the interosseous membrane and ligament.[31] Growth plate fractures are more common during the first year and during the rapid growth phases in early teens.[53] The growth plate fuses at different rates in males and females, and the method of closure in the distal tibia is important in understanding fracture patterns. Fusion of the distal tibial epiphysis begins at age 12 in girls and at age 13 in boys. Fusion does not occur symmetrically. Closure of the growth plate occurs over a period of approximately 18 months (Fig. 4-23). The process begins centrally with the medial portion of the physis closing before the lateral portions. The medial fused portion becomes less susceptible to fracture than the lateral physis, a situation that results in the juvenile Tillaux's and triplane fracture patterns seen in patients of this age group.[43,47]

Most growth plate fractures are secondary to varus, valgus, shearing, or crushing forces that lead to opening, shifting, or compression of the physis.[27,35,39,52,53] The physis is involved in half of tibial fractures and in about 75% of fibular fractures.[48]

The most commonly used classification of physeal injuries was described by Salter and Harris (Fig. 4-24).[53] This classification is useful because of its prognostic significance and easy-to-use radiographic patterns.[46,47,53] Type I fractures are caused by separation of the epiphysis with the fracture line confined to the growth plate. The fracture usually extends through the hypertrophic zone and does not involve the epiphysis or metaphysis.[53] In Rogers series of 118 physeal fractures, 6% were type I.[52] This type of injury may be subtle radiographically. Comparison radiographs of the uninjured ankle may be helpful (Figs. 4-25 and 4-26). Type I injuries

(Text continues on page 186)

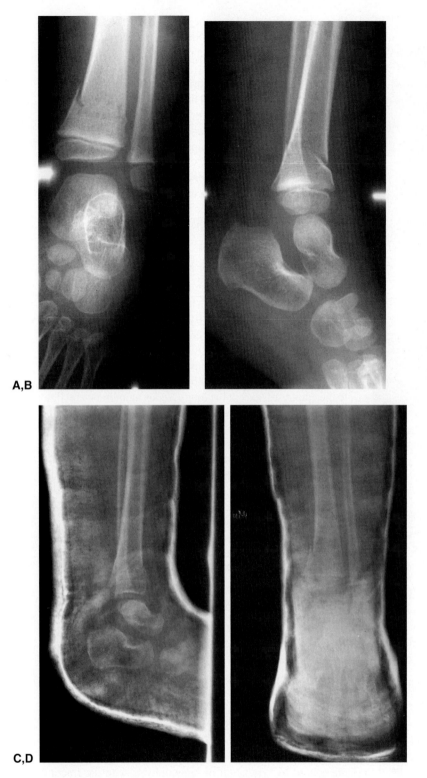

A,B

C,D

FIG. 4-20. AP (**A**) view of the ankle demonstrates a complete cortical back medially with buckling of the lateral cortex. The lateral view (**B**) shows buckling anteriorly. AP (**C**) and lateral (**D**) radiographs taken with cast immobilization, which is the usual treatment for this injury.

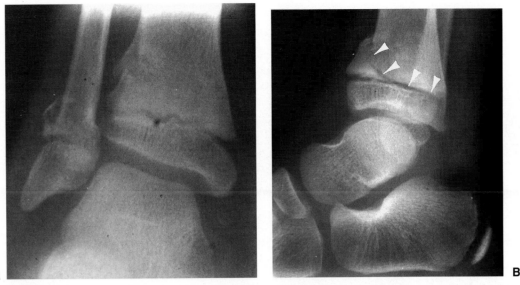

FIG. 4-21. AP (**A**) and lateral (**B**) radiographs of the ankle demonstrate Salter-Harris II fractures of the tibia and fibula. The *arrowheads* in **B** demonstrate the fracture entering the physis.

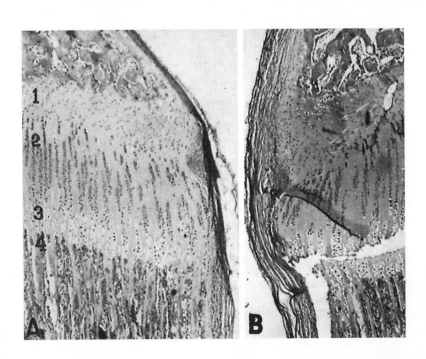

FIG. 4-22. A: Normal physis in rabbit. *1,* resting zone; *2,* proliferating zone; *3,* hypertrophic zone; *4,* zone of provisional calcification. **B:** Fracture experimentally produced through the hypertrophic zone. (From Rogers, ref. 52, with permission.)

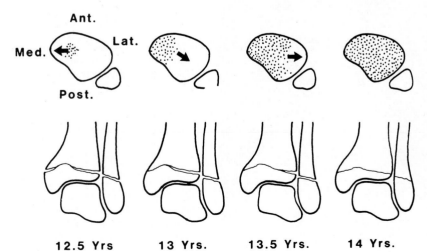

12.5 Yrs   13 Yrs.   13.5 Yrs.   14 Yrs.

FIG. 4-23. Illustration of growth plate closure in the distal tibia. Fusion occurs asymmetrically medially to laterally. (From MacNealy et al., ref. 47, with permission.)

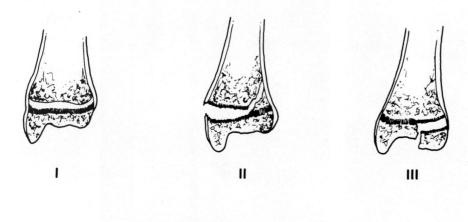

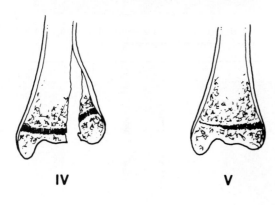

FIG. 4-24. Illustration of the five types of growth plate fracture described by Salter and Harris.

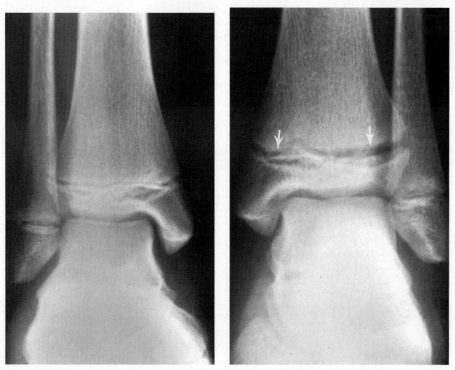

FIG. 4-25. AP radiographs of the normal right (**A**) and injured left (**B**) ankles. Note the growth plate widening on the left (*arrows*) resulting from a Salter-Harris I fracture.

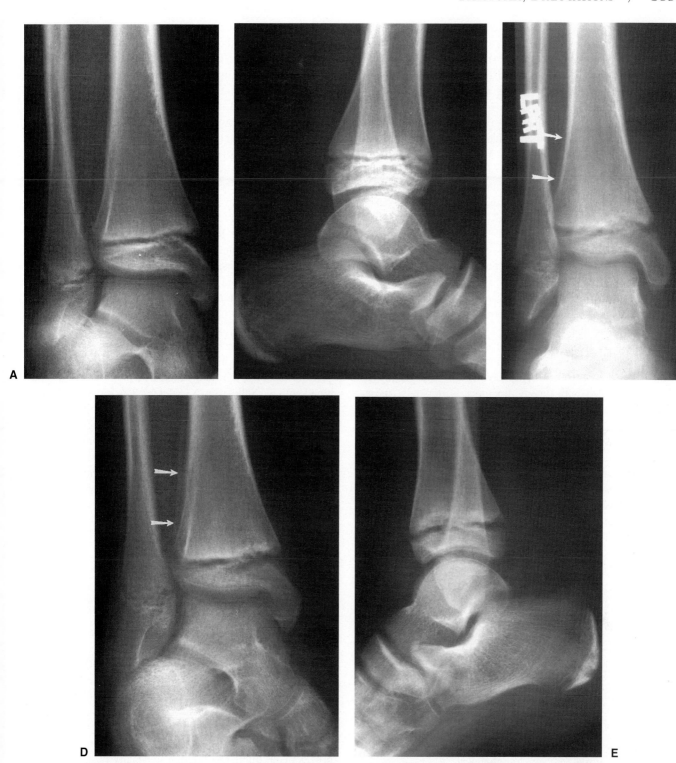

FIG. 4-26. Mortise (**A**) and lateral (**B**) radiographs of the injured right ankle. Is there widening of the tibial physis? AP (**C**), mortise (**D**), and lateral (**E**) views 3 weeks later show a healing Salter-Harris I fracture of the tibia with irregularity of the growth plate and periosteal new bone (*arrows*) along the tibia.

tend to occur more commonly in children less than 5 years of age. The prognosis is generally excellent.[31,53]

Type II fractures (see Fig. 4-24) are the most common, (75% in Rogers series).[52] Type II fractures extend through the growth plate for a variable distance before exiting through the metaphysis.[53] Type II fractures occur more commonly in patients older than 10 years of age. Eversion or inversion injuries with forced abduction or adduction of the foot have been implicated in this ankle fracture.[31,53]

Type III fractures (see Fig. 4-24) are intraarticular, extending through the epiphysis and entering the growth plate, where they exit through the hypertrophic zone. The metaphysis is spared.[53] This injury is usually caused by an intraarticular shearing force.

Type IV fractures (see Fig. 4-24) extend from the articular surface of the epiphysis through the growth plate and exit through the metaphysis. Complete reduction of this fracture is essential to prevent growth disturbances. This fracture type makes up 10% of Salter-Harris fractures and is most common in the distal humerus.[53]

Type V fractures (see Fig. 4-24) are the result of compression injuries that cause impaction of the growth plate. The ankle and knee are commonly involved.[53] The prognosis is more guarded with type V fractures. Fortunately, these fractures are uncommon (1% of 118 fractures in Rogers' series).[52]

Other classifications have also been applied to growth plate fractures.[28,32,33,47,52] Bishop[25] classified pediatric ankle injuries according to the direction of the force producing the injury. Crenshaw[32] proposed a similar classification that is frequently used because of its simplicity. Injuries were categorized according to forces applied: external rotation, abduction, adduction, plantar flexion, and direct violence. The incidence and radiographic appearance of these injuries are summarized in Table 4-2. Using this approach, the pattern

of injury can be used to reduce fractures gently. Fractures are reduced by gently reversing the direction of the mechanism of injury as noted radiographically.[32]

External rotation injuries occur when the foot is supinated and subjected to external rotation forces. This stress leads to fracture of the posterolateral tibial physis (usually Salter-Harris II) and often a fracture of the fibula above the growth plate.[32,47] Abduction (eversion) injuries result in Salter-Harris I or II fractures of the anterolateral tibia (see Fig. 4-21). The direction of stress and of talar shift usually displaces the fragment laterally. Talar forces may lead to associated fibular fractures.[32,49] Adduction forces are similar to inversion injuries placing tension on the lateral ligament complex. This results in avulsion or distal fibular physeal fractures. The force, if continued, causes impaction of the talus against the medial malleolus, leading to a Salter-Harris III or IV fracture of the medial malleolus (Fig. 4-27). Plantar-flexion injuries lead to posterior epiphyseal injuries. By definition, there is no external rotation force, and therefore no associated fibular fracture is evident (Fig. 4-28).[32] The Crenshaw fracture patterns are most common during the twelfth year, with a significantly higher incidence in males.[32,47]

More recently, the Lauge-Hansen system has been combined with the Salter-Harris system.[34] The former is an accurate method commonly applied to adult ankle injuries.[44] Dias and Tachdjian[34] studied 71 patients using their combined classification system, and only 4 patients (5.6%) did not properly fit their categories. This classification, like the Lauge-Hansen system, is based on the position of the foot during the injury and the direction of the abnormal force (see Fig. 4-28).

Two stages of injury are described with supination-inversion fractures (Fig. 4-29A to C) (Table 4-3).[34,38] If an inversion force is applied with the foot supinated a Salter-Harris I or II of the distal fibula, rarely a lateral ligament injury (mimics Lauge-Hansen supination-abduction stage I in adults) occurs (Fig. 4-30).[44] This injury comprised 39% of cases in the series of Dias and Tachdjian series.[34] If the force continues, the talus will impact medially, producing a Salter-Harris III or IV fracture of the medial malleolus (mimics Lauge-Hansen supination-adduction stage II) (Fig. 4-31).[34] This injury accounted for 22.5% of ankle injuries. Therefore, supination inversion injuries combined accounted for 61% of ankle injuries.[33–35,38]

Supination–plantar-flexion injuries (see Fig. 4-29D and Table 4-4) generally lead to Salter-Harris II fractures of the posterodistal tibia. The fracture is usually best seen on the lateral view (see Fig. 4-28). No matching Lauge-Hansen pattern exists for this fracture.

Two stages of injury are also described with supination–external rotation fractures (see Fig. 4-29E).[34,38] Initially, a Salter-Harris II fracture of the distal tibia occurs. This fracture has a spiral component extending proximally into the tibia. Differentiation from a supination–plantar-flexion injury is most easily accomplished on the anteroposterior (AP) view as the spiral fracture can be seen extending lat-

TABLE 4-2. *Pediatric ankle fractures: Crenshaw classification[a]*

Type	Appearance	Incidence[b]
External rotation	Salter-Harris II of tibia with posterior metaphyseal fragment; associated fibular fracture common; juvenile Tillaux's triplane	39.7%
Abduction	Salter-Harris I or II, anterolateral metaphyseal fragment with type II; distal fibular shaft fracture may be associated	14.2%
Plantar flexion	Posterior displacement of epiphysis or metaphyseal fragment; no fibular fracture	18.6%
Adduction	Avulsion of fibular tip or physeal fracture; Salter-Harris III or IV of medial malleolus	22.1%

[a] Data from references 32 and 52.
[b] Total <100%; approximately 5% did not fit categories.

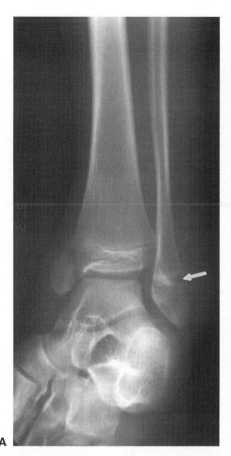 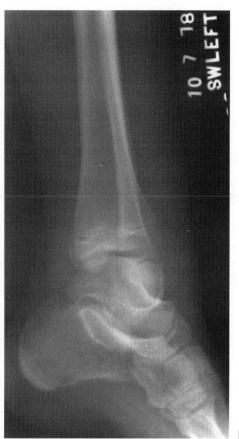

FIG. 4-27. Mortise (**A**) and external oblique (**B**) views of the ankle demonstrating a Salter-Harris IV medial malleolar fracture and a Salter-Harris I fracture (*arrow*) of the fibular growth plate.

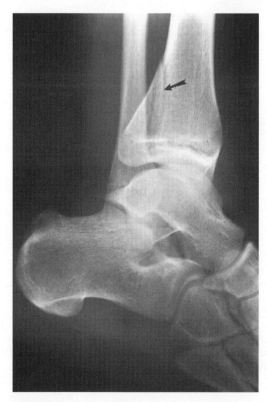

FIG. 4-28. Lateral view of the ankle demonstrating a Salter-Harris II fracture of the posterior tibia (*arrow*) resulting from a plantar-flexion injury.

TABLE 4-3. *Ankle growth plate fractures in children: Dias-Tachdjian classification[a]*

Supination–inversion	
Stage I	Traction on lateral ligaments leads to Salter-Harris I or II of fibula, rarely ligament tear or avulsion fracture of the fibula occurs (Figs. 4-29A and 4-30).
Stage II	Greater inversion force leads to Salter-Harris III or IV of the medial tibia in addition to stage I changes (Figs. 4-29C and 4-31)
Supination–plantar flexion	Salter-Harris I or II of distal tibia; metaphyseal fragment best seen on the lateral view (Figs. 4-29D and 4-28)
Supination–external rotation	
Stage I	Salter-Harris II of distal tibia with spiral component similar to supination–plantar flexion (Fig. 4-29E)
Stage II	Grade I plus spiral fibular fracture above the growth plate (Figs. 4-29E and 4-32)
Pronation–eversion–external rotation	Tibial and fibular physes fracture simultaneously Salter-Harris II of the tibia with fibular fracture above the growth plate (5 to 6 cm) (Figs. 4-29F and 4-33)

[a] Data from references 33 to 35 and 44.

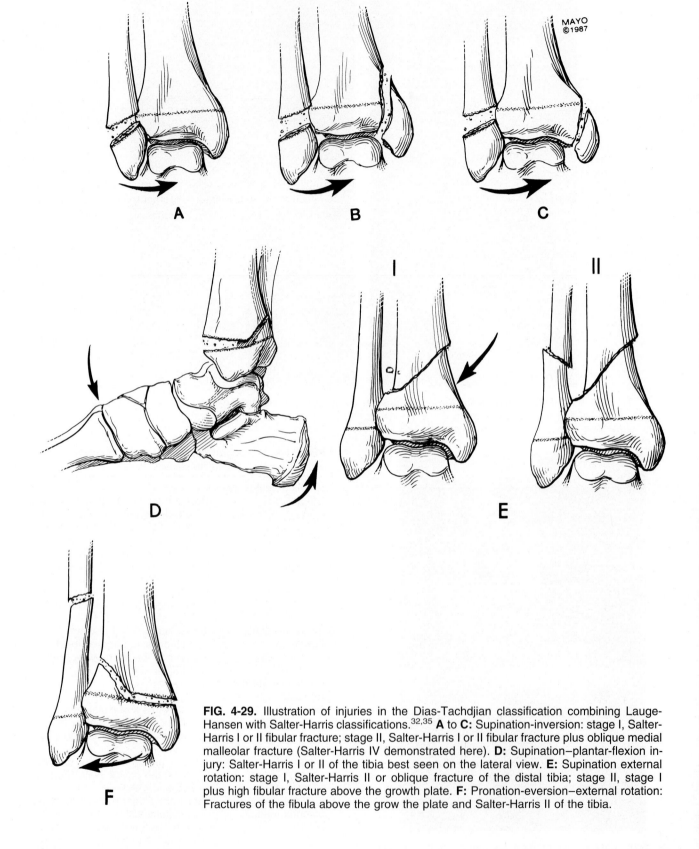

FIG. 4-29. Illustration of injuries in the Dias-Tachdjian classification combining Lauge-Hansen with Salter-Harris classifications.[32,35] **A** to **C:** Supination-inversion: stage I, Salter-Harris I or II fibular fracture; stage II, Salter-Harris I or II fibular fracture plus oblique medial malleolar fracture (Salter-Harris IV demonstrated here). **D:** Supination–plantar-flexion injury: Salter-Harris I or II of the tibia best seen on the lateral view. **E:** Supination external rotation: stage I, Salter-Harris II or oblique fracture of the distal tibia; stage II, stage I plus high fibular fracture above the growth plate. **F:** Pronation-eversion–external rotation: Fractures of the fibula above the grow the plate and Salter-Harris II of the tibia.

FRACTURES/DISLOCATIONS / 189

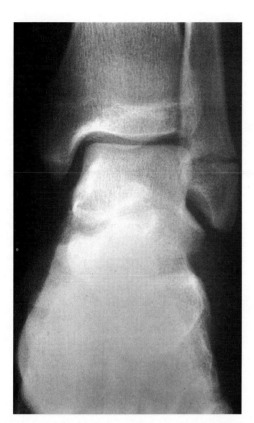

FIG. 4-30. AP view of the left ankle demonstrating a fracture through the fibular growth plate in an adolescent. The tibial growth plate is nearly fused.

TABLE 4-4. *Pediatric ankle fractures: indications for open reductions^a*

Open Fractures
Inability to obtain reduction
Inability to maintain reduction
Displaced physeal fractures
Articular fractures
Extensive soft tissue injury

^{a} Data from references 32, 45, 51, and 55.

erally to medially.[34] If the force continues, the second stage, a fibular fracture, occurs above the growth plate (Fig. 4-32).

When pronation-eversion–external rotation forces are applied to the foot and ankle, simultaneous fractures develop in the tibial and fibular physis. A lateral Salter-Harris II fracture of the tibia is usually noted along with a fibular fracture that is 5 to 7 cm above the growth plate (Fig. 4-33).[34,38] This fracture is similar to the stage III Lauge-Hansen pronation–lateral rotation injury. This injury accounts for approximately 18% of pediatric ankle fractures.[39]

Several ankle fractures do not fit into this classification. A Salter-Harris III of the distal tibia is usually caused by external rotation forces. This fracture is generally seen in the lateral portion of the tibia.[40] Triplane fractures do not fit the original Dias-Tachdjian classification (Fig. 4-34). This fracture was described by Marmor in 1970,[49] and it has subsequently been reported by other authors.[29,41,46,51] The injury

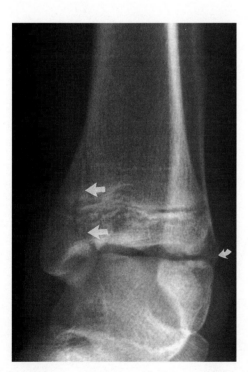

FIG. 4-31. Oblique view of the ankle demonstrating a Salter-Harris IV fracture medially (*arrows*) and a Salter-Harris II (*curved arrow*) of the fibular growth plate. Supination–inversion stage II.

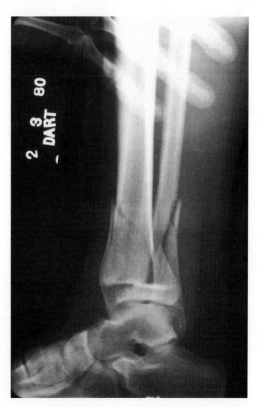

FIG. 4-32. Lateral view of the ankle demonstrating a stage II supination–external rotation injury.

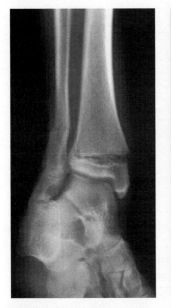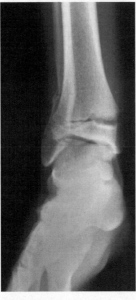

FIG. 4-33. Oblique view of the ankle demonstrating a pronation-eversion–external rotation injury with a Salter-Harris II fracture of the tibia and a high fibular fracture.

is believed to be caused by external rotation with or without associated plantar flexion.[29,38] The fracture consists of three fragments instead of the two fragments seen with most growth plate fractures. The first fragment involves the anterolateral portion of the tibial epiphysis and looks like a Salter-Harris III injury. The second fragment is the remainder of the tibial epiphysis with the metaphyseal attachment. The third fragment is the tibial metaphysis.[29,33,49,51] The fracture has a characteristic radiographic appearance. On the AP view, it has the appearance of a Salter-Harris III fracture, and on the lateral view, it resembles a Salter-Harris II fracture of the distal tibia (see Fig. 4-17).[50] Triplane fractures are not uncommon. Cooperman and associates[30] noted an incidence of 6% in a series of 237 patients with epiphyseal fractures of the ankle. However, because of increased awareness of this injury, more recent studies report an incidence of up to 17%.[51] In reality, the fracture behaves like a Salter-Harris IV, and since its original description, many authors believe that it is often only a two-part fracture.[42] The medial malleolus and anteromedial portion of the epiphysis remain attached to the tibial metaphysis and form one fragment. The

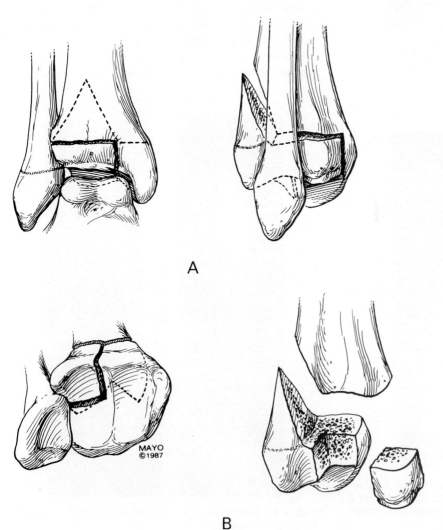

A

B

MAYO ©1987

FIG. 4-34. Illustration of the three-part (triplane) fracture. **A:** AP and lateral. **B:** Axial and separated.

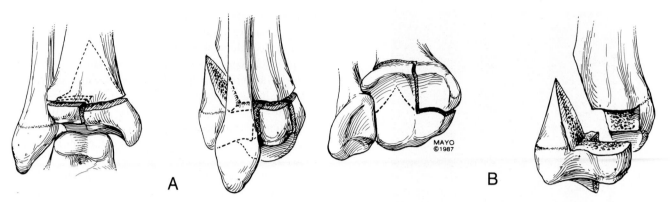

FIG. 4-35. Illustration of a two-part to triplane fracture. **A:** AP and lateral. **B:** Axial and separated.

second fragment is the lateral portion of the epiphysis with the lateral metaphyseal attachment.[25,44] Other variations of the triplane fracture have also been described (Fig. 4-35).[29]

The so-called juvenile Tillaux's fracture is a Salter-Harris III fracture of the distal lateral tibia.[35,53,55] The fragment is displaced by the distal tibiofibular ligaments when the foot is externally rotated (Fig. 4-36). This injury does not clearly fit into the categories of injury described by Dias and Tachdjian.[34] It was not originally included in Crenshaw's classification, but it could be placed in the external rotation category.[32,48]

Radiographic Evaluation

Most epiphyseal injuries can be clearly defined using the routine ankle trauma series AP, lateral, and mortise views.[54]

In most cases, the entire tibia and fibula should be included on the films so a high fibular fracture is not overlooked. Fractures of the fibular physis, the most common ankle fracture, may be subtle (see Figs. 4-25 and 4-26).[34] Usually, Salter-Harris I or, more commonly, II fractures are best seen on the mortise view. When the foot is internally rotated 15° to 20°, the fibula is viewed clear of the tibia. However, this fracture should be suspected in any child with swelling and point tenderness over the growth plate. When no other fractures are evident (supination-inversion grade I, see Table 4-3), the patient can be splinted, and a repeat study in 10 to 14 days often demonstrates the fracture line more clearly. Slight periosteal callus may also be evident at this time (Figs. 4-37 and 4-38). Ligament injury is much less common in children compared with adults. Salter-Harris I and II fractures of the distal tibia may also present with subtle radio-

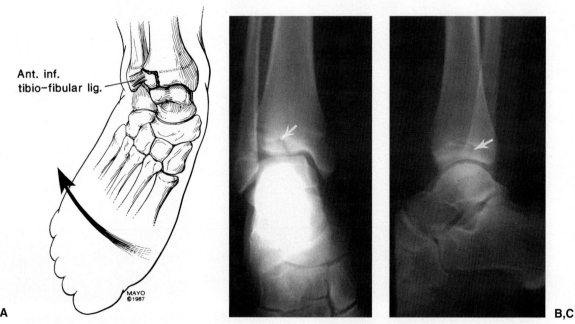

Ant. inf.
tibio–fibular lig.

FIG. 4-36. A: Illustration of juvenile Tillaux's fracture. A Salter-Harris III fracture of the lateral tibial epiphysis. AP (**B**) and lateral (**C**) views of juvenile Tillaux's fracture (*arrow*).

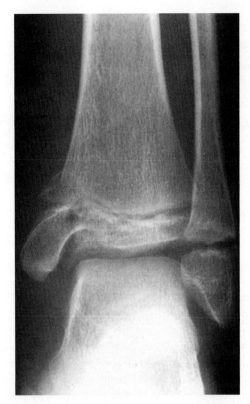

FIG. 4-37. AP view of the ankle with a Salter-Harris IV medially and a Salter-Harris I of the fibular supination-inversion stage II.

graphic findings. Comparison views (see Figs. 4-25 and 4-26) on an approach similar to the one described earlier can be used to evaluate these fractures.

More complex physeal injuries, especially triplane fractures or comminuted epiphyseal fractures, can be better evaluated using computed tomography (CT) (Fig. 4-39) or magnetic resonance imaging (MRI).[29,36,45,55] MRI using T2-weighted sequences is especially useful to detect subtle physeal fractures. The healing phases can also be followed with MRI. These techniques clearly demonstrate the epiphyseal fragmentation and distal tibiofibular relationships. As in adults, it is important to define the degree of articular involvement, to note any articular irregularity, and clearly to define the degree of separation of the fracture fragments. Displacement of the physis or fracture fragments by more than 2 mm has significant treatment implications.[30,32,33,41,55]

Treatment

Proper application of the classifications of ankle injuries will assist in determining the mechanism of injury. This knowledge permits gentle reduction, generally achieved by reversing the forces that caused the injury.[33] I prefer the Dias-Tachdjian classification because it is similar to the Lauge-Hansen system that is so useful in adults. By using similar classifications for children and adults, it is easier to maintain a consistent approach to ankle injuries. Using these classifications, the injury is more completely evaluated, and multiple injuries are less likely to be overlooked. For exam-

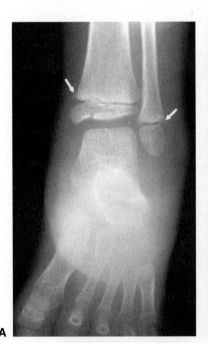
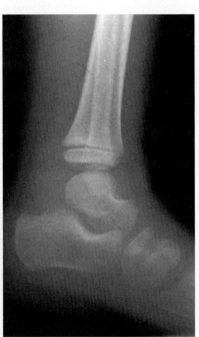
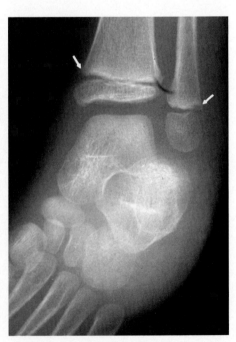

A   B,C

FIG. 4-38. Young child with an ankle injury. AP (**A**), lateral (**B**) and mortise (**C**) views show a Salter-Harris IV medially and a Salter-Harris II of the fibula. Note the small metaphyseal fragments (*arrows*). There is also marked swelling and an effusion.

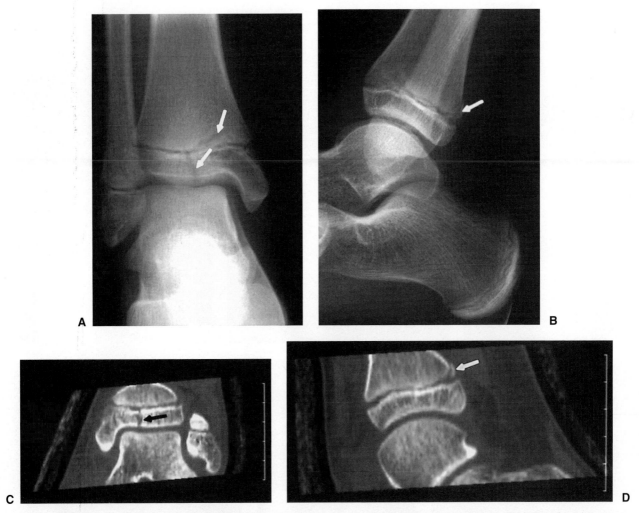

FIG. 4-39. AP (**A**) and lateral (**B**) radiographs demonstrate a triplane fracture (*arrows*). The tibial fragment on the lateral view (*arrow*) is subtle. Coronal (**C**) and sagittal (**D**) CT images clearly define the physes and the degree of displacement.

ple, when a Salter-Harris III or IV fracture of the medial malleolus is present, there is a ligament tear, an avulsion fracture, or a Salter-Harris I or II fracture of the fibula (see Fig. 4-37).[33,34,53]

Fractures involving the growth plates should be reduced gently to avoid increasing the damage to the growth plate. The treatment can usually be accomplished with closed techniques and casting, but there are exceptions. Considerations include the patient's age, the type of injury (use of classifications important in assessing mechanism of injury and prognosis), and the degree of displacement.

Most Salter-Harris I and II injuries of the distal tibia and fibula can be treated with closed reduction (Fig. 4-40). Fibular fractures are treated with a short leg walking cast for 4 weeks. Tibial fractures are treated with a long leg cast for 3 weeks followed by a short leg walking cast for an additional 3 weeks.[32,33,37,56] Occasionally, reduction cannot be achieved or maintained. Soft tissue or periosteum may become trapped between the fragments, or ligament traction

may make it difficult to maintain reduction. Open or percutaneous K-wire or cannulated screw fixation may be needed in this setting (Fig. 4-41).[32] Following cast removal, radiographs should be repeated to be certain that healing is progressing normally. AP, lateral, and mortise views are generally sufficient. However, unlike the original diagnostic films, the AP and lateral views should be taken in the standing position when the patient is allowed to bear weight. This series will serve as a baseline for possible growth plate complications and articular complications such as talar asymmetry or tilt.

Undisplaced Salter-Harris III and IV fractures may also be treated with closed reduction. However, the potential for deformity is greater.[32,56] Displacement of 2 mm or more or articular deformity is unacceptable and usually indicates the need for open reduction.[32,33,51,56] The incidence of growth plate deformities after healing of Salter-Harris III and IV fractures is approximately 14%.[33]

Tillaux's and triplane fractures are generally treated using

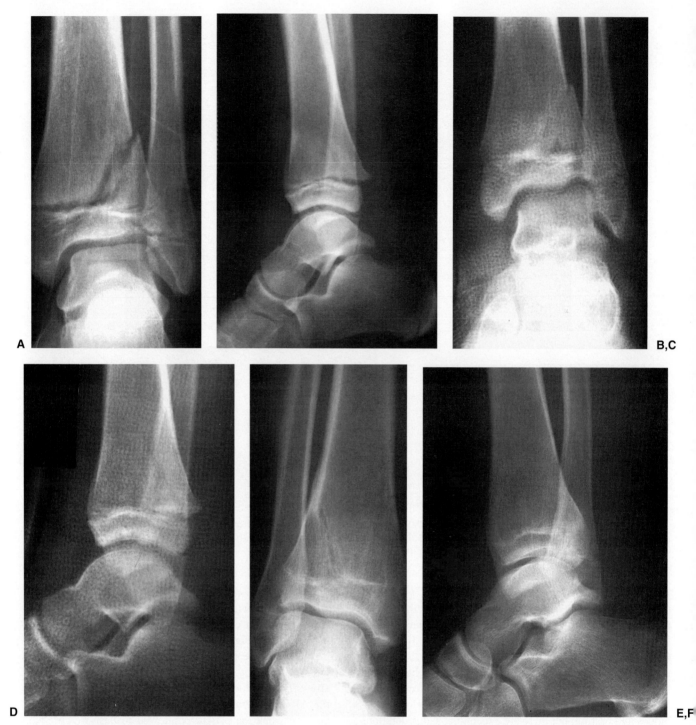

A

B,C

D

E,F

FIG. 4-40. AP (**A**) and lateral (**B**) views of a slightly displaced Salter-Harris II fracture of the tibia. AP (**C**) and lateral (**D**) views taken after reduction and cost immobilization show slightly improved position. AP (**E**) and lateral (**F**) radiographs 6 months later show a healed fracture with slight talar tilt.

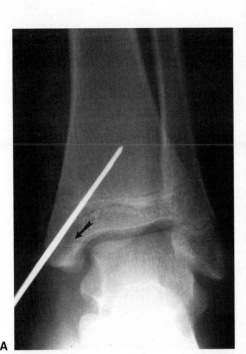
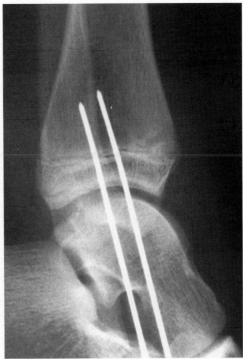

FIG. 4-41. AP (**A**) and lateral (**B**) views taken during K-wire fixation of a medial malleolar fracture (*arrow*). The reduction is excellent. The growth plate is almost fused. Therefore, instrumentation across the growth plate should not cause significant complications.

the approaches described earlier. The main difference is the potential for more complex articular involvement, especially with triplane fractures. If closed reduction is used, CT should be considered as a postreduction technique to be certain that fragments are optimally positioned.[28,32,36,43] If internal fixation is required, routine radiographs may provide the necessary information. Important considerations include fragment position, joint alignment, and confirmation that fixation devices do not cross the growth plate, especially in young children with years of growth remaining. Small-caliber K-wires can be put through the growth plate if they are not left in position too long, but screws and larger fixation devices can lead to early asymmetric growth plate healing (Fig. 4-42).[33]

Imaging of patients with internal fixation devices is more difficult. Conventional tomography is still useful when performed in two planes, usually AP and lateral. However, trispiral tomography may cause more metal artifact than linear tomography. Artifacts from metal on CT images may cause some degree of image degradation, especially in the ankle, where the metal is adjacent to the fracture line. Table 4-4 summarizes the indications for open reduction and internal fixation.[32,45,51,55]

Complications

The most common problem encountered after growth plate fractures is premature or asymmetric closure.[32,33,53] Fractures pass through the hypertrophic cartilage zone of the growth plate. If the blood supply is intact, healing can progress normally without affecting the growth potential. The fibrin that forms in the fracture line is typically resorbed in approximately 21 days.[52] Endochondral ossification continues normally after this process is completed, and healing is usually complete in 3 weeks.[53]

When the fracture line crosses the growth plate, Salter-Harris III and IV fractures, bone can form in the growth plate at the fracture site (see Fig. 4-42). Growth can progress on either side of the fracture, asymmetrically, or the growth plate can close.[53] Adequate reduction and the age of the patient obviously affect the degree of deformity that develops. Spiegel and colleagues[56] identified three groups of patients using the Salter-Harris classification (Table 4-5). The low-risk group (6.7% complications) included all type I and II fibular fractures, all type I tibial fractures, and type III and IV tibial fractures with more than 2 mm of displacement. The high-risk group included patients with type III and IV tibial fractures with more than 2 mm of displacement, juvenile Tillaux's fractures, triplane fractures, comminuted epiphyseal fractures, and type V fractures. The complication rate was 32% in this group. The third group was unpredictable. Type II tibial fractures were the only fractures included, and a complication rate of 16.7% was noted. Growth plate deformity caused by growth arrest may not be evident for 6 months to 1 year. Therefore, follow-up radiographs (standing AP and lateral preferred) are needed for at least 1 year to be certain that deformity has not developed.[32,56]

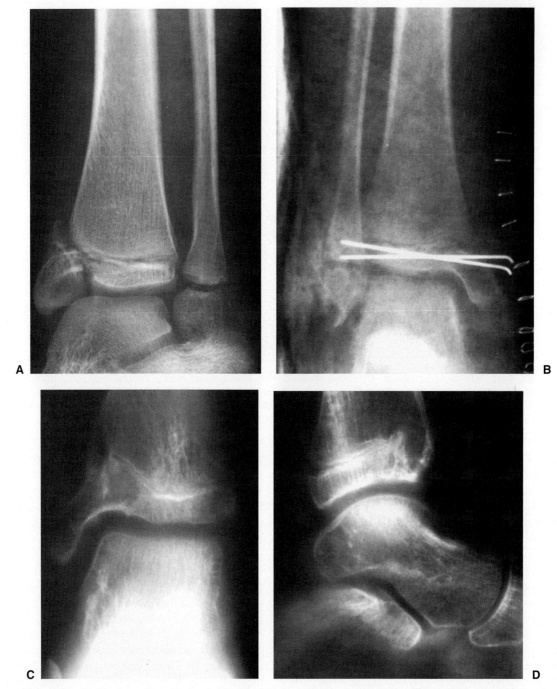

FIG. 4-42. A: Mortise view demonstrating a displaced Salter-Harris IV medial malleolar fracture and Salter-Harris I of the fibula. In this setting, K-wires can be used to reduce the fracture and crossing the growth plate is avoided (**B**). AP (**C**) and lateral (**D**) tomograms 6 months later show deformity and premature closure of the medial growth plate. Less than 50% of the growth plate was involved. *(continued)*

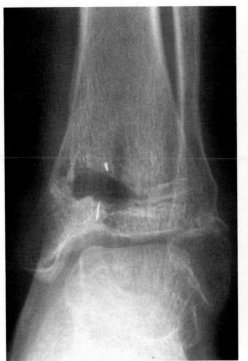 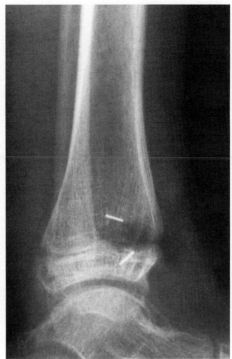

FIG. 4-42. *Continued.* AP (**E**) and lateral (**F**) radiographs after resection of the bony bar.

Deformities caused by growth plate fracture may lead to leg length discrepancy, or angular deformity (varus or valgus).[32,33,53,56] The type of deformity can be assessed on conventional ankle films (standing PA, lateral, and mortise views) and with leg length scanograms.

Excision of the osseous bar can be performed if less than 50% of the growth plate is involved (see Fig. 4-42E and F). If

TABLE 4-5. *Pediatric ankle fractures: incidence of complications[a]*

Patient group	Type of injury	Incidence of complications
Low risk	Salter-Harris I and II fibular fractures Salter-Harris I tibial fracture Salter Harris III and IV fractures <2 mm displacement Epiphyseal avulsion fractures	6.7%
High risk	Salter-Harris III and IV fractures >2mm displacement Salter-Harris V fractures Comminuted epiphyseal fractures Juvenile Tillaux's fractures	32%
Risk uncertain	Salter-Harris II tibial fractures	16.7%

[a] Data from references 32 and 56.

greater than 50% of the growth plate is affected, contralateral epiphysiodesis is generally performed. These procedures are generally reserved for younger patients who have at least 1 year of their growth remaining. When angular deformities are greater than 10°, surgeons may consider performing a wedge osteotomy at the same time the bar is resected (Fig. 4-43). Before planning the surgical procedure, a tomogram, CT with reformatting in appropriate image planes, or MRI of the affected growth plate is useful to determine the degree of closure better (see Fig. 4-42).

Leg length discrepancy occurs in 10 to 30% of patients; obviously, it is more common in high-risk groups (see Table 4-4).[28,32,33,56] Treatment of this problem depends on growth potential and the degree of leg length discrepancy. Length differences less than 2 cm may not require surgery. If growth projections indicate that the deformity will exceed 2 cm but will be less than 5 cm, an epiphysiodesis of the normal extremity may be indicated.[33] If the discrepancy may exceed 5 cm, a leg lengthening procedure may be indicated.[33,56]

Other complications include rotational deformity, delayed or nonunion, malunion, and avascular necrosis (AVN).[30,38,53,56] Rotational deformities are more common with triplane injuries. The deformity may be significant, requiring derotational osteotomy.[30] Assessment of this problem radiographically may be most easily accomplished using CT or MRI, which allows the degree of rotation to be more easily assessed. Nonunion may be obvious on routine radiographs. However, in certain cases, CT may be helpful. The areas of nonbone contact can be clearly seen. MRI is most useful in demonstrating if nonunion is fibrous or if there is still active healing potential. Fibrous tissue in the fracture line has low

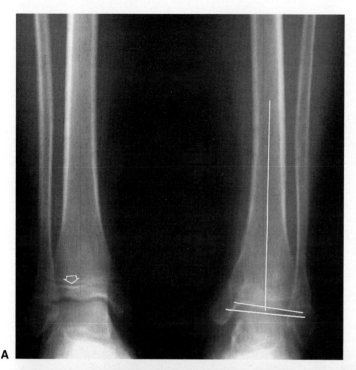

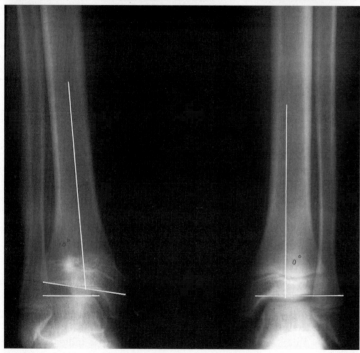

FIG. 4-43. Scanograms in two patients with Salter-Harris IV tibial fractures. **A:** There is joint space narrowing on the injured left side. The growth plate is closed (*arrow*). The lateral physis is open in the normal right ankle (*open arrow*). There is a minimal tilt line on the left. **B:** There is premature fusion on the right with overgrowth medially and an incongruent joint space.

intensity on both T1- and T2-weighted sequences. MRI is also useful in detection of early AVN. The MRI features of AVN are more specific than isotope scans, which can be difficult to interpret in areas with posttraumatic deformity.

Adult Fractures

Complete evaluation of ankle fractures in adults includes assessment of the fracture fragments and accurate descrip-

tion of associated ligament injuries. Bone and soft tissue involvement is important in determining the mechanism of injury, which, in turn, has significant treatment implications.[59,60,63,68,90,111]

When evaluating ankle fractures, it is common to consider the bones and ligaments as a ring-like structure in the coronal plane (Fig. 4-44). This concept has been popularized by Neer and other authors.[64,95,99] The ring is made up of the medial malleolus, tibial plafond, distal tibiofibular ligaments and

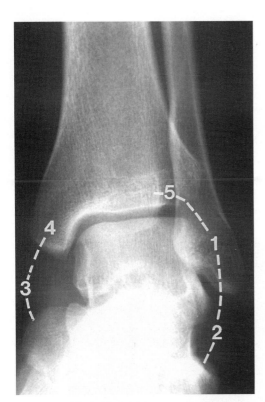

FIG. 4-44. AP radiographs demonstrating the ring concept created by the osseous and ligamentous structure of the ankle. Common breaks in the ring are (*1*) lateral malleolus, (*2*) lateral ligaments, (*3*) medial ligaments, (*4*) medial malleolus, and (*5*) syndesmosis.

syndesmosis, lateral malleolus, lateral ligaments, talus, and medial ligaments.[64,95,99] Breaks in the ring commonly occur at five sites either alone or in combination. Shift of the talus indicates disruption of the ring at more than one site. The five common sites of injury are (1) lateral malleolus, (2) lateral ligaments, (3) deltoid ligaments, (4) medial malleolus, and (5) syndesmosis.[95] Fractures of the tibial plafond occur after axial loading with varying degrees of plantar flexion.[63,93,95]

Clinical Features

After ankle injury, patients generally present with varying degrees of pain, swelling, and ecchymosis, depending to some degree on the significance of the injury. The incidence of swelling and the presence of ecchymosis are higher when fractures are present, but this is not a reliable clinical finding. With incomplete injuries and stable fractures (single break in the "ring"), weight bearing is usually still possible. Weight bearing is more difficult or impossible with unstable fractures.[63,93,90,95]

Classifications

Most ankle fractures occur as a result of inversion or eversion forces.[59,68] However, the mechanism of injury is rarely pure. Most often, abduction, adduction, lateral rotation,

or axial loading occurs in addition to eversion or inversion.[63,68,72,90,122]

The value of classifications for ankle fractures is that they have a significant impact on treatment, prognosis, and establishing the mechanism of injury. Classifications must also be workable and easy to remember. With this in mind, various classifications have been developed for ankle fractures.[81,90, 95,100,126–129] Ashhurst and Bromer[60] classified ankle fractures based on mechanism of injury. Most of their 300 patients (95%) sustained fractures after abduction, adduction, or external rotation of the foot. In the remaining cases, injuries were caused by axial loading. This classification did not include the ligament injuries associated with fractures and was limited by describing the fracture mechanism as the result of a single force. Most fractures are caused by force vectors from more than one direction.[81,95]

The more commonly used classifications are those proposed by Lauge-Hansen,[81] Weber, and the Arbeitsgen Einschaft für Osteogynthesefragen/Association for Study of Internal Fixation (AO/ASIF) group.[75,116] The former is accurate in predicting the mechanism of injury and the extent of ligament involvement. Therefore, it is recommended to radiologists to improve the accuracy when describing the injury.[59,81] The Weber classification is not as complex. This system is frequently used by orthopedic surgeons in planning appropriate therapy.[75,90,95] The AO classification is more detailed than the Weber system.[116]

Lauge-Hansen Classification

The Lauge-Hansen classification was devised using cadaver specimens. It is based on the position of the foot at the time of injury (first word) and the direction of the injuring force (second word or phrase). Using this system, four basic categories of injury are described. The classification considers different levels of injury in each category, based on the degree and length of time the force is applied (Table 4-6). Supination-adduction injuries (inversion) (Fig. 4-45) cause traction on the lateral ligaments resulting in either a ligament tear or an avulsion fracture of the lateral malleolus (stage I). The fracture is generally transverse and below the joint level (Figs. 4-46 to 4-48).[59,81,90,95] If the force is sufficient, the talus can impact against the medial malleolus (stage II) (Fig. 4-49; see Table 4-6). If an oblique fracture of the medial malleolus is evident, but no fracture is seen in the lateral malleolus, one can assume that the lateral ligaments are disrupted. This has to be the case if the talus is shifted (two breaks in the ring). Supination-adduction injuries account for 18 to 21% of ankle fractures fitting the Lauge-Hansen classification.[129,130]

Supination–lateral rotation injuries cause medial tension, with the talus causing posterior displacement of the lateral malleolus.[59,90] This causes disruption of the anterior distal tibiofibular ligament (stage I) (Figs. 4-50 and 4-51). As the force continues, a spiral fracture of the lateral malleolus occurs at or just above the tibiotalar joint. This fracture is best seen on the lateral view (see Fig. 4-51). This stage II injury

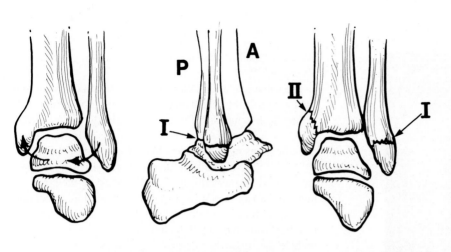

FIG. 4-45. Illustration of supination-adduction injury. Stage I, transverse fracture of the lateral malleolus below the ankle joint or ligament injury. Stage II, steep oblique medial malleolar fracture. (From Berquist et al., ref. 1, with permission.)

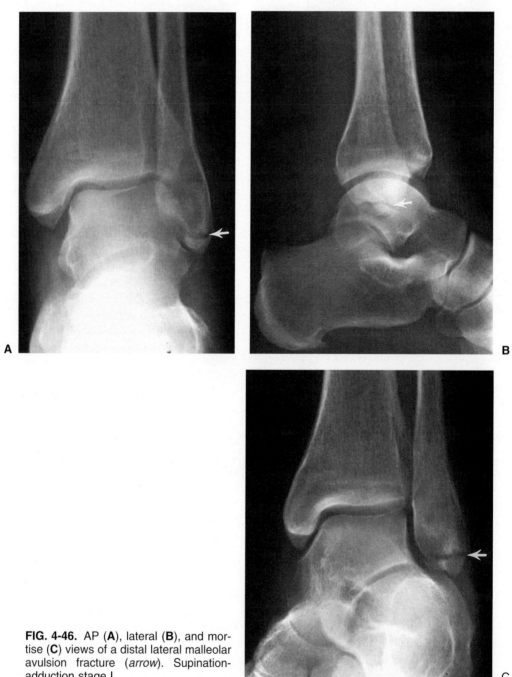

FIG. 4-46. AP (**A**), lateral (**B**), and mortise (**C**) views of a distal lateral malleolar avulsion fracture (*arrow*). Supination-adduction stage I.

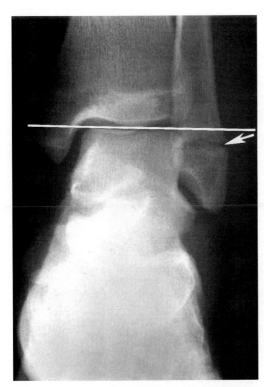

FIG. 4-47. AP view of the ankle demonstrating a transverse fibular fracture (*arrow*) below the ankle joint (*line*). Supination-adduction stage I.

TABLE 4-6. *Lauge-Hansen classification*[a]

Pronation abduction	
Stage I	Ruptured deltoid ligament or transverse medial malleolar fracture
Stage II	Disruption of the distal tibiofibular ligaments (anterior and posterior)
Stage III	Oblique fibular fracture[b] at the joint level (best seen on AP view)
Pronation–lateral rotation	
Stage I	Rupture of the deltoid ligament or transverse medial malleolar fracture
Stage II	Disruption of the anterior tibiofibular ligament and interosseous membrane
Stage III	Fibular fracture[b] above the joint space (usually 6 cm or more above the joint line
Stage IV	Posterior tibial chip fracture or rupture of posterior tibiofibular ligament
Supination–adduction	
Stage I	Lateral ligament injury or transverse lateral malleolar fracture[b] below the ankle joint
Stage II	Steep oblique fracture of the medial malleolus
Supination–lateral rotation	
Stage I	Disruption of the anterior tibiobular ligament
Stage II	Spiral fracture[b] of the distal fibular near the joint (best seen on the lateral view)
Stage III	Rupture of the posterior tibiofibular ligament
Stage IV	Transverse fracture of the medial malleolus

[a] Data from references 59 and 81
[b] Fibular fracture appearance is key to determining mechanism of injury.

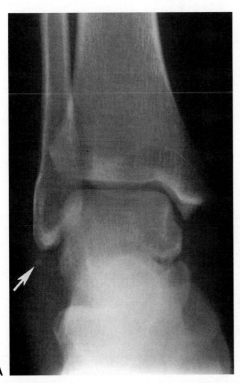
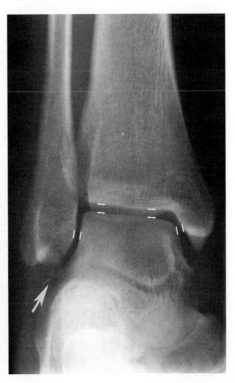

A   B

FIG. 4-48. AP (**A**) and mortise (**B**) view demonstrate avulsed fragments from the lateral malleolar tip (*arrow*) with marked swelling. The ankle mortise (*lines*) is intact with no talar shift. Supination-adduction stage I.

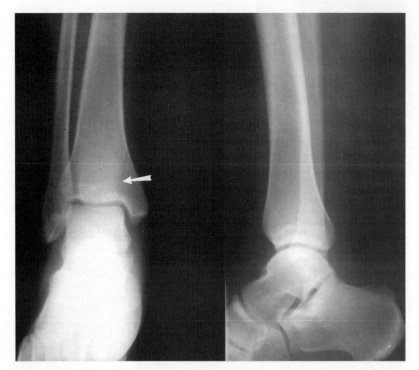

FIG. 4-49. AP (**A**) and lateral (**B**) radiographs of a supination-adduction stage II injury with no obvious fracture of the lateral malleolus and a steep oblique medial malleolar fracture (*arrow*).

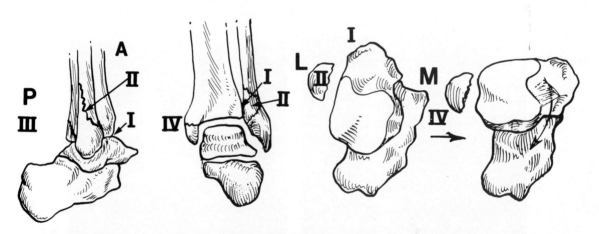

FIG. 4-50. Illustration of Lauge-Hansen supination–lateral rotation injuries. Stage I, disruption of the anterior distal tibiofibular ligaments. Stage II, an oblique fibular fracture best seen on the lateral view. Stage III, posterior tibial fracture. Stage IV, transverse medial malleolar fracture (From Berquist et al., ref. 1, with permission.)

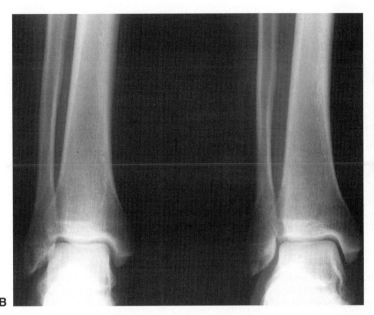
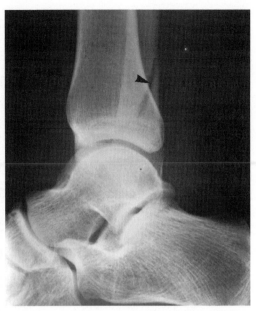

A,B   C

FIG. 4-51. AP (**A**) and mortise (**B**) views of the right ankle are negative. The lateral view (**C**) shows the oblique fibular fracture (*black arrowhead*). Supination–lateral rotation stage II.

is the most common ankle fracture.[59,129,130] When the force and talar rotation continue, a small posterior malleolar fracture occurs (stage III); and if the force continues, an avulsion fracture of the medial malleolus or rupture of the deltoid ligament occurs (stage IV) (Fig. 4-52). Supination–lateral rotation injuries account for 55 to 58% of ankle fractures.[130]

Pronation-abduction injuries (eversion) result in abduction of the talus in the ankle mortise placing tension on the medial structures. This leads to a transverse avulsion fracture of the medial malleolus or rupture of the deltoid ligament (stage I) (Fig. 4-53). With continued force, the anterior and posterior distal tibiofibular ligaments are torn, or avulsion fractures of the anterior and posterior tibial attachments occur (stage II) (Fig. 4-54). With further force, an oblique fibular fracture develops at or just above the tibiotalar joint.[72,81] This fracture is best seen on the AP view (see Fig. 4-54), which differentiates from the spiral fracture seen with supination–lateral rotation injuries. The latter is seen best

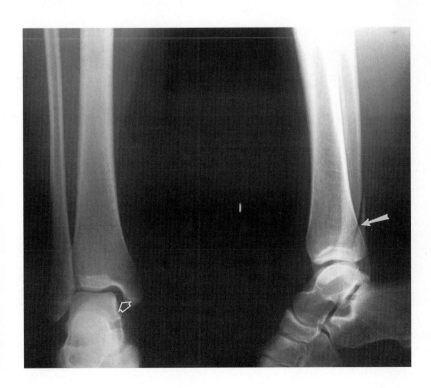

FIG. 4-52. Stage IV supination lateral rotation injury. The fibular fracture (*white arrow*) is best seen on the lateral view. The talus is shifted on the AP view resulting from a medial ligament injury (*open arrow*).

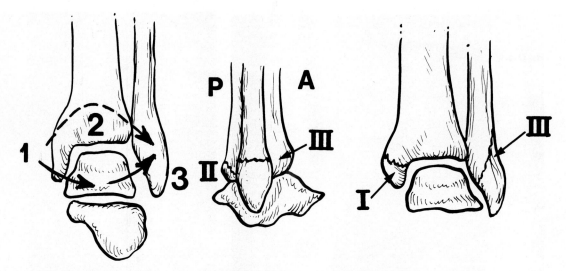

FIG. 4-53. Illustration of pronation-abduction injury. Stage I, transverse medial malleolar fracture below the joint level or medial ligament tear. Stage II, disruption of the distal tibiofibular ligaments. Stage III, oblique fibular fracture near the joint line best seen on the AP view.

on the lateral view.[59] When an oblique lateral malleolar fracture is noted on the AP view, one should assume that the tibiofibular ligaments and deltoid ligaments are ruptured even though no obvious talar shift may be noted.[59] Stress views may be needed to confirm this finding.

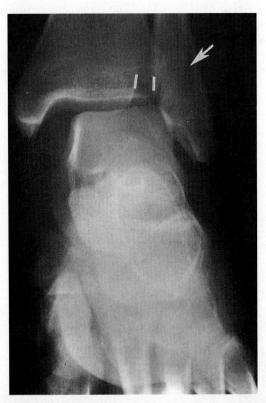

FIG. 4-54. AP view of the ankle demonstrating talar shift resulting from medial ligament injury. The distal tibiofibular space (*lines*) is widened and there is an oblique fibular fracture (*arrow*) pronation-abduction stage III injury.

Pronation–lateral rotation injuries cause medial tension as the talus rotates laterally (Fig. 4-55). Initially, the medial ligaments rupture or an avulsion fracture of the medial malleolus occurs (stage I). As the force continues, the injury progresses clockwise around the ankle in the axial plane. The anterior distal tibiofibular ligament and interosseous membrane rupture (stage II), followed by a fibular fracture. This fracture (stage III is typical in that it occurs well above the joint space at greater than or equal to 5 to 6 cm), a feature that allows differentiation of this injury from the others on the basis of the radiograph (Fig. 4-56). When the force continues, the posterior distal tibiofibular ligament ruptures or

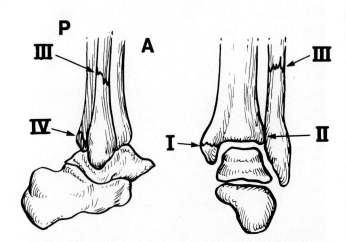

FIG. 4-55. Illustration of pronation–lateral rotation injuries. Stage I, transverse fracture of the medial malleolus or ligament rupture. Stage II, rupture of the anterior distal tibiofibular ligaments. Stage III, fibular fracture well above (at least 6 cm) the joint space. Stage IV, posterior tibial avulsion fracture or rupture of posterior tibia fibular ligaments. (From Berquist et al., ref. 1, with permission.)

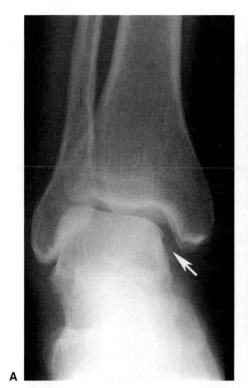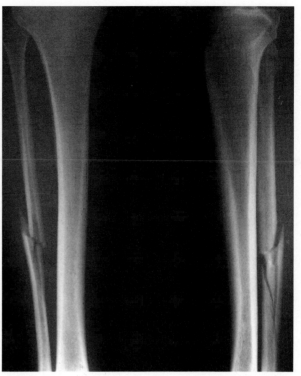

FIG. 4-56. Pronation–lateral rotation stage III injury. **A:** AP view of the ankle shows widening of the ankle mortise medially (*arrow*) resulting from a ligament injury. In this setting, the entire tibia and fibular should be imaged. **B:** Radiographs of the leg demonstrate the high fibular fracture.

a posterior tibial avulsion fracture is noted (stage IV) (see Fig. 4-55). Pronation injuries (abduction lateral rotation) account for approximately 20% of ankle fractures.[130]

In his original series, Lauge-Hansen found that 75% of injuries were either supination-adduction or supination–lateral rotation injuries.[81] The classification is accurate in detection of fracture and ligament components of ankle injuries in 90 to 95% of cases.[59] There are exceptions, most notably fractures of the tibial plafond owing to axial loading or plantar-flexion injuries. However, the characteristic appearance of the fibular fracture and orderly progression of the injuries make this classification ideal for radiologists. Accurate reporting of ankle injuries is greatly facilitated.[59,95,128]

Weber Classification

The Weber classification is commonly used by orthopedic surgeons.[59,90,95,128] This classification is much simpler using the level of fibular fracture in predicting the degree of syndesmosis injury and mortise displacement.[58,75,95,102,106,114]

Type A injuries cause fractures below the tibiotalar joint and do not involve the syndesmosis (similar to Lauge-Hansen supination-adduction).[59,81] Type B fractures occur at the joint level producing an oblique fibular fracture (similar to Lauge-Hansen pronation-abduction) that is seen best on the AP view (see Fig. 4-54).[75,90,95] Two categories of type C fractures are described. Type C1 is an oblique fibular frac-

ture above the level of the distal tibiofibular ligaments. Type C2 lesions present with higher fibular fractures and therefore more extensive rupture of the syndesmosis (Fig. 4-57). Treatment of type A injuries can usually be accomplished closed, whereas type B and C injuries usually require internal fixation. The Weber classification is useful for treatment purposes but is not as useful in understanding the mechanism of injury and ligament involvement as the Lauge-Hansen system.[58,75,90,95,102,106,114,125]

AO Classification

The AO classification for malleolar fractures is similar to, but more complex than, the Weber system.[116] This system (Fig. 4-58) also relates fracture level and syndesmotic and interosseous ligament and membrane injury. Type A fractures are below the syndesmosis and may involve the fibula (see Figs. 4-57 and 4-58A) or fibula and medial malleolus (type A2) or medial malleolus and tibia articular surface (type A3). Type B fractures are at the level of the syndesmosis and may involve the fibular (type B1), fibula, and medial malleolus (type B2) or both malleoli and with tibiofibular avulsions anteriorly and posteriorly (type B3). Type C fractures are above the syndesmosis (see Figs. 4-57C and 4-58). Type C1 fractures involve the medial and distal ligaments tibiofibular ligaments. Type C2 fractures are associated with distal tibiofibular ligament rupture and medial malleolar

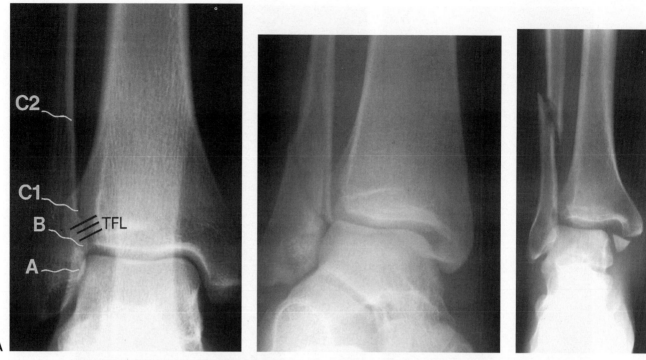

FIG. 4-57. Radiographs demonstrating the Weber classification. **A:** Radiographs demonstrating the level of fracture: type A fracture at or below the joint line; type B fracture near joint level; type C1 fracture just above the distal tibiofibular ligaments (*TFL*); type C2 high fibular fracture. **B:** Mortise view demonstrating a Weber type B fibular fracture. **C:** AP radiographs demonstrating a Weber C2 fracture (AO C2 also).

fracture similar to the case shown in Figure 4-57C, which is a Weber C2 fracture. Type C3 fractures are near the fibular head and involve more of the interosseous ligament in addition to the tibiofibular ligaments and medial malleolus.[116]

Fractures of the tibial plafond do not fit neatly into the foregoing classifications. Most occur in patients less than 50 years of age (77%).[74,77,101] These injuries, although uncommon, are difficult to manage.[62,65,82,83,95,108,117,125] Fractures are caused by axial loading and generally occur in association with falling from a significant height or during motor vehicle accidents when the foot becomes trapped against the floor.[77,82,95] Fractures usually extend up the tibial shaft in an oblique or spiral manner. Severe comminution with multiple articular fragments (pilon fracture) is common.[58,65,101,117] Twenty percent of plafond fractures are open.[101] Ovadia and Beals[101] classified plafond fractures based on radiographic evidence of displacement and metaphyseal and articular involvement (Fig. 4-59). Type I fractures are nondisplaced. Type II fractures showed minimal displacement. Type III fractures have articular surface displacement with several large bone fragments. Type IV and V fractures have comminuted articular components with displacement of the articular fragments. Fibular fractures were not considered in this classification. Type I and II fractures are usually caused by less severe trauma. Internal fixation is required for type III to V fractures.[101]

The AO classification is slightly different and considers intra- and extraarticular distal tibial fractures. Type A fractures are extraarticular (Fig. 4-60). Type B fractures involve a portion of the articular surface, and type C fractures have more complex articular involvement (see Fig. 4-60).[116]

Isolated dislocations of the ankle without associated fractures are rare. Moehring and associates[92] reported 14 cases over an 11-year period. The injury occurred most often in young patients (average age, 28 years; range, 18 to 41 years). All but 1 case resulted in an open injury. The mechanism of injury was considered to be marked plantar flexion followed by inversion resulting in disruption of the anterolateral capsule, anterior talofibular ligament, calcaneofibular ligament, and lateral retinacula.[92] These unusual dislocations are almost always posteromedial. Despite the open injury and severe soft tissue disruption, infection and chronic instability are not common.[92]

Radiographic Evaluation

As noted early in this chapter, ankle injuries are common. The Ottawa ankle rules were developed to reduce unnecessary ankle radiographs. Although controversial in the United States because of legal issues, these rules are helpful. If there is no tenderness over the malleoli or distal fibula and the patient can bear weight, a radiograph may not be necessary.

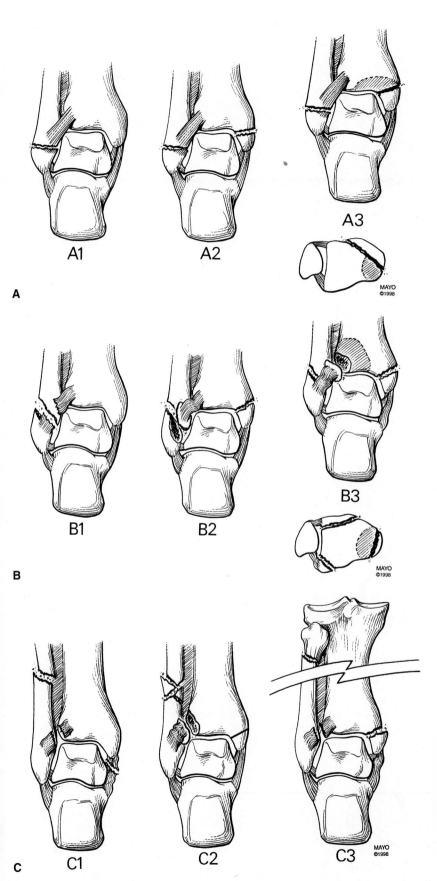

A

A1 A2 A3

MAYO
©1998

B

B1 B2 B3

MAYO
©1998

C

C1 C2 C3

MAYO
©1998

FIG. 4-58. Illustration of the AO classification system. **A:** Type A OA injuries: *A1,* fibular fracture below the syndesmosis and tibiofibular ligament; *A2,* A1 plus associated low medial malleolar fracture; *A3,* A2 plus tibial articular fracture. **B:** AP type B injuries: *B1,* isolated transyndesmotic fibular lesion; *B2,* A1 with medial malleolar fracture; *B3,* A2 with tibial articular or tibiofibular avulsion injuries. **C:** AO type C injures: *C1,* high fibular fracture with distal ligament injury; *C2,* high fibular fracture with associated medial malleolar fracture (see Fig. 4-57); *C3,* distal tibiofibular ligament and medial malleolar fracture with fibular fracture just below the fibular head.

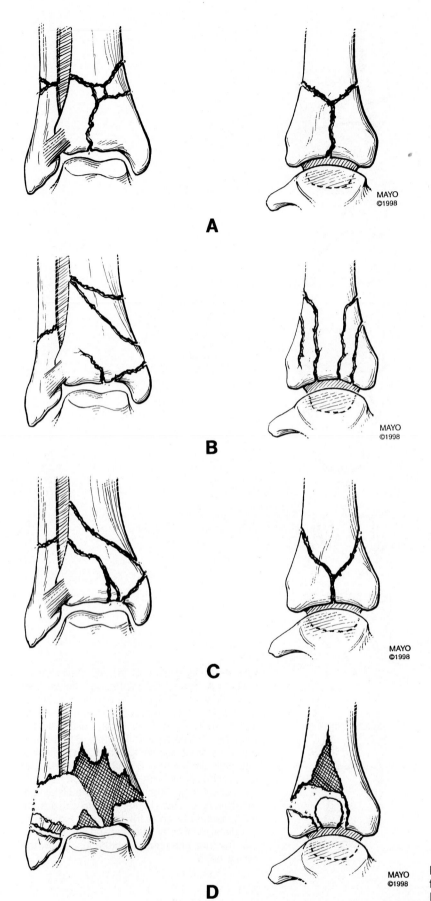

FIG. 4-59. Ovadia classification of the tibial plafond fractures. **A:** Type I. **B:** Type II. **C:** Type III. **D:** Type IV. *(continued)*

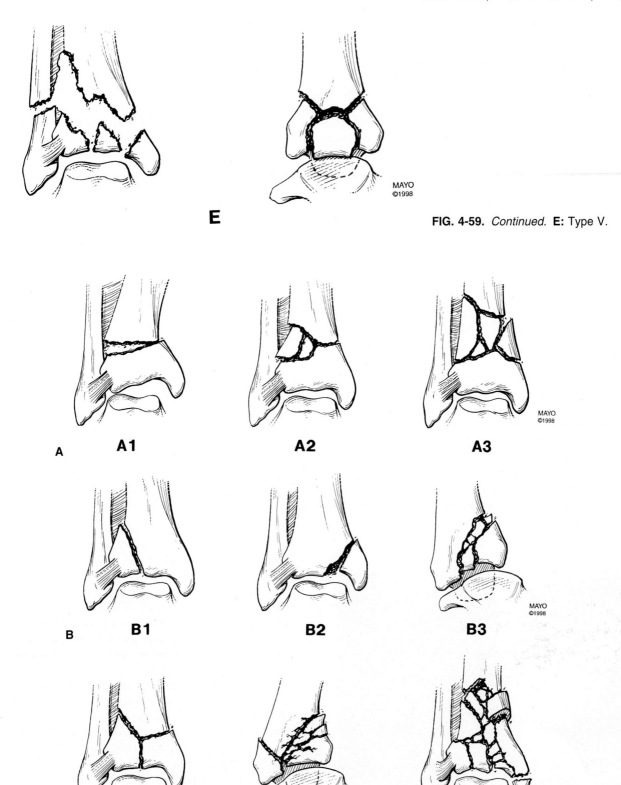

E

FIG. 4-59. *Continued.* **E:** Type V.

FIG. 4-60. AO classification of distal tibial (pilon) fractures. **A:** Type A injuries: *type A1,* simple extraarticular fracture; *type A2,* comminuted metaphyseal fracture; *type A3,* complex comminuted fracture with no articular involvement. **B:** Type B injuries: *type B1,* undisplaced articular fracture line; *type B2,* displaced articular fracture; *type B3,* comminution of a portion of the articular surface. **C:** Type C injuries: complete articular involvement with varying degrees (*C1* to *C3*) of articular fragmentation.

Following these rules, Verma and colleagues[120] found an overall sensitivity of 99% and specificity of 22%. The need for radiographs was reduced 16%. For purposes of this section, I emphasize appropriate imaging techniques to image ankle injuries optimally.[61,89]

AP, lateral, and mortise views are obtained in patients with ankle fractures. I also routinely obtain the external oblique view (see Chapter 2).[95,111] In most cases, these views provide sufficient information regarding the degree of bone and soft tissue involvement.[68,72,95,111] This is especially true in patients with fractures that fit the Lauge-Hansen classification (more than 95%). It is also essential to include the entire tibia and fibula when studying patients with ankle fractures. The fibular fracture, which is key to classifying the injury, may be just below the fibular head.[59,95] The AP view is useful in evaluating soft tissue swelling that may lead the interpreter to a subtle fracture. The oblique fracture of the fibula (pronation-abduction stage III) is best seen on the AP view. Avulsion fractures of the tibia and fibular can also be seen on this view.[59,72,95,111]

The mortise view (foot internally rotated 15° to 20°) is critical for evaluating the position of the talus and the syndesmosis. The space between the talar margin and the medial malleolus, plafond, and lateral malleolus should be equal.[95] The distance between the distal tibia and fibular should not exceed 4.5 mm.[69,84] Talar asymmetry indicates the presence of two injuries, whether two ligaments, two fractures, or a combination of fracture and ligament rupture (see Figs. 4-48 and 4-54).[95,99,111,128–130]

The lateral view is most useful for detecting anterior and posterior tibial chip or avulsion fractures (Fig. 4-61). In addition, the fibular fracture seen with supination–lateral rotation stage II injuries is best seen on the lateral view.[59] The presence of an ankle effusion or Achilles tendon injury (obliteration of the pre-Achilles fat triangle) is also most easily noted on the lateral view (see Fig. 4-1).[61]

We routinely obtain a 45° external oblique view in addition to the foregoing radiographs. This protocol provides added information, especially when subtle posterior tibial fractures are present. Because of the frequency of associated fractures in the foot and foot fractures that may mimic ankle injury, it may also be wise to obtain routine (AP, lateral, oblique) views of the foot in patients presenting with ankle injury.

Occasionally, special studies are needed before planning conservative (closed) or operative therapy. Tomography (AP and lateral projections) is useful in evaluating the degree of articular involvement in complex plafond fractures and may also be necessary to exclude articular involvement. The position of fragments, especially articular fragments, can be better demonstrated using thin (1.5- to 3-mm) section CT.[76] This technique offers the capability of three-dimensional reconstruction, which can be useful in planning surgical approaches for complex fractures.[67,76,95]

Treatment

The goals of treatment should be accurate anatomic reduction and a parallel articular surface. Early motion is also essential to prevent reduced motion or adhesive capsulitis.[114] Decisions regarding open or closed reduction can be based on the type of fracture (single versus bimalleolar or trimalleolar) and the degree of displacement.[58,62,65,70,74,85,86,95,102,106,115,118,125]

Fractures of the medial or lateral malleolus without a second fracture or ligament injury may be treated conservatively if displacement does not exceed 2 mm.[64,69,76,80,85,95] Immobilization with a cast for 6 weeks is generally adequate. If the fracture is displaced more than 2 mm, internal fixation is indicated. The medial malleolus can usually be reduced with one or two malleolar screws; fibular fractures may require multiple lag screws, plate and screw fixation, or a Rush rod (Figs. 4-62 to 4-65). Percutaneous threaded screws may also produce excellent results.[107]

Most bimalleolar and trimalleolar fractures require internal fixation.[85,95,102] These injuries are, by definition, unstable. Medial malleolar fractures are treated with screw fixation. The fibular fracture can also be reduced with multiple screws (see Fig. 4-62) if it is spiral. Short oblique or transverse fractures are reduced with plate and screws or intramedullary fixation (see Figs. 4-63 to 4-65).[95,107] It is important that the fibular and syndesmosis be reduced, to avoid chronic instability.[102,115,125] This is especially true with supination–lateral rotation and pronation–lateral rotation injuries.[84,97,110,121] In patients with extensive syndesmosis disruption, a syndesmosis screw may be needed to reduce the ankle mortise (see Fig. 4-65).[95,97,102] Syndesmotic screws must be properly positioned and not placed too tightly or complications may result. If the screw is placed too high,

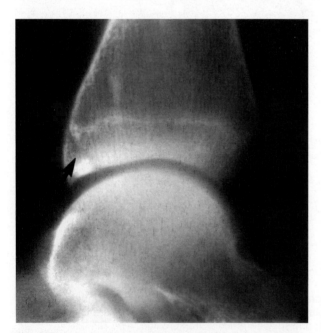

FIG. 4-61. Lateral tomogram of the ankle demonstrating a posterior tibial avulsion fracture (*arrow*).

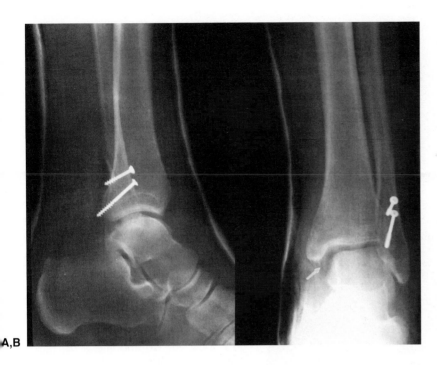

FIG. 4-62. Lateral (**A**) and AP (**B**) radiographs of a spiral fibular fracture reduced with two lag screws. The medial ankle mortise is widened (*arrow*), but the syndesmotic region is stabilized.

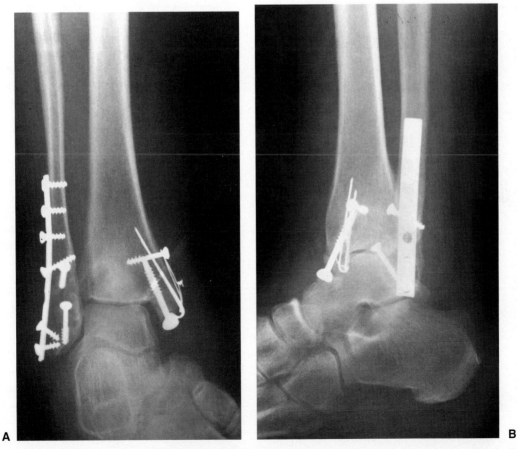

A   B

FIG. 4-63. Fractures of the medial and lateral malleoli. The medial malleolus is reduced anatomically with a tension band and a malleolar screw. The fibular fracture is reduced with a one-third tubular plate and two leg screws. AP (**A**) and lateral (**B**) radiographs demonstrate fixation devices.

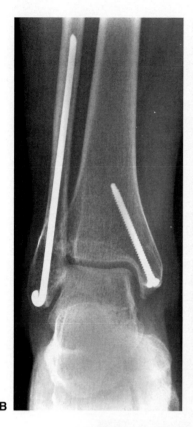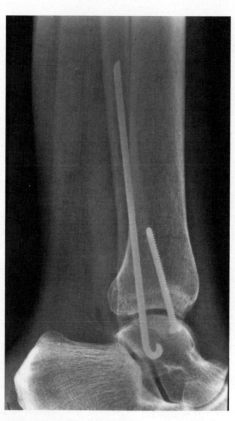

A,B

FIG. 4-64. AP (**A**) and lateral (**B**) radiographs demonstrate healed fractures. The fibular fracture was internally fixed with a Rush rod and the medial malleolar fracture with a single fully threaded screw. The ankle mortise is normal.

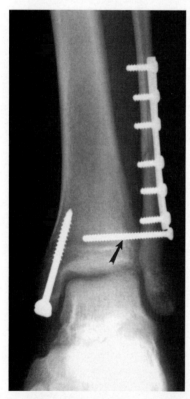

FIG. 4-65. Mortise view of a stage III pronation–lateral rotation injury. There are two medial malleolar screws. The fibular fracture is internally fixed with a one-third tubular plate and cortical screws. The syndesmosis is reduced with a fully threaded syndesmotic screw (*arrow*).

the distal tibia may displace laterally. When screws are placed too low, the syndesmotic ligament may be injured, resulting in cross union and reduced motion (Fig. 4-66). When the screw is too tight, foot dorsiflexion may be restricted or the talus may sublux anteriorly and inferiorly.[97] Internal fixation of the posterior tibial fragment is generally required if more than 25% of the articular surfaces involved.[129]

Fractures of the tibial plafond are particularly difficult to manage.[62,74,88,101,117,119] Considerable separation of fragments and loss of articular cartilage may be present (Figs. 4-67 and 4-68). Three-dimensional CT may be particularly useful in planning reconstruction of these fractures. The fragments need to be repositioned and the articular surface restored as completely as possible. Bone grafting is useful to support the articular surface and to fill in areas of dead space or bone loss.[62] Severely comminuted fractures may require calcaneal traction for several weeks. This helps to reduce the ankle mortise and perhaps allows fibrous ingrowth that reduces posttraumatic arthritis. In certain cases, arthrodesis is necessary. Twenty-one of 145 patients with plafond fractures required arthrodesis in Ovadia's series.[101] Regardless of the treatment, type I fractures have excellent results. Only 22% of patients with type V (Ovadia classification, see Fig. 4-59) had good results. Radiographs are necessary for 4 to 8 weeks after reduction to be certain that fragments do not change position. In certain cases, more complex studies (tomography, CT, or MRI) are needed if the fracture pattern is unclear.[61]

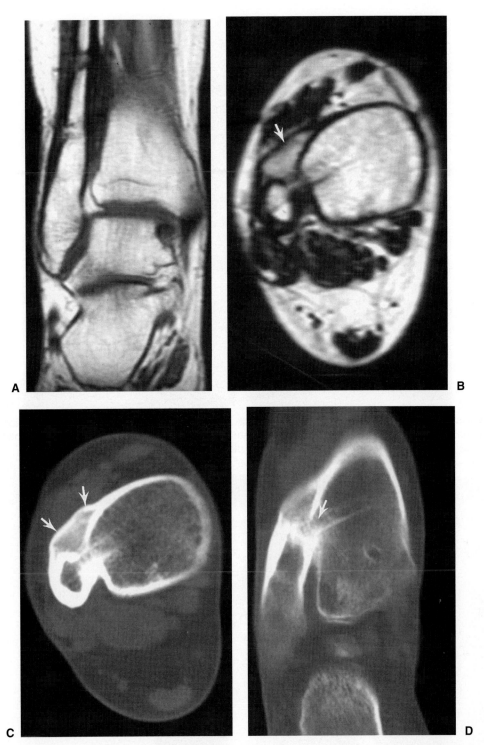

FIG. 4-66. Posttraumatic ankle pain and restricted motion. The syndesmotic screw and fibular hardware have been removed. Coronal (**A**) and axial (**B**) T1-weighted MRI images show the screw tracts and bony cross union (*arrow*) anteriorly. Axial (**C**) and coronal (**D**) CT images are superior to demonstrate syndesmotic bone changes (*arrows*) and cross union.

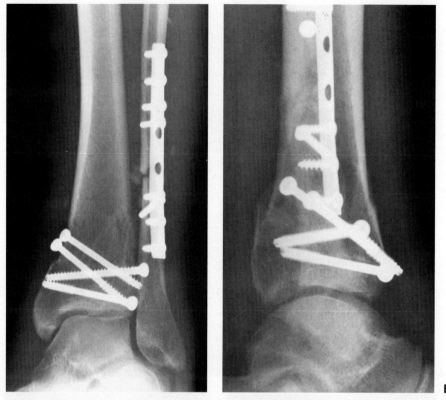

A   B

FIG. 4-67. Pilon fracture of the distal tibia with high fibular fracture. AP (**A**) and lateral (**B**) radiographs demonstrate screw fixation of the tibial fracture. There is minimal residual articular deformity. The fibular fracture is internally fixed with a one-third tubular plate and cortical screws.

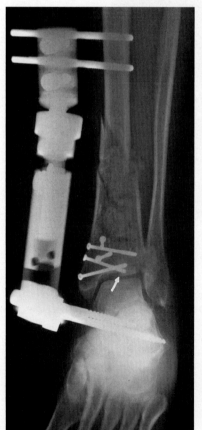

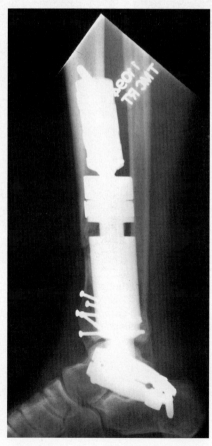

A,B

FIG. 4-68. Complex pilon fracture (AO C3, Ovadia IV or V). AP (**A**) and lateral (**B**) radiographs show multiple tibial screws and a lateral frame external fixator. There is residual articular step-off (*arrow*) seen on the AP view (**A**).

TABLE 4-7. *Complications of ankle fractures[a]*

Osteoarthritis
Chronic instability
Nonunion
Malunion
Reflex sympathetic dystrophy
Infection
Adhesive capsulitis
Tendon rupture or dislocation
Synovial chondromatosis
Tarsal tunnel syndrome
Neurovascular injury
Pes cavovarus deformity

[a] Data from references 66, 73, 82, 91, 95, 101, and 104.

Complications

Complications may result from the initial injury or may be related to treatment (Table 4-7).[73,78,79,102,103] Loss of reduction generally occurs with closed reduction but can occur after internal fixation as well.[95] Reduction may be difficult or impossible to maintain using closed manipulation in certain cases. For example, the fibula can become trapped behind the tibia. In addition, soft tissue underposition or tendon entrapment may make it impossible to reduce

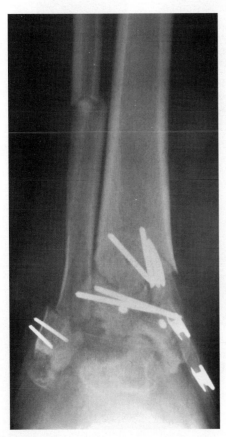

FIG. 4-69. Complex Ovadia type I fracture with K-wire fixation. The reduction could not be maintained.

fractures.[66,80,103] Usually, routine radiographs are adequate to evaluate change in position of fragments (Fig. 4-69). Failure to maintain reduction because of soft tissue interposition can be easily diagnosed using CT or MRI. If these techniques are not available, tenography can be performed.[61]

Degenerative arthritis is the most common long-term complication, occurring in up to 30 to 40% of patients regardless of the treatment method used.[123] The incidence is higher with displaced plafond fractures (types III to V), when the syndesmosis is poorly reduced or with chronic instability, and in older patients.[87,101,104,123] Radiographic findings of arthritis may not become obvious for 3 to 8 years (Fig. 4-70). Pain symptoms may lead to operative intervention with ankle fusion or, in certain cases, ankle arthroplasty.[91,95]

Malunion and nonunion are uncommon when adequate reduction is obtained. Nonunion occurs most commonly after avulsion of the medial malleolus (Fig. 4-71). The incidence (10 to 15%) is much higher after closed than open (0.5%) reduction.[80,123] displaced fragments with well-defined sclerotic margins indicate obvious nonunion radiographically (Fig. 4-72). Subtle cases can be detected tomographically or more accurately with MRI. On T2-weighted sequences, there is increased signal in the fracture line with nonunion. Fibrous union is seen as a dark area in the fracture line on both T1- and T2-weighted sequences.

Patients with internal fixation are more prone to infection. Fortunately, except for open fractures, the incidence is low, and infections are usually superficial.[123]

Reflex sympathetic dystrophy is a syndrome of refractory pain, neurovascular changes of swelling, and vasomotor instability, as well as trophic changes involving soft tissues and bone.[71,105] The cause is unclear, but the syndrome has been attributed to trauma, infection, and cervical arthritis, for example. The severity of trauma does not correlate with the severity of the symptoms. Most authors believe that the syndrome is caused by posttraumatic reflex spasm leading to loss of vascular tone and aggressive osteoporosis.[105] Osteoporosis may have a diffuse or patchy appearance involving both medullary and cortical bone. Prompt diagnosis can lead to more effective therapy. Isotope scans may demonstrate multiple articular changes earlier, suggesting the diagnosis and permitting treatment to be instituted more promptly.

Neurovascular injury can occur during the injury or because of inadequate treatment (Fig. 4-73). In the acute setting, angiography is most often used to evaluate vascular occlusion. Doppler techniques can also be used to evaluate vascular patency.

Ossification of the syndesmosis can occur after ankle fracture.[123] Most often, it is incomplete. However, complete bony fusion can occur (see Fig. 4-66), usually when a syndesmosis screw has been used. These changes are usually obvious on routine radiographs. However, scarring and stenosis may be purely fibrous, in which case CT (see Fig. 4-66) or MRI is more useful.

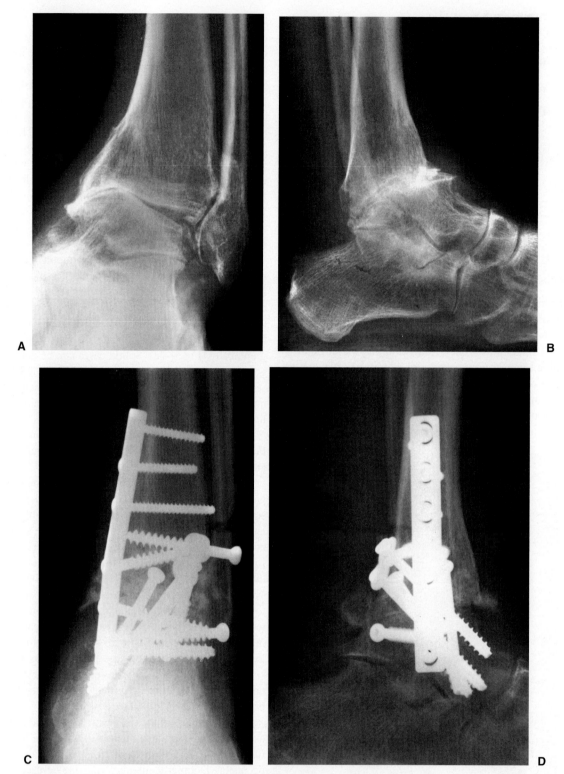

FIG. 4-70. Old ankle fracture with advanced degenerative arthritis and instability. AP (**A**) and lateral (**B**) radiographs demonstrate advanced arthritis with multiple bone fragments laterally and joint asymmetry. The patient was treated with arthrodesis. AP (**A**) and lateral (**B**) radiographs show fusion with multiple screws and a medial compression plate.

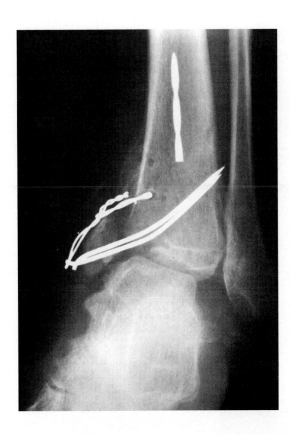

FIG. 4-71. AP radiograph with failed fixation of the medial malleolus using K-wire and tension-band technique.

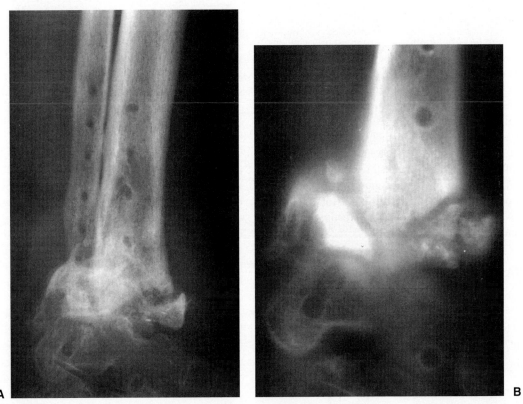

A

B

FIG. 4-72. Lateral radiograph (**A**) and tomogram (**B**) demonstrating nonunion of a distal tibial fracture. Note the sclerotic margins and fragmentation (**B**). The fixation devices have been removed.

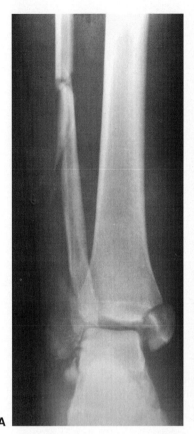
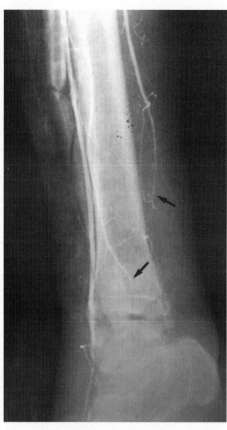
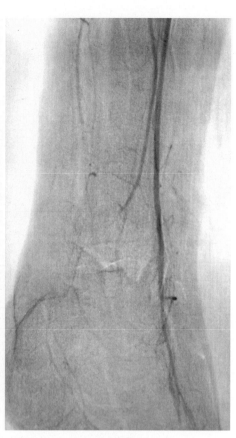

A   B

FIG. 4-73. AP (**A**) radiograph of complex ankle fracture with midfibular comminution. Routine (**B**) and subtracted (**C**) angiographic images show occlusion (*arrows* in **B**) of the peroneal and posterior tibial arteries.

When treatment of initial injuries is unsuccessful or when severe arthritis develops, further surgery may be required. Arthrodesis is an accepted technique for posttraumatic ankle problems (see Fig. 4-70).[96,98] Multiple techniques have been described, with good results reported in over 75% of patients.[98] Imaging is helpful to confirm bony union and to detect complications. Routine radiographs are usually sufficient to follow union of fusions. Tomography or CT is useful in detection of bony fusion and sequestra in cases of infection (Fig. 4-74). MRI may prove to be most useful, depending on the type and amount of metal in place for fixation. Pseudarthrosis can develop in 10 to 25%, infection in up to 23%, and malunion in 12% of patients.[94,96,109]

TALAR FRACTURES AND DISLOCATIONS

Fractures and fracture dislocations of the talus are rare in children.[138,154,186,196] Therefore, adult and pediatric injuries are discussed together, emphasizing differences in diagnosis and treatment when they are significant.

Anatomy

The talus is a unique and important functional unit of the hindfoot. It serves to support the body weight and to distribute the forces to the foot. The talus ossifies from a single primary center with ossification beginning in the neck. The posterior aspect ossifies last, with maturation completed 16 to 20 years after birth.[160] Articular cartilage covers 60% of the talar surface, and there are no direct tendon or muscle attachments.[159,174] Therefore, the blood supply is vulnerable.[157,162,181,183]

Superiorly, the trochlear surface articulates with the tibia. This articular surface is wider anteriorly. Medially and laterally, there are articular facets for the medial and lateral malleoli. Bony processes are present posteriorly and laterally. The posterior process is divided into medial and lateral tubercles by a groove for the flexor hallucis longus tendon.[140] This tendon in its fibrous tunnel is the closest anatomically to a tendinous attachment.[140,157,162,185] In up to 50% of patients, the os trigonum is present as a secondary ossification center. This lies just posterior to the lateral tubercle of the posterior process.

Inferiorly, the talus articulates with the calcaneus via the larger posterior, and smaller middle and anterior facets. The talus forms the roof of the tarsal tunnel between the middle and posterior facets. The talar head articulates with the navicular. Articular stability is maintained by articular capsules and ligaments (Fig. 4-75).[162,173,185] Movements in the subtalar joint include eversion (lateral rotation of the hindfoot), inversion (medial rotation of hindfoot), and slight flexion and extension.[185]

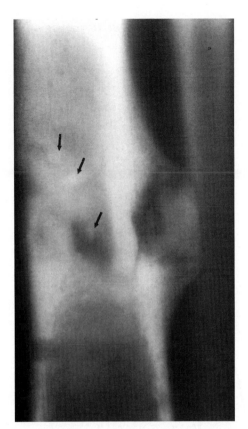

FIG. 4-74. Tomogram of an old infected nonunion with sclerotic sequestra (*arrows*).

The blood supply to the talus is limited by the significant articular surface area and its lack of muscle and tendon insertions. The main blood supply enters the talus via the tarsal canal as a branch of the posterior tibial artery. This artery supplies the inferior neck and most of the body. Branches of the dorsalis pedis artery enter the superior aspect of the talar neck and supply the dorsal portion of the neck and head of the talus. The peroneal artery supplies a portion of the lateral talus (Figs. 4-76 and 4-77).[162,174]

Talar Neck Fractures

Fractures of the talar neck are uncommon in adults and rare in children. Letts and Gibeault[164] identified 12 pediatric fractures over an 18-year period. The largest series of talar fractures was reported by Coltart.[143] He noted 228 talar injuries in a total of 25,000 fractures and dislocations (0.9%). Talar injuries accounted for only 6% of all foot and ankle injuries. Fractures of the talar neck are the second most common talar injury (Table 4-8).[143,155,166] The injury usually occurs during abrupt dorsiflexion of the forefoot. This is most often associated with motor vehicle accidents or after significant falls.[145,161] Direct trauma from an object striking the top of the foot may also lead to fracture of the talar neck.[145,166] As usual, the mechanism of injury is rarely pure. Adduction or external rotation forces are also implicated.[145,155,162] Talar neck fractures have also been reported with other ankle injuries implicating supination, supination–lateral rotation, and less commonly pronation injuries.[162]

Management of talar neck fractures and fracture-dislocation depends on accurate demonstration of the bone and soft tissue injury. The most commonly used classification of these injuries was devised by Hawkins[155] and was modified by Canale and Kelly[138] to include four categories of injury. This classification is useful in determining the prognosis of the injury, specifically in predicting the incidence of AVN.[155,166] The types of fracture or fracture dislocation are summarized in Table 4-9.

Talar neck fractures must be undisplaced to be considered type I. These fractures enter the subtalar joint between the middle and posterior facets and may extend into the body. Type II fractures are displaced with subluxation or dislocation of the subtalar joint. The ankle joint is normal. In this setting, two and occasionally all three sources of blood supply are disrupted.[138,145,174] Type III fractures are displaced with dislocation of the body from both the tibiotalar and subtalar joints; all three sources of blood supply are interrupted. Type IV fractures have associated talonavicular subluxation or dislocation.[138] Twenty-four percent of type

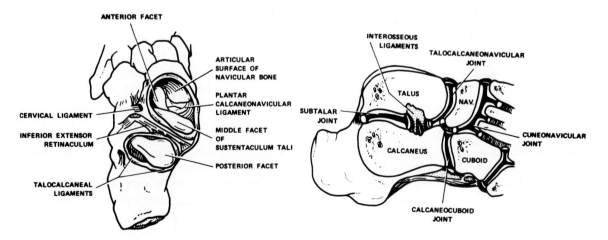

FIG. 4-75. Illustration of the ligaments and articulations of the hindfoot (From Resnick, ref. 185, with permission.)

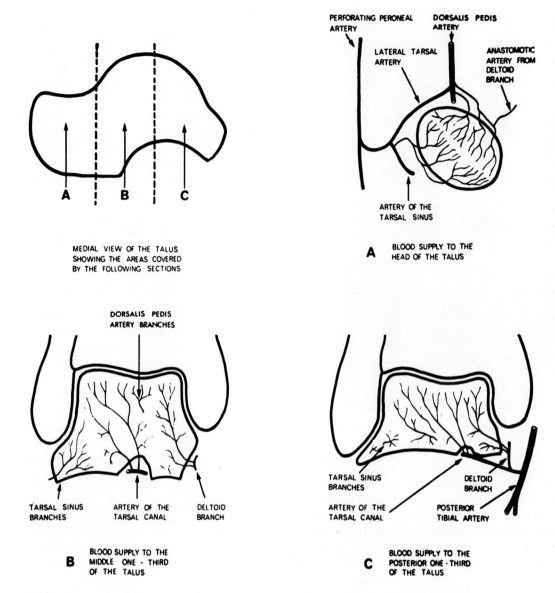

MEDIAL VIEW OF THE TALUS
SHOWING THE AREAS COVERED
BY THE FOLLOWING SECTIONS

A BLOOD SUPPLY TO THE
HEAD OF THE TALUS

PERFORATING PERONEAL ARTERY

DORSALIS PEDIS ARTERY

LATERAL TARSAL ARTERY

ANASTOMOTIC ARTERY FROM DELTOID BRANCH

ARTERY OF THE TARSAL SINUS

DORSALIS PEDIS ARTERY BRANCHES

TARSAL SINUS BRANCHES

ARTERY OF THE TARSAL CANAL

DELTOID BRANCH

B BLOOD SUPPLY TO THE MIDDLE ONE - THIRD OF THE TALUS

TARSAL SINUS BRANCHES

ARTERY OF THE TARSAL CANAL

DELTOID BRANCH

POSTERIOR TIBIAL ARTERY

C BLOOD SUPPLY TO THE POSTERIOR ONE - THIRD OF THE TALUS

FIG. 4-76. Coronal illustration of the talus showing the entry of blood supply demonstrated in **A, B,** and **C,** which show the blood supply to the head, middle third and posterior talus respectively. (From Mulfinger and Trueta, ref. 174, with permission.)

II and III injuries were open fractures in Hawkins' series.[155,187]

Radiographic Diagnosis

Routine AP, lateral, and mortise views of the ankle, and AP, lateral, and oblique views of the foot are obtained in patients with suspected talar fracture. Talar neck fractures, especially undisplaced (Hawkins type I) can be subtle and easily overlooked on routine views. The presence of an ankle injury should alert one to search for a talar neck fracture. Too frequently, the more obvious ankle injury provides too much interest for the unwary observer, and a subtle talar fracture may be overlooked. Up to 20% of patients have associated medial malleolar fractures, which are often more obvious.[155,159] Sixteen percent of patients have fractures in the ipsilateral foot. Conventional tomography or CT may be needed to confirm subtle fractures or to confirm a suspected injury (Fig. 4-78).

Displaced talar neck fractures or fractures with dislocation are usually easily detected on routine views (Fig. 4-79). Detection of subluxation may require that joint spaces and articular relationships be more carefully assessed. Stress views may be helpful. However, the risk of displacing a talar fracture, when present, is significant, and therefore stress views are not always suggested in this setting. If the tarsal relationships are not clear, CT or conventional tomography should be obtained.[154]

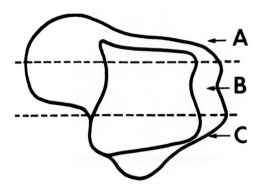

DORSAL VIEW OF THE TALUS
SHOWING THE AREAS COVERED
BY THE FOLLOWING SECTIONS·

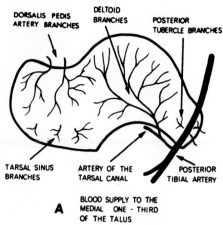

A BLOOD SUPPLY TO THE
MEDIAL ONE - THIRD
OF THE TALUS

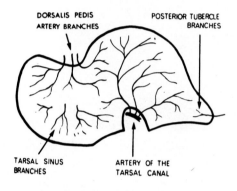

B BLOOD SUPPLY TO THE
MIDDLE ONE - THIRD
OF THE TALUS

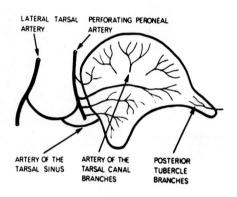

C BLOOD SUPPLY TO THE
LATERAL ONE - THIRD
OF THE TALUS

FIG. 4-77. Dorsal illustration of the talus demonstrating the good supply to the medial talus (**A**), medial one-third (**B**), and lateral one-third (**C**). (From Mulfinger and Trueta, ref. 174 with permission.)

TABLE 4-8. *Talar fractures*[a]

Fracture type	Incidence[b]
Chip or avulsion fracture	40–49%
Neck fracture	28–32%
Body fracture	11–14%
Compression fracture	5–10%
Fracture dislocations	
Neck fracture with subtalar dislocation	45–50%
Neck fracture with posterior body dislocation	30–40%
Body fracture with subtalar dislocation	9–12%
Total dislocation	3–12%

[a] Data from references 113, 135, 148, 154, 158, and 174.
[b] Variable, owing to multiple series.

TABLE 4-9. *Talar neck fractures and fracture dislocations*[a]

Type	Definition	Incidence[b]
I	Undisplaced vertical neck fracture	11–21%
II	Displaced vertical neck fracture with subtalar subluxation or dislocation	40–42%
III	Displaced vertical neck fracture with subluxation or dislocation of both tibiotalar and subtalar joints	23–47%
IV	Displaced vertical fracture of the talus with subtalar or tibiotalar dislocation and subluxation or dislocation of the talonavicular joint	5%

[a] Data from references 138, 139, 155, and 166.
[b] Incidence >100% because of multiple series.

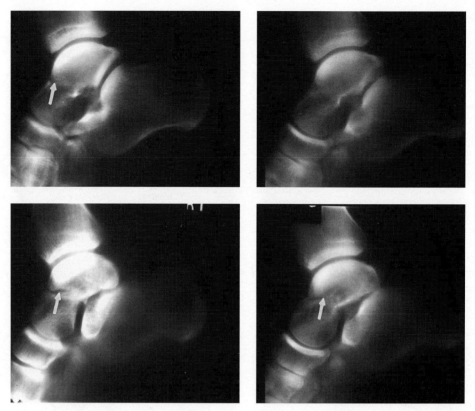

FIG. 4-78. Lateral tomograms of an undisplaced Hawkins type I talar neck fracture (*arrows*). Routine radiographs were normal.

Treatment

Treatment should be instituted as soon as possible after radiographs have been assessed and the fracture has been properly classified.[145,154] Undisplaced (Hawkins type I) fractures can be treated with a below-the-knee cast for 8 to 12 weeks and non-weight bearing for up to 5 months.[138,145]

Fractures that are minimally displaced may be reduced using closed techniques and cast immobilization. However, open reduction with lag screws or K-wires is often needed to

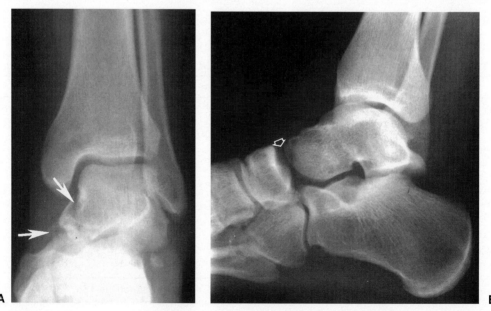

FIG. 4-79. AP (**A**) and Lateral (**B**) views of the ankle demonstrate a comminuted talar neck fracture (best seen on the AP view) (*arrows*) with subluxation (*open arrow*) of the talonavicular and subtalar joints.

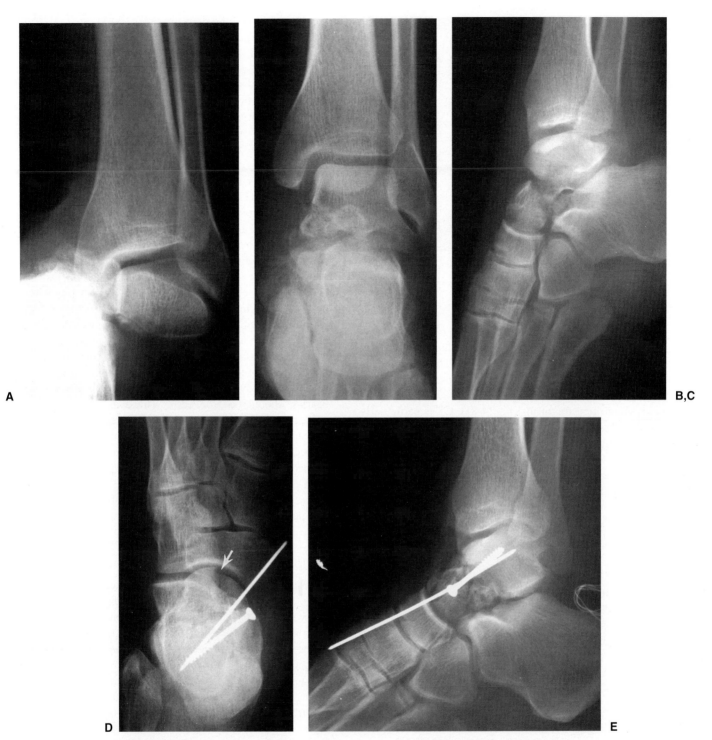

FIG. 4-80. A: AP view of the ankle demonstrating a displaced talar fracture with subtalar dislocation (Hawkins type II). AP (**B**) and lateral (**C**) views after closed manipulation show communication of the talar neck with residual displacement. AP (**D**) and lateral (**E**) radiographs after screw and K-wire fixation show the fracture. The fracture enters the talar head with irregularity of the articular surface (*arrow*).

maintain reduction in type II to IV injuries (Fig. 4-80).[138,155] Even slight displacement can lead to varus malunion.[157] Prognosis is improved in types II to IV if adequate open reduction can be obtained.[161] Although most patients have some residual disability, good results can be achieved in 75% of type I fractures. Good results are obtained in 42% of type II and III fractures.[180]

During reduction, routine radiographs or monitoring with a C-arm fluoroscopic unit can be used to be certain that adequate position of the fragments has been achieved (see

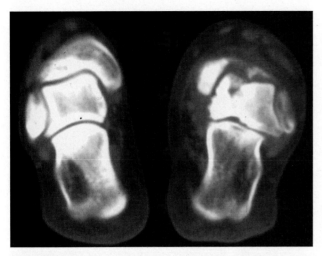

FIG. 4-81. Coronal CT images after talar fracture demonstrating irregularity of the subtalar joint and a large defect with fragmentation of the trochlea.

Fig. 4-80). Canale and Kelley[138] recommend that more than 5 mm displacement and more than 5° malalignment on the AP view should not be accepted. In certain cases, tomography or CT may be needed to evaluate articular alignment and residual joint fragments (Fig. 4-81). CT is particularly useful in this regard. Follow-up radiographs should be obtained for up to 2 years after the injury to exclude AVN. In children, monthly radiographs should be obtained for 6 months because AVN is usually evident by that time.[154] MRI may be indicated when symptoms suggest AVN or as an initial baseline study in patients with type II to IV injuries where the risk for AVN is significant.[133]

Complications

Complications are particularly common after displaced talar neck fractures (Hawkins types II to IV).[138,145,155,166,170] Table 4-10 summarizes the common complications associated with talar neck fractures.

Avascular Necrosis

If untreated, AVN progresses through stages. Changes are based on radiographic features and similar to those described in the hip. Stage I AVN shows slight increased density of the talar body with no deformity (Fig. 4-82). Stage II AVN presents with increased sclerosis with moderate deformity of the trochlea. Stage III AVN presents with more severe deformity and sequestration. Fragmentation of the talus occurs in stage IV AVN (Fig. 4-83).[166] The incidence of AVN increases significantly in type II to IV fractures (see Table 4-10).[140,155,166] An exception appears with pediatric injuries. Although rare, type I fractures developed AVN in 7 of 22 patients reported by Canale and Kelly[138] and Letts and Gibeault.[164]

AVN usually becomes evident on routine radiographs in 6 to 8 weeks (Fig. 4-84). During this non–weight-bearing period, disuse osteoporosis develops that leads to subchondral lucency in the talar dome. This finding (Hawkins' sign) was described by Hawkins and indicates intact vascular supply.[155] The finding is most easily identified on AP or mortise views of the ankle. Canale noted this sign in 23 patients, and only 1 developed AVN. Twenty of 26 patients with a negative Hawkins sign developed AVN.[138]

Although routine radiographic features are well described, changes are evident earlier with radionuclide bone scans and MRI.[133] Interosseous phlebography is not commonly used for diagnosis at this time.[178] Technetium-99m isotope studies have been advocated to assist in determining when weight bearing should be allowed.[138] However, compared with MRI, bone detail is inferior. MRI is the technique of choice for early detection or follow-up evaluation of patients with suspected AVN (Fig. 4-85).[133,190] T1- and T2-weighted sequences (see Fig. 4-85) are usually adequate for detection of AVN. Short T1 inversion recovery (STIR) images or, rarely, gadolinium scans are useful in subtle cases or high-risk patients with equivocal findings.[133]

Arthritis

Posttraumatic arthritis is common after talar neck fractures. The incidence, as expected, increases with the severity of the injury (see Table 4-10).[145] Peterson and associates[180] reported that 97% of patients developed osteoarthritis. Most series show a lower incidence but indicate that degenerative changes developed in nearly two-thirds of type II and III injuries.[138,144,155,166] The incidence of arthritis is also higher in the subtalar joint than in tibiotalar joint (Fig. 4-86).[139,166]

Early radiographic changes may show only slight narrowing of the joint space. This feature may be too subtle to detect without comparison views or CT. In certain cases,

TABLE 4-10. *Complications of talar neck fractures*[a]

Type	Avascular necrosis	Tibiotalar arthritis	Subtalar arthritis	Malunion	Nonunion
I	0–4%	15%	25%	0	0
II	24–42%	36%	66%	28%	6%
III	75–100%	69%	63%	18%	12%

[a] Data from references 138, 139, 155, and 166.

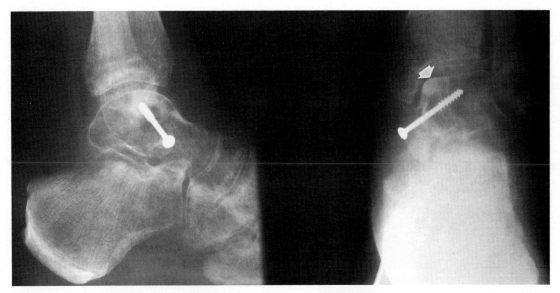

FIG. 4-82. Old talar neck fracture with a single screw for fixation. There is sclerosis (*arrow*) in the medial talar dome resulting from stage I avascular necrosis. The remainder of the talus is osteopenic.

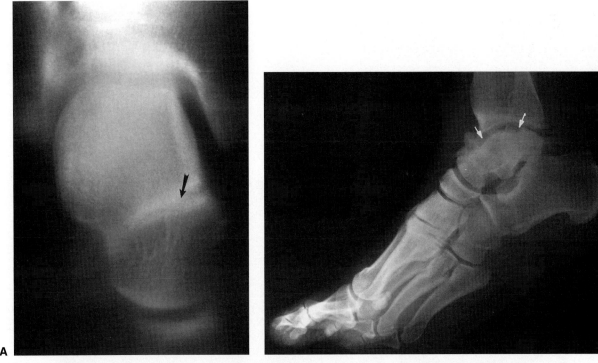

A

B

FIG. 4-83. A: AP tomogram demonstrating a healing talar neck fracture (*arrow*). **B:** Progressive avascular necrosis results in articular collapse (*arrows*) demonstrated on the lateral radiograph of the foot.

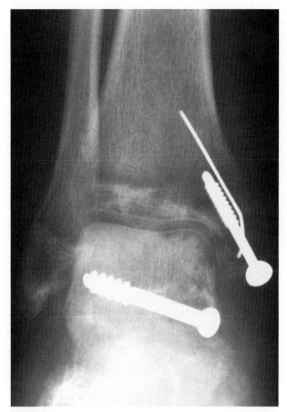

FIG. 4-84. Talar neck fracture with associated medial malleolar fracture. The lateral talus is sclerotic resulting from avascular necrosis. There is normal subchondral lucency medially.

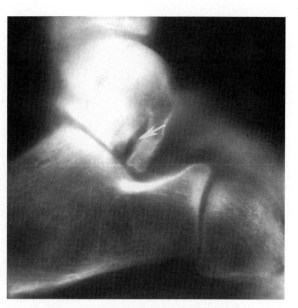

FIG. 4-86. Lateral tomogram demonstrating incomplete bony union (*arrow*) of a talar neck fracture with arthrosis in the posterior facet joint.

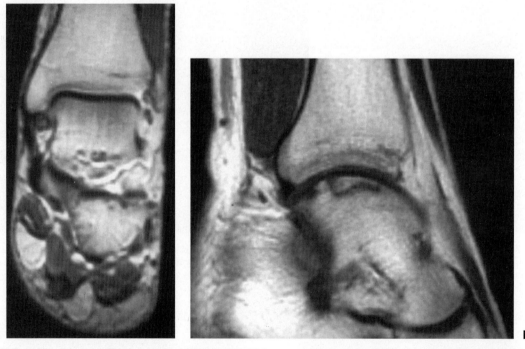

A   B

FIG. 4-85. Coronal (**A**) and sagittal (**B**) SE 500/20 images of the ankle. There is a geographic defect in the posterior talus (*arrow* in **B**) resulting from early avascular necrosis. Radiographs were normal.

ankle or subtalar arthrography is useful for diagnosing early changes. This also permits injection of anesthetic for diagnostic purposes or a combination of steroid and anesthetic for treatment (Fig. 4-87). MRI, especially with intraarticular gadolinium, is useful for assessing early changes in articular cartilage.[133]

Malunion and Nonunion

Delayed healing is not uncommon after talar neck fractures (15%).[180] Delayed union is considered in fractures that have not healed by 6 months.[145] It is not unusual for fractures to take more than 1 year to heal in adults. This is partially because of their intraarticular nature, lack of periosteum, and decreased blood supply.[157] Nonunion occurs in only approximately 4% of cases overall.[157,164] However, the incidence of nonunion is higher in Hawkins type II and III fractures.[166]

Malunion is also more common in complex injuries (Hawkins types II to IV). Lorentzen and associates[166] reported malunion in 15% of all cases, but none occurred in patients with Hawkins type II and III fractures. Canale and Kelly[138] noted varus deformity in 47% of type II fractures. This resulted in increased stress in the lateral subtalar joint.[138,158]

Radiographic diagnosis of malunion or nonunion can be difficult. Serial radiographs may demonstrate widening, sclerosis, and irregularity of the fracture line if nonunion has occurred.

Tomography and CT may be useful, but both have difficulty clearly defining nonunion from fibrous union or early pseudarthrosis. MRI is particularly useful in this situation. T2-weighted sequences demonstrate high intensity (fluid) in the fracture line if nonunion is present and low signal (black) if a fibrous union is present.[133]

Malunion is most easily demonstrated using AP and lateral radiographs that allow measurements to be obtained and compared with the uninjured side. CT may be particularly useful in evaluating the degree of malunion and resulting articular deformities of the complex subtalar joint (see Fig. 4-81).[172]

Other complications include associated fractures (see Fig. 4-84), infection, skin necrosis, and neurovascular damage. Ipsilateral foot and ankle fractures have been reported in 16% of patients.[144] Patients with Hawkins type IV fractures have associated fractures of the medial malleolus in 15%, a finding indicating that complex forces including pronation and rotation were also present (see Fig. 4-84).[138] Fractures distant from the involved foot and ankle are noted in approximately 22% of patients.[144]

Skin necrosis is particularly common after complex (types II to IV) open fractures. This group of patients is also more prone to infection.[138,149,150]

Treatment of complications depends on the patient's age, activity level, and severity of symptoms. Even patients with AVN may have satisfactory results with conservative treatment. Alternatives to treatment of AVN, malunion, nonunion, infection, and talar break formation include triple arthrodesis, tibiocalcaneal fusion, and resection of dorsal talar breaks.[138,147,150] Talectomy alone has not proven to be a successful treatment method in most authors' experience.[138,147] Talectomy with an interposed bone graft has been more successful.

Imaging techniques also play an important role in evaluating surgical procedures. Follow-up studies are needed to be

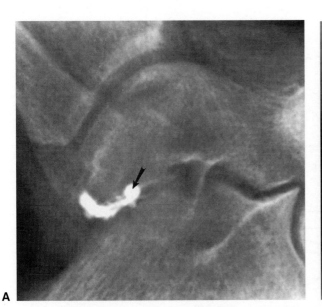 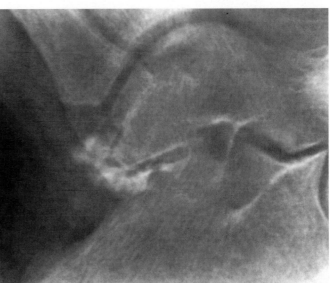

FIG. 4-87. Subtalar joint injection for diagnostic anesthetic injection to confirm the source of pain before subtalar arthrodesis. **A:** Needle in place (*arrow*) with a small test injection of contrast. **B:** Contrast is dispersed with anesthetic injection.

certain that fusion occurs properly without loss of position. Complications such as infection and pseudarthrosis also require careful diagnostic evaluation. To date, routine AP, lateral, and oblique views have been used to evaluate the various fusion procedures. CT is frequently needed to evaluate the complex anatomy. External and internal fixation devices do interfere with CT and MRI. Therefore, conventional tomography may be used in this setting.[133,172]

Early infection may be identified with gallium-67- or indium-111–labeled white blood cells. In addition, the extent of infection can be easily demonstrated with MRI.[133]

Diagnostic anesthetic injection of suspected pseudarthrosis can be accomplished fluoroscopically. This technique may be helpful in localizing the patient's symptoms. This information is particularly useful if further surgery is considered.[172]

Talar Body, Head, and Process Fractures

Fractures of the talar body and posterior and lateral processes are uncommon in adults and rare in children.[157,160,168,175,183] Although the incidence is lower than talar neck fractures, complications are similar for body and neck fractures.

Most talar body fractures are caused by significant falls or motor vehicle accidents that lead to axial compression of the talus between the tibial plafond and calcaneus. Fractures of the lateral process count for only 1% of ankle injuries.[168] Fractures of the lateral process usually occur with the foot dorsiflexed and inverted.[156] The calcaneus causes shearing of the lateral process. Medial process fractures are rare. Most are associated with avulsion of the talotibial ligament. Patients may present with tarsal tunnel syndrome.[195] Sneppen and associates[193] described six basic fracture patterns (Fig.

4-88). These included simple compression fractures, vertical fractures in the coronal and sagittal planes, posterior tubercle fractures, lateral tubercle fractures, and comminuted crush fractures. In addition, chip or avulsion fractures may also occur. Fractures of the head generally involve the talonavicular joint. Many body fractures, especially those caused by shearing forces, are displaced and associated with subluxation.[157]

McCrory and Bladin[168] further classified lateral process fractures into three types. A type 1 fracture is a nonarticular avulsion of the anterior inferior portion of the lateral process. This may be related to anterior talofibular ligament avulsion. The type 2 fracture is a larger single fragment that involves the talofibular articular surface. This fracture may be undisplaced (type 2A) or displaced (type 2B). Type 3 fractures are comminuted and involve the articular surface.[168]

Radiographic Diagnosis

AP, lateral, and mortise views of the ankle are usually adequate for diagnosis of displaced fractures. Lateral process fractures are most easily appreciated on the AP view.[168] More subtle fractures (chip, avulsion, or undisplaced body fractures) require conventional or CT for detection (Fig. 4-89). Views of the foot should also be obtained because multiple injuries are common.[193] Treatment planning is facilitated by CT or conventional tomography in many cases. MRI may also be helpful to assess associated soft tissue injury.[133]

Avulsion fractures dorsal and distal to the neck are not common. Bone fragments are avulsed by the articular capsule and talonavicular ligament. These fractures are best seen on the lateral view of the ankle and should not be confused with the normal talar ridge (Fig. 4-90).[184]

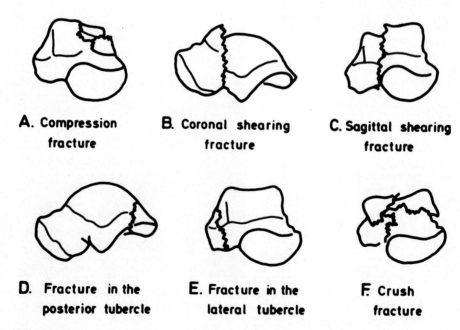

A. Compression fracture

B. Coronal shearing fracture

C. Sagittal shearing fracture

D. Fracture in the posterior tubercle

E. Fracture in the lateral tubercle

F. Crush fracture

FIG. 4-88. Illustration of talar body fracture types. (From Sneppen et al., ref. 193, with permission.)

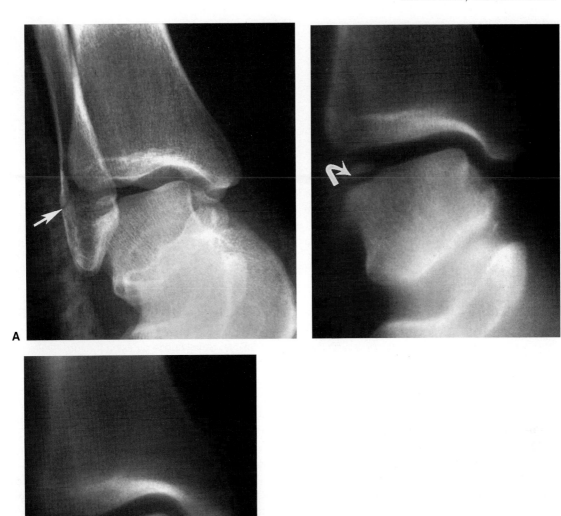

FIG. 4-89. Inversion injury with an undisplaced lateral malleolar fracture (*arrow*) seen on the AP view of the ankle (**A**). Tomograms (**B** and **C**) demonstrate a displaced lateral talar dome fracture (*curved arrow* in **B**) and small medial avulsion fractures (*arrows* in **C**).

Treatment

Treatment principles are similar to those applied to talar neck fractures. Anatomic reduction is necessary and is accomplished using operative techniques for displaced fractures. Although process fractures are uncommon (0.86% of 1,500 patients presenting with ankle sprains), there is often significant cartilage loss leading to osteoarthritis.[168,169] Posterior and lateral process fractures can be treated with cast immobilization if they are not displaced.[159,168,171,193] In patients with displaced process fractures, either early internal fixation or late removal of the fragment is preferred.[172]

Complications are similar to talar neck fractures, with almost all patients eventually developing arthrosis. The incidence is somewhat lower with posterior and lateral process fractures. Sneppen and colleagues[193] reported malunion in one-third of patients and AVN in 16% of cases. When complications developed, a second procedure such as tibiocalcaneal fusion or tibiotalar (Blair) fusion may be indicated.[134,150,172]

Talar Dome Fractures

Osteochondral fractures of the talar dome differ from other chip or avulsion fractures in that they are more difficult to detect and prognosis is potentially worse than that of a nonarticular chip or avulsion fracture.[172,177] Talar dome fractures are the most common talar fracture. This injury is much

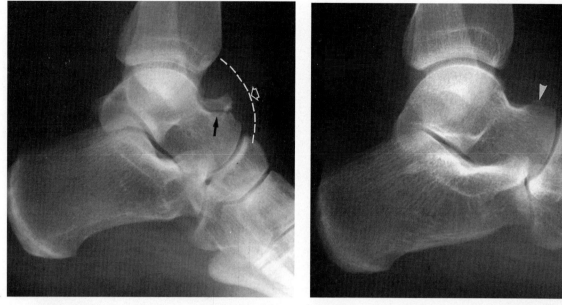

FIG. 4-90. Lateral views of the ankle demonstrating dorsal talar avulsion fractures. **A:** Large avulsed fragment (*arrow*) with effusion (*white broken line, open arrow*). **B:** Small subtle avulsion fracture (*white arrowhead*).

more common in adults. Only 8% (16 of 201) of patients in the series of Berndt and Harty series were less than 16 years of age.[132]

The origin of the lesion is controversial. Suggested mechanisms include ischemic necrosis, abnormal vascular anatomy, congenital disorders, spontaneous necrosis, and trauma.[132,172,176] Most agree that trauma is responsible for

most fractures, especially those occurring laterally. Eighty-four to 90% of patients describe a definite traumatic event that precipitated their symptoms. Males outnumbered females by nearly 2:1.[132,172]

The mechanism of injury and radiographic appearance of medial and lateral talar dome fracture differs significantly. Lateral fractures are caused by inversion or inversion-dorsi-

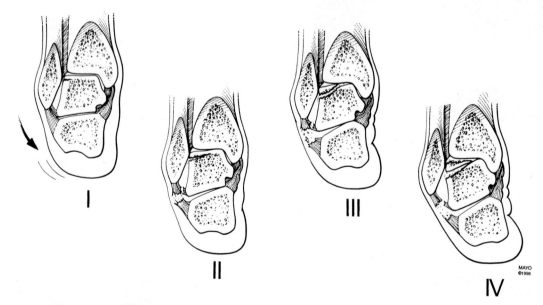

FIG. 4-91. Illustration of mechanism of lateral talar dome fracture. Inversion injury causes the lateral talar dome to impact the fibular. Stage I, compression injury. Stage II, incomplete fracture with partial elevation. Stage III, complete fracture without displacement. Stage IV, complete fracture with displacement. (Data from refs. 132 and 139.)

flexion injuries (Fig. 4-91). The fracture is shallow, with a flake-like fragment.[132,139] Medial lesions are deeper, not always clearly associated with trauma, and are often less symptomatic.[139] Traumatic lesions are caused by lateral rotation of the plantar-flexed ankle (Fig. 4-92).[132]

The most commonly used classification for talar dome fractures was devised by Berndt and Harty (see Figs. 4-91 and 4-92).[132] Stage I lesions are compressions of the talar dome with no associated ligament ruptures and intact cartilage. These lesions are the most subtle and are rarely symptomatic. Stage II lesions are incomplete fractures with the fragment remaining partially attached. Stage III lesions are complete fractures but not displaced. Stage IV lesions are detached.[132] Stage II to IV lesions can be overlooked because of the significant ligament injuries that accompany them (Figs. 4-91 and 4-92).[132,139,165]

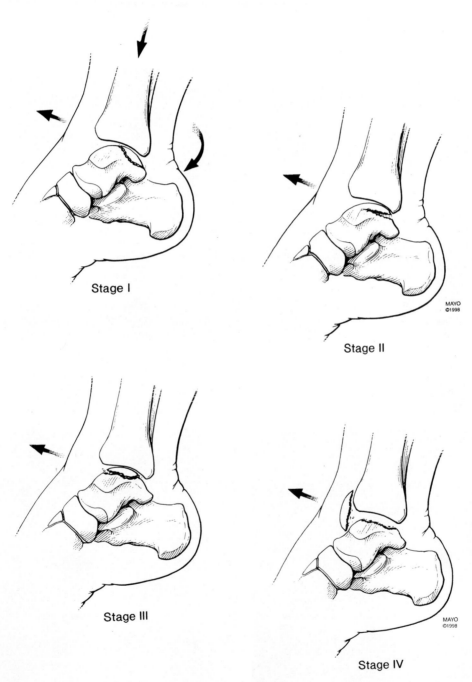

FIG. 4-92. Illustration of mechanism of injury for medial talar dome fractures. The injury occurs with plantar flexion, axial loading and inversion lateral rotation. Stage I, compression. Stage II, fracture with partial elevation. Stage III, complete fracture with no significant displacement. Stage IV, displaced fracture. (Data from refs. 132 and 139.)

Diagnosis

Routine AP, lateral, and mortise views of the ankle are taken in patients with suspected fracture or ligament injury. Talar dome fractures are most easily detected on mortise or occasionally the AP view (Fig. 4-93). The lateral view is rarely useful for identification of this fracture. However, the lateral view should be carefully evaluated for the presence of an effusion. The presence of an effusion should lead one to search more carefully for a talar dome fracture.[142] Stage I lesions can be especially subtle. The only finding on routine views may be a subtle change in bone density at the margin (usually lateral) of the talar dome. If an effusion is present or if clinical suspicion is high, CT should be performed (Figs. 4-94 and 4-95).[165] Tomograms should be obtained in the AP and lateral projections and CT images reformatted (thin sections up to 3 mm) to demonstrate the size and position of the fragment. It is not uncommon to overlook this lesion on the initial examination (see Fig. 4-93). Patients are commonly treated for an ankle sprain. It is imperative to keep this lesion in mind in all patients with ankle sprains. When a history of inversion injury, exercise-related ankle pain, clicking, or catching, and persistent swelling is present, one should definitely pursue the possibility of an osteochon-

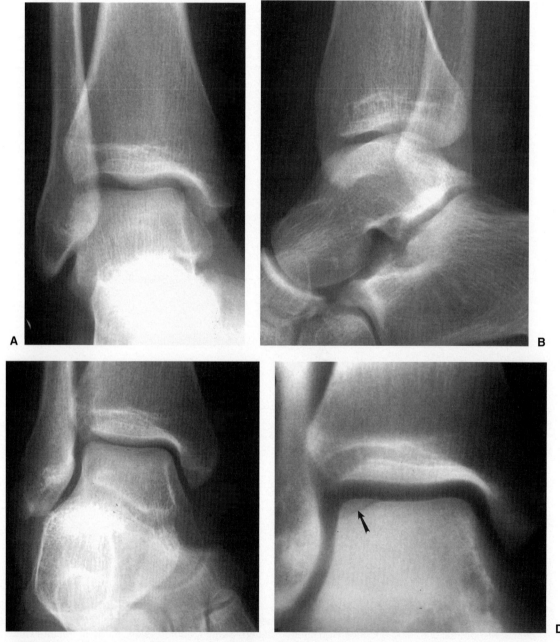

FIG. 4-93. AP (**A**), lateral (**B**) and mortise (**C**) views after ankle injury presenting as a sprain. Tomogram (**D**) clearly demonstrates a talar dome fracture (*arrow*). Berndt and Harty stage III.

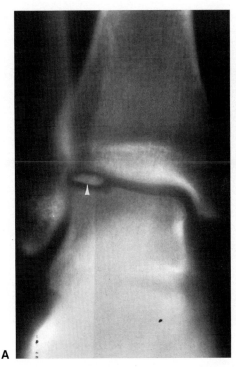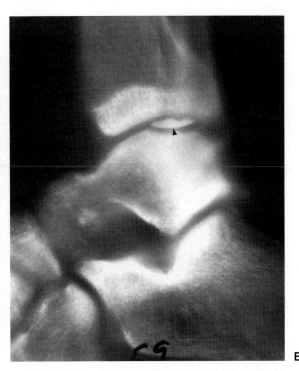

FIG. 4-94. AP (**A**) and lateral (**B**) tomograms demonstrate a stage IV lateral talar dome fracture. The articular surface (*arrowhead*) is reduced.

dral fracture.[179,197] More than 20% of lesions are missed when additional studies (tomography, CT, bone scans) are not performed.[137,172,179]

Once the lesion is detected, it is important to determine its exact site and size. This can be determined with CT or tomography (see Fig. 4-94).[191] The cartilage over the lesion may be intact or interrupted. Articular cartilage can be evaluated using arthrography (CT or conventional). However, MRI is more commonly used today (Fig. 4-96 and 4-97). Subtle changes may be more evident if MR arthrography is performed.[133]

Treatment

Opinions vary on the optimal treatment for talar dome lesions.[132,141,152,182] Berndt and Harty[132] reviewed 201 cases—43.7% lateral and 56.3% medial. The lateral lesions most often involved the middle third of the dome and the medial fractures the posterior portion of the articular surface. Fifteen percent were stage I, 36% were stage II, 28% were stage III, and 21% were stage IV lesions. One hundred forty-nine of the patients were treated conservatively, and 73.9% had poor results. Patients treated surgically had good results in 78.6% of cases. Alexander and Lichtman[131] found better results with drilling and curettage, followed by non-weight bearing and early range-of-motion exercises. Their results were also excellent in chronic lesions. Canale and Belding[139] recommended conservative treatment for stage I and II lesions and reserved surgery for patients in whom this earlier treatment was unsuccessful. Surgery was recommended for all stage III and IV lesions. More recently, arthroscopy has been used to evaluate the articular cartilage and to determine whether arthroscopic or conventional surgery is required.[141,182]

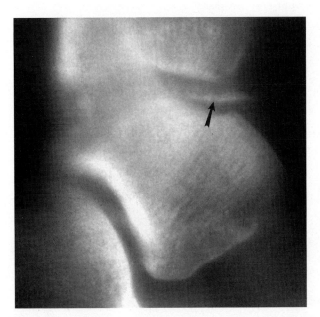

FIG. 4-95. Lateral tomogram of a stage IV medial talar dome fracture (*arrow*).

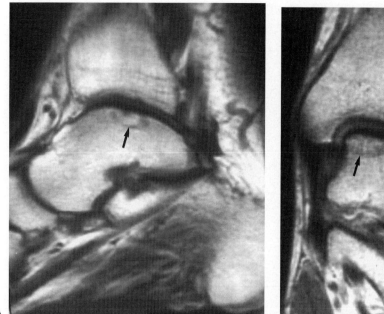
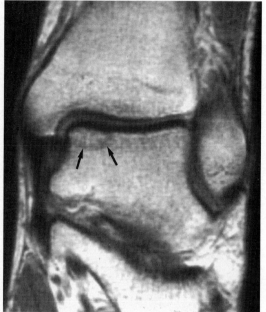

FIG. 4-96. Sagittal (**A**) and coronal (**B**) SE 500/20 MRI images demonstrate an undisplaced medial talar dome fracture (*arrows*).

Complications

Symptoms are often more prolonged and displacement of lateral lesions more common. The most common complication is osteoarthritis (Figs. 4-98 and 4-99).[139,167] This is evident in 50% of patients regardless of the treatment used.[139] Displaced fragments lose their blood supply and are susceptible to AVN. Subchondral cyst formation has also been reported, presumably because of intrusion of synovial fluid through defects in the articular cartilage and subchondral bone (Fig. 4-100).[198]

Talar and Subtalar Dislocations

The majority of eversion and inversion motion occurs at the subtalar joint. Inversion is limited by the interosseous ligament, peroneal tendons, and lateral ankle ligaments.

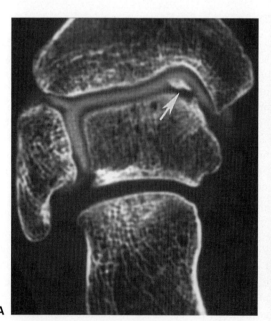
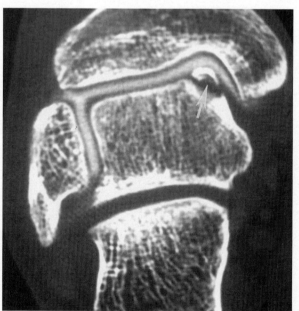

FIG. 4-97. Stage III medial talar dome fracture. CT arthrogram with bone (**A**) and soft tissue (**B**) setting shows the fracture. Contrast does not extend between the talus and fragment (*arrow*). *(continued)*

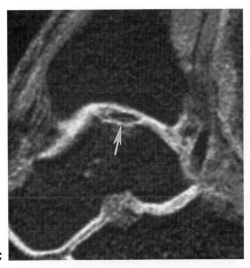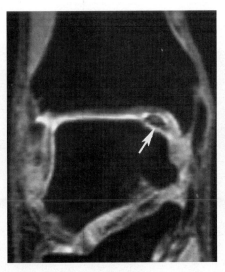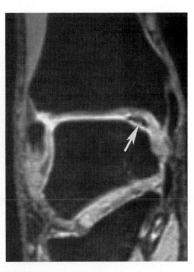

C

D,E

FIG. 4-97. *Continued.* Sagittal (**C**) and coronal (**D** and **E**) images show high signal between the fragment and the talus indicating that fluid (*arrow*) extends between the fragment and the talus.

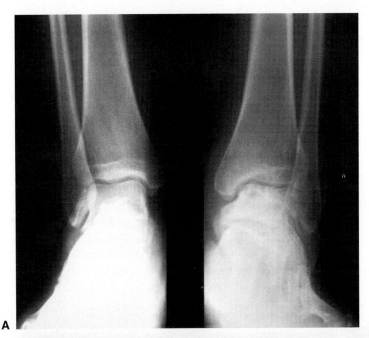

A

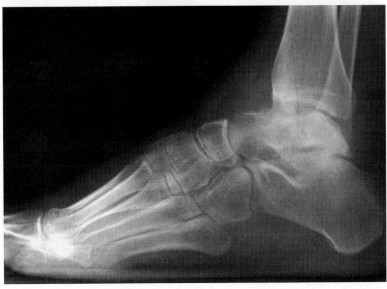

B

FIG. 4-98. Standing AP views of the ankles (**A**) and standing lateral of the left foot (**B**) demonstrate tibiotalar and subtalar arthrosis after medial talar dome fracture.

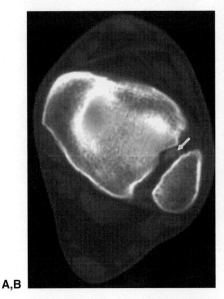 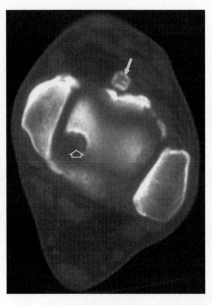

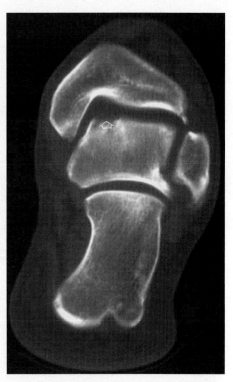

FIG. 4-99. Axial (**A** and **B**) and coronal (**C**) CT images of a stage IV medial talar dome fracture (*open arrow*) with multiple displaced joint fragments (*arrows*) and degenerative arthritis.

Eversion is limited by the deltoid ligament, posterior tibial tendon, and anterior tibial tendon.[160,171]

The talus and calcaneus are connected by joint capsules and the lateral, medial, interosseous, and cervical ligaments (see Fig. 4-75). The talonavicular ligament provides less support than the talocalcaneal group.[151,157,160]

Pure subtalar dislocations occur with simultaneous dislocation of the talocalcaneal and talonavicular joints. Total talar dislocation occurs when the talus is dislocated from the ankle mortise in addition to the foregoing joints.[136,140,148,157,171]

Subtalar dislocations are uncommon (1.3 to 2% of all dislocations).[146,158,188] Fifteen percent of all talar injuries are caused by dislocation.[179] Most injuries occur during significant falls with inversion forces, motor vehicle accidents, or landing on the inverted ankle in sporting events.[146,188,192] Bilateral dislocations have been reported with Ehlers-Danlos syndrome.[158] The injury is rare in chldren.[149] DeLee and Curtis[146] reported the average age to be 33.6 years. The incidence of subtalar dislocations in males is 6 to 10 times higher than in females.[151]

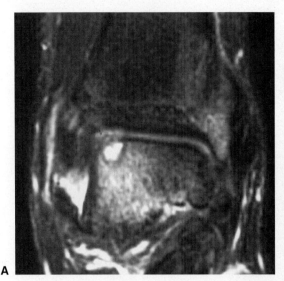 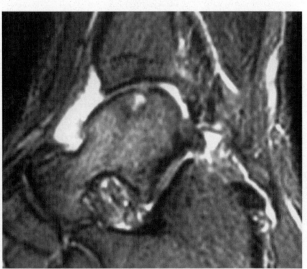

FIG. 4-100. Old missed medial talar dome injury. MRI images in the coronal (**A**) and sagittal (**B**) planes using SE 2000/80 sequences demonstrate marrow edema with a cystic lesion medially.

Subtalar dislocations may be medial (56%), lateral (34%), posterior (6%), or anterior (4%).[192] With medial dislocations, the talus remains in the ankle mortise, and the calcaneus and navicular are dislocated medially (inversion force). Lateral dislocations occur with eversion injuries.[146] DeLee and Curtis[146] reported a higher incidence of associated fractures with lateral dislocations. Articular fractures of the talus, navicular, or calcaneus occurred in 75% of patients with lateral dislocation compared with 45% with medial dislocations. Lateral dislocations are also more commonly open injuries. Associated malleolar fractures or fractures of the

fifth metatarsal base can occur with any subtalar dislocation.[146,157]

Total dislocation is uncommon but potentially one of the worst hindfoot injuries.[188] Detenbeck and Kelly[148] noted only nine cases of total talar dislocations from 1959 to 1967. Seven of nine cases were open injuries and required open reduction. Despite aggressive reduction and adequate position, seven of these nine patients eventually required talectomy because of infection (Fig. 4-101). Most infections were severe enough to require open drainage or irrigation.

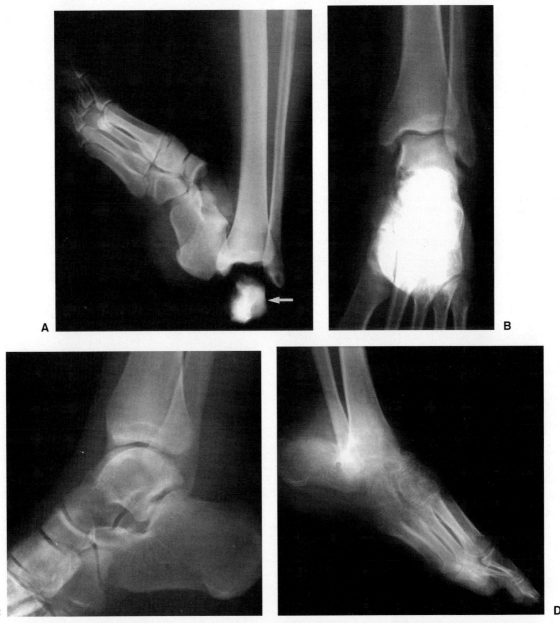

FIG. 4-101. A: AP radiograph of the leg and ankle after total talar dislocation. The talar dome (*arrow*) is directed laterally. AP (**B**) and lateral (**C**) radiographs after reduction show the talus in normal position. Because of chronic infection and persistent drainage, a talectomy (**D**) was performed 1 year later. (From Detenbeck and Kelly, ref. 148, with permission.)

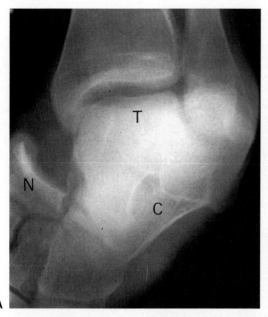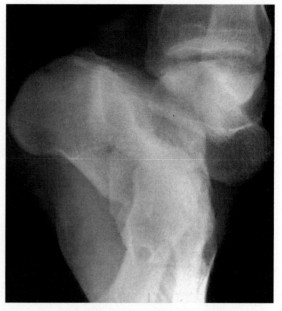

FIG. 4-102. Subtalar and talonavicular dislocation. **A:** AP view of the ankle shows the navicular (*N*), talus (*T*), and calcaneus (*C*), which is rotated under the talus. **B:** Oblique view of the hindfoot shows the talus lateral to the calcaneus.

Diagnosis

Routine radiographs of the foot and ankle are usually sufficient to diagnose subtalar or total talar dislocation (Fig. 4-102). In certain cases, stress views may be useful. Associated fractures should be looked for carefully after reduction.[188] CT is best for this purpose.[153,159,172,189,194]

Treatment

Prompt reduction and early motion (3 weeks after injury) should be the goals of treatment. The latter is particularly important to maintain subtalar motion. Medial dislocations can more often be reduced using closed techniques than lateral subtalar dislocations. When there are associated fractures, immobilization in casts leads to poorer results.[148,149,157,160] Inability to reduce dislocations has been reported. The posterior tibial tendon becomes entrapped, making it impossible to reduce lateral dislocations.[146,163,166]

Because of the high incidence of infection and the need for eventual talectomy, Detenbeck and Kelly[148] suggested early talectomy. The morbidity and problems with infection and AVN are reduced. AVN almost always accompanies total talar dislocation.[148]

CALCANEAL FRACTURES

The calcaneus is the largest tarsal bone, and because of its complex anatomy, it can be difficult to image with routine radiographic techniques (see Chapter 2). It is composed of a thin cortical shell with sparse trabecular bone, especially in adults.[211,226] The superior surface has three facets, which articulate with the anterior, medial, and posterior talar facets (see Fig. 4-75). The middle facet is located on the sustentaculum tali and lies anterior to the sinus tarsi. There is a groove on the inferior surface of the sustentaculum for the flexor hallucis longus tendon. The posterior facet (largest of the three) forms the posterior border of the sinus tarsi.[204,209,221,233]

The calcaneus is the most commonly fractured bone in the adult foot, accounting for 60% of foot fractures and 2% of all skeletal fractures.[200,203,204,209,221] Fractures occur most commonly in males. Calcaneal fractures in children are much less common (5% of all calcaneus fractures), and the patterns differ from adult calcaneal fractures.[208,230,234] Most calcaneal fractures in children are less extensive, and compression is less likely to occur because of the cancellous bone.[230,234] Moreover, unlike in adults, calcaneal fractures in children are generally extraarticular. Overall, 63% of pediatric fractures are extraarticular and 37% are intraarticular. In patients less than 7 years of age, 92% of fractures are extraarticular.[230] In adults, 70 to 75% of calcaneal fractures are intraarticular and 25 to 30% are extraarticular. The adult calcaneus is more susceptible to axial loading, resulting in frequent compression and displacement of the fractured fragments.[201,221,226,229]

Mechanism of Injury and Classification

Most severe adult calcaneal fractures are caused by falls or motor vehicle accidents resulting in axial loading of the calcaneus. Bilateral fractures occur in up to 10% of patients with falls from significant height. Associated vertebral

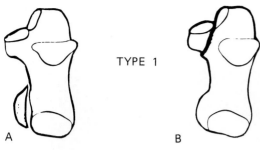

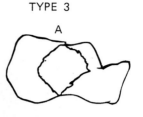

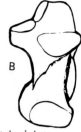

TYPE 1

A   B

Fracture of tuberosity   Fracture of sustentaculum tali

TYPE 3

A   B

Oblique fracture not involving sub-talar joint

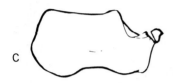

C

Fracture of anterior process

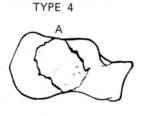

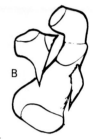

TYPE 4

A   B

Fracture involving sub-talar joint

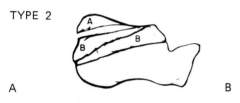

TYPE 2

A   B

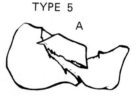

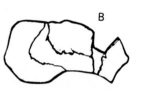

TYPE 5

A   B

FIG. 4-103. Illustration of the Rowe classification for calcaneal fractures. (From Rowe et al., ref. 228, with permission.)

compression fractures are also reported in 10% of these patients.[215] Less severe avulsion and extraarticular fractures occur with twisting injuries or muscle pulls.[207,221,229] The mechanism of injury differs somewhat in children. Although falls and motor vehicle accidents still account for many injuries, direct trauma from lawn mower injury is the third most common mechanism of injury in children. This obviously results in an open fracture with a prognosis that is much worse than the usual benign prognosis of pediatric calcaneus fractures.[230]

The classification of calcaneal injuries has been proposed by Rowe and associates[228] and Essex-Lopresti.[204,205] The Rowe classification (Fig. 4-103) is less commonly used. Using this classification, type I and II fractures are caused by avulsion injuries. These may be subtle radiographically, especially anterior process fractures, and if there is articular involvement, management is more difficult. Type III to IV fractures are more extensive with more complex treatment considerations.[221,228] The Essex-Lopresti classification (Table 4-11) is more popular than the Rowe classification. This classification divides fractures into two major categories, intraarticular (involving subtalar joint) and those not involving the subtalar joint.[204,205,221] Types IIB and IIC are the most common intraarticular fractures.[205] To provide a more general classification that can be used for both adults and children, Schmidt and Weiner[230] proposed a combined

classification using both the Rowe and colleagues[228] and Essex-Lopresti[205] classifications (Table 4-12). A separate type 6 fracture was added because of the significant soft tissue injury seen with this fracture in children (Fig. 4-104).

Type I fractures generally have a benign course and are caused by avulsion or twisting injuries.[205,221,228] However, types IB, C, and D do involve articular surfaces resulting in different treatment consideration. Apophyseal fractures (type IA) only occur in children. Anterior process fractures (15% of calcaneal fractures) (type 1C) can be particularly subtle.[211,225] Patients often present with symptoms of an

TABLE 4-11. *Essex-Lopresti classification of calcaneal fractures[a]*

I. No subtalar joint involvement
  A. Tuberosity fractures
    1. Beak type
    2. Medial avulsion
    3. Vertical
    4. Horizontal
  B. Calcaneocuboid joint involvement
II. Involving subtalar joint
  A. Undisplaced
  B. Displaced
  C. Gross comminution

[a] Data from references 204 and 205.

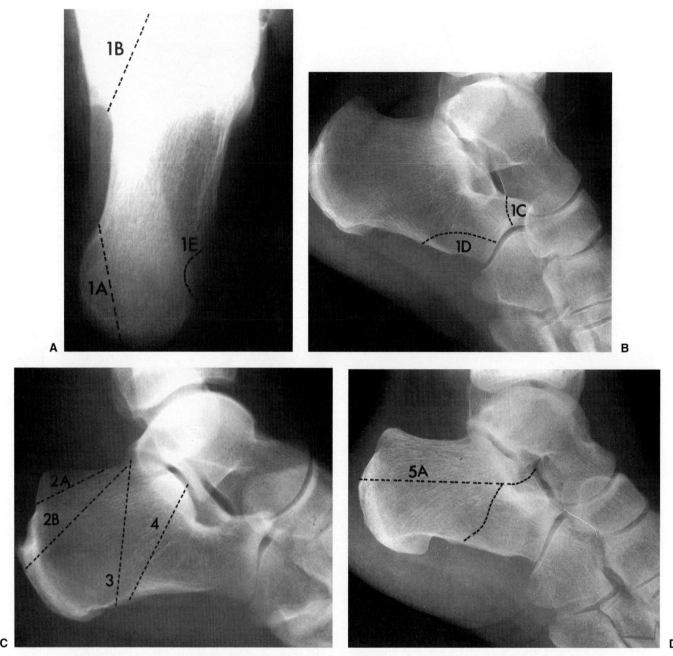

FIG. 4-104. Schmidt and Weiner[230] classification, which modifies the Rowe[228] and Essex-Lopresti[204,205] classifications for calcaneal fractures. **A:** Axial view of the calcaneus demonstrating type 1A (tuberosity or apophysis fracture), type 1B (fracture of the sustentaculum), and type 1E (avulsion fractures). **B:** Lateral view of the calcaneus demonstrating type 1C (anterior process fracture) and type 1D (inferior articular fracture). **C:** Lateral view demonstrating type 2A (beak fracture), type 2B (Achilles avulsion fracture), type 3 (undisplaced extraarticular fracture), and type 4 (linear intraarticular fracture). **D:** Lateral view demonstrating a type 5A (tongue-type compression fracture of the subtalar joint). *(continued)*

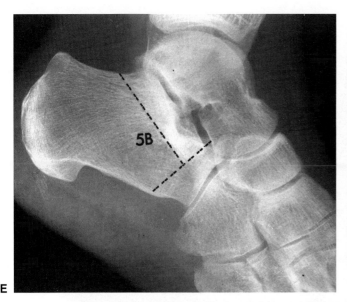

E

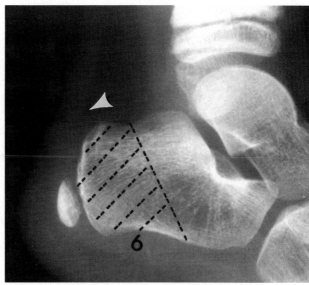

F

FIG. 4-104. *Continued.* **E:** Lateral view demonstrating a type 5B (joint depression type fracture). **F:** Lateral view of the calcaneus in a child demonstrating the extent of a type 5 fracture with loss of the Achilles tendon insertion (*white arrow*).

ankle sprain.[225] The most common mechanism of injury is inversion with internal rotation of the foot with the anterior process avulsed by the bifurcate ligament.[221,225] A less common mechanism is a compression fracture (''nutcracker injury'') with the foot dorsiflexed during varus stress leading to compression of the anterior process (Fig. 4-105). Other inversion fractures affecting the dorsal lateral calcaneus can be confused with sprain, anterior process fracture, or the os peroneum (a normal variant). Norfay and colleagues[222] noted this small, flake-like fracture in 10% of patients with suspected ankle fracture.

Type 2 fractures are caused by direct trauma (2A) usually with abrupt contraction of the Achilles tendon (2B) when the ankle is in a fixed position. These fractures account for only approximately 4% of calcaneal injuries.[217, 228]

Type 3 to 5 injuries are usually caused by axial loading.

TABLE 4-12. *Calcaneal fractures: classification and incidence[a]*

Type	Schmidt and Weiner modification of Rowe and Essex-Lopresti classification	Incidence
1C	Anterior process	15%
1A	Tuberosity	6%
1B	Sustentaculum tali	3%
1D and 1E		1%
2	A beak or B Achilles avulsion	3–4%
3	Linear extraarticular	19%
4	Intraarticular, linear	10–24%
5A	Tongue-type	5%
5B	Joint depression or comminution	43–60%

[a] Data from references 205, 208, 221, and 228.

This may be a direct vertical force or posterior force directed toward the base of the posterior facet (Fig. 4-106). Generally, the fracture also involves the sustentaculum tali, which is commonly involved because of associated shearing forces (Fig. 4-107).[207] Type 3 fractures account for approximately 19% of calcaneal fractures, and types 4 and 5 (intraarticular) account for 70 to 75% of calcaneal fractures.[208,221,228]

Type 6 fractures involve the posterior calcaneus, tuberosity, and Achilles tendon. There is extensive posterior soft tissue injury. This injury commonly occurs with lawn mower accidents in children (see Fig. 4-104F).[230] More recently, Paley and Hall developed a fracture classification based on lateral radiographic features (Fig. 4-108).[224] This system is a modification of the Essex-Lopresti and Soeur-Remy classifications.[205,224] Type a fractures result in a two-part intraarticular fracture (see Fig. 4-108, a). Type b fractures are tongue fractures with secondary anterior and posterior fracture lines (type b1) or with comminution (type b2) (see Fig. 4-108, b1 and b2). Type c fractures are depression injuries with anterior and posterior fracture lines (type c1) or with comminution (type c2) (Fig. 4-108, c1, and c2). Type d fractures are complex comminuted fractures (see Fig. 4-108, d).[224]

Radiographic Diagnosis

Routine radiographs in patients with suspected calcaneal fractures should include lateral, oblique, and axial views (see Chapter 2). Routine views are generally adequate for detection of displaced fractures (Fig. 4-109). Care should be taken to measure Böhler's angle and to assess the degree of articular involvement. The latter problem and the need to detect more subtle injury usually require further studies.

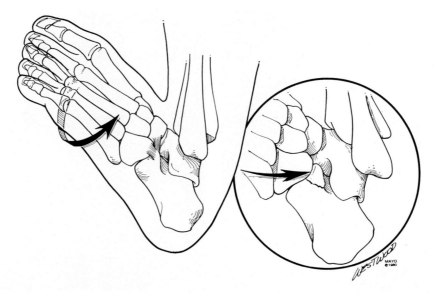

FIG. 4-105. Illustration of compression injury of the anterior calcaneal process. (From Morrey et al., ref. 221, with permission.)

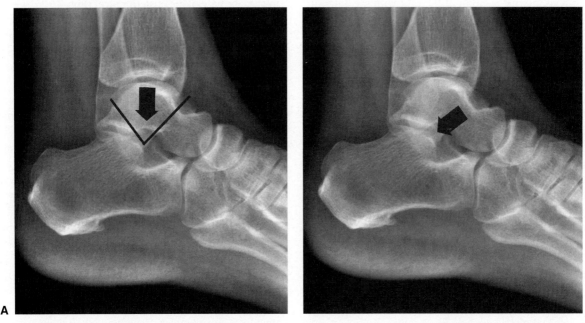

FIG. 4-106. A and B: Lateral radiographs demonstrating the forces leading to intraarticular tongue and compression fractures of the calcaneus.

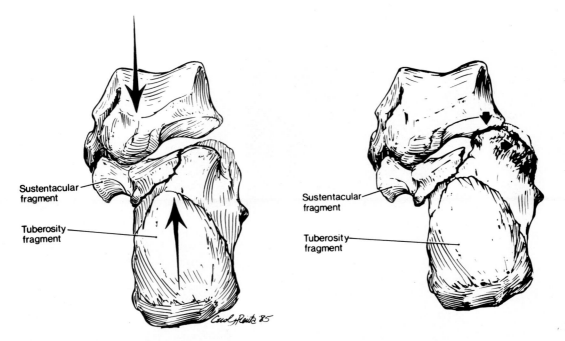

FIG. 4-107. Illustration of vertical forces leading to calcaneal fracture and sustentacular involvement. (From Gilmer et al., ref. 207, with permission.)

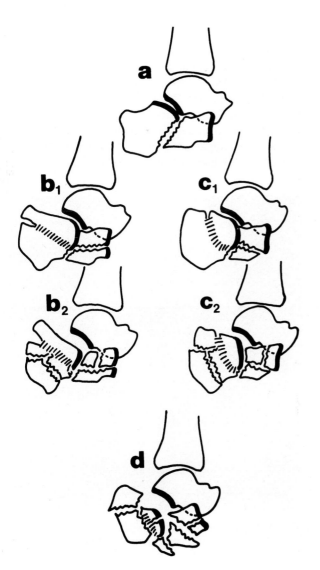

FIG. 4-108. Illustration of Paley and Hall modification of Essex-Lopresti and Soeur-Remy calcaneal fracture classifications. The classification is based on fracture identified on lateral radiographs. (From Paley D and Hall H, ref. 224, with permission.)

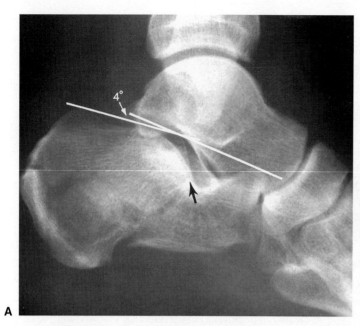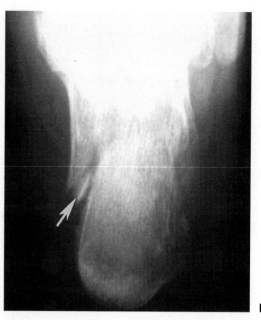

FIG. 4-109. A: Lateral view of the calcaneus demonstrating an intraarticular fracture (*arrow*) with multiple posterior fragments (Böhler's angle measures 4°; normal is 20° to 40°). **B:** Axial view shows medial impaction and comminution (*arrow*).

Special oblique views for the subtalar joint and anterior process have been described (see Chapter 2).[204,205] In the acute setting, fluoroscopically positioned spot views are more easily obtained. CT has replaced conventional tomography as the technique of choice for defining more complex fractures and foot anatomy. This approach is important not only for diagnoses but also to assist in determining the type of therapy.[201,207,209,221,223] Undisplaced type 1 fractures are frequently missed. Schmidt and Weiner[230] noted that 81% of fractures overlooked radiographically fell into the type 1 category. These fractures can be easily detected using conventional tomography or CT (Figs. 4-110 and 4-111).[206,211] Conventional tomograms can also be used in patients with

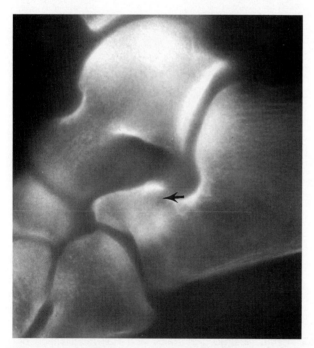

FIG. 4-110. Lateral tomogram demonstrating a slightly displaced anterior process fracture (*arrow*). Type 1C, up to 50% of these fractures are overlooked if tomograms or CT scans are not obtained.

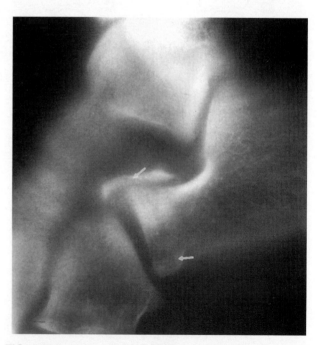

FIG. 4-111. Lateral tomogram demonstrating type 1C (*upper arrow*) and 1D (*lower arrow*) fractures of the anterior calcaneus.

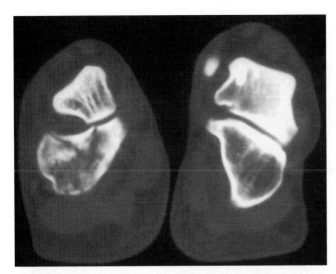

FIG. 4-112. Coronal CT image demonstrating a minimally displaced intraarticular fracture. Type 1.

intraarticular fractures. However, generally CT is preferred. CT provides advantages in defining joint alignment and in detecting intraarticular fragments and the integrity of the sustentacular portion of the calcaneus.[201,202,219]

Several CT classification systems have been devised in recent years.[201,219] Corbett and colleagues[201] devised a five-part CT classification system using CT features of calcaneal fractures. The classification was based on conventional 4-mm thick axial and coronal CT images. Most intraarticular fractures result in three major fragments consisting of the tuberosity, the sustentaculum, and a superolateral fragment.[205,224,230] These fragments may involve the posterior facet and may result in loss of calcaneal height (see Fig. 4-

109) and increased width. The lateral fragments may cause peroneal impingment.[201] Displacement of fragments by more than 2 mm or angulation of more than 10° is considered significant by more orthopedic surgeons.[201,228]

Based on these data, Corbett and associates[201] divided calcaneal fractures into types 1 to 5. Type 1 fractures are minimally displaced or undisplaced without significant articular deformity. There is no lateral wall blowout or comminution (Fig. 4-112). Type 2 fractures have widening of the calcaneus, but the primary fracture line involves less than 10% of the posterior subtalar joint (Fig. 4-113). Type 3 fractures result in three major fragments with blowout of the lateral calcaneus (Fig. 4-114). Type 4 fractures have both

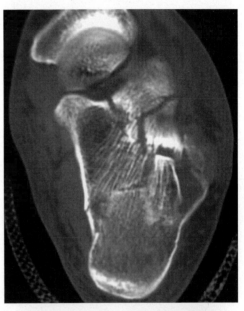

A

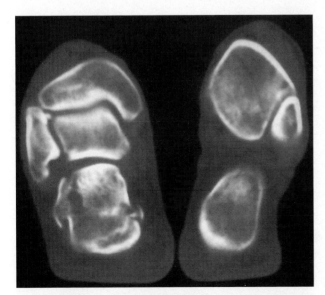

FIG. 4-113. Coronal CT image demonstrating a type 2 fracture with widening of the calcaneus but only marginal involvement of the subtalar joint.

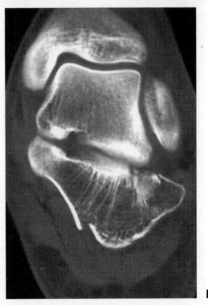

B

FIG. 4-114. CT images of a type 3 fracture with lateral displacement (A) and a displaced sustentacular fragment on the coronal image (B).

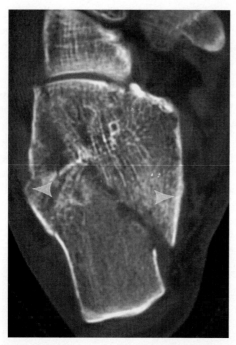

FIG. 4-115. Axial CT image demonstrating a type 4 fracture with outward displacement of the medial and lateral walls (*arrowheads*).

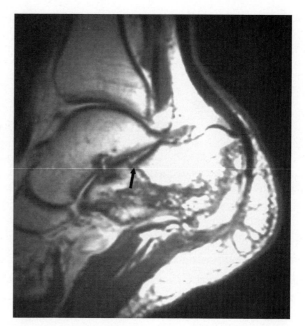

FIG. 4-117. Sagittal SE 500/20 image of a complex calcaneal fracture involving the posterior facet (*arrow*).

medial and lateral wall displacement. The posterior facet is not significantly displaced, so reconstruction is possible (Fig. 4-115). Type 5 fractures have comminution of the posterior facet into at least three fragments. All fracture classes are given a (+) or (−) depending on involvement (+) or

sparing (−) of the calcaneocuboid articulation.[201] These are key factors in therapy planning.[201,212,219,223,231]

Soft tissue injury can also be assessed using CT.[207,223–225] However, when tendon and ligament complications are suspected, MRI may provide better information. MRI can also identify fractures (Figs. 4-116 and 4-117). However, we generally reserve MRI for soft tissue or osseous complications.

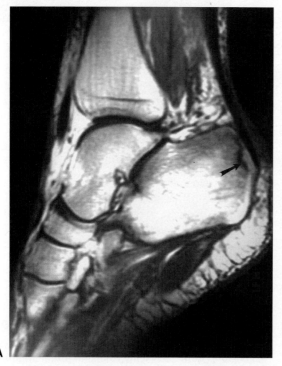

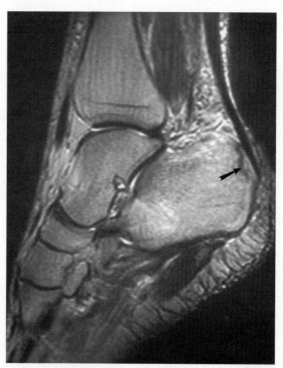

FIG. 4-116. Sagittal SE 400/11 (**A**) and SE 2000/80 (**B**) images of a subtle calcaneal fracture (*arrow*).

Treatment

Treatment of simple or extraarticular calcaneal fractures is much less controversial than management of complex intraarticular fractures.[200,215–220,224,232] The goals of treatment are to reestablish the articular alignment, particularly the posterior facet (Böhler's angle[199]) and to maintain normal calcaneal width.[201,227,232] Early motion is also important to maintain normal function. Fulfilling these criteria is more difficult with complex fractures. The importance of pretherapy imaging to define the extent of injury clearly cannot be overstated.[201,221]

Type 1 (Rowe or Schmidt and Weiner) fractures (see Figs. 4-103 and 4-104) are generally not difficult to treat if recognized. Diagnoses, as mentioned earlier, can be a problem, especially in children (81% of extraarticular fractures overlooked on initial radiographs).[230,234] Most extraarticular (type 1A and 1E) fractures can be treated with cast immobilization for approximately 6 weeks.[221] Fractures of the sustentaculum tali (type 1B) and those involving the calcaneocuboid joint (types 1C and 1D; see Fig. 4-104) may require more aggressive therapy.[205,214,221,228] Undisplaced fractures can still be treated with cast immobilization, although up to 12 weeks may be required for fractures with larger fragments. Displaced fragments may require internal fixation or excision, depending on their size and position. CT is useful if the latter treatment decision is being entertained.[219]

Type 2 and 3 fractures (see Figs. 4-103 and 4-104) can also be treated conservatively. Occasionally, the Achilles avulsion fractures are significantly displaced, in which case internal fixation may be necessary.[221,228]

Treatment of patients with type 4 and 5 fractures is more controversial. Vertical forces applied to the talus via the tibia lead to an initial fracture in the coronal plane that is located just anterior to the posterior calcaneal facet (see Figs. 4-105 and 4-106). If the force continues, the calcaneus becomes divided into three major fragments. The first fragment consists of the tuberosity and lateral portion of the posterior facet, the second portion includes the sustentaculum and anteromedial calcaneus, and the third portion consists of the anterolateral calcaneus with the calcaneocuboid articulation. With tongue-type fractures (type 5A), the fracture line may extend medial to the posterior facet, through it, or lateral to the facet.[227] The exact location of this is critical in planning the operative approach. This further points out the need for CT in preoperative evaluation of intraarticular fractures (Fig. 4-118). The talocalcaneal joints are best seen on coronal scans, and the talonavicular and calcaneocuboid articulations are most clearly demonstrated on axial scans.[201,209,227] Lateral radiographs are also important in demonstrating the degree of displacement of the posterior facet and reduction in Böhler's angle (see Figs. 4-109 and 4-118).[221]

Multiple approaches to treatment of these fractures have been proposed. Subtalar arthrodesis and triple arthrodesis were considered appropriate for comminuted fractures at one time. Open reduction with accurate reduction and fixation has become more popular (Fig. 4-119). If comminution is too severe and adequate reduction cannot be achieved, closed treatment with early motion may be the only option.[220,221,227,228]

The results achieved by the various treatment methods are more closely related to the fracture pattern than to the treatment method. Although somewhat controversial, subtalar arthrodesis has been successful in certain series. Hall and Pennal[210] and Johannson and associates[214] both reported that 90% of patients treated with subtalar arthrodesis had satisfactory results with return to work or normal activity in 6 to 7 months. Immediate motion without specific reduction is no longer advocated, although certain authors reported that 50 to 68% of patients have satisfactory results.[220,221] Open reduction and internal fixation result in good to satisfactory results in 68 to 100% of patients.[221] Corbett and associates[201] reported good results, except in patients with comminution of the posterior facet.

Complications

The most common problems after calcaneal fracture are prolonged pain and disability.[221] These occur most commonly after type 5 fractures. The average period of disability is several months, but pain may persist for 2 years or more. Slatis and colleagues[232] reported that 2 to 6 years after fracture, only 28 of 86 patients (32.5%) were pain free. The cause of the pain varies. Loss of motion was noted in 74 to 89% of patients. Early in the postfracture period, pain may be related to altered hindfoot anatomy. Pain may also occur because of peroneal tendinitis or incomplete disruption of these tendons, plantar nerve entrapment, and, in the later stages, degenerative arthritis (Fig. 4-120).[218–221,223] Fibulocalcaneal abutment syndrome may develop owing to widening of the calcaneus with fracture (see Fig. 4-118). Compartment syndrome and tarsal tunnel syndrome can also result in persistent hindfoot pain.[213,221]

CT is particularly useful in defining articular and certain soft tissue changes. However, because of its unparalleled soft tissue contrast and multiplanar imaging, MRI is better suited to evaluate soft tissue (nerve and tendon) injury and compartment syndromes. Imaging with CT and MRI is more difficult in patients with metal fixation devices.

Associated fractures are common with calcaneal injury (Fig. 4-121). Bilateral calcaneal fractures occur in 10% of patients because of the mechanism of injury (e.g., falling and landing on both feet).[200,215,229]

Lower extremity fractures in the ipsilateral extremity have been reported in 20 to 46% of patients.[200,232] Spine injuries, usually lumbar compression fractures, are associated with calcaneal fractures in 10 to 30% of adults.[212,218,221,232] The incidence of associated fractures or soft tissue injuries in children approaches 57%.[230] As expected, associated fractures are more common in children older than 12 years of age (50%) compared with younger children (20% less than 12 years of age). Twenty-five percent of children have asso-

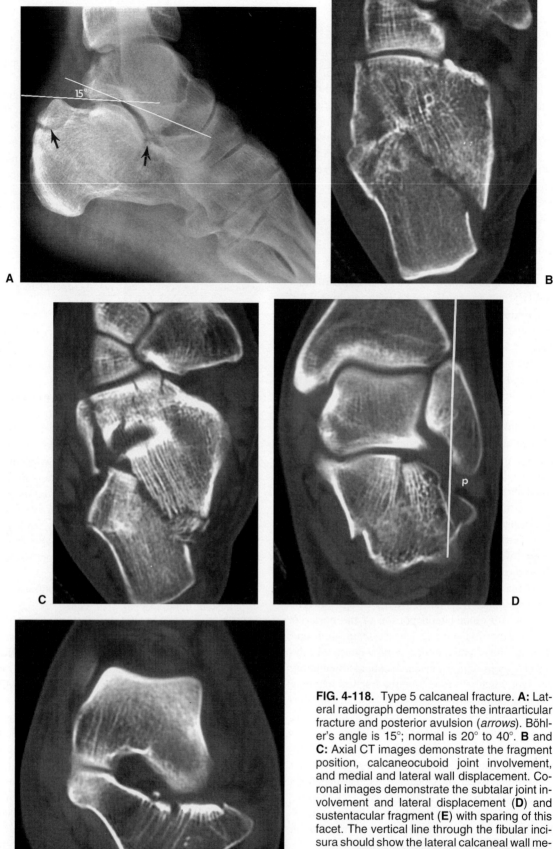

FIG. 4-118. Type 5 calcaneal fracture. **A:** Lateral radiograph demonstrates the intraarticular fracture and posterior avulsion (*arrows*). Böhler's angle is 15°; normal is 20° to 40°. **B** and **C:** Axial CT images demonstrate the fragment position, calcaneocuboid joint involvement, and medial and lateral wall displacement. Coronal images demonstrate the subtalar joint involvement and lateral displacement (**D**) and sustentacular fragment (**E**) with sparing of this facet. The vertical line through the fibular incisura should show the lateral calcaneal wall medial to the line and the peroneal tendons and nerve laterally. In this case, the fragments project lateral to the line, increasing the chances for impingement. *P,* peroneal tendons).

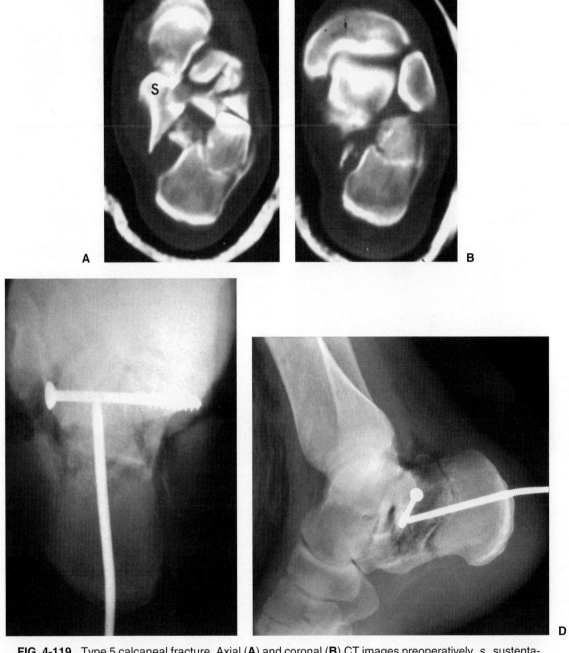

FIG. 4-119. Type 5 calcaneal fracture. Axial (**A**) and coronal (**B**) CT images preoperatively. *s,* sustentaculum. Intraoperative reduction (**C** and **D**). *(continued)*

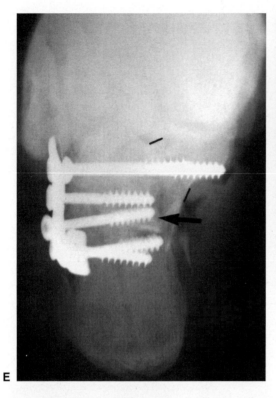

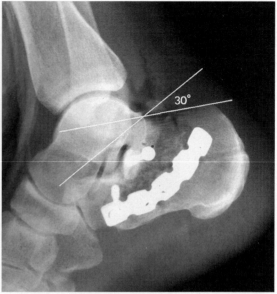

FIG. 4-119. *Continued.* Postoperative axial (**E**) and lateral (**F**) views with screw and reconstruction plate fixation show reduction of calcaneal width (*arrow*) and a Böhler's angle of 30°.

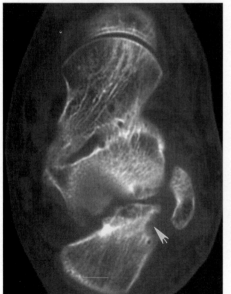

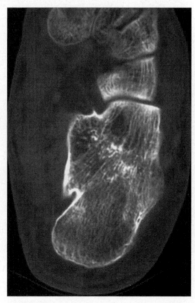

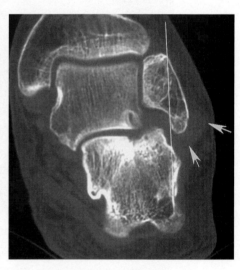

FIG. 4-120. Axial (**A** and **B**) and coronal (**C**) CT images in a patient with a healed type 5 calcaneal fracture. One sees subtalar joint arthrosis with lateral displacement and soft tissue swelling (*arrows*) resulting from impingement. Note the bone erosion in **A** (*arrow*).

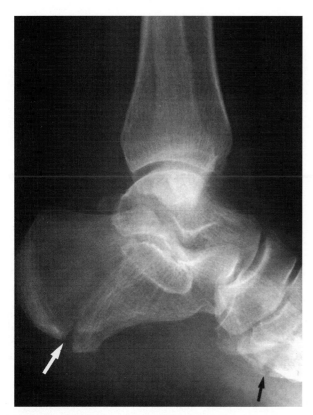

FIG. 4-121. Lateral view of the calcaneus demonstrating an intraarticular calcaneal fracture (*white arrow*) and fracture of the fifth metatarsal base (*black arrow*).

ciated lacerations caused by lawn mower injury or direct trauma. The incidence of associated spine fracture is lower in children (5.4%) than in adults.[230]

Surgically related complications include skin infection, osteomyelitis, loss of reduction, and paresthesias that may develop in up to 10% of patients.[221] Infection, after surgical reduction with metal fixation devices, causes problems in imaging patients with suspected osteomyelitis. Metal artifact can cause problems with CT, conventional tomography, and MRI (nonferromagnetic metal). Indium-111–labeled white blood cells may be particularly useful in detecting subtle postoperative infection.[221]

MIDFOOT AND FOREFOOT INJURIES

Midfoot Fractures and Fracture Dislocations

The midfoot is made up of the lesser tarsal bones (navicular, cuboid, and three cuneiforms). There is minimal motion in the articulations of these bones, and stability is greater laterally than medially.[250] Additional plantar support is because of stronger ligaments and tendon reinforcement. The major joint (Chopart's joint) is formed by the combination of the talonavicular and calcaneocuboid articulations.[250,258]

The tarsometatarsal joint (Lisfranc's) is a complex group of articulations involving the midfoot and forefoot. The first

through third metatarsals articulate with the cuneiforms, and the fourth and fifth metatarsals articulate with the cuboid.[266]

Mechanism of Injury and Classifications of Midfoot Fracture Dislocations

Injuries to the bones and midtarsal joints have been classified by Main and Jowett.[258] Their classification is based on the deforming force and resulting displacement. Five categories of injury were established: 1, medial (30% of injuries); 2, longitudinal (41% of injuries); 3, lateral (17% of injuries); 4, plantar (7% of injuries); and 5, crush injury (5% of injuries).[258] When forces are applied medially, the following injuries can occur: 1, inversion resulting in dorsal avulsion fractures of the talus or navicular and lateral margins of the calcaneus or cuboid (Fig. 4-122); 2, medial subluxation of the forefoot; and 3, rotational dislocation of the talonavicular joint, leaving the calcaneo-cuboid articulation intact (Fig. 4-123). This is less common than subtalar dislocation.[258]

Longitudinal forces cause compression of the metatarsals with forces transmitted to the cuneiforms, compressing the navicular between the cuneiform and talar head. This injury causes lines of force and fractures to occur parallel to the articular margins of the cuneiforms.[258]

Lateral forces are usually caused by falls causing medial distraction that may lead to avulsion fractures of the navicular or talus and lateral impaction that causes compression of the calcaneus and cuboid. Lateral subluxation of the talonavicular joint may also occur (Fig. 4-124).[250,258]

Plantar forces result in talonavicular or calcaneocuboid subluxation or dislocation, with associated periarticular avulsion fractures (Fig. 4-125). Crush injuries have no consistent pattern of injury.[250,258]

Isolated Tarsal Fractures

Isolated fractures of the tarsal bones without associated joint involvement are uncommon. These injuries are especially unusual in children and can only be diagnosed when subluxation or dislocation have been excluded.[248,250,253] The navicular articulates with the talar head proximally, and three facets on the distal surface articulate with the cuboid and cuneiforms. There are ligament and tendon attachments on both the dorsal and plantar surfaces. The posterior tibial tendon attaches, in part, to the tuberosity of the navicular.[243,248,250] Eichenholtz and Levene[243] described several categories of navicular fracture. In their study, 47% of navicular injuries were avulsion fractures, 29% involved the body, and 24% were tuberosity fractures. Stress fractures are discussed in the last section of the chapter. Avulsion fractures are caused by twisting or eversion forces, with fragment avulsion caused by the pull of the talonavicular capsule or anterior fibers of the deltoid. These fractures should not be confused with the well-marginated cortex that is seen on secondary ossification centers. Tuberosity fractures are also,

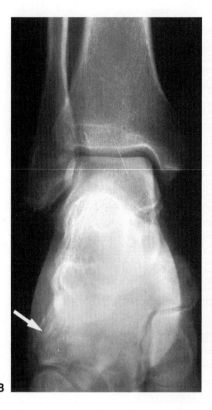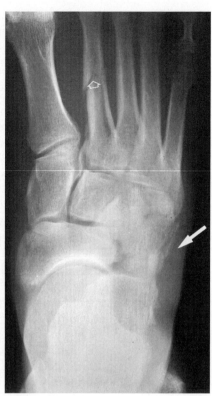

A,B

FIG. 4-122. A: AP view of the ankle demonstrating a cuboid avulsion fracture (*arrow*). **B:** AP view of the foot demonstrating the avulsion fracture (*arrow*) and a second metatarsal fracture (*open arrow*). Tarsal and metatarsal articulations are difficult to evaluate in the AP view, especially laterally.

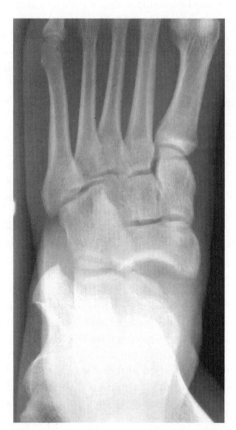

FIG. 4-123. AP view of the foot demonstrating a swivel injury with fracture dislocation of the talonavicular.

in a sense, avulsion fractures (see Fig. 4-124) because either the posterior tibial tendon or anterior deltoid fibers are implicated during eversion of the foot.[250] Most body fractures are associated with fracture dislocations of the midfoot.[250] In children, the normal irregularity of the navicular ossification center should not be confused with the fracture. This can be avoided by comparison radiographs with the normal extremity and clinical findings.[248] Isolated fractures of the cuneiforms and cuboid are uncommon in children and adults (Fig. 4-126).[248,250]

Radiographic Diagnosis of Midfoot Injuries

Imaging of the midfoot begins with routine AP, lateral, and oblique views of the foot (Fig. 4-127). In many cases, subtle subluxations, avulsion fractures, or undisplaced fractures are difficult to identify. Main and Jowett[258] reported delay in diagnosis in more than 41% of patients using routine views. One should carefully study the soft tissues. Swelling or hemorrhage that causes distortion of the fat planes may provide a valuable clue to the location of a fracture or subtle subluxation. The articular surfaces of all bones should be parallel (see Fig. 4-127).

If routine views are normal or if a questionable area is identified, further studies should be performed. Fluoroscopically positioned spot films (Fig. 4-128) may be useful in the acute setting and can be performed quickly. CT is preferred to more clearly demonstrate osseous and articular anatomy (see Fig. 4-126).

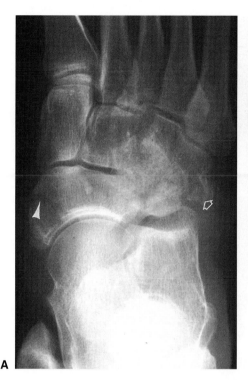

A

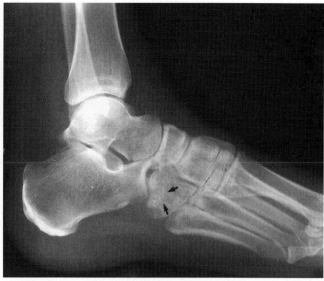

B

FIG. 4-124. A: AP radiograph shows a medial navicular fracture (*arrowhead*) and a compression fracture of the cuboid (*open arrow*). **B:** Lateral view shows increase density in the cuboid (*arrows*) resulting from compressed overlying fragments.

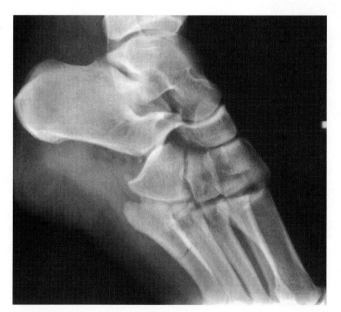

FIG. 4-125. Oblique view of the foot shows a calcaneocuboid dislocation with avulsed fragments. There is also Lisfranc's injury.

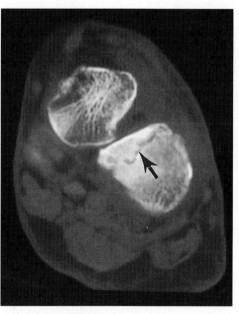

FIG. 4-126. Isolated tarsal fracture (*arrow*) seen only on CT.

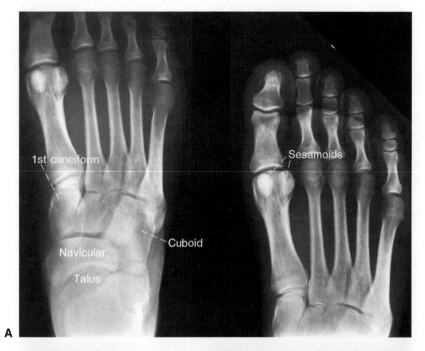

A

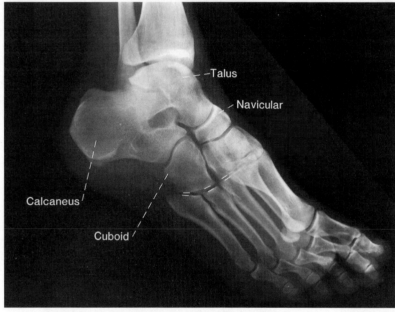

B

FIG. 4-127. AP (**A**) and oblique (**B**) views of the normal foot alignment of the articulations of each joint, which are difficult to evaluate with routine views.

Treatment

Most subluxations and minimally displaced fractures (less than or equal to 2 mm) are treated conservatively with closed reduction and casting. The prognosis of lateral injuries is more guarded than that of medial injury and may require calcaneocuboid arthrodesis. Triple arthrodesis is an excellent procedure in complex injury or when conservative treatment is unsuccessful.[258]

Isolated tarsal fractures, if nondisplaced, can be treated with elastic support or cast immobilization for 4 to 6 weeks.[243,250] Treatment of displaced fractures is more controversial, but open reduction with either triple arthrodesis or talonavicular cuneiform arthrodesis is advocated by most authors.[242,243,250,256,258,264]

Tarsometatarsal Fracture Dislocations

Tarsometatarsal fracture dislocations are commonly referred to as Lisfranc's injuries. This injury is based on the description of amputation through these joints by a surgeon of the same name during the Napoleonic wars.[236] Whether Lisfranc ever described the dislocation is uncertain, but the joint has become known as Lisfranc's joint based on his surgical description.[241,253] The injury is uncommon, accounting for less than 1% of fracture dislocations.[235,244]

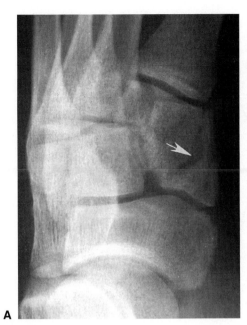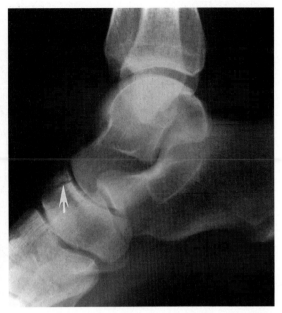

FIG. 4-128. Fluoroscopically positioned spot views demonstrate a fracture of the medial cuneiform (**A**) and dorsal navicular fracture (**B**).

The four lateral metatarsals (second through fifth) are connected at the bases by transverse metatarsal ligaments (Fig. 4-129). This is not the case at the base of the first and second metatarsal. Here the transverse ligament is absent. The second metatarsal is situated in a mortise formed by the medial

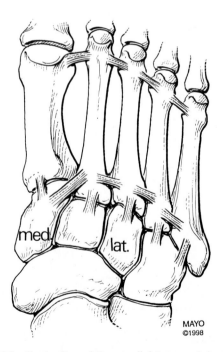

FIG. 4-129. Illustration of the medial tarsometatarsal joints and ligaments. There is no transverse ligament between the first and second metatarsal bases. An oblique ligament extends from the medial cuneiform to the second metatarsal base. The second metatarsal base is situated in a mortise formed by the medial (*med.*) and lateral (*lat.*) cuneiforms.

and lateral cuneiform and its ligamentous support is via the transverse ligament laterally and the medial and second cuneiform proximally (see Fig. 4-129).[235,236,266,268] The oblique ligament from the medial cuneiform to the base of the second metatarsal is implicated in avulsion fractures of the second metatarsal base. The plantar ligaments and tendons provide more support than the dorsal soft tissues, a feature that explains why most dislocations occur dorsally.[236] The dorsalis pedis artery passes between the proximal first and second metatarsals as it enters the plantar aspect of the foot to form the plantar arch. Therefore, it is susceptible to injuries of fracture dislocations in this region.[250]

The mechanism of injury is similar in children and adults.[268] Typically, the injury occurs with forced plantar flexion of the forefoot with or without associated rotation.[267,268] This can occur during a fall, such as from the upper bunk (bunk bed fracture in children), or landing on the toes, an action that forces the forefoot into plantar flexion (Fig. 4-130). Other mechanisms include falls with the forefoot fixed (Fig. 4-131) or compression of the foot from a heavy object striking the heel when the patient is kneeling (Fig. 4-132). In adults, motor vehicle and motorcycle accidents are more commonly implicated, but the forces producing the injury are similar.[236,250] The injury that occurs takes several different patterns.[235,236,250] The homolateral pattern (total incongruity) occurs when all five metatarsals are displaced. The displacement is almost always in the lateral direction (Fig. 4-133). The alignment of both the first and second metatarsal bases is abnormal. Fractures of the second metatarsal are common with this pattern because of its position in the mortise formed by the cuneiforms (see Figs. 4-129 and 4-133).[235,236,249,268] Partial incongruity (see Fig. 4-133) occurs when the first metatarsal fractures at the base

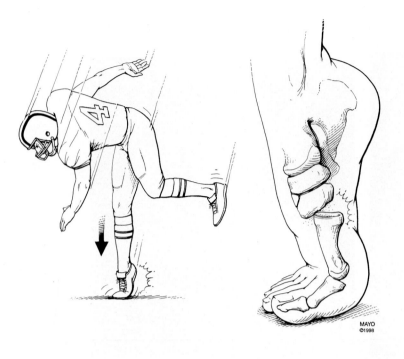

FIG. 4-130. Illustration of tip-toe landing leading to Lisfranc's injury.

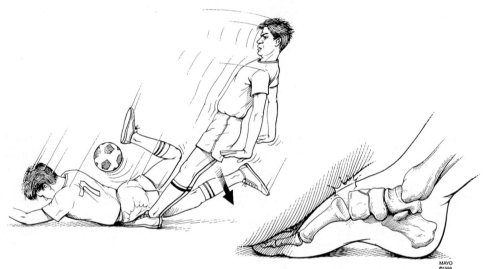

FIG. 4-131. Illustration of fixed forefoot injury leading to Lisfranc's injury.

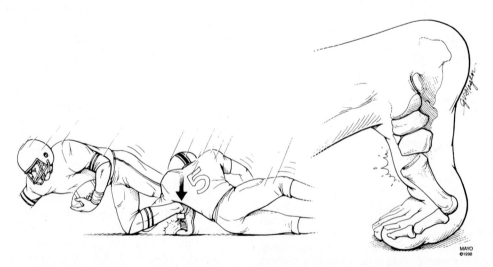

FIG. 4-132. Illustration of mechanism for Lisfranc's injury in the kneeling position.

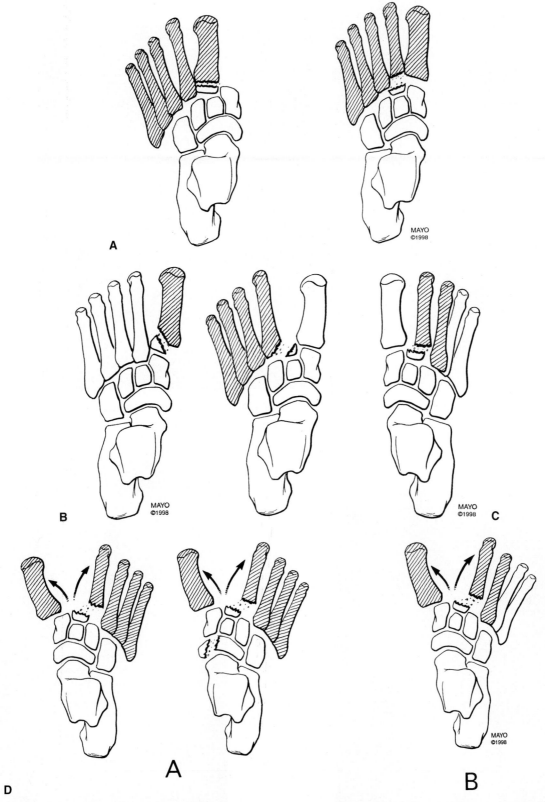

FIG. 4-133. Illustration of the patterns of Lisfranc's fracture dislocations. **A:** Type A, total incongruity. **B:** Type B, partial incongruity. **C:** Lateral dislocation. **D:** Divergent or type C with total displacement (**A**) and partial displacement (**B**).

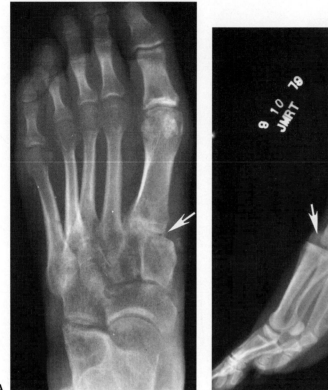
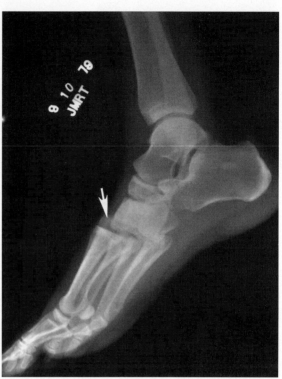

FIG. 4-134. PA (**A**) and lateral (**B**) radiographs of obvious Lisfranc's injuries (*arrows*).

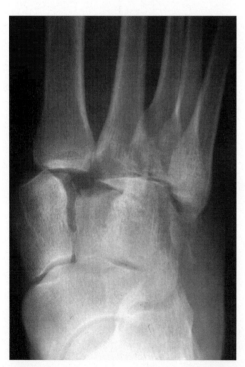

FIG. 4-135. Severe Lisfranc's fracture dislocation seen on the AP radiograph. There is abnormal shift of the metatarsals laterally.

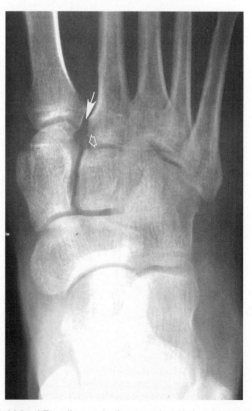

FIG. 4-136. AP radiograph shows only subtle widening of the space (*arrow*) between the first and second metatarsal bases with a small marginal fracture (*open arrow*).

and the shaft displaces medially, accompanied with lateral displacement of the second through fifth metatarsals.[249] A third pattern of injury (divergent) occurs when the base of the first metatarsal subluxes or dislocates medially and the second metatarsal or a combination of the second through fifth metatarsals displaces laterally.[235,236,249,268] The significance of this injury is the associated cuneiform and navicular fractures. Rarely, an isolated tarsometatarsal dislocation can occur.[257]

Radiographic Evaluation

Radiographic evaluation must start with careful evaluation of the tarsometatarsal relationships. Routine views of the foot are usually sufficient for diagnosis of obvious fracture dislocations of the tarsometatarsal joint (Figs. 4-134 and 4-135). However, subtle ligament injuries may be easily overlooked (Figs. 4-136 and 4-137). These injuries may spontaneously reduce so that nonstress radiographs appear normal. On the AP view, the medial margin of the second metatarsal base should align with the margin of the second cuneiform (Fig. 4-138). The space between the first and second metatarsal bases should be assessed, but it is less useful than the foregoing relationship (see Fig. 4-136).[245] However, the lateral margins of the first metatarsal and cuneiform should align. The medial base of the fourth metatarsal should align with the medial margin of the cuboid. The bases of the remaining metatarsals are more difficult to evaluate because of bony overlap and the overlapping tuberosity of the fifth metatarsal. However, the metatarsal bases should be parallel to the tarsal articular surfaces.[245,259,260] On the lateral view, the second metatarsal and cuneiform should be aligned such that an uninterrupted line can be drawn along their dorsal surfaces. In children, care must be taken so that

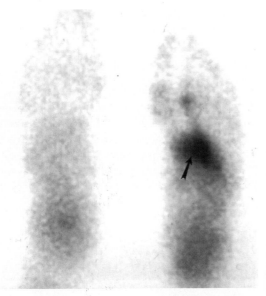

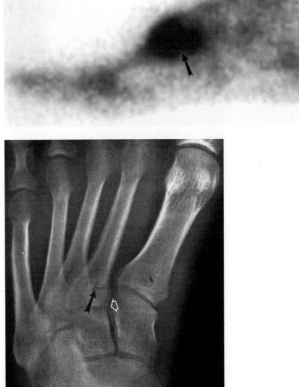

FIG. 4-137. Radionuclide bone scan images (**A** and **B**) show intense increased tracer in the medial tarsometatarsal region (*arrow*) in a patient with persistent posttraumatic foot pain. Initial radiographs were interpreted as normal. Repeat radiograph (**C**) shows subtle joint space widening (*open arrow*) and a fracture of the second metatarsal base (*arrow*).

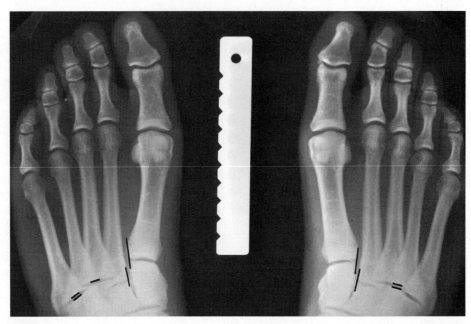

FIG. 4-138. Normal standing AP views of the foot. Note the normal alignment of the first and second metatarsals and the cuneiforms (*vertical lines*). Joint spaces are symmetric bilaterally. The tarsometatarsal joints (*lines*) are parallel.

subtle fractures of the first metatarsal base are not overlooked. This injury is associated with ligamentous disruption, and the subtle first metatarsal fracture may be the only clue radiographically (Fig. 4-139). Comparison views with the uninvolved foot are useful in children.[251,253]

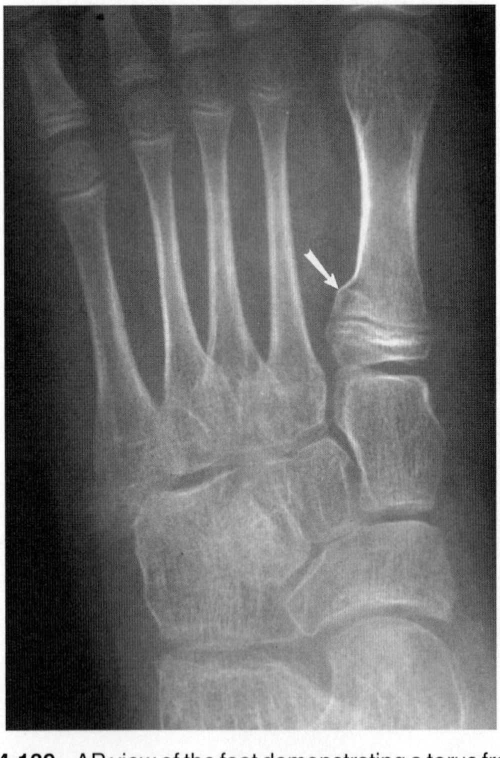

On occasion, fluoroscopically positioned spot views or stress views may be indicated to detect subtle ligament injury. Conventional tomography or CT with reformatted images in the tarsometatarsal planes can also be useful to evaluate the bony relationships more fully and to exclude cuneiform and navicular fractures.[247] Conventional tomograms should be obtained in the AP and lateral planes (Fig. 4-140).

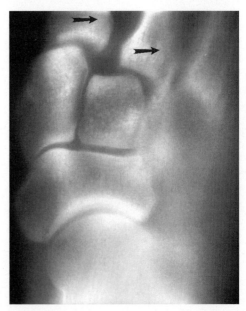

FIG. 4-139. AP view of the foot demonstrating a torus fracture of the first metatarsal base (*arrow*). Bunkbed fracture.

FIG. 4-140. AP tomogram demonstrating lateral displacement (*arrows*) of the first and second metatarsal bases. The medial and intermediate cuneiforms are in normal position.

Treatment

Closed reduction can be used for patients with subtle injury or displacement less than 2 to 3 mm.[248] With more significant fracture dislocation, reduction can be more difficult. The anterior tibial and peroneal tendons may interfere with reduction.[241,248] If reduction is difficult, MRI may be useful to determine whether tendons (specifically tibialis anterior) have become entrapped between fragments.[250] Open reduction with accurate realignment and internal fixation should be used in these patients.[238,255,264,269] During surgery, AP views of the foot should be obtained to determine whether satisfactory realignment of the second metatarsal base has been achieved.[238] Follow-up routine films should be obtained to be certain that the reduction is maintained. In problem cases, CT or tomography is useful to define the complex bony relationships better.

Complications

The most common problems include degenerative arthritis and persistent pain. These problems may occur in 20 to 30% of patients.[270] Vascular injury has been reported, but it is generally uncommon.[239,261] Gissane[246] reported gangrene of the foot in three patients that led to below-the-knee amputations. AVN of the second metatarsal head has also been reported.[241,267,269] This was believed to be caused by the relationship of the dorsalis pedis artery and interosseous branch with the bases of the first and second metatarsals.[257]

Metatarsal and Phalangeal Fractures

Metatarsal fractures are common in adults and children. Injuries are usually the result of direct trauma from a heavy object striking the foot. However, twisting or shearing injuries may also lead to fracture.[236,248,250] The neck of the metatarsal is weaker than the shaft, a feature that explains the higher incidence at this location, especially in children.[248] Patients generally present with pain, swelling, and ecchymosis over the injured metatarsals. Fractures may be incomplete (torus or green-stick) in children (Fig. 4-141).[253] In adults, complete fractures are most common.[236,248]

Fractures of the fifth metatarsal base are common in children and adults. Two basic fracture patterns with differing prognosis can be distinguished. Avulsion of the proximal tuberosity is most common. This is caused by an abrupt pull of the peroneus brevis (Fig. 4-142). The adductor digiti minimi and lateral cord of the plantar fascia also insert on the fifth metatarsal base.[248] This fracture must be distinguished from the normal tuberosity in children (Fig. 4-143). The growth plate runs parallel to the shaft, whereas fractures are perpendicular to the shaft (see Fig. 4-143).[253] Avulsion of the epiphyses is uncommon, but if suspected, comparison with the normal extremity should be obtained. Differentiation of this fracture from the os peroneum or os vesalianum is usually not difficult because of their smooth cortical margins.

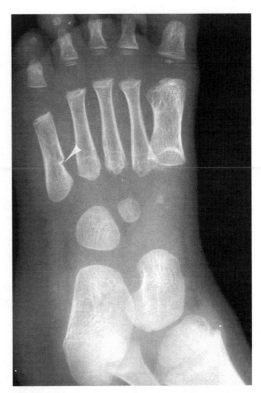

FIG. 4-141. Oblique view of the foot in a child demonstrating a torus fracture (*arrowhead*) of the fifth metatarsal.

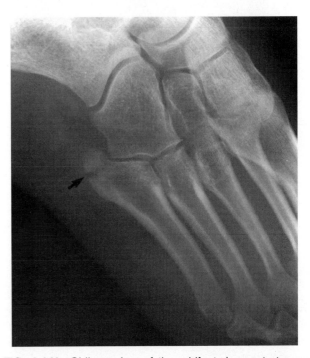

FIG. 4-142. Oblique view of the midfoot demonstrates an avulsion fracture (*arrow*) of the fifth metatarsal base.

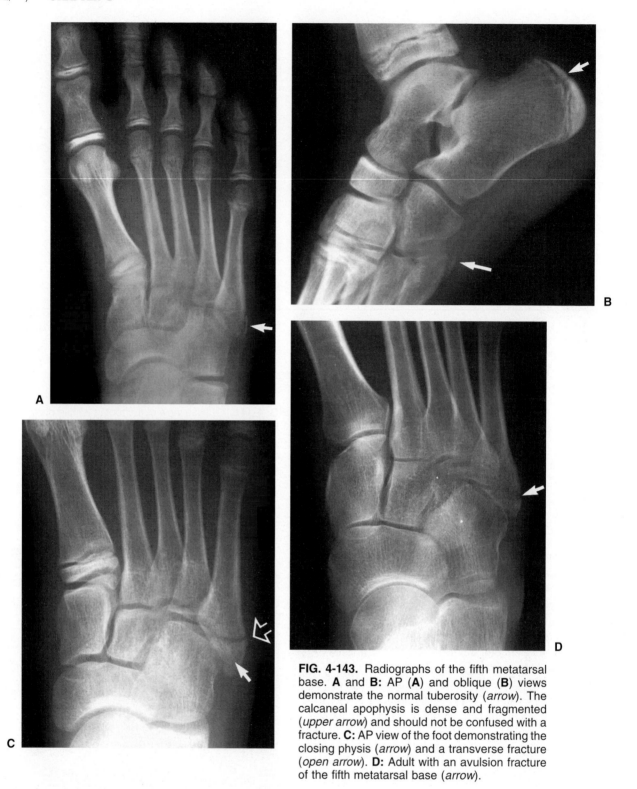

FIG. 4-143. Radiographs of the fifth metatarsal base. **A** and **B**: AP (**A**) and oblique (**B**) views demonstrate the normal tuberosity (*arrow*). The calcaneal apophysis is dense and fragmented (*upper arrow*) and should not be confused with a fracture. **C**: AP view of the foot demonstrating the closing physis (*arrow*) and a transverse fracture (*open arrow*). **D**: Adult with an avulsion fracture of the fifth metatarsal base (*arrow*).

The second type of fifth metatarsal base fracture is often referred to as the Jones fracture.[252,254] This fracture involves the proximal diaphyses or metaphysis (Fig. 4-144). Treatment of this fracture can be more difficult and may require internal fixation.[240]

Fractures of the metatarsal bases may be difficult to detect because of bone overlap on conventional views. Serial images usually increase the ability to detect these subtle fractures because of resorption along the fracture line (Fig. 4-145). Bone scans or CT may be required in subtle cases.

Phalangeal fractures occur when the bare toe strikes a hard object or when a heavy object lands on the toe. Most frac-

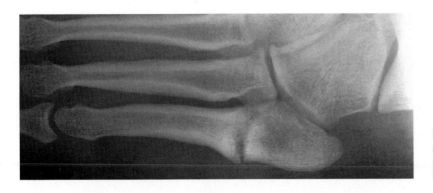

FIG. 4-144. Jones fracture of the proximal fifth metatarsal with early hypertrophic nonunion. Note the sclerosis along the fracture line and hypertrophic callus.

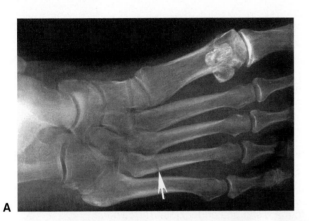

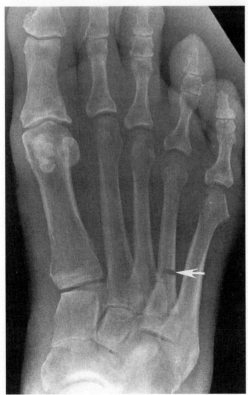

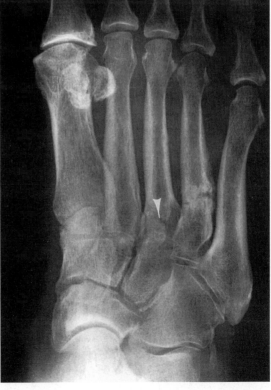

FIG. 4-145. Serial images of the foot in a patient with midfoot pain after trauma. **A:** Initial oblique view shows a linear transverse fracture of the proximal fourth metatarsal (*arrow*) the second and third metatarsal bases overlap. **B:** Several weeks later, the fracture line (*arrow*) is wider. **C:** Six weeks after injury, there is sclerosis along the fourth metatarsal fracture. The subtle fracture of the third metatarsal (*arrowhead*) is now evident.

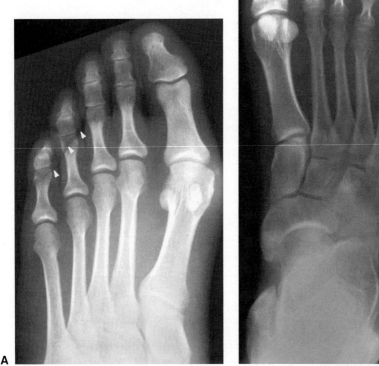
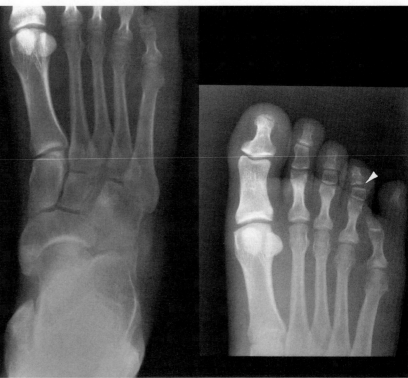

A

B

FIG. 4-146. A: Normal AP view of the forefoot. Soft tissue shadow created by the skin cleft at the base of the toes overlies the phalanges (*arrowheads*) and should not be mistaken for a fracture. Look at all views and note that this line extends beyond the cortex (*arrowheads*). **B:** AP views of the midfoot and forefoot. There is a fracture subluxation of the fourth distal phalangeal joint (*arrowhead*).

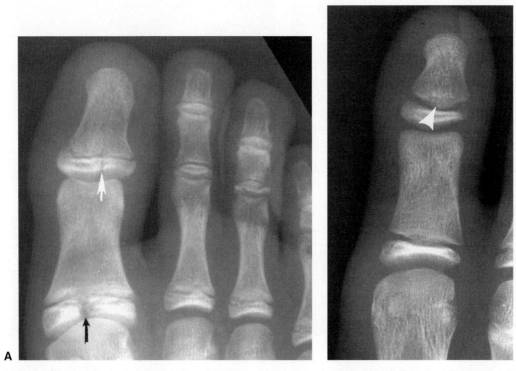

A

B

FIG. 4-147. A: AP view of the forefoot demonstrating a normal epiphyseal cleft in the phalanges of the great toe (*arrows*). *(continued)*

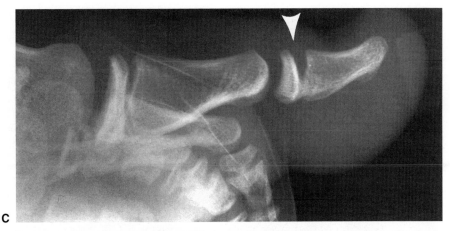

FIG. 4-147. *Continued.* AP (**B**) and lateral (**C**) views of a distal phalangeal growth plate fracture (*arrowhead*). Note the physeal with compared with the other physis.

tures are minimally displaced. Care must be taken to carefully evaluate all radiographs or these fractures can be overlooked. It is important to determine whether fractures are intraarticular (Fig. 4-146). In children, the injuries may be subtle and may involve the growth plate. Differentiation from normal variants is also a problem (Fig. 4-147).[253]

Dislocations of the metatarsophalangeal and interphalangeal joints may be isolated or associated with fracture (see Fig. 4-146). Metatarsophalangeal dislocations are usually caused by hyperextension, with the proximal phalanx forced dorsally over the metatarsal tearing the plantar capsule (Fig. 4-148).[236,253] The great toe is most commonly involved. Medial and lateral dislocations are less common.

Similar forces lead to dislocations of the interphalangeal joints.[236,253,262]

Radiographic Evaluation

AP, oblique and lateral radiographs of the foot are routinely obtained. The AP and oblique views are most useful as bony overlap makes evaluation more difficult on the lateral view (Fig. 4-149). The lateral view is useful in determining fracture angulation and the direction of dislocations. After reduction of dislocations, it is important to obtain the same views to be certain there is no associated fracture or soft tissue interposition (wide joint space). Tomography, CT

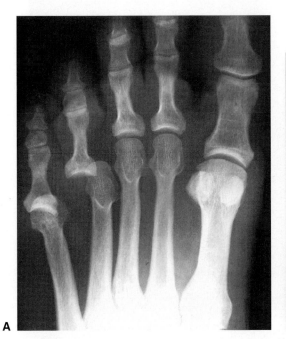
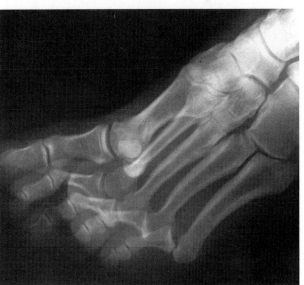

A   **B**

FIG. 4-148. AP (**A**) and oblique (**B**) views of the foot demonstrating dorsal dislocations of the fourth and fifth metatarsophalangeal joints. The fourth joint is also displaced laterally.

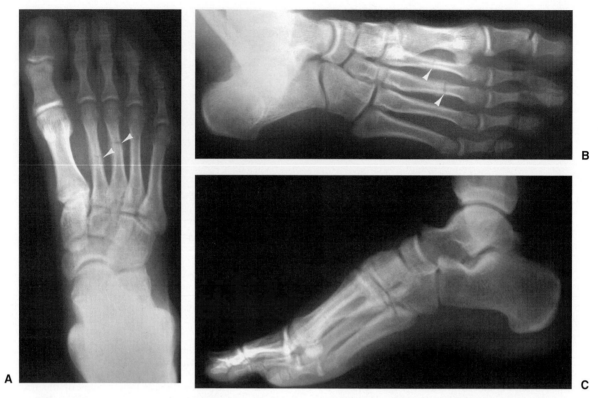

FIG. 4-149. AP (**A**) and oblique (**B**) views of the foot demonstrate transverse healing fractures of the second and third metatarsals (*arrowheads*). The fracture lines are obscured on the lateral view (**C**).

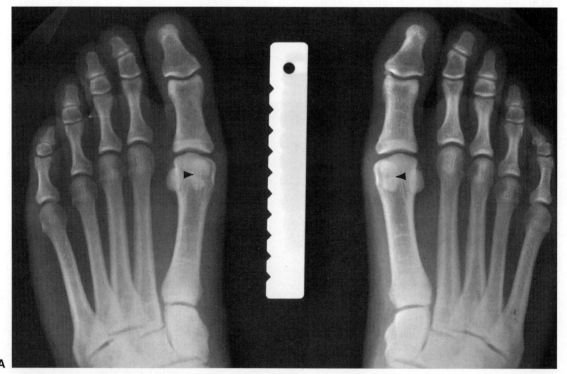

FIG. 4-150. AP standing (**A**) and sesamoid views (**B**) of the left foot demonstrating normal sesamoids. The medial sesamoids are bipartite (*arrowheads*). *L*, lateral; *M*, medial; *m*, second portion of bipartite sesamoid. *(continued)*

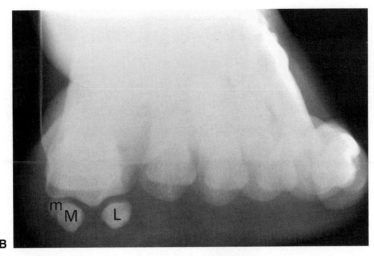

FIG. 4-150. *Continued.*

or MRI are useful on occasion, especially for sesamoid fractures (Figs. 4-150 and 4-151).[270]

Treatment

Treatment of most closed fractures and dislocations is conservative. Undisplaced metatarsal fractures are treated with walking casts for 4 to 6 weeks.[236,237,250,263] Displaced fractures (Fig. 4-152) or open fractures are better managed with internal fixation. This reduces the problem of malposition, which can result in uneven weight bearing on the metatarsal heads. Debridement and parenteral antibiotics are needed after reduction of open wounds.[236,248] Differentiation of tuberosity and Jones fractures is important. Jones fractures can be more difficult to manage. Torg and associates[265] classified these fractures according to their radiographic appearance: acute fractures with a narrow fracture line (Fig. 4-153); fractures with medullary sclerosis and widening of the fracture line; and nonunion with sclerosis of the fracture line and obliteration of the medullary canal (see Fig. 4-144).

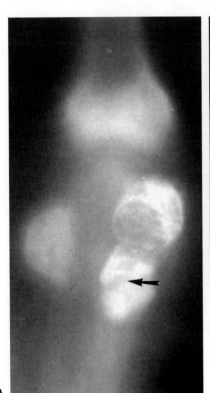

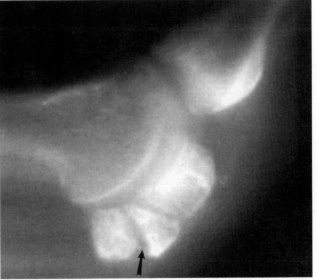

FIG. 4-151. AP (**A**) and lateral (**B**) tomograms of a fractured sesamoid (*arrow*).

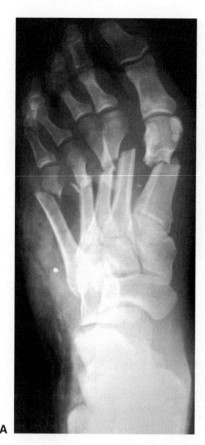

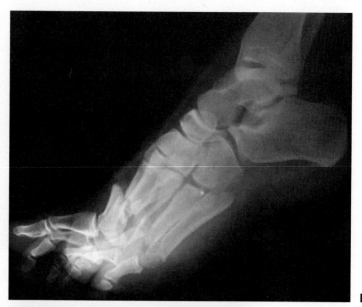

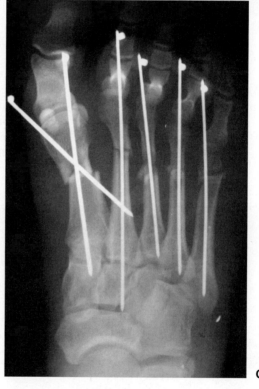

FIG. 4-152. AP (**A**) and oblique (**B**) views demonstrating comminuted metatarsal fractures with tarsometatarsal subluxations. *(continued)*

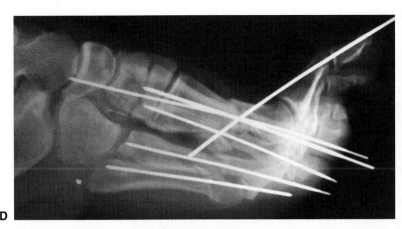

D

FIG. 4-152. *Continued.* AP (**C**) and lateral (**D**) views after K-wire reduction show improved position with residual angular deformity of the first metatarsal. AP view (**E**) after healing and K-wire removal.

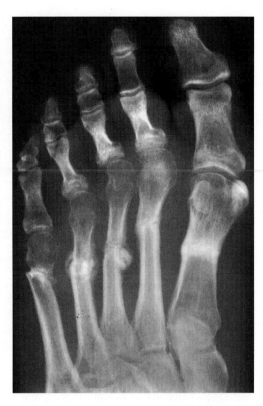

E

Acute fractures healed with a non–weight-bearing knee-to-toe cast. If the fracture line was widened with sclerosis, curettage and bone grafting are most successful.[265] Others choose to use internal fixation early (Figs. 4-154 and 4-155).

Most dislocations and phalangeal fractures can also be reduced and treated conservatively. Buddy taping of the injured phalanx to the adjacent toe may be all that is required. Articular involvement may require K-wire reduction.[264]

STRESS FRACTURES

The term stress fracture is used to describe fractures that occur after repetitive stress that is insufficient to cause an acute fracture. Daffner[274] reported that most stress fractures are caused by muscular activity rather than direct bony trauma. Most stress fractures involve the lower extremity and are actually fatigue fractures caused by muscle tension on normal bone.[272–274,276,283,295] These fractures have been

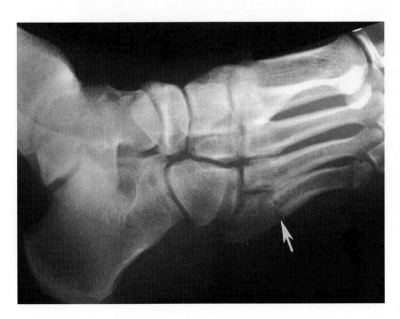

FIG. 4-153. Oblique view of the foot demonstrating a Jones fracture (*arrow*) with a thin fracture line and no sclerosis.

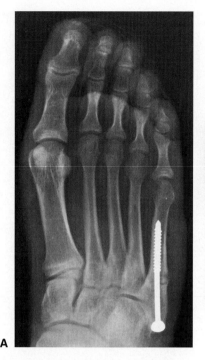

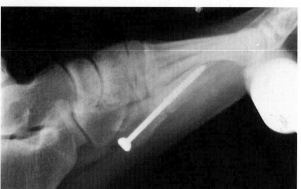

FIG. 4-154. AP (**A**) and lateral (**B**) views demonstrate fixation of a Jones fracture with a long partially threaded screw.

seen most frequently in military recruits but can occur in children and adults in the civilian population. [271–279,281,282] Insufficiency fractures occur when normal stresses, usually caused by muscle tension, act on bone with abnormal elastic resistance or mineral content.[274,276,279,295,297]

Civilians with stress fractures usually give a history of initiating a new activity, such as running. Symptoms develop several weeks after starting this activity, are usually relieved by rest, but progress if activity is continued. Table 4-13 lists common stress fractures of the foot and ankle and the associated activity.

Physical examination may reveal tenderness and slight

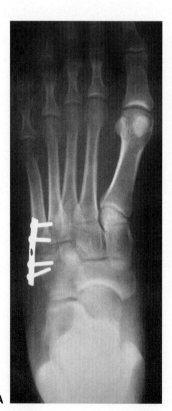

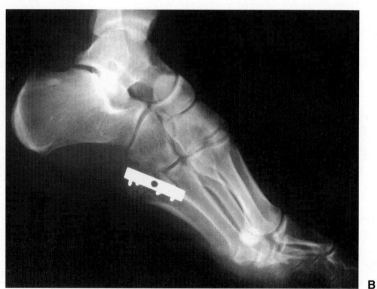

FIG. 4-155. AP (**A**) and lateral (**B**) views show internal fixation with a one-third minitubular plate and cortical screws.

TABLE 4-13. *Stress fractures*

Location	Causes	References
Metatarsals	Marching	271, 274, 280, 282, 286
	Running	271, 290, 296
	Ballet	288
	Prior surgery	279
	Rheumatoid arthritis	297
Tarsals	Long-distance running	274, 281, 284, 292
	Marching	274, 282
Calcaneus	Jumping	285
	Running	271, 274, 282, 296
	Recent immobilization	271
Sesamoids	Marching, standing, skiing, cycling	271, 276, 287
Distal tibia	Running	271, 274, 276, 292, 293, 296
Distal fibula	Running	271
	Parachute jumping	271

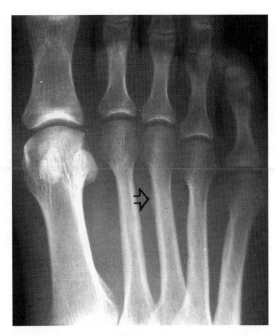

FIG. 4-156. AP view of the forefoot demonstrating callus (*open arrow*) resulting from a healing third metatarsal stress fracture.

swelling. Children may have slight temperature elevation. Symptoms and radiographic features (exuberant callus or periosteal reaction) simulate infection, neoplasm, gout, pseudogout, claudication, or ligament injury.[271]

Distribution of Fractures

More than 80% of adult stress fractures involve the tibia, fibula, metatarsals, and calcaneus.[273,278,287,296] Stress fractures in children have a different distribution and clinical presentation. Most pediatric stress fractures involve the upper tibia, although the lower fibula is more commonly involved than the upper fibula. Fibular stress fractures may occur in infants. Metatarsal stress fractures occur less frequently in children.[277,289]

Stress fractures of the long bones in children can mimic malignancy. Patients present with pain, tenderness, and elevated temperature. Radiographically, there may be extensive callus and periosteal reaction, suggesting a more aggressive process.[276]

Studies in adult military and civilian populations have reviewed distribution and identification of stress fractures. A total of 642 patients were reported by Wilson and Katz,[296] Greaney and colleagues,[282] and Orava's group.[290] Most of metatarsal stress fractures involve the second and third metatarsals (Fig. 4-156). Fractures of the first metatarsal account for up to 7 to 8%, and fractures of the fourth and fifth metatarsals account for 3% of metatarsal stress fractures.[286] Most military stress fractures are caused by marching in new recruits. Stress fractures in civilians are more commonly caused by new footwear or a new activity (e.g., running, standing for long periods).[271,273,274,276,288]

Calcaneal stress fractures are nearly as common as metatarsal fractures, and in the series of Greaney and colleagues, these fractures were more common (Figs. 4-157 and 158).[282,296] Associated upper tibial stress fractures were noted in 60% of military recruits.[280] Bilateral calcaneal stress fractures were noted in 24% of patients reported by Meurman.[287] Calcaneal stress fractures are less common in civilians and again related to footwear in many cases. Pain is often medial or lateral, rather than on the plantar surface. Physical examination reveals pain when the examiner squeezes the patient's heel from the sides.[271]

Stress fractures of the navicular, other tarsal bones, and sesamoids occur less frequently than in the metatarsals and calcaneus. However, the exact incidence of these fractures, especially the navicular, may be higher, because they are easily misdiagnosed. Most navicular fractures occur in the sagittal plane and involve the medial third of the navicular (Fig. 4-159).[281,284,292,294]

Stress fractures more commonly involve the tibia than the fibula. Any portion of the bone can be involved. Typically, tibial stress fractures are more common proximally and involve the posteromedial cortex at the metaphyseal-diaphyseal junction.[271]

Radiographic Diagnosis

Detection of stress fractures in the early stages is difficult, except with isotope studies (see Fig. 4-157). Radiographs are usually normal in the acute phase.[271,274,276] Metabolic changes at the site of fracture allow isotope bone scans to detect the injury as early as 24 hours later. Bone changes are usually not evident for 10 to 21 days.[271,282]

Blickenstaff and Morris[272] described the phases of stress fractures that at least partially explain the changes seen using

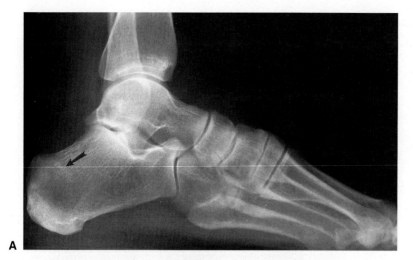

A

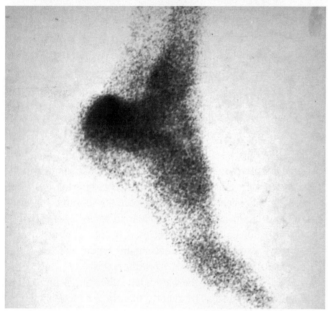

B

FIG. 4-157. **A:** Lateral view of the foot was interpreted as normal. There is subtle bone condensation (*arrow*) in the calcaneus. **B:** Because of the patient's symptoms, a bone scan was performed 1 day later that shows intense calcaneal uptake resulting from stress fracture.

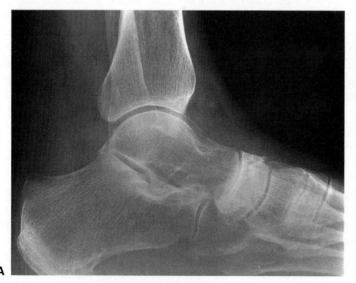

A

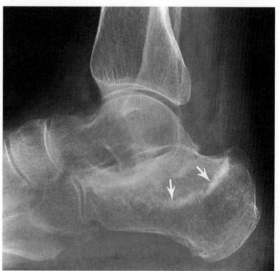

B

FIG. 4-158. **A:** Normal hindfoot radiograph. **B:** Bone condensation (*arrows*) in the opposite calcaneus resulting from stress fracture.

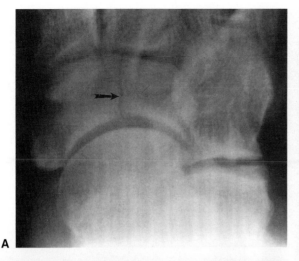

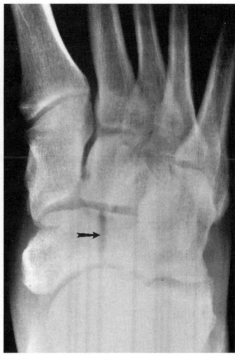

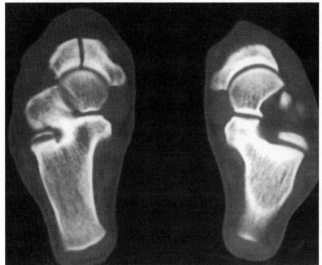

FIG. 4-159. National Basketball Association basketball player with chronic midfoot pain. A: AP view shows a sagittal linear line in the center of the navicular (arrow). B: AP view 2 months later shows widening of the fracture line (arrow). C: Axial CT image shows widening with slight articular deformity.

imaging techniques. Osteoclastic resorption occurs 5 to 14 days after the initial injury. This is followed by increased vascularity, which accompanies endosteal and periosteal callus formation. With continued activity, fracture occurs. Fractures may be primarily cortical or medullary, depending on the fracture site. In the series by Greaney and colleagues,[282] 77% of fractures were cancellous and 23% cortical. Routine radiographs were more useful in cortical fractures.

Classification of stress fractures has been proposed by several authors. Devas[276] divided stress fractures into compression and distraction categories. Compression fractures occur most commonly in the elderly and young children. Distraction fractures may be oblique, transverse, or longitudinal and can become complete. Wilson and Katz[296] described fractures according to their radiographic appearance. Type I fractures present with a lucent line, whereas one sees sclerosis of cancellous bone or endosteal callus with type II fractures. Type III fractures present with external callus; type IV fractures have features of types I to III (Fig. 4-160).

Stress fractures differ in their appearance at different locations. Calcaneal fractures tend to present with a curvilinear area of condensation radiographically (Fig. 4-161). Metatarsal fractures, when visible radiographically, typically present with either slight callus (type II) (see Fig. 4-156) or simply a subtle lucent line in the cortex (type I). Fractures in the first metatarsal tend to involve the cancellous bone proximally and periosteal reaction is minimal.[286] Tarsal navicular stress fractures may present with a lucent line or sclerosis involving the medial third (see Fig. 4-159). Typically, isotope studies and tomography or CT scans are required to confirm the suspected stress fracture.

MRI may be useful in selected cases (Figs. 4-162 and 4-163). However, MRI is most useful in atypical cases to exclude other pathologic features.[271]

Treatment

Unlike more proximal lower extremity fractures, those in the distal tibia, fibula, and foot rarely become complete.

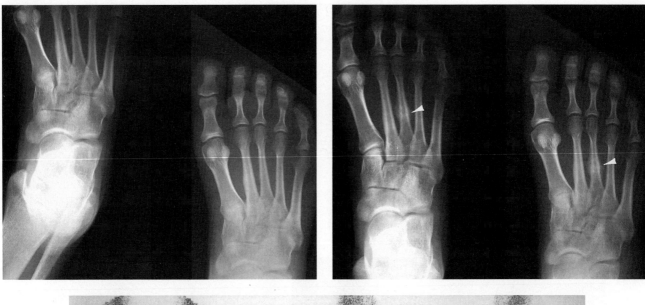

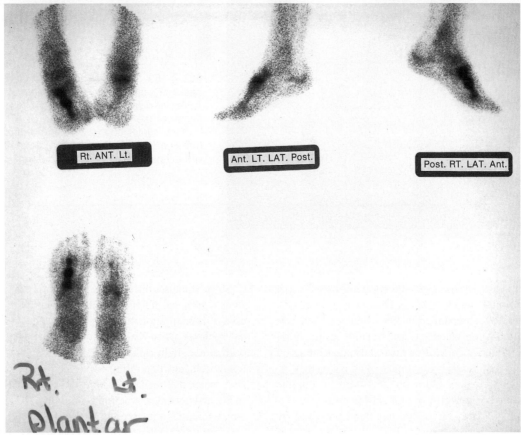

FIG. 4-160. Metatarsal stress fractures. **A:** Initial AP radiographs are normal. **B:** Bone scan shows increased tracer in the metatarsals bilaterally. **C:** Radiograph 3 weeks later shows abundant callus at the third metatarsal fracture site (*arrowhead*).

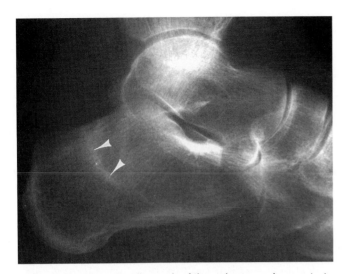

FIG. 4-161. Lateral radiograph of the calcaneus demonstrating a dense line of condensation (*arrowheads*) resulting from a stress fracture.

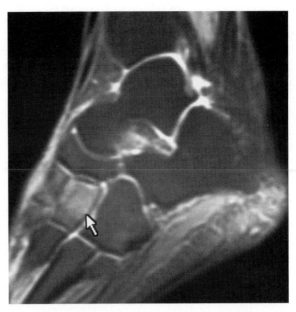

FIG. 4-163. Stress fractures result in significant arrow edema. In the tarsal bones, the entire structure may have abnormal signal intensity, as in this lateral cuneiform stress fracture (*arrow*).

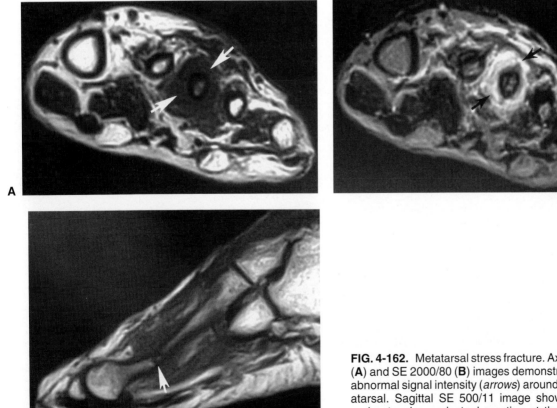

FIG. 4-162. Metatarsal stress fracture. Axial SE 500/11 (**A**) and SE 2000/80 (**B**) images demonstrate extensive abnormal signal intensity (*arrows*) around the third metatarsal. Sagittal SE 500/11 image shows angulation and extensive periosteal reaction at the fracture site (*arrow*).

Therefore, once the diagnosis is established, conservative treatment is sufficient.[271] Restriction from weight bearing is all that is required for metatarsal stress fractures. Calcaneal fractures are treated with a plastic heel cup and a 4-inch foam pad. Navicular stress fractures may respond to restriction of activity, but if weight bearing is allowed, nonunion may develop in a significant percentage of patients (see Fig. 4-159). Torg and colleagues[294] reported nonunion in seven of nine patients treated with activity restriction only.

Tibial stress fractures were graded by Hallet and colleagues.[283] Grade I fractures have periosteal reaction involving one cortex, grade II fractures have periosteal reaction that is circumferential, and grade III has a displaced fracture. Grade I fractures can be treated with non-weight bearing, but cast immobilization is required for grade II or higher to prevent complete fracture or displacement.[283]

REFERENCES

Introduction to Fractures

1. Berquist TH, Morrey BF, Cass JR, Johnson, KA. The Foot and Ankle. In Berquist TH, ed. Imaging of Orthopedic Trauma. 2nd Ed. New York, Raven Press, 1992; pp. 453–578.
2. Bosworth DM. Fracture-dislocation of the ankle with fixed displacement of the fibula behind the tibia. J. Bone Joint Surg. Am. 1947; 29:130–135.
3. Chande VT. Decision rules for roentgenography of children with acute ankle injuries. Arch. Pediatr. Adolesc. Med. 1995; 149:255–258.
4. Cotton FJ. Ankle fractures. A new classification and a new class. N. Engl. J. Med. 1929; 201:753–760.
5. Cotton FJ. A new type of ankle fracture. JAMA 1915; 64:318–321.
6. Destot E. Traumatismes du pied et rayons. V. Malleoles, astragale, calcaneum, avant-pied. Paris, Masson, 1911.
7. Jones R. Fracture of the fifth metatarsal bone. Med. Chir. J. 1902; 22:103–107.
8. Kavanah JH, Brower TD, Mann RV. The Jones fracture revisited. J. Bone Joint Surg. Am. 1978; 60:776–782.
9. Kelikian H, Kelikian AS. Disorders of the Ankle. Philadelphia, W.B. Saunders, 1985.
10. Kerr L, Kelly AM, Grant J, O'Donovan P, Basivek, Graham R. Failed validation of a clinical decision rule for the use of radiography in acute ankle injury. N. Z. Med. J. 1994; 107:294–295.
11. Marmor L. An unusual fracture of the tibial epiphysis. Clin. Orthop. 1970; 73:132–135.
12. McBride KL. Validation of the Ottawa ankle rules. Can. Fam. Physician 1997; 43:459–465.
13. Ovadia DN, Beals RK. Fractures of the tibial plafond. J. Bone Joint Surg. Am. 1986; 68:543–551.
14. Peiro A, Araal J, Martos F, Mat T. Triplane distal tibial epiphyseal fracture. Clin. Orthop. 1981; 160:196–200.
15. Pentecost RL, Murry RA, Brindley HH. Fatigue, insufficiency and pathologic fractures. JAMA 1964; 187:1001–1004.
16. Perry CR, Rice S, Aswath R, Burdge R. Posterior fracture-dislocation of the distal part of the fibula. J. Bone Joint Surg. Am. 1983; 65:1149–1157.
17. Pitt MJ, Speer DP. Radiologic reporting of orthopedic trauma. Med. Radiogr. Photogr. 1982; 58:14–18.
18. Rand JA, Berquist TH. Fracture healing. In Berquist TH, ed. Imaging of Orthopedic Trauma and Surgery. Philadelphia, W.B. Saunders, 1986; pp. 51–90.
19. Sartoris DJ. Radiographic review. Eponymic fractures of the ankle. J. Foot Ankle Surg. 1993; 32(2):239–241.
20. Schultz RJ. The Language of Fractures. Baltimore, Williams & Wilkins, 1972.
21. Torg JS, Baldini FC, Zelko RR, Pavlov H, Peff TC, Dos M. Fractures of the base of the fifth metatarsal distal to the tuberosity. J. Bone Joint Surg. Am. 1984; 66:209–214.
22. Tornetta P III, Weiner L, Bergman M, Watnek N, Steuer J, Kelley M, Yang E. Pilon fractures. Treatment with combined internal and external fixation. J. Orthop. Trauma 1993; 7:489–496.
23. Towbin R, Dimbar JS, Towbin J. Teardrop sign. Plain film recognition of ankle effusion. AJR Am. J. Roentgenol. 1980; 134:985–990.
24. Verma S, Hamilton K, Hawkins HH, Kothari R, Surgal B, Buncher R, Nguyen P, O'Neill M. Clinical application of the Ottawa ankle rules for the use of radiography in acute ankle injuries. An independent site assessment. AJR Am. J. Roentgenol. 1997; 169:825–827.

Pediatric Ankle Fractures

25. Bishop PA. Fractures and epiphyseal separations of the ankle. AJR Am. J. Roentgenol. 1932; 67:28–49.
26. Busconi BD, Pappas AM. Chronic, painful ankle instability in skeletally immature athletes. Ununited osteochondral fractures of the distal fibula. Am. J. Sports Med. 1996; 24(5):647–651.
27. Cameron HU. A radiologic sign of lateral subluxation of the distal tibial epiphysis. J. Trauma 1975; 15(11):1030–1031.
28. Carothers CO, Crenshaw AH. Clinical significance of a classification of epiphyseal injuries at the ankle. Am. J. Surg. 1955; 89:879–889.
29. Cone RO III, Nguyen V, Flournoy JG, Guerra J. Triplane fracture of the distal tibia epiphysis. Radiologic and CT studies. Radiology 1984; 153:763–767.
30. Cooperman DR, Spiegel PG, Laros GS. Tibial fractures involving the ankle in children. J. Bone Joint Surg. Am. 1978; 60:1040–1045.
31. Crawford AH. Ankle fractures in children. J. Orthop. Trauma 1994; 8(4):328–331.
32. Crenshaw AH. Injuries of the distal tibial epiphysis. Clin. Orthop. 1965; 41:98–107.
33. Dias LS. Fractures of the tibia and fibula. In Rockwood CA, Wilkins KE, King RE. Fractures in Children. Vol. 3. Philadelphia, J.B. Lippincott, 1984; pp. 983–1042.
34. Dias LS, Tachdjian MO. Physeal injuries of the ankle in children. Clin. Orthop. 1956; 136:230–233.
35. Dias LS, Giegerich CR. Fractures of the distal tibia epiphysis in adolescence. J. Bone Joint Surg. Am. 1983; 65:438–444.
36. Ferries JS, DeCoster TA, Froozbakhsh RK, Garcia JR, Miller RA. Plain radiographic interpretation in trimalleolar ankle fractures poorly assesses posterior fragment size. J. Orthop. Trauma 1994; 8(4):328–331.
37. Goldberg VM, Aadalen R. Distal tibial epiphyseal injuries. The role of athletics in 53 cases. Am. J. Sports Med. 1978; 6(5):263–268.
38. Harsh WN. Effects of trauma upon epiphyses. Clin. Orthop. 1957, 10:140–147.
39. K(rrholm J, Hansson LI, Laurin S. Pronation injuries of the ankle in children. Acta Orthop. Scand. 1983; 54:1–17.
40. Kleiger B, Mankin JJ. Fracture of the lateral portion of the distal tibial epiphysis. J. Bone Joint Surg. Am. 1964; 46:25.
41. King TF, Bright RW, Hensinger RN. Distal tibial physeal fractures in children that may require open reduction. J. Bone Joint Surg. Am. 1984; 66:647–657.
42. Kump WL. Vertical fractures of the distal tibial epiphysis. AJR Am. J. Roentgenol. 1966; 97:676–681.
43. Laer LU. Classification diagnosis, and treatment of transitional fractures of the distal part of the tibia. J. Bone Joint Surg. Am. 1985; 67:687–698.
44. Lauge-Hansen N. Fractues of the ankle II. Combined experimental-surgical and experimental-radiological investigations. Arch. Surg. 1950; 60:957–985.
45. Lintecum N, Blasier RD. Direct reduction with indirect fixation of distal tibial physeal fractures. A report of a technique. J. Pediatr. Orthop. 1996; 16:107–112.
46. Lynn MD. The triplane distal tibial epiphyseal fractures. Clin. Orthop. 1972; 86:187–190.
47. MacNealy GA, Rogers LF, Hernandez R, Pozanski AK. Injuries of the distal tibial epiphysis. Systematic radiographic evaluation. AJR Am. J. Roentgenol. 1982; 138:683–689.
48. Mann DC, Rajmaira S. Distribution of physeal and non-physeal fractures in 2,650 long bone fractures in children aged 10–16 years. J. Pediatr. Orthop. 1990; 10:713–716.

49. Marmor L. An unusual fracture of the tibial epiphyseal. Clin. Orthop. 1970; 73:132–137.
50. Peiro A, Araal J, Mortos F, Mut T. Triplane distal tibial epiphyseal fracture. Clin. Orthop. 1981; 160:196–200.
51. Rapariz JM, Gonzalez-Herranz P, Lopez-Mondejar JA, Domenech J, Burgos J, Amaya S. Distal tibial triplane fractures. Long term follow-up. J. Pediatr. Orthop. 1996; 16:113–118.
52. Rogers LR. Radiology of epiphyseal injuries. Radiology 1970; 96: 289–299.
53. Salter RB, Harris WR. Injuries involving the epiphyseal plate. J. Bone Joint Surg. Am. 1963; 45:587–622.
54. Sartoris DJ. Diagnosis of ankle injuries. The essentials. J. Foot Ankle Surg. 1994; 33(1):102–107.
55. Schlesinger I. Wedge JH. Percutaneous reduction and fixation of dis-placed juvenile Tillaux fractures. A new surgical technique. J. Pediatr. Orthop. 1993; 13:389–391.
56. Spiegel PG, Cooperman DR, Laros GS. Epiphyseal fractures of the distal ends of the tibia and fibula. J. Bone Joint Surg. Am. 1978; 60: 1046–1050.
57. Trueta J, Morgan JD. The vascular contribution to osteogenesis. I. Studies by the injection method. J. Bone Joint Surg. Br. 1960; 42: 97–109.

Adult Ankle Fractures

58. Albers GHR, deKort AFC, Middendorf PRJM, Van Dijk CN. Distal tibiofibular synostosis after fracture. A 14 year follow-up study. J. Bone Joint Surg. Br. 1996; 78:250–252.
59. Arimoto HR, Forrester DM. Classification of ankle fractures. An algo-rithm. AJR Am. J. Roentgenol. 1970; 135:1057–1063.
60. Ashhurst APC, Bromer RS. Classification and mechanism of fractures of the leg bones involving the ankle. Arch. Surg. 1922; 4:51–129.
61. Berquist TH, Morrey BF, Cass JR, Johnson KA. The Foot and ankle. In Berquist TH. Imaging of Orthopedic Trauma. 2nd Ed. New York, Raven Press, 1992; pp. 453–578.
62. Brumback RJ, McGarvey WC. Fractures fo the tibial plafond. Evolv-ing treatment concepts for the pilon fracture. Othop. Clin. North Am. 1995; 26:273–285.
63. Charnley J. The Closed Treatment of Common Fractures. Baltimore, Williams & Wilkins, 1963.
64. Coonrad RW. Fracture dislocation of the ankle joint with impaction injury of the lateral weight bearing surface of the tibial. J. Bone Joint Surg. Am. 1970; 52:1337–1344.
65. Crutchfield EH, Seligson D, Henry SL, Warnholtz A. Tibial pilon fractures. A comparative clinical study of managment techniques and results. Orthopedics 1995; 18(7):613–617.
66. DeZwart DF, Davidson JSA. Rupture of the posterior tibial tendon associated with fractures of the ankle. J. Bone Joint Surg. Am. 1983; 65:260–262.
67. Dihlman W. Computed tomography of the ankle joint. Chirurg 1982; 53:123–126.
68. Edeiken J, Cotler JM. Ankle trauma. Semin. Roentgenol. 1978; 13(2): 145–155.
69. Edwards GS, DeLee JC. Ankle diastasis without fracture. Foot Ankle 1984; 4(6):305–312.
70. Eventon I, Salama R, Goodwin DRA, Weissman SL. An evaluation of surgical and conservative treatment of fractures of the ankle in 200 patients. J. Trauma 1978; 18(4)271–274.
71. Genant HK, Kozin F, Bekerman C, McCarty DJ, Sims J. The reflex sympathetic dystrophy syndrome. Radiology. 1975; 117:21–32.
72. Griffiths HJ. Trauma to the ankle and foot. CRC Crit. Rev. Diagn. Imaging 1979; 26(1):45–105.
73. Griffiths HJ, Utz R, Burke J, Bonfiglio T. Adhesive capsulitis of the hip and ankle. AJR Am. J. Roentgenol. 1985; 144:101–105.
74. Griffiths GP, Thordarson DB. Tibial plafond fractures. Limited inter-nal fixation and an hybrid external fixator. Foot Ankle Int. 1996; 17(8):444–448.
75. Hall H. A simplified workable classification of ankle fractures. Foot Ankle 1980; 1:5–10.
76. Harper MC. The short oblique fracture of the distal fibula without medial injury. An assessment of displacement. Foot Ankle Int. 1995; 16(4):181–186.
77. Helfet DL, Koval K, Pappas J, Sanders RW, DiPasquale T. Intra-articular pilon fracture of the tibia. Clin. Orthop. 1994; 298:221–228.
78. Horne G. Pes cavovarus following ankle fracture. Clin. Orthop. 1984; 184:249–251.
79. Jenkins D, Campbell LG. Synovial chondromatosis of the ankle. J. Am. Podiatry Assoc. 1981; 71(12):666–670.
80. Kelikian H, Kelikian AS. Disorders of the Ankle. Philadelphia. W.B. Saunders, 1985.
81. Lauge-Hansen N. Fractures of the ankle. II. Combined experimental-surgical once experimental roentgenologic investigations. Arch. Surg. 1950; 60:957–985.
82. Leach RE. Fractures of the tibia and fibula. In Rockwood CA, Green DP, eds. Fractures in Adults. Vol. II. Philadelphia, J.B. Lippincott, 1984; pp. 1593–1663.
83. Leach RE. Fractures of the tibial plafond. AAOS Instruct Course Lect 1979; 28:88–93.
84. Leeds HC, Erlich MG. Instability of the distal tibiofibular syndesmosis after bimalleolar and trimalleolar fractures. J. Bone Joint Surg. Am. 1984; 66:490–503.
85. Lim SL, Lim HH. Review of results of ankle fracture fixation in Alexandra Hospital (Singapore) between January 1987 April 1990. Singapore Med. J. 1995; 36(2):139–142.
86. Low YP. Treatment of ankle fractures. Singapore Med J. 1995; 36: 136–137.
87. Mabit C, Pecout C, Arnaud JP. Ilizarov's technique in correction of ankle malunion. J. Orthop. Trauma 1994; 8(6):520–523.
88. Marsh L, Bonar S, Nepola JV, Decoster TA, Hurwitz SR. Use of an articulated external fixator for fractures of the tibial plafond. J. Bone Joint Surg. Am. 1995; 77:1498–1509.
89. Michelson JD, Ahn H, Magid D. Economic analysis of roentgenogram use in the closed treatment of stable ankle fracture. J. Trauma 1995; 39(6):1119–1122.
90. Michelson JD. Fractures about the ankle. J. Bone Joint Surg. Am. 1995; 77:142–152
91. Miller SD. Late reconstruction after failed treatment for ankle frac-tures. Orthop. Clin North Am. 1995; 26(2):363–373.
92. Moehring HD, Tan RT. Marder RA, Lian G. Ankle dislocation. J. Orthop. Trauma 1994; 8(2):167–172.
93. Montague AP, McQuillan RF. Clinical assessment of apparently sprained ankle and detection of fracture. Injury 1985; 16:545–546.
94. Morgan CD, Henke JA, Bailey RW, Kaufer H. Long-term results of tibiotalar arthrodesis. J. Bone Joint Surg. Am. 1985;67:546–550.
95. Morrey BF, Cass JR, Johnson KA, Berquist TH. Foot and ankle. In Berquist TH, ed. Imaging of Orthopedic Trauma. 2nd Ed. New York, Raven Press, 1992; pp. 453–578.
96. Morrey BF, Weedeman GP. Complications and long term results of ankle arthrodesis following trauma. J. Bone Joint Surg. Am. 1980; 62:777–784.
97. Mosheiff R, Libergail M, Margulies JY, Peyser A, Longdon E, Segal D. Technical complications of the tibiofibular syndesmotic screw. J. Foot Ankle Surg. 1993; 32(5):462–466.
98. M(ller ME, Allgower M, Willenegger H. Manual of Internal Fixation. New York, Springer-Verlag, 1970.
99. Neer CS II. Injuries of the ankle joint. Evaluation. Conn. State Med. J. 1953; 17:580–583.
100. Olerud C. Supination-eversion ankle fractures sustained during down-hill skiing. Acta Orthop. Trauma Surg. 1985; 104:129–131.
101. Ovadia DN, Beals RK. Fractures of the tibial plafond. J. Bone Joint Surg. Am. 1986; 68:543–551.
102. Parfenchuck TA, Frix JM, Bertrand SL, Corpe RS. Clinical use of a syndesmosis screw in stage IV pronation-external rotation ankle fractures. Orthop. Rev. 1994; Aug: 23–28.
103. Perry CR, Rice S, Rao A, Burdge R. Posterior fracture-dislocation of the distal part of the fibula. J. Bone Joint Surg. Am. 1983; 65: 1149–1157.
104. Pettrone FA, Gail M, Pee D, Fitzpatrick T, Van Herpe LB. Quantita-tive criteria for prediction of the results after displaced fracture of the ankle. J. Bone Joint Surg. Am. 1983; 65:667–677.
105. Poplawski ZJ, Wiley AM, Murry JF. Post-traumatic dystrophy of the extremities. J. Bone Joint Surg. Am. 1983; 66:642–654.
106. Port AM, McVie JL, Naylor G, Kreibich DN. Comparison of two conservation methods of treating an isolated fracture of the lateral malleolus. J. Bone Joint Surg. Br. 1996; 78:568–572.
107. Ray TD, Nimityougashul P, Anderson LD. Percutaneous intramedul-lary fixation of lateral malleolar fractures. Technique and report of early results. J. Trauma 1994; 36(5):669–675.

108. Ruedi T. Fractures of the lower end of the tibia into the ankle joint. Results of 9 years after open reduction and internal fixation. Injury 1973; 5:130–134.
109. Said F, Hunka L, Siller TN. Where ankle fusions stand today. J. Bone Joint Surg. Am. 1978; 60B:211–214.
110. Sarkisian JS, Cody GW. Closed treatment of ankle fractures. A new criteria for evaluation. A review of 250 cases. J. Trauma 1976; 16(4): 323–326.
111. Sartoris DJ. Diagnosis of ankle injuries. The essentials. J. Foot Ankle Surg. 1994; 33(1):102–107.
112. Sartoris DJ. Eponymic fractures of the ankle. Am. J. Foot Ankle Surg. 1993; 32(2):239–241.
113. Schutzer SF, Gosslurg HR. The treatment of reflex sympathetic dystrophy sundrome. J. Bone Joint Surg. Am. 1984; 66:625–629.
114. Segal D, Wiss DA, Whitelaw GP. Functional bracing and rehabilitation of ankle fracutres. Clin. Orthop. 1985; 199:39–45.
115. Slawski DP, West C. Maisonneuve fracture with an associated distal fibular fracture. Clin. Orthop. 1995; 317:193–198.
116. Texhammer R, Colton C. AO/ASIF Instruments and Implants. A Technical Manner. 2nd Ed. Berlin, Springer-Verlag, 1994.
117. Tornetta P, Weiner L, Bergmann M, Watnik N, Steuer J, Kelley M, Yang E. Pilon fractures. Treatment with combined internal and external fixation. J. Orthop. Trauma 1993;7(6)489–496.
118. Tropp H, Norlin R. Ankle performance after ankle fracture. A randomized study of early mobilization. Foot Ankle Int. 1995; 16(2):79–83.
119. Velkovski G. The value of osteosynthesis in the threatment of bimalleolar fractures. Ann. Chir. Gynaecol. 1995; 84:403–416.
120. Verma S, Hamilton K, Hawkins HH, Kothari R, Singal B, Buncher R, Nguyen P, O'Neill M. Clinical application of the Ottawa Ankle Rules for the use of radiography or acute ankle injuries. An independent assessment. AJR Am. J. Roentgenol. 1997; 169:825–827.
121. Weber BG, Simpson LA. Corrective lengthening osteotomy of the fibular. Clin Orthop. 1985; 199:61–67.
122. Wilson FC. Fractures and dislocations of the ankle. In Rockwood CA, Green DP, eds. Fractures in Adults. Vol. II. Philadelphia, J.B. Lippincott, 1984; pp. 1665–1702.
123. Wilson FC, Skibred LA. Long-term results in the treatment of displaced bimalleolar fractures. J. Bone Joint Surg. Am. 1966; 48: 1065–1078.
124. Woersdoefer O, Weber BG. Diaphyseal fracture of both bones of the lower leg with associated injury of the ankle mortise. Arch. Orthop. Trauma Surg. 1981; 98:293–296.
125. Xenos JS, Hopkinson WJ, Mulligan ME, Olson EJ, Popovic NA. The tibiofibular syndesmosis J. Bone Joint Surg. Am. 1995; 77:847–856.
126. Yablon IG, Heller FG, Shouse L. The key role of the lateral malleolus in displaced fractures of the ankle. J. Bone Joint Surg. Am. 1977; 59: 169–173.
127. Yablon IG, Wasilewski S. Management of unstable ankle fractures. Foot Ankle 1980; 1:11–19.
128. Yde J. The Lauge-Hansen Classification of malleolar fractures. Acta Orthop. Scand. 1980; 51:181–192.
129. Yde J, Kristensen KD. Ankle fractures. Supination eversion fractures of stage IV. Acta Orthop. Scand. 1980; 51:981–990.
130. Yde J, Kristensen KD. Ankle fractures. Supination eversion fractures stage II. Primary and late operative and non-operative treatment. Acta Orthop. Scand. 1980; 51:695–702.

Talar Fractures and Dislocations

131. Alexander AH, Lichtman DM. Surgical treatment of transchondral talar dome fractures. J. Bone Joint Surg. Am. 1980;62:646–652.
132. Berndt AL, Harty M. Transchondral fractures (osterochondritis dissecans) of the talus. J. Bone Joint Surg. Am. 1959;41:988–1020.
133. Berquist TH. MRI of the Musculoskeletal System. 3rd Ed. New York, Lippincott–Raven, 1996.
134. Blair HC. Comminuted fractures and fracture dislocations of the body of the talus. Am J. Surg. 1943; 59:37–43.
135. Bonnin JG. Injuries of the Ankle. New York, Grune & Stratton, 1950.
136. Brewester NT, Maffulli N. Re-implementation of the totally extruded talus. J. Orthop. Trauma 1997; 11(1):42–45.
137. Burkus JK, Sella FJ, Southwick WO. Occult injuries of the talus diagnosed by bone scan and tomography. Foot Ankle 1984; 4(6): 316–324.
138. Canale ST, Kelly FB. Fractures of the neck and the talus. J. Bone Joint Surg. Am. 1978; 60:143–156.
139. Canale ST, Belding RH. Osteochondral lesions of the talus. J. Bone Joint Surg. Am. 1980; 62:97–102.
140. Chen Y-J, Hsu RW-W. Fracture of the posterior process of the talus associated with subtalar dislocation. J. Formos. Med. Assoc. 1994; 93(9):802–805.
141. Chin JW, Mitra AK, Lun GH, Tan SK, Tay BS. Arthroscopic treatment of osteochondral lesion of the talus. Ann. Acad. Med. Singapore 1996; 25:236–240.
142. Clark TWI, Janzen DL, Kendall H, Grunfeld A, Connell DG. Detection of radiographically occult ankle fractures following acute trauma. Positive predictive value of ankle effusion. AJR Am. J. Roentgenol. 1995; 164:1185–1189.
143. Coltart WD. Aviators astragalus. J. Bone Joint Surg. Br. 1952; 34: 545–566.
144. Cooper RR, Capillo W. Talectomy. Clin. Orthop. 1985; 201:32–35.
145. Daniels TR, Smith JW. Talar neck fractures. Foot Ankle 1993; 14(4): 225–234.
146. DeLee J, Curtis R. Subtalar dislocation of the foot. J. Bone Joint Surg. Am. 1982; 64:433–437.
147. Dennis DM, Tullas HS. Blair tibiotalar arthrodesis for injuries of the talus. J. Bone Joint Surg. Am. 1980; 62:103–107.
148. Detenbeck LC, Kelly PJ. Total dislocation of the talus. J. Bone Joint Surg. Am. 1969; 51:283–288.
149. Dimentberg R, Rosman M. Peritalar dislocations in children. J. Pediatr. Orthop. 1993; 13:89–93.
150. Eddman Rd, Fizber GR. Tibio calcaneal arthrodesis of a failed ankle fusion. J. Foot Ankle Surg. 1993; 32(2):197–203.
151. El-Khoury GY, Yousefzadek DH, Mulligan GM, Moore TE. Subtalar dislocation. Skletal Radiol. 1982; 8:99–103.
152. Flick AB, Gould N. Osteochondritis dissecans of the talus. Review of the literature and a new surgical approach for medial dome lesions. Foot Ankle 1985; 5(4)165–185.
153. Floyd FJ, Ransom RA, Dailey JM. Computed tomography scanning of the subtalar joint. J. Am. Podiatry Assoc. 1984; 14(1):533–537.
154. Gross RH. Fractures and dislocations of the foot. In Rockwood CA, Wilkins KE, King RE, eds. Fractures in Children. Vol. 3. Philadelphia, J.B. Lippincott, 1984; pp. 1043–1103.
155. Hawkins LG. Fractures of the neck of the talus. J. Bone Joint Surg. Am. 1970; 52:991–1002.
156. Hawkins LG. Fractures of the lateral process of the talus. J. Bone Joint Surg. Am. 1965; 47:1170–1175.
157. Heckman JD. Fractures and dislocations of the foot. In Rockwood CA, Green DP, eds. Fractures in Adults. 2nd Ed. Philadelphia, J.B. Lippincott, 1984; pp. 1703–1832.
158. Janssen T, Kopta J. Bilateral recurrent subtalar dislocation. J. Bone Joint Surg. Am. 195; 67:1432–1433.
159. Karasick D. Fractures and dislocations of the foot. Semin. Roentgenol. 1994; 29(2):152–175.
160. Kelikian H, Kelikan AS. Disorders of the Ankle. Philadelphia, W.B. Saunders, 1985.
161. Kenwright J, Taylor RG. Major injuries of the talus. J. Bone Joint Surg. Br. 1970; 52:36–48.
162. Kleiger B, Ahmed M. Injuries of the talus and its joints. Clin. Orthop. 1976; 121:243–262.
163. Leitner B. Obstacles to reduction of subtalar dislocation. J. Bone Joint Surg. Am. 1954; 39:299–306.
164. Letts RM, Gibeault D. Fractures of the neck of the talus in children. Foot Ankle 1980; 1(2):74–77.
165. Loomer R, Fisher C, Lloyd-Smith R, Sisler J, Cooney T. Osteochondral lesions of the talus. Am. J. Sports. Med. 1993; 21(1):13–19.
166. Lorentzen JE, Christensen SB, Krogsoe O, Sneppen. Fractures of the neck of the talus. Acta Orthop. Scand. 1977; 48:115–120.
167. Mankin HJ. The response of articular cartilage to mechanical injury. J. Bone Joint Surg. Am. 1982; 64:460–466.
168. McCrory P, Bladin C. Fractures of the lateral process of the talus. A clinical review. Snowboarders ankle. Clin. J. Sports Med. 1995; 6: 124–128.
169. McDougall A. The os trigonum. J. Bone Joint Surg. Br. 1955; 37: 257–265.
170. Mindell EB, Cisek EE, Kartalian G, Dziob JM. Late results or injuries of the talus. J. Bone Joint Surg. Am. 1963; 45:221–245.
171. Monson ST, Ryan JR. Subtalar dislocation. J. Bone Joint Surg. Am. 1981; 63:1156–1158.
172. Morrey BF, Cass JR, Johnson KA, Berquist TH. Foot and ankle. In

Berquist TH, ed. Imaging of Orthopedic Trauma and Surgery. Philadelphia, W.B. Saunders, 1980; pp. 407–498.

173. Mukhergee SK, Pringle RM, Baxter RM. Fracture of the lateral process of the talus. J. Bone Joint Surg. Br. 1974; 56:263–273.

174. Mulfinger GL, Trueta JC. The blood supply of the talus. J. Bone Joint Surg. Br. 1970; 52:160–167.

175. Mulligan ME. Horizontal fracture of the talar head. Am. J. Sports Med. 1986; 14(2):176–177.

176. Naumetz VA, Schweigel JF. Osteocartilagenous lesions of the talar dome. J. Trauma 1980; 20(11):924–927.

177. Newberg AH. Osteochondral fractures of the dome of the talus. Br. J. Radiol. 1979; 52:105–109.

178. Nyari T, Kazar G, Frenyo S, Balla I. The role of interosseous phlebography in the prognosis of injuries of the talus. Injury 1982; 13: 317–323.

179. Pennal GF. Fractures of the talus. Clin. Orthop. 1963; 30:53–64.

180. Peterson L, Goldie IF, Irstam L. Fracture of the neck of the talus. Acta Orthop. Scand. 1977; 48:696–707.

181. Peterson L, Goldie I, Lindell D. The arterial supply of the talus. Acta Orthop. Scand. 1974; 45:260–270.

182. Pritsch M, Horoshovski H, Farine I, Tel-hanormer O. Arthroscopic treatment of osteochondral lesions of the talus. J. Bone Joint Surg. Am. 1986; 68:862–864.

183. Quirk R. Talar compression syndrome in dancers. Foot Ankle 1982; 3(2):65–68.

184. Resnick D. Talar ridges, osteophytes and beaks. A radiologic commentary. Radiology 1984; 151:329–332.

185. Resnick D. Radiology of the talocalcaneal articulations. Radiology 1974; 111:581–586.

186. Rijsbosch JKC. Fractures of the talus. Arch. Chir. Nierland. 1956; 8: 163–173.

187. Scott JE. Dislocatios of the ankle without fracture. J. Bone Joint Surg. Am. 1974; 39:299–306.

188. Segal D, Waselewski S. Total dislocation of the talus. J. Bone Joint Surg. Am. 1980; 62:1370–1372.

189. Seltzer SE, Weissman BN, Braunstein EM, Adams DF, Thomas WH. Computed tomography of the hind foot. J. Comput. Assist. Tomogr. 1984; 8(3):488–497.

190. Sierra A, Potchen EJ, Moore J, Smith GH. High-field magnetic resonance imaging of aseptic necrosis of the talus. J. Bone Joint Surg. Am. 1986; 68:927–928.

191. Smith GR, Winquist RA, Allan NK, Northrop CH. Subtle transchondral fractures of the talar dome. A radiological perspective. Radiology 1977; 124:667–673.

192. Smith H. Subastragalar Dislocation. J. Bone Joint Surg. 1937; 19: 373–380.

193. Sneppen O, Christensen SB, Krogsoe O, Lorentzen J. Fracture of the body of the talus. Acta Orthop. Scand. 1977; 48:317–324.

194. Solomon MA, Gilula LA, Oloff LM, Oloff J, Compton J. CT scanning of the foot and ankle. Normal anatomy. AJR Am. J. Roentgenol. 1986; 146:1192–1203.

195. Stefko RM, Lauerman WC, Heckman JD. Tarsal tunnel syndrome caused by unrecognized fracture of the posterior process of the talus (Cedell fracture). J. Bone Joint Surg. Am. 1994; 76:116–118.

196. Stephens NA. Fracture-dislocation of the talus in childhood. Br. J. Surg. 1956; 43:600–604.

197. Thompson JP, Loomer RL. Osteochondral lesions of the talus in a sports medicine clinic. Am. J. Sports Med. 1984; 12(6):460–463.

198. Yuan HA, Cody RB, DeRosa C. Osteochondritis dissecans of the talus associated with subchondral cysts. J. Bone Joint Surg. Am. 1979; 61: 1249–1251.

Calcaneal Fractures

199. Böhler L. Diagnosis, pathology, and treatment of fractures of the os calcis. J. Bone Joint Surg. 1931;13:75–89.

200. Cave EF. Fracture of the os calcis. The problem in general. Clin. Orthop. 1963; 30:64–66.

201. Corbett M, Levy A, Abramowitz AJ, Whitelaw GP. A computed tomographic classification for the displaced intra-articular fracture of the os calcis. Orthopedics 1995; 18(8):705. 710.

202. Crosby LA, Fitzgibbons I. Computerized tomographic scanning of acute intra-articular fractures of the calcaneus. J. Bone Joint Surg. Am. 1990;72:852–859.

203. DuVries HL. Surgery of the foot. 4th Ed. St. Louis, C.V. Mosby, 1978.

204. Essex-Lopresti P. The mechanism, reduction technique and results in fractures of the os calcis. Clin. Orthop. 1993; 290:3–16.

205. Essex-Lopresti P. The mechanism, reduction technique, and results in fractures of the os calcis. Br. J. Surg. 1952; 39:395–419.

206. Gellman M. Fractures of the anterior process of the calcaneus. J. Bone Joint Surg. 1931; 13:877–879.

207. Gilmer PW, Herzenberg J, Frank JL, Silverman P, Morteney S, Goldner JL. Computerized tomographic analysis of acute calcaneal fractures. Foot Ankle 1986; 6:184–193.

208. Gross RH. Fractures and dislocations of the foot. In Rockwood CA, Wilkins KE, King RE, eds. Fractures in Children. Vol. 3. Philadelphia, J.B. Lippincott, 1984; pp. 1043–1103.

209. Guyer BH, Levinsuhn EM, Fredrickson BE, Bailey GL, Formikell M. Computed tomography of calcaneal fractures. Anatomy, pathology, dosimetry, and clinical relevance. AJR Am. J. Roentgenol. 1985; 145: 911–919.

210. Hall MC, Pennal GF. Primary subtalar arthrodesis in treatment of severe fractures of the calcaneus. J. Bone Joint Surg. Br. 1960; 42: 336–343.

211. Heckman JD. Fractures and dislocations of the foot. In Rockwood CA, Green DP, eds. Fractures in Adults. Vol. 2. Philadelphia, J.B. Lippincott, 1984; pp. 1703–1832.

212. Heger L, Wolff K. Computed tomography of the calcaneus. Normal anatomy. AJR Am. J. Roentgenol. 1985; 145:123–129.

213. Isbister JF. Calcaneofibular abutment following crush fractures of the calcaneus. J. Bone Joint Surg. Br. 1974; 56:274–278.

214. Johannson J, Harrison J, Greenwood GAH. Subtalar arthrodesis for adult arthritis. Foot Ankle 1982; 2:294–298.

215. Karasick D. Fractures and dislocations of the foot. Semin. Roentgenol. 1994; 29:152–175.

216. Kitaoka HB, Schaap EJ, Chao EYS, An K-N. Displaced intra-articular fractures of the calcaneus treated non-operatively. J. Bone Joint Surg. Am. 1994; 76:1531–1540.

217. Korn R. Der Bruch durch Lintere obere Drittel des Fersenbeines. Arch. Orthop. 1942; 47:189.

218. Lance EM, Corey EJ, Wase PA. Fractures of the os calcis. J. Trauma 1964; 4:15–56.

219. Laughlin RT, Carson JG, Calhoun JH. Displaced intra-articular calcaneal fractures treated with the Galveston Plate. Foot Ankle Int. 1996; 17(2):71–78.

220. Low CK, Mesenas S, Lam KS. Results of closed intra-articular calcaneal fractures treated with early mobilization and without reduction. J. Trauma 1995; 38(5):713–716.

221. Morrey BF, Cass JF, Johnson KA, Berquist TH. Foot and ankle. In Berquist TH, ed. Imaging of Orthopedic Trauma and Surgery. Philadelphia, W.B. Saunders, 1986; pp. 407–498.

222. Norfay JF, Rogers LF, Adams GP, Graves HC, Herser WJ. Common calcaneal avulsion fracture. AJR Am. J. Roentgenol. 1980; 134: 119–123.

223. Pablot SM, Daneman A, Strurger DA, Carroll N. The value of computed tomography or early assessment of comminuted calcaneal fractures. J. Pediatr. Orthop. 1985; 5:435–438.

224. Paley D, Hall H. Intra-articular fractures of the calcaneus. A critical analysis of results and prognostic factors. J. Bone Joint Surg. Am. 1993; 75:342–354.

225. Renfrew DL, El-Khoury GY. Anterior process fractures of the calcaneus. Skeletal Radiol. 1985; 14:121–125.

226. Rosenberg ZS, Feldman F, Surgson RD. Intra-articular calcaneal fractures. Computed tomographic analysis. Skeletal Radiol. 1987; 16: 105–113.

227. Ross SDK, Sowerby RR. The operative treatment of fractures of the os calcis. Clin. Orthop. 1985;199:132–143.

228. Rowe CR, Sakillarides HT, Freeman PA. Fractures of the os calcis. A long term follow-up study in 146 patients. JAMA 1963; 184:920–924.

229. Sartoris DJ. Diagnosis of foot trauma, The essentials. J. Foot Ankle Surg. 1993; 32(5):539–550.

230. Schmidt TL, Weiner DS. Calcaneal fractures in children. An evaluation of the nature of injury in 56 children. Clin. Orthop. 1982; 171: 150–155.

231. Segal D, Marsh JL, Leiter B. Clinical application of computerized axial tomography scanning of calcaneal fractures. Clin. Orthop. 1985; 199:114–123.

232. Slatis P, Kroduoto O, Santavista S, Laasonen EM. Fractures of the calcaneus. J. Trauma 1979; 19(12):939–943.

233. Stephenson JR. Displaced fractures of the os calcis involving the subtalar joint. The key role of the superomedial fragment. Foot Ankle 1983; 4:91–101.
234. Trott AW. Fractures of the foot in children. Orthop. Clin. North Am. 1976; 7:677–686.

Midfoot and Forefoot Fractures

235. Aitken AP, Paulsen D. Dislocation of the tarsometatarsal joints. J. Bone Joint Surg. Am. 1963; 45:246–260.
236. Anderson LD. Injuries of the forefoot. Clin. Orthop. 1977; 122:18–27.
237. Bonutti PM, Bell GR. Compartment syndrome of the foot. J. Bone Joint Surg. Am. 1986; 68:1449–1450.
238. Cain PR, Seligson D. Lisfranc's fracture-dislocation with intercuneiform dislocation. Foot Ankle 1981; 2(3):156–160.
239. Campbell WB, Flectcher EL, Hands LD. Assessment of the distal lower limb arteries: a comparison of arteriography and Doppler ultrasound. Ann. R. Coll. Surg. Engl. 1986; 68:37–39.
240. Carp L. Fracture of the fifth metatarsal bone with special reference to delayed union. Ann. Surg. 1927; 86:308–320.
241. Cassebaum WH. Lisfranc fracture dislocations. Clin. Orthop. 1963; 30:116–129.
242. Dick IL. Impacted fracture of the tarsal navicular. Proc. R. Soc. Med. 1941; 35:760.
243. Eichenholtz SN, Levene DB. Fracture of the tarsal navicular bone. Clin. Orthop. 1964; 34:142–157.
244. English TA. Dislocation of the metatarsal bone and adjacent toe. J. Bone Joint Surg. Br. 1964; 46:700–704.
245. Foster SC, Foster RR. Lisfranc's tarsometatarsal fracture dislocation. Radiology 1976; 120:79–83.
246. Gissane W. A dangerous type of fracture of the foot. J. Bone Joint Surg. Br. 1951; 33:535–538.
247. Goiney RC, Connell DG, Nichols DM. CT evaluation of tarsometatarsal fracture-dislocation injuries. AJR Am. J. Roentgenol. 1985; 144:985–990.
248. Gross RH. Fractures and dislocation of the foot. In Rockwood CA, Wilkins KE, King RE, eds. Fractures in Children. Vol. 3. Philadelphia, J.B. Lippincott, 1984; pp. 1043–1103.
249. Hardcastle PH, Reschauer R, Kutscha-Lissberg E, Schoffman W. Injuries of the tarsometatarsal joint. Incidence classification, and treatment. J. Bone Joint Surg. Br. 1982; 64:349–356.
250. Heckman JD. Fractures of the foot and ankle. In Rockwood CA, Green DP, Bucholz RW, Heckman JD, eds. Rockwood and Green Fractures in Adults. Philadelphia, Lippincott–Raven, 1996; pp. 2267–2405.
251. Johnson GF. Pediatric Lisfranc injury. Bunkbed fracture. AJR Am. J. Roentgenol. 1981; 137:101–1044.
252. Jones R. Fracture of the base of the fifth metatarsal bone by indirect violence. Ann. Surg. 1902; 35:697–700.
253. Karasick D. Fracture and dislocation of the foot. Semin. Roentgenol. 1994; 29(2):152–175.
254. Kavanaugh JH, Borower TD, Mann RV. The Jones fracture revisited. J. Bone Joint Surg. Am. 1978; 60:776–782.
255. Lewis AG, DeLee JC. Type I complex dislocation of the 1st metatarsophalangeal joint. Open reduction through a dorsal approach. J. Bone Joint Surg. Am. 1978; 60:1120–1123.
256. Littlejohn SG, Line LL, Yerger LB. Complete cuboid dislocation. Orthopedics 1996; 19(2):175–176.
257. Macy NJ, de Voer P. Mid-tarsal dislocation of the first ray. J. Bone Joint Surg. Am. 1983; 65:265–266.
258. Main BJ, Jowett RL. Injuries of the mid-tarsal joint. J. Bone Joint Surg. Br. 1975; 57:89–97.
259. Nielsen S, Agnholt J, Christensen H. Radiologic findings in lesions of the ligamentum bifurcatum of the mid foot. Skeletal Radiol. 1987; 16:114–116.
260. Norfray JF, Feline RA, Steinberg RI, Galinski AW, Gilula LA. Subtleties of Lisfranc fractures-dislocations. AJR Am. J. Roentgenol. 1981; 137:1151–1156.
261. Rodersheimer LR, Feins R, Green RM. Doppler evaluation of the pedal arch. Am. J. Surg. 1981; 142:601–604.
262. Sartoris DJ. Diagnosis of foot trauma. The essentials. Foot Ankle Surg. 1993; 32(5):539–550.
263. Silas SI, Herzenberg JE, Myerson MS, Sponseller PD. Compartment syndrome of the foot in children. J. Bone Joint Surg. Am. 1995; 27:356–561.
264. Tan YH, Chin TW, Mitra AK, Tan SK. Tarsometatarsal (Lisfranc's) injuries. Results of open reduction and internal fixation. Ann. Acad. Med. Singapore 1995; 24(6):8160–819.
265. Torg JS, Balduini FC, Selko RR, Povlov LT, Peff TC, Das M. Fractures of the base of the fifth metatarsal distal to the tuberosity. J. Bone Joint Surg. Am. 1984; 66:209–214.
266. Trevino SG, Kodros S. Controversies in tarsometatarsal injury. Orthop. Clin. North Am. 1995; 26(2):229–238.
267. Wiley JJ. Tarso-metatarsal joint injuries in children. J. Pediatr. Orthop. 1981; 1:255–260.
268. Wiley JJ. The mechanism of tarsometatarsal joint injuries. J. Bone Joint Surg. Br. 1971; 53:474–482.
269. Wilppula E. Tarsometatarsal fracture-dislocation. Acta Orthop. Scand. 1973; 44:335–345.
270. Zinman H, Keret Q, Reis ND. Fracture of the medial sesamoid bone of the Hallus. J. Trauma 1981; 21(7):581–582.

Stress Fractures

271. Berquist TH, Cooper KL, Pritchard DJ. Stress fractures. In Berquist TH, ed. Imaging of Orthopedic Trauma. 2nd Ed. New York, Raven Press, 1992, pp. 891–894.
272. Blickenstaff LD, Morris JM. Fatigue fracture of the femoral neck. J. Bone Joint Surg. Am. 1966; 48:1031–1047.
273. Chowchuen P, Resnick D. Stress fractures of the metatarsal heads. Skeletal Radiol. 1998; 27:22–25.
274. Daffner RH. Stress Fractures. Skeletal Radiol. 1987; 2:221–229.
275. Darby RE. Stress fractures of the os calcis. JAMA 1967; 200:1183–1184.
276. Devas MB. Stress Fractures. Churchill Livingstone, Edinburgh, 1975.
277. Devas MB. Stress fractures in children. J. Bone Joint Surg. Br. 1963; 45:528–541.
278. Eisele SA, Sammarco GJ. Fatigue fractures of the foot and ankle in the athlete. J. Bone Joint Surg. Am. 1993; 75:290–298.
279. Ford LT, Filula LH. Stress fractures of the middle metatarsals following Keller operation. J. Bone Joint Surg. Am. 1977; 59:117–118.
280. Gilbert RS, Johnson HA. Stress fractures in military recruits. A review of 12 years experience. Milit. Med. 1966; 131:716–721.
281. Goergen TG, Rossman DJ, Gerber KH. Tarsal navicular stress fractures in runners. AJR Am. J. Roentgenol. 1981; 136:201–203.
282. Greaney RB, Gerber FH, Laughlin RL. Distribution and natural history of stress fractures in U.S. Marine recruits. Radiology 1983; 146:339–346.
283. Hallet T, Amit S, Segal D. Fatigue fractures of the tibial and femoral shaft in soldiers. Clin. Orthop. 1976; 118:35–43.
284. Hunter LY. Stress fractures of the tarsal navicular. More frequent than we realize? Am. J. Sports Med. 1981; 9(4)217–219.
285. Kroening PM, Shelton ML. Stress fractures. AJR Am. J. Roentgenol. 1963; 89:1281–1286.
286. Levy JM. Stress fractures of the first metatarsal. AJR Am. J. Roentgenol. 1978; 130:679–681.
287. Meurman KOA. Less common stress fractures of the foot. Br. J. Radiol. 1981; 54:1–7.
288. Micheli LJ, John RS, Solomon R. Stress fractures of the second metatarsal involving Lafranc's joint in ballet dancers. J. Bone Joint Surg. Am. 1985; 67:1372–1375.
289. Nicastro JF, Haupt HA. Probable stress fracture of the cuboid in an infant. J. Bone Joint Surg. Am. 1984; 66:1106–1108.
290. Ovara S, Puranen J, Ala-Ketala L. Stress fractures caused by physical exercise. Acta Orthop. Scand. 1978; 49:19–27.
291. Orvara S, Karpakka J, Taimela S, Hulkko A, Permi J, Kujala U. Stress fracture of the medial malleolus. J. Bone Joint Surg. Am. 1995; 77:362–365.
292. Pavlov H, Torg JS, Freeberger RH. Tarsal navicular stress fractures. Radiology 1983; 148:641–645.
293. Reider B, Falconiero R, Yurkofsky J. Nonunion of a medial malleolus stress fracture. Am. J. Sports Med. 1993; 21(3):478–481.
294. Torg JS, Pavlou H, Cooley LH. Stress fractures of the tarsal navicular. J. Bone Joint Surg. Am. 1982; 64:700–712.
295. Umans H, Pavlov H. Stress fractures of the lower extremities. Semin. Roentgenol. 1994; 29(2):176–193.
296. Wilson ES, Katz FN. Stress fractures. An analysis of 250 consecutive cases. Radiology 1969; 92:481–486.
297. Young A, Kinsella P, Boland P. Stress fractures of the lower extremity in patients with rheumatoid arthritis. J. Bone Joint Surg. Br. 1981; 63:239–342.

Radiology of the Foot and Ankle, Second Edition,
edited by Thomas H. Berquist.
© 2000 by Mayo Foundation.
Published by Lippincott Williams & Wilkins, Philadelphia.

CHAPTER 5

Arthritis

Laura Wasylenko Bancroft and Richard A. McLeod

DEGENERATIVE JOINT DISEASE

The radiologic hallmarks of degenerative arthritis are osteophytes, subchondral sclerosis, asymmetric joint space narrowing, subchondral cysts, and loose bodies. Degenerative joint disease is the most common radiographic abnormality seen in the skeleton. Osteoarthritis is the degenerative change of fibrous, cartilaginous, and synovial articulations. Primary degenerative joint disease occurs in the absence of any obvious underlying abnormalities, whereas secondary osteoarthritis is the result of alterations from a preexisting disorder, such as other arthritides.[21] One of the earliest radiographic signs is the formation of new bone at the margins of the articular surface. The osteophytes are composed of both cancellous and cortical bone, which blends imperceptibly with the normal adjacent bone.[21] This is an extremely important radiographic sign, because bone production is rare in rheumatoid arthritis. Because the protective cushion of cartilage is lost, trauma to the articular bone surface stimulates osteoblastic activity, resulting in eburnation or subchondral sclerosis. These changes are most prominent at the points of maximal weight bearing. Nonuniform joint space narrowing may occur either early or late during the course

L. W. Bancroft: Mayo Medical School, Mayo Clinic Jacksonville, Jacksonville, Florida 32224; St. Luke's Hospital, Jacksonville, Florida 32216.

R. A. McLeod: Mayo Medical School (Emeritus), Rochester, Minnesota 55905.

of the disease. In contrast to that seen in rheumatoid arthritis, thinning of the joint space in this condition is almost invariably nonuniform or asymmetric.[8] Subchondral cysts may form but alone, they are of little diagnostic value. Osteocartilaginous loose bodies commonly form within the joint.

Probably the most common site of degenerative joint disease of the foot and ankle is the first metatarsophalangeal (MTP) joint (Fig. 5-1A). The usual changes consist of asymmetric joint space narrowing, osteophyte formation, and subchondral sclerosis (see Fig. 5-1B). The osteophytes are largest dorsally and laterally. They frequently cause painful limitation of dorsiflexion of the great toe, referred to as hallux rigidus (see Fig. 5-1C and D). Flattening and deformity of the metatarsal head, subchondral cysts, and loose bodies also may be seen. These changes are often superimposed on hallux valgus deformity. Osteoarthritis of the second through fifth MTP joints is unusual, but it can be seen in any MTP joint that becomes the primary weight-bearing joint.[8] Interphalangeal (IP) degenerative joint disease usually involves the first digit. Involvement of other digits is unusual and is usually asymptomatic (Fig. 5-2A).[7] It can result in *claw toe, hammer toe, mallet toe* (flexion of the distal IP [DIP] joint), and *curly toe* (flexion of the proximal IP [PIP] and DIP joints) (see Chapter 10)[21]. Degenerative joint disease also occurs throughout the tarsometatarsal (TMT) and intertarsal joints (see Fig. 5-2B). The changes in the TMT joints are more common medially, especially at the first TMT joint. In this location, joint space narrowing and sclerosis may

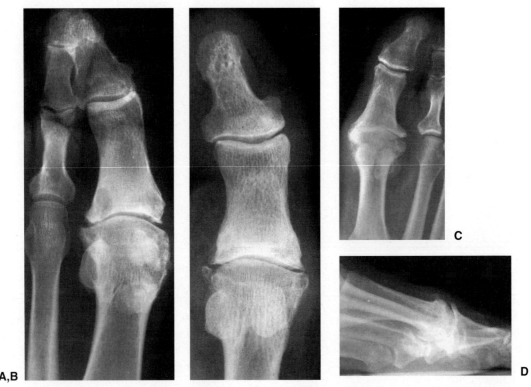

FIG. 5-1. Osteoarthritis involving the first MTP joint, the most common location in the foot. **A** and **B:** AP radiographs of the first MTP joint demonstrate asymmetric joint space loss, osteophyte formation, and subchondral sclerosis. Also note the loose body lateral to the joint in **B** and the subchondral cysts in the lateral aspects of the proximal phalanx and metatarsal head in **A** and in the medial metatarsal head in **B**. **C** and **D:** AP and lateral radiographs of the first ray demonstrate hallux rigidus.

simulate gout (see Fig. 5-2C).[21] When the degenerative changes are generalized, they may be superimposed on an inflammatory condition. Degenerative changes of the midfoot may also be secondary to previous trauma or abnormal motion related to tarsal coalition or surgical fusion. The talonavicular portion of the anterior talocalcaneonavicular joint is the most common hindfoot joint affected by osteoarthritis, resulting from previous trauma or, rarely, occurring spontaneously.[21] Early neurotrophic arthropathy may also be confused with degenerative joint disease of the midfoot.

Plantar and posterior calcaneal enthesophytes at the attachment of the Achilles tendon, plantar aponeurosis, and long plantar ligament are commonly seen and are often clinically silent.[21] The enthesophytes are almost always well defined and reflect ligamentous or tendinous traction.

Primary degenerative joint disease of the ankle is unusual (Fig. 5-3). Findings include joint space narrowing, subchondral sclerosis, and talar beaking resulting from capsular traction. These changes can be distinguished from those of tarsal coalition because the osteoarthritic dorsal talar spur is posterior to the talonavicular joint, osteophytes can involve the anterior tibia, and joint space loss is usually noted.[7] Therefore, when degenerative changes are seen at this site, an underlying cause should be sought. The most common of

these are trauma, disease in the knees or feet, and other arthritides.

RHEUMATOID ARTHRITIS

The radiologic hallmarks of rheumatoid arthritis are joint effusions, periarticular soft tissue swelling, symmetric joint space narrowing, marginal cortical erosions, osteoporosis, subchondral cysts, and subluxations.

Rheumatoid arthritis is a systemic inflammatory arthropathy that commonly involves the foot in 90% of cases at some time.[4] The radiographic changes in the soft tissues, cartilage, and bone are a result of inflammation of the synovia, bursae, and tendon sheaths. Perivascular synovitis leads to synovial hypertrophy, joint effusion, and edema of adjacent soft tissues. These changes combine to result in fusiform periarticular swelling and increased soft tissue density, which are early and important radiographic findings in rheumatoid arthritis. Early disease can be appreciated on low–peak kilovolt (kVp) imaging.[7] Experimental studies with gadolinium-enhanced T1-weighted images have been shown to be sensitive for differentiating active synovitis from fibrosis and joint effusions in the early stages of rheumatoid arthritis, although studies have focused on the hands and wrists.[26]

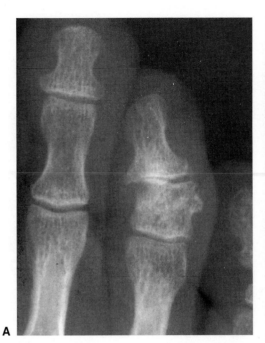

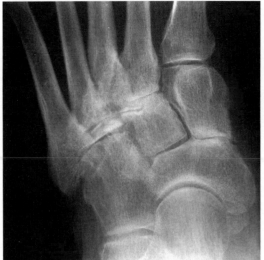

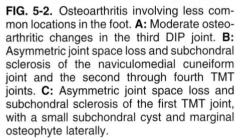

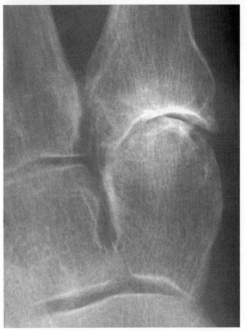

FIG. 5-2. Osteoarthritis involving less common locations in the foot. **A:** Moderate osteoarthritic changes in the third DIP joint. **B:** Asymmetric joint space loss and subchondral sclerosis of the naviculomedial cuneiform joint and the second through fourth TMT joints. **C:** Asymmetric joint space loss and subchondral sclerosis of the first TMT joint, with a small subchondral cyst and marginal osteophyte laterally.

The pattern or distribution of involvement is of diagnostic significance. The foot not only is a common site of involvement, but also is involved early in the disease process; it may be the initial site affected. The fifth MTP joint is often the earliest joint affected (Fig. 5-4), more so than the other MTP joints (Fig. 5-5A and B). The IP joint of the great toe is also a commonly affected joint (see Fig. 5-5C), whereas the IP joints of the remaining toes are frequently spared. The midfoot is often involved in rheumatoid arthritis, but soft tissue changes are difficult to appreciate. Swelling, increased density of the soft tissues, and bursitis also may be seen at the insertion of the Achilles tendon and near the insertion of the plantar aponeurosis onto the calcaneus. Soft tissue swelling of the ankle joint occurs but less frequently than it does in the foot.

Osteoporosis occurs early and is nearly always present in rheumatoid arthritis, although the exact cause is not well understood. The radiographic detection of osteoporosis is difficult and possible only when the demineralization is advanced. The radiodensity of bone is so variable that it alone is of little diagnostic value. Cortical thinning, however, is a reliable indicator of bone loss, as is the accentuation of the cortical bone and remaining trabecular, which results from the preferential resorption of transverse trabecular.

Articular cartilage is destroyed in a uniform manner in rheumatoid arthritis, resulting in uniform symmetric joint space narrowing.[8] Symmetric joint space loss occurs earliest and most frequently at the MTP joints (Fig. 5-6), although the IP joint of the great toe is also frequently affected. The other IP joints sometimes may be affected, with the proximal

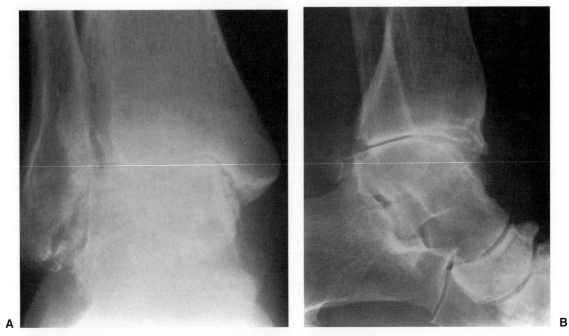

FIG. 5-3. Osteoarthritis of the ankle. AP (**A**) and lateral (**B**) radiographs of the ankle demonstrate the typical subchondral sclerosis and marginal osteophytes of osteoarthritis; however, the fairly uniform joint space loss is atypical. Degenerative change of the ankle is unusual in the absence of prior trauma, disease in the knees or feet, or other arthritides.

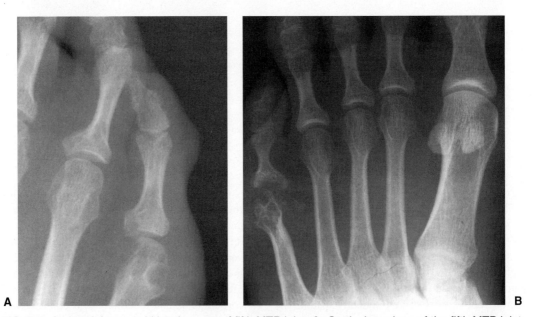

FIG. 5-4. Isolated rheumatoid involvement of fifth MTP joint. **A:** Cortical erosions of the fifth MTP joint, with soft tissue swelling lateral to the MTP and PIP joints. **B:** Advanced destruction of the fifth MTP joint, associated with lateral soft tissue swelling.

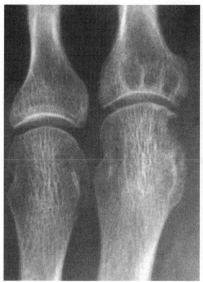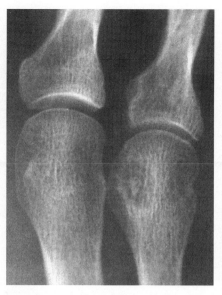

A,B

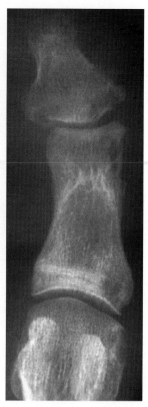

C

FIG. 5-5. Rheumatoid arthritis of the forefoot. **A:** Mild symmetric joint space loss, marginal erosions and multiple subchondral cysts involving the second MTP joint. **B:** Subtle periarticular osteopenia and erosive changes of the metatarsal head and base of the third proximal phalanx. **C:** Minimal joint space narrowing and marginal erosions of the first MTP and IP joints.

joints being more commonly involved. Rheumatoid arthritis frequently involves the midfoot (Fig. 5-7A), and uniform joint space narrowing is characteristic. The entire midfoot is diffusely affected. When involvement is more localized, the most frequently affected articulations are the talonavicular (see Fig. 5-7B), TMT, subtalar, and cuneonavicular

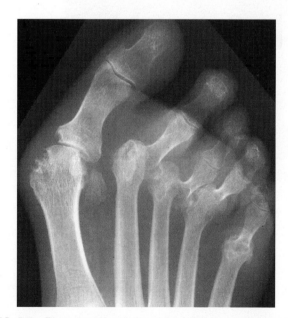

FIG. 5-6. Rheumatoid arthritis of the MTP joints. Destructive changes of the MTP joints, hallux valgus deformity, and fibular deviation and dislocation of the second through fifth toes.

joints. Ankle involvement usually results in symmetric narrowing of the tibiotalar joint (Fig. 5-8).

Hypertrophied synovium or pannus can result in cortical erosions, typically located at the joint margin between the articular cartilage and the synovium. The erosions have poorly defined margins, and although varied in size, they are usually small. Like other manifestations, rheumatoid erosions arise most frequently at the MTP joints (Fig. 5-9A) and the IP joint of the great toe (see Fig. 5-9B). They predominate along the medial aspect of the metatarsal heads and the head of the proximal phalanx of the great toe. The lateral aspect of the fifth metatarsal head is frequently affected in rheumatoid arthritis before other sites (see Fig. 5-9C), and involvement may occur early when findings elsewhere may be lacking and the diagnosis is in question. Synovial inflammation at the junction of the first metatarsal and its sesamoid can result in sesamoid erosion. Erosions are less common in the second through fifth PIP and are unusual in the second through fifth DIP joints. Cortical erosions in the midfoot are either lacking or are small, despite an advanced loss of cartilage. Calcaneal erosions adjacent to the Achilles tendon (Fig. 5-10) can be associated with retrocalcaneal bursitis and inflammatory changes of the Achilles tendon. Erosions and enthesophytes at the plantar surface of the calcaneus can be associated with plantar fasciitis. After uniform cartilage loss occurs in the ankle, small erosions may be present, but they are usually not a prominent finding in this joint.

Cysts are common in rheumatoid arthritis and are usually

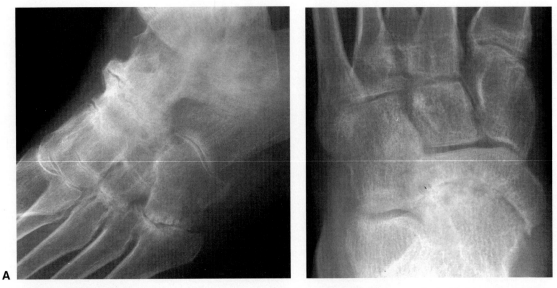

FIG. 5-7. Rheumatoid arthritis of the midfoot. **A:** Oblique radiograph demonstrates fairly uniform joint space loss throughout the midfoot, with both indistinct and sclerotic margins. **B:** Advanced rheumatoid involvement of the talonavicular joint, which is one of the most frequently involved sites of localized disease.

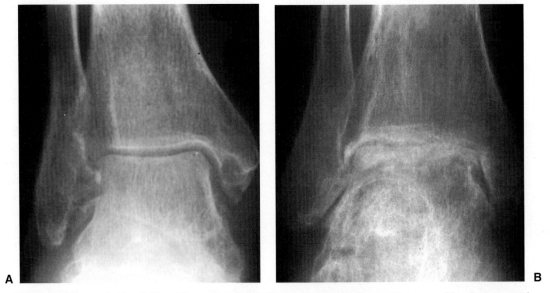

FIG. 5-8. Rheumatoid arthritis of the ankle. **A:** Uniform loss of articular cartilage resulting in symmetric joint space narrowing and subchondral cyst in the medial malleolus. **B:** Advanced rheumatoid changes of severe joint space loss, irregularity, and sclerosis of the articular bone.

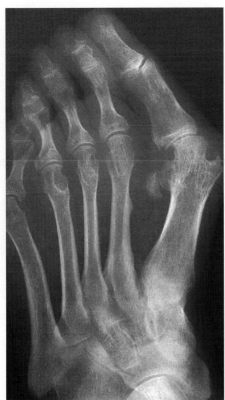

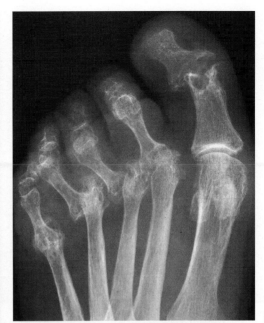

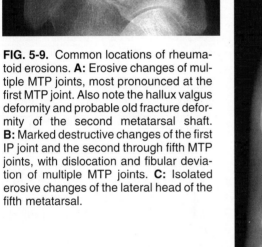

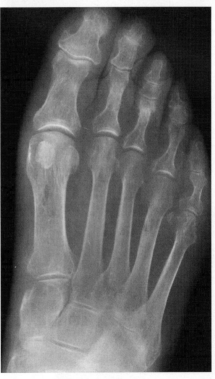

FIG. 5-9. Common locations of rheumatoid erosions. **A:** Erosive changes of multiple MTP joints, most pronounced at the first MTP joint. Also note the hallux valgus deformity and probable old fracture deformity of the second metatarsal shaft. **B:** Marked destructive changes of the first IP joint and the second through fifth MTP joints, with dislocation and fibular deviation of multiple MTP joints. **C:** Isolated erosive changes of the lateral head of the fifth metatarsal.

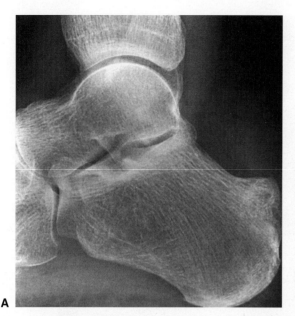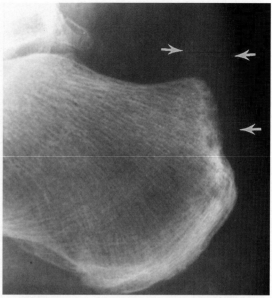

A   **B**

FIG. 5-10. Posterior calcaneal erosions in rheumatoid arthritis. **A:** Typical location of erosive changes in the calcaneus adjacent to the insertion of the Achilles tendon. **B:** Irregular erosive changes of the calcaneus, associated with abnormal soft tissue density (*arrows*) indicative of inflammatory changes of the Achilles tendon and possibly retrocalcaneal bursitis.

subcortical. Some erosions can simulate cysts when viewed in a different obliquity. Rheumatoid cysts are variable in size and can become quite large (Fig. 5-11).[1] Cysts are not specific for rheumatoid arthritis and can be seen in other arthritides, such as gout and degenerative arthritis. When they occur alone, cysts are of little diagnostic significance.

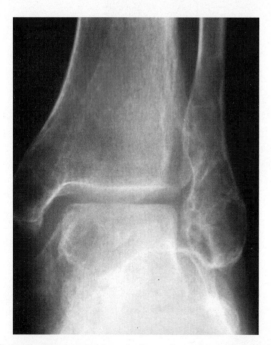

FIG. 5-11. Rheumatoid cysts throughout the ankle. Multiple subchondral cysts involve the medial malleolus, distal fibula, and medial talus.

Periosteal new bone formation is extremely rare in rheumatoid arthritis. When it occurs, it favors another diagnosis, such as infection or one of the seronegative arthropathies.

Inflammatory changes of the synovium, joint capsules, ligaments, and bursae can lead to malalignment and subluxations. Hallux valgus deformity and fibular deviation of the second through fourth toes are common (Fig. 5-12A).[19] Claw toes, hammer toes, forefoot spread, and dorsal dislocation of the toes (see Fig. 5-12B) are also common. Rupture of the posterior tibial tendon is a known cause of flatfoot deformity in patients with rheumatoid arthritis.[4] Joint ankylosis is a late manifestation of rheumatoid arthritis, usually involving the tarsal bones (Fig. 5-13), nearly always sparing the IP and MTP joints. Synovial cysts are unusual in the foot and ankle, although they can arise from any joint. Insufficiency-type stress fractures occur in the foot and ankle, and they are probably related to osteoporosis and alterations in the weight-bearing forces (Fig. 5-14).[21]

Rheumatoid nodules are commonly located subcutaneously, but they can involve bursae, joints, tendons, and ligaments.[24] Subcutaneous rheumatoid nodules occur commonly in advanced cases of rheumatoid arthritis, but only about 1% of all nodules occur in the feet (Fig. 5-15A and B).[24] Nodules have been reported in the dorsal soft tissues of the feet, adjacent to the Achilles tendon, on the toes, and in the heel pad. Lesions in the plantar aspect of the foot can become painful and may erode adjacent bone. Magnetic resonance imaging (MRI) findings are nonspecific, but when combined with the clinical history of rheumatoid arthritis, they are suggestive of rheumatoid nodules (see Fig. 5-15C and D). Masses may be slightly heterogeneously isointense to mus-

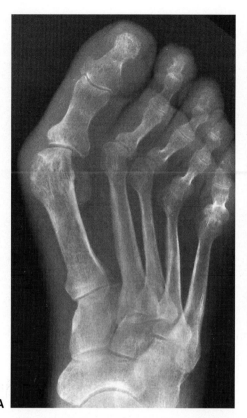

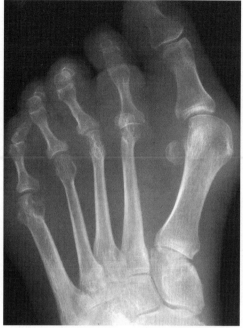

FIG. 5-12. Malalignment and subluxations due to rheumatoid arthritis. **A:** Hallux valgus deformity and fibular deviation of the second through fourth toes. Also note the erosive changes of the head of the first metatarsal bone and adjacent soft tissue swelling. **B:** Hallux valgus deformity and dislocation of the second toe. Also note the marginal cortical erosions of multiple MTP and TMT joints and the soft tissue swelling adjacent to the first and fifth MTP joints.

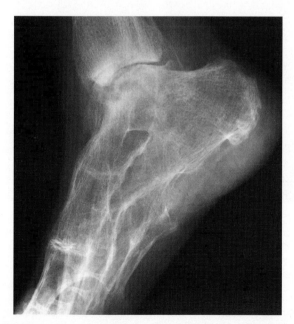

FIG. 5-13. Advanced rheumatoid arthritis. Lateral radiograph demonstrates extensive tarsal ankylosis, which is a late manifestation of rheumatoid arthritis, as well as advanced changes in the ankle and calcaneal erosions.

cle on T1-weighted images and slightly hyperintense on T2-weighted images, and they may demonstrate intense heterogeneous enhancement.[24]

JUVENILE CHRONIC ARTHRITIS

Chronic inflammatory arthritides in children can be subdivided into juvenile rheumatoid arthritis (JRA) and juvenile spondyloarthropathies. The radiologic hallmarks of juvenile chronic arthritis are changes similar to those of the adult disease, except for possible severe extraarticular manifestations, late or absent cartilage loss and cortical erosions, more frequent periosteal new bone, altered bone growth, common and possibly extensive joint ankylosis, and possibly asymmetric and either oligoarticular or monoarticular involvement.

Juvenile Rheumatoid Arthritis

The three categories of JRA are distinguished by their clinical characteristics at the onset of disease.[28] *Pauciarticular* JRA is the most common type, with involvement of four or fewer joints at disease onset. There are two subdivisions within the pauciarticular type: type 1 occurs in young fe-

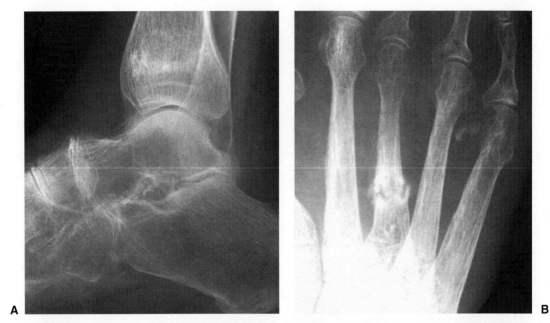

FIG. 5-14. Insufficiency-type stress fractures in rheumatoid arthritis. **A:** Linear condensation in the distal tibial metaphysis, indicative of a stress fracture. **B:** Healing insufficiency stress fracture of the third metatarsal shaft and typical rheumatoid changes of the MTP joints.

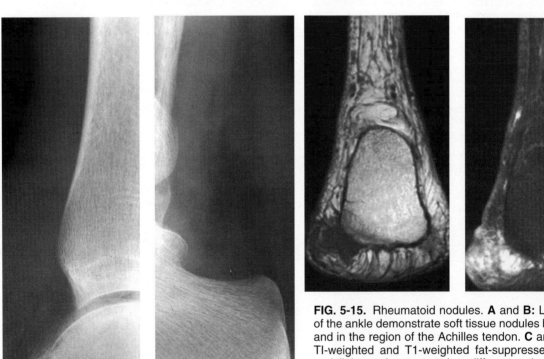

FIG. 5-15. Rheumatoid nodules. **A** and **B:** Lateral images of the ankle demonstrate soft tissue nodules both anteriorly and in the region of the Achilles tendon. **C** and **D:** Coronal Tl-weighted and T1-weighted fat-suppressed image with gadolinium enhancement in a different patient display a biopsy-proven rheumatoid nodule. The low signal intensity on T1-weighted imaging and intense heterogeneous enhancement have been reported in rheumatoid nodules, but these findings are nonspecific and must be correlated with the clinical history.

males and has a high association with antinuclear antibodies and iridocyclitis, and type II occurs in older boys and is associated with spondyloarthropathies. The second category of JRA is the *polyarticular* type, which involves five or more joints at disease onset. This group can be divided into seropositive and seronegative subtypes. Finally, *systemic-onset* JRA is characterized by fever, skin rash, lymphadenop-athy, organomegaly, pericarditis, and other systemic findings.[28]

The feet and ankles are commonly involved in JRA, and after the knee, the ankle is the second most frequent site for monoarticular disease (Fig. 5-16). Juvenile-onset adult-type (seropositive) rheumatoid arthritis closely resembles the adult type of rheumatoid arthritis, with common involvement

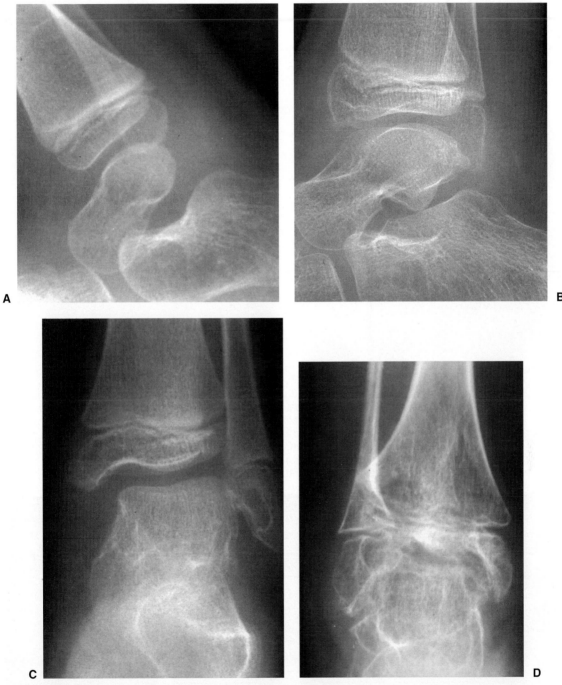

FIG. 5-16. Juvenile rheumatoid arthritis of the ankle. **A** and **B:** Lateral images of the ankle in the same patient over a 4-year span demonstrate soft tissue swelling in the posterior ankle resulting from synovitis. No other rheumatoid changes are evident. **C:** Erosive changes of the lateral malleolus and medial talus, with preservation of the joint spaces. **D:** More advanced changes consist of joint space irregularity, cortical erosions, and synovitis.

of the hand, wrist, knee, and foot. There is a female predominance, and patients usually present at less than 10 years of age. Patients commonly have soft tissue swelling secondary to joint effusion and synovitis, periarticular osteoporosis, periostitis, and erosions.

Still's disease (seronegative rheumatoid arthritis) is the largest subtype of JRA (about 70%) in which patients may either have the classic systemic disease described previously, polyarticular, pauciarticular, or monoarticular disease. The systemic and polyarticular forms have no sex predilection; the systemic form affects patients less than 5 years of age, whereas the polyarticular type presents at variable ages. The pauciarticular and monoarticular subtypes have a female predilection, and patients present at a young age.[21] Still's dis-

ease primarily affects the ankle, intertarsal, MTP, and IP joints when the foot is involved (Fig. 5-17A and B). Asymmetric involvement is more common than is seen in adult rheumatoid arthritis.

Joint space narrowing and cortical erosions are often absent or develop late in JRA (see Fig. 5-17C). These changes are presumably related to the thick articular and epiphyseal cartilage overlying the ossified bone ends.[15] Periosteal new bone is common in JRA, and the small tubular bones of the feet are a favored site (Fig. 5-18A). This new bone is often thick and is seen early during the course of the disease (see Fig. 5-18B). The new bone may blend imperceptibly with the normal cortex, resulting in rectangular bones.

Because JRA occurs during bone growth, there may be

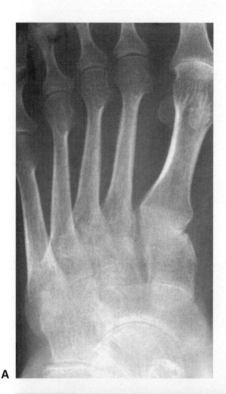

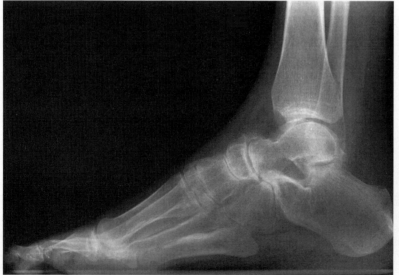

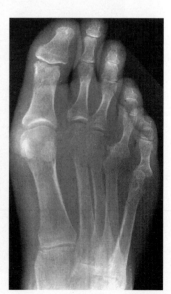

FIG. 5-17. Changes of juvenile rheumatoid arthritis (JRA), evident in the adult foot. **A:** Joint space narrowing of the MTP, TMT, and intertarsal joints without significant erosion. Joint space narrowing and cortical erosions are often absent or develop late in JRA, as opposed to the adult variety. **B:** Lateral image of the foot demonstrates rheumatoid changes throughout the midfoot. **C:** Destructive changes in the fourth and fifth MTP joints and narrowing of multiple TMT joints.

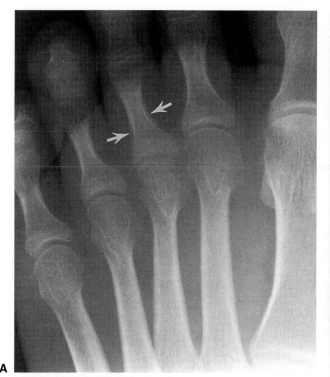
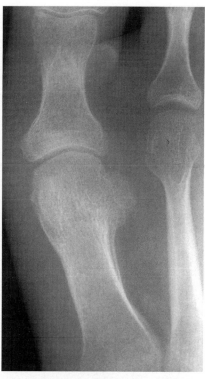

A

B

FIG. 5-18. Periosteal new bone in JRA. **A:** Periosteal new bone of the proximal third phalanx and joint space narrowing of the third MTP joint. Periosteal new bone is a common finding in JRA, as opposed to the adult variety. **B:** Well-organized periosteal new bone formation of the first metatarsal, mild symmetric joint space narrowing, and subtle erosive changes of the first MTP joint.

superimposed changes in bone maturation, bone growth, and epiphyseal fusion. Bone growth may be accelerated. This overgrowth is most frequently seen in the epiphysis and is believed to be related to hyperemia. Bone growth may be retarded secondary to premature epiphyseal fusion. Alteration in bone growth may result in many different types of deformity.

Joint ankylosis often occurs late in the disease process and may be diffuse, a finding seldom seen in other arthritides (Fig. 5-19). Some cases progress to extreme destruction (Fig. 5-20).

Juvenile Spondyloarthropathies

The seronegative spondyloarthropathies—ankylosing spondylitis, psoriatic arthritis, arthritis associated with inflammatory bowel disease and Reiter's syndrome—are referred to as juvenile spondyloarthropathies when they present in patients less than 16 years old.

Juvenile-onset ankylosing spondylitis is just like the adult-onset variety, but it involves the peripheral skeleton more preferentially. This disorder usually presents in late childhood or adolescence in a 7:1 male-to-female ratio.[3] This entity rarely presents with the classic sacroiliitis and spondylitis typical of the adult form of AS. Extraaxial arthritis is more common than in the adult form and usually involves the lower extremities. Enthesitis of the foot commonly involves the Achilles tendon and plantar fascia.

Juvenile psoriatic arthritis occurs at a peak age of 10 years with a 1.2:1 female-to-male ratio.[3] The diagnosis can be made even in the absence of a psoriatic rash by relying on nail pitting, dactylitis, a family history of psoriasis, and an atypical rash.[23] This disorder most commonly is an asymmetric, pauciarticular arthritis of large and small joints, which can be indistinguishable from pauciarticular JRA.[3] DIP joint destruction, phalangeal tuft resorption, and enthesitis occur, but they are seen less commonly than in juvenile ankylosing spondylitis.

Arthritis associated with inflammatory bowel disease is associated most commonly with either ulcerative colitis or Crohn's disease. The overall incidence of inflammatory arthritis of inflammatory bowel disease is between 13 and 17%, and there is no sex predilection. Two distinct patterns exist—the more common peripheral arthritis and the sacroiliitis/spondylitis type.[3] Most cases are pauciarticular and can involve the ankles.

SERONEGATIVE ARTHROPATHIES

Psoriatic Arthritis

The radiologic hallmarks of psoriatic arthritis are equal involvement of the hands and feet, asymmetric involvement without osteoporosis, consistent involvement of DIP joints, IP ankylosis, and joint space widening and distal phalangeal tuft erosion. Psoriasis is sometimes accompanied by charac-

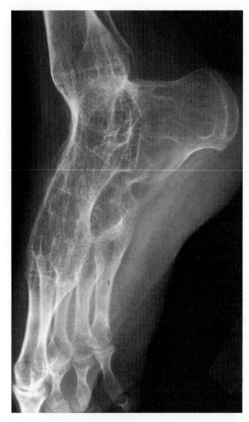

FIG. 5-19. Juvenile rheumatoid arthritis (JRA) of the foot, resulting in complete ankylosis of the ankle, hindfoot, and midfoot. Intraarticular bony ankylosis is a common finding in JRA, as opposed to adult-onset rheumatoid arthritis.

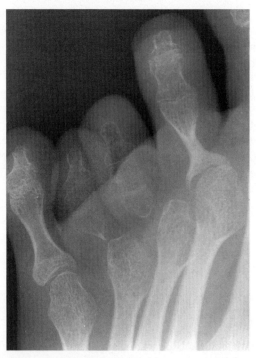

FIG. 5-20. Juvenile rheumatoid arthritis of the toes. Extreme destruction of the proximal phalanges, resulting in toe shortening.

teristic arthritis. Perhaps 3 to 5% of psoriatic patients develop such an arthritis. In most patients, the skin changes precede the articular abnormalities by some months, or more commonly years. Occasionally, however, psoriatic arthritis occurs before the skin disease develops. Psoriatic arthritis is almost always accompanied by nail changes consisting of subungual keratosis, lateral onycholysis, thickening, and irregularity.

Psoriatic arthritis generally affects the hands and feet to the same extent, a finding that is useful in distinguishing this entity from Reiter's syndrome, which has a pronounced tendency to spare the hands.[18] Any of the foot joints may be affected, as can the ankle joint and the sesamoid bones. Psoriatic arthritis can be bilateral, asymmetric, or unilateral, with or without a ray-like pattern. Asymmetric joint involvement is more common in psoriasis than in rheumatoid arthritis. Psoriatic arthritis characteristically strikes the IP joints of the feet, especially the DIP joints, whereas in rheumatoid arthritis, MTP involvement is more common and DIP involvement is rare (Fig. 5-21A). Distal phalangeal tufts and the calcaneus are also common sites affected by psoriatic arthritis.

The toes are commonly affected in psoriatic arthritis (see Fig. 5-21B). Destruction of the first IP joint is greater than any of the other arthritides (see Fig. 5-21C and D). Periarticular soft tissue swelling is often seen, although more diffuse swelling of the entire toe may occur. Narrowed joint spaces are typical, but sometimes the joint space may be widened secondary to replacement of the joint by fibrotic material (Fig. 5-22).[7] Although uncommon, this appearance is characteristic of psoriasis. Cortical erosions are usually located at the margins initially (Fig. 5-23A) but later grow to involve the remainder of the articular cortex.[15] This bone destruction may become profound (see Fig. 5-23B). As seen in Reiter's syndrome and ankylosing spondylitis, bone proliferation is usually present in combination with the destructive changes. Irregular osseous production combined with the erosive changes gives the involved surface a fuzzy, irregular, or spiculated appearance (Fig. 5-24A). Acroosteolysis and reparative periosteal new bone formation may occur and sometimes can result in sclerosis of the involved bones, referred to as "ivory phalanges."[7] Some workers believe that these changes are most characteristic when they occur at the IP joint of the great toe (see Fig. 5-24B).[2] Osteolysis with pencil-and-cup deformity occurs more commonly in psoriatic arthritis than in Reiter's syndrome, and this is characterized by a pointed bone projecting into an expanded base of the articulating bone (Fig. 5-25A). The absence of osteoporosis and the lack of fibular deviation, despite significant arthritic changes, are two additional signs that are suggestive of psoriatic arthritis (see Fig. 5-25). In advanced disease, IP ankylosis is a common finding and is rarely the result of rheumatoid arthritis (see Fig. 5-25C).

Resorption of the distal phalangeal tufts may be an important diagnostic finding (see Fig. 5-25D). These patients almost always have nail changes. Tuft erosion in association

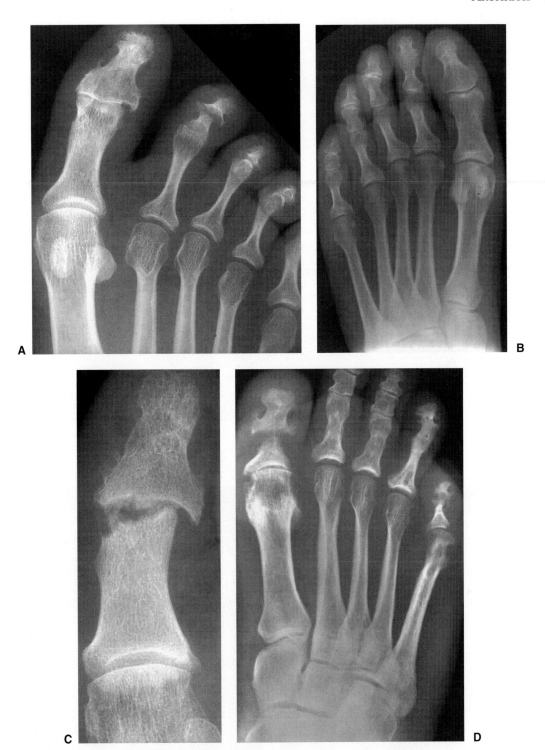

FIG. 5-21. Psoriatic arthritis of the toes. **A:** Joint space narrowing and erosions of multiple DIP joints, characteristic of psoriatic arthritis. **B:** Irregular joint space narrowing of the third and fourth DIP joints and ankylosis of the second DIP joint. **C:** Asymmetric destruction of the first IP joint and bony proliferation of the base of the distal phalanx. The combination of destructive and proliferative changes is classic for the seronegative spondyloarthropathies. (**D**) The ray-like distribution of joint space narrowing, erosions, and ankylosis in the first, fourth, and fifth rays are classic for psoriatic arthritis.

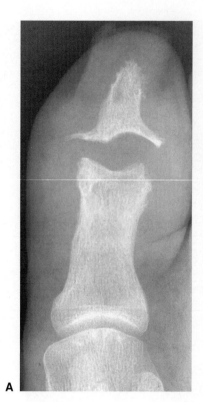

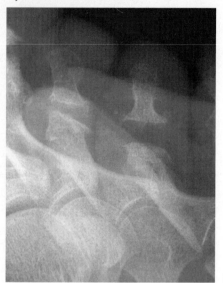

FIG. 5-22. Joint space widening in psoriatic arthritis. **A:** Joint space widening of the first IP joint, associated soft tissue swelling, bony proliferation at the base of the distal phalanx, and tuft resorption. Joint space widening can be secondary to fibrotic material replacing the joint. **B:** Joint space widening in multiple DIP joints.

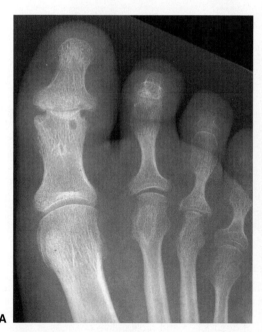

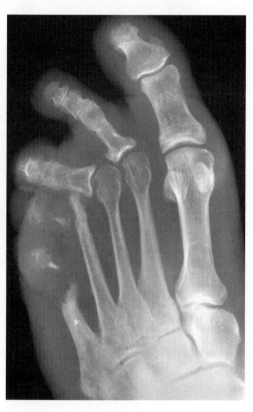

FIG. 5-23. Erosive destruction in psoriatic arthritis. **A:** Erosive destruction of the first IP joint and several MTP joints. Note the ankylosis of the second and third PIP joints. **B:** Marked destruction of the fourth and fifth rays in a patient with advanced disease. The fibular deviation of the second and third toes is uncommon in psoriatic arthritis.

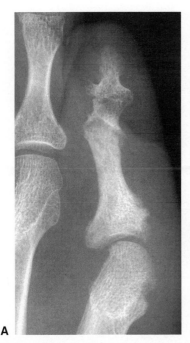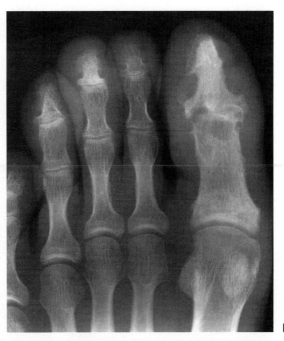

FIG. 5-24. Reparative periosteal new bone formation in psoriatic arthritis. **A:** Destruction of the joints of the fifth toe and proliferative changes of the proximal phalanx give the base a fuzzy appearance. **B:** Osteolysis and reparative new bone formation of the first and third distal phalanges result in ivory phalanges. Note the destructive changes of the first IP joint, which is a common location for affliction by psoriatic arthritis.

with the IP arthritic changes is practically diagnostic of psoriatic arthritis.

As in Reiter's syndrome and ankylosing spondylitis, calcaneal changes may occur. The changes are similar to those seen in Reiter's syndrome (see Fig. 5-26). Soft tissue swelling, osseous erosion, and osseous proliferation constitute the main findings, whereas the unusual sites are the posterior and plantar surfaces of the calcaneus. Coarse, broad-based enthesophytes or fluffy bone proliferation can arise from the plantar aspect of the bone at the insertion of the plantar fascia.[9] Occasionally, the entire inferior calcaneus can be eburnated.[21] The Achilles tendon can become thickened and associated with irregular osteophytes at its attachment.[21]

Reiter's Syndrome

The radiologic hallmarks of Reiter's syndrome are as follows: calcaneal, phalangeal, and sacroiliac joint involvement; oligoarticular with asymmetric involvement; sparing of the upper extremities; and combined destruction and productive changes. Reiter's syndrome is considered a reactive arthritis and usually is seen after an infection of the lower genitourinary tract (*Chlamydia*) or the bowel (*Shigella, Salmonella, Yersinia*).[6] The disease usually begins 2 to 4 weeks after the infection. Most patients with Reiter's syndrome are males between the ages of 20 and 40 years. One-third of patients present with the classic clinical triad of conjunctivitis, urethritis, and arthritis, whereas 40% of patients only

develop the arthritis.[12] In addition, diarrhea and mucocutaneous lesions are seen. There is a prevalence of a positive HLA-B27 in 63 to 75% of patients, a finding suggesting a genetic predisposition.[12]

Although arthritis is often the last of the triad to appear in Reiter's syndrome, the arthritis eventually becomes the most prolonged and disabling clinical manifestation in most patients. There are three patterns of Reiter's disease: (1) disease primarily affecting the DIP and PIP joints; (2) arthritis affecting all the joints of a single or several digits; and (3) arthritis simulating rheumatoid arthritis.[7] Asymmetric or unilateral involvement is characteristic, and typically fewer joints are affected in Reiter's syndrome than with rheumatoid arthritis or psoriatic arthritis. Soft tissue swelling is an important radiographic finding because it occurs early and frequently. Swelling results not only from fluid and synovitis but also from periarticular edema, bursitis, and tendinitis. The swelling may be diffuse and may involve the entire digit, the so-called "cocktail sausage digit," similar to psoriasis. (Fig. 5-27). In contrast, swelling in rheumatoid arthritis tends to be limited to the periarticular region.

In Reiter's syndrome, joint space narrowing generally occurs and tends to be symmetric. Marginal erosions with proliferation can be seen in early stages of disease.[21] Cortical erosions are usually seen first at the joint margin, but they may develop to involve any or all of the articular bone. Unlike patients with rheumatoid arthritis, these patients frequently have osseous proliferation, even as the destructive

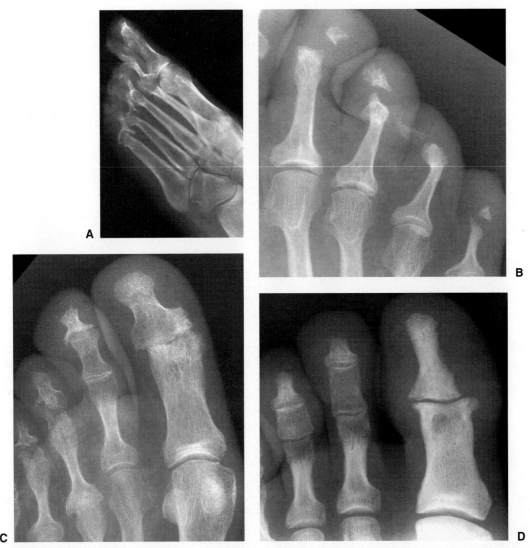

FIG. 5-25. Psoriatic arthritis of the toes. **A:** Osteolysis with pencil-and-cup deformity of the fifth MTP joint, which occurs more commonly in psoriatic arthritis than in Reiter's syndrome. **B:** Despite advanced changes of psoriatic arthritis of the IP joints, no osteoporosis is present. **C:** Mixed destructive and proliferative arthritis of the IP joints and ankylosis of the third and fourth PIP joints. **D:** Acroosteolysis of the first, second, and third digits. Osteosclerosis of the distal phalanges and first proximal phalanx result in ivory phalanges. Also note the medial destruction and lateral proliferative spurs of the first IP joint.

erosions occur (Fig. 5-28). This combination of bone erosion and proliferation is characteristic of Reiter's syndrome, psoriatic arthritis, and ankylosing spondylitis and is useful in distinguishing these rheumatoid variants from rheumatoid arthritis. Periosteal new bone formation may occur in more than half of cases and is especially common about the phalanges and metatarsals adjacent to the involved joints (Fig. 5-29).[12] New bone may occur in the absence of articular abnormalities and is also another feature distinguishing Reiter's syndrome from rheumatoid arthritis. Periostitis and enthesitis can involve the shafts of the phalanges, metatarsals, base of the fifth metatarsal, medial navicular, or any site of ligamentous attachment.[7] Periostitis can be indistinct during early stages of disease, but later it may become better defined and associated with a thickened cortex.[12] Hyperostosis is another form of bone production seen in Reiter's syndrome. Osteoporosis may be present, but the relative absence of osteoporosis despite extensive joint destruction is more common.[12]

The toes are the major sites of foot involvement by Reiter's syndrome (Fig. 5-30A and B). Any or all of the IP and MTP joints may be involved (see Fig. 5-30C to E), but there is a predilection for the joints of the great toe. Acroosteolysis, pencil-and-cup deformity, and subluxation, and deformity of the MTP joints can be observed. Ankylosis of the small joints in the feet occurs in Reiter's syndrome, but far

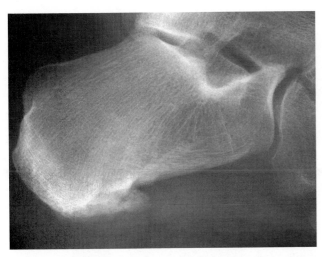

FIG. 5-26. Psoriatic arthritis of the calcaneus. The coarse, broad-based enthesophyte with fluffy bony proliferation of the plantar aspect of the calcaneus is characteristic for both psoriatic arthritis and Reiter's syndrome.

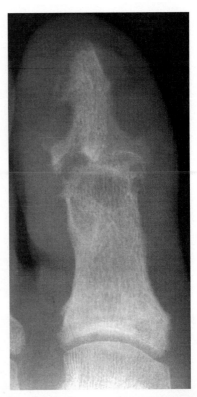

FIG. 5-28. Reiter's syndrome of the great toe. The combination of bone destruction and proliferation of the first IP joint is characteristic of both Reiter's syndrome as well as the remainder of the seronegative spondyloarthropathies.

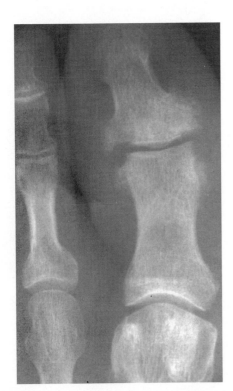

FIG. 5-27. Sausage digit in Reiter's syndrome. Soft tissue swelling in Reiter's syndrome may be diffuse and may involve the entire digit, the so-called "cocktail sausage digit," similar to psoriasis. Also note the erosive and proliferative changes in the IP joint.

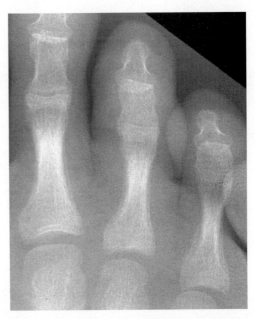

FIG. 5-29. Periosteal new bone in Reiter's syndrome. Linear periosteal new bone along the proximal phalanges. Periosteal new bone may occur in over half of cases in Reiter's syndrome and is especially common about the phalanges and metatarsals adjacent to the involved joints[17].

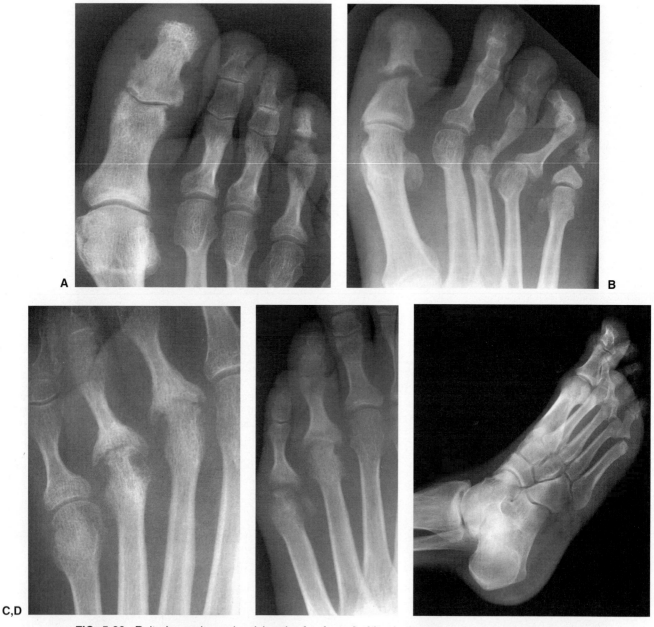

FIG. 5-30. Reiter's syndrome involving the forefoot. **A:** Marginal erosive changes of the first IP and fourth DIP joints and diffuse soft tissue swelling of the first and fourth toes. **B:** Despite advanced changes in the feet, this patient had no involvement of the hands, elbows, shoulders, or hips. **C:** Considerable loss of articular cartilage, marginal erosions, osseous proliferation, and hyperostosis of the MTP joints. Also note the ankylosis of the fourth PIP joint. **D:** Periarticular soft tissue swelling, joint space narrowing, and marginal cortical erosions of the fourth and fifth MTP joints. **E:** Oblique radiograph accentuates the destructive changes of the fourth and fifth MTP joints and the fifth PIP joint.

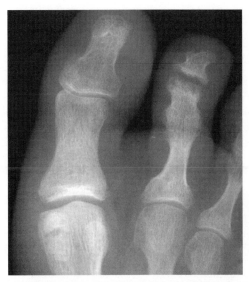

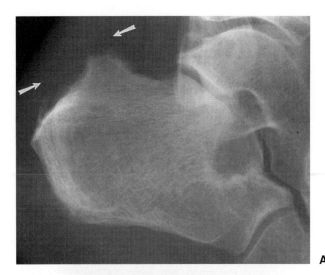

FIG. 5-31. Ankylosis of the second PIP joint in Reiter's syndrome. Ankylosis of the small joints in the feet occur in Reiter's syndrome, but far less commonly than in ankylosing spondylitis or psoriatic arthritis. Also note the widening of the second DIP joint.

less commonly than in ankylosing spondylitis or psoriatic arthritis (Fig. 5-31).[21] Any of the foot joints may be affected by Reiter's syndrome, but the dorsal midfoot and medial midfoot are favored sites. The affected surface most often has an irregular or fluffy appearance secondary to the typical combination of bone erosion and proliferation.

Some of the more characteristic findings occur in the calcaneus (Fig. 5-32A). The changes most often occur near the attachment of the plantar aponeurosis and are less likely at the posterior calcaneus. The radiographic changes at these sites consist of soft tissue swelling, osseous erosion, and osseous proliferation (see Fig. 5-32B). The synovial-lined retrocalcaneal bursa enlarges with fluid and hypertrophied synovium, which raises the density of the fat that is normally seen anterior to the Achilles tendon. The tendon itself may also be thickened. Soft tissue swelling and increased density are also seen adjacent to the plantar surface of the calcaneus, when this area is involved. Poorly defined and sometimes subtle surface resorption or erosion is frequent, and this is sometimes seen in combination with hyperostosis and

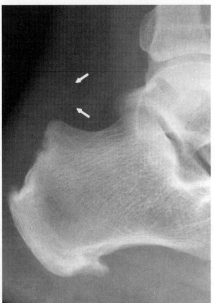

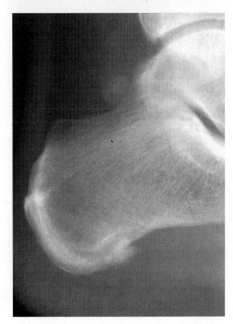

FIG. 5-32. Reiter's syndrome of the calcaneus. **A:** Lateral image demonstrates poorly defined erosive changes of the posterior, superior, and plantar surfaces of the calcaneus. In addition, there is marked thickening of the Achilles tendon (*arrows*), obliteration of the radiolucency of the pre-Achilles fat pad suggestive of retrocalcaneal bursitis, and a small amount of osseous proliferation. **B:** Posterior calcaneal and plantar enthesophytes and erosion of the posterior and superior aspect of the calcaneus are noted. The Achilles tendon is also thickened, and there is evidence of distension of the retrocalcaneal bursa (*arrows*). **C:** Poorly defined spur at the insertion of the plantar aponeurosis.

osseous proliferation (see Fig. 5-32C). Ill-defined erosions, whiskering, and periosteal new bone formation at the insertion of the plantar aponeurosis are the hallmarks of disease for both Reiter's syndrome and psoriatic arthritis.

Involvement of the ankle joint is common and most frequently consists of soft tissue swelling, although any of the changes seen in the foot may also occur in the ankle. Soft tissue swelling and linear or fluffy periostitis of the medial and lateral malleoli can be observed.[21]

Ankylosing Spondylitis

The radiologic hallmarks of ankylosing spondylitis are bilateral symmetric sacroiliitis, oligoarticular and asymmetric involvement, and calcaneal changes. Males between the ages of 15 and 40 years are usually affected.

Ankylosing spondylitis is a chronic inflammatory disorder of unknown origin that occurs between puberty and 35 years of age, with a peak in the middle to late twenties.[12] Ninety

FIG. 5-33. Ankylosing spondylitis of the forefoot. **A:** Marginal erosions of the fifth metatarsal head, similar to changes seen in rheumatoid arthritis. **B:** Destructive changes predominate in the fourth and fifth MTP joints. **C:** Advanced changes in the first IP joint, with fluffy proliferation of new bone superimposed on erosive changes. **D:** Ankylosis of the second DIP joint and minimal destructive and proliferative changes in the second PIP and second and third MTP joints.

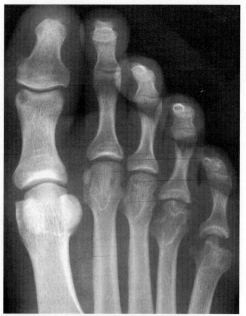

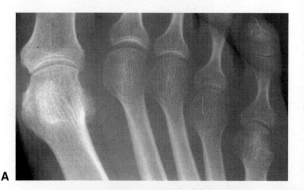

A

B

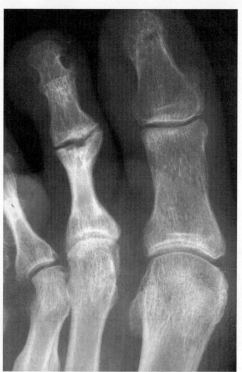

C

D

percent of patients are males, and there is an increased association with HLA-B27. Ankylosing spondylitis, along with Reiter's syndrome and psoriatic arthritis, comprises the three rheumatoid variant disorders. Like them, ankylosing spondylitis is a systemic disorder with widespread manifestations. Unlike them, however, involvement predominates in the axial skeleton, where bilateral symmetric sacroiliitis occurs frequently. Between 5 and 50% of the patients have peripheral manifestations, which are most common in the hips and shoulder. Involvement tends to be oligoarticular and asymmetric. When ankylosing spondylitis involves the foot, it affects the MTP, first TMT, and first IP joints preferentially, with infrequent and mild involvement of the second through fifth IP joints (Fig. 5-33). However, these changes are seldom specific, so evaluation of the sacroiliac joints and correlation with the clinical findings usually leads to the diagnosis.[5] Subluxation of the MTP joints is also observed.

Calcaneal changes are frequent when the foot is involved by ankylosing spondylitis, and these changes are indistinguishable from those seen in Reiter's syndrome and psoriatic arthritis (Fig. 5-34). Retrocalcaneal bursitis can result in osseous erosions in the posterior and superior calcaneus: although these findings may resemble rheumatoid arthritis, there will typically be more prominent reactive bone formation.[21] Well-defined enthesophytes occur at the insertion of the Achilles tendon. At the plantar aspect of the calcaneus, there can be poorly marginated erosions, reactive sclerosis, and poorly defined enthesophytes.[21] Ankle joint changes may also occur.

Hypertrophic synovitis in the foot can lead to adjacent soft tissue masses, which, in turn, can be associated with

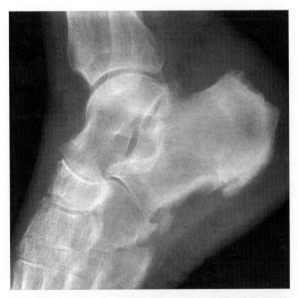

FIG. 5-34. Ankylosing spondylitis of the calcaneus. The proliferative and destructive changes of the posterior and plantar surfaces of the calcaneus are indistinguishable from those changes seen in Reiter's syndrome and psoriatic arthritis.

tarsal tunnel syndrome. In one series, 10% of patients with AS had unilateral tarsal tunnel syndrome, characterized by burning pain, tingling, numbness or sensory loss in the foot, paresthesias on eversion, a positive Tinel's sign at the ankle, weakness of toe flexion, atrophy of the abductor hallucis muscle, and positive electrodiagnostic tests.[13]

Neuropathic Osteoarthropathy

Neuropathic osteoarthropathy is believed to be the result of repetitive trauma resulting from sensory impairment.[14] The proposed sequence of events leading to neuropathic arthropathy begins with a loss of deep sensation and proprioception, leading to relaxation of supporting structures, resulting in recurrent injury, malalignment, erosions of chondral surfaces, subchondral sclerosis, fractures, fragmentation, and joint disorganization.[21] Disorders of the central nervous system (i.e., syphilis, meningomyelocele, trauma, multiple sclerosis), peripheral nervous system (i.e., diabetes mellitus, alcoholism, infection), or congenital insensitivity to pain are the most common causes of neuropathic joints.[21] Although diabetes is the most common cause for this disorder, the actual incidence of neuropathic joints in diabetic patients is low (0.1 to 0.5%). The distribution of neuropathic joints in the lower extremity in diabetic arthropathy is as follows: 11%, ankle (Fig. 5-35); 24%, tarsus (Fig. 5-36); 30%, TMT joints (Fig. 5-37); 30%, MTP (Fig. 5-38); and 4%, IP joints.[10] Injuries involving the TMT joints often result in painless Lisfranc's fracture-dislocations; radiographic findings are marked and evolve rapidly. Osseous changes in the navicular, cuneiform, and head and neck of the talus are less common.[14] Avascular necrosis, infection, crystal-induced arthritis, hemophilia, and rheumatoid arthritis can all radiographically resemble neuropathic osteoarthropathy.

The two forms of neuropathic osteoarthropathy are the acute resorptive or hyperemic phase (Fig. 5-39) and the hypertrophic reparative or sclerotic phase (Fig. 5-40).[25] The hypertrophic, reparative form tends to predominate. The radiographic findings of the hypertrophic form have been likened to osteoarthritis with a vengeance. They include (1) dissolution of the joint, (2) sclerosis with osteophyte formation, (3) continued dislocation and subluxation, (4) extensive fractures with debris, often resulting from minor trauma, and (5) joint distension.[25] MRI demonstrates decreased signal intensity on all sequences, consistent with osteosclerosis, as well as cyst-like lesions; these findings serve to differentiate this entity from osteomyelitis. Associated subcutaneous edema and joint effusions in either the ankle or subtalar joints can also be detected with MRI.[14]

The acute, resorptive form predominantly involves the forefoot, and, less so, the midfoot. There can be bizarre abnormalities, including osteolysis of the distal metatarsal and proximal phalanges with tapering of the osseous contours and collapse of the metatarsal heads that resembles Frei-

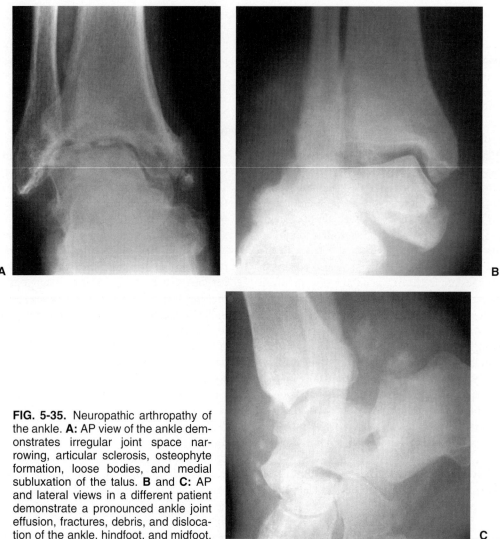

FIG. 5-35. Neuropathic arthropathy of the ankle. **A:** AP view of the ankle demonstrates irregular joint space narrowing, articular sclerosis, osteophyte formation, loose bodies, and medial subluxation of the talus. **B** and **C:** AP and lateral views in a different patient demonstrate a pronounced ankle joint effusion, fractures, debris, and dislocation of the ankle, hindfoot, and midfoot.

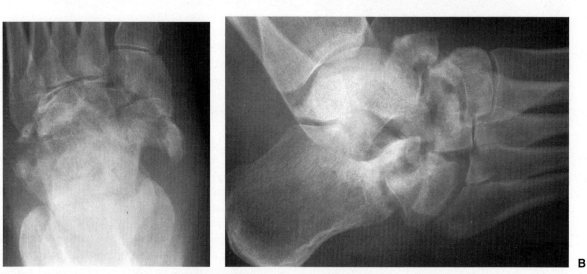

FIG. 5-36. Neuropathic arthropathy of the tarsus. AP (**A**) and lateral (**B**) radiographs demonstrate extensive neuropathic changes, primarily involving the intertarsal joints.

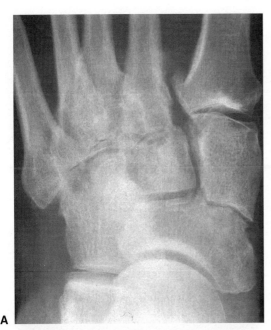

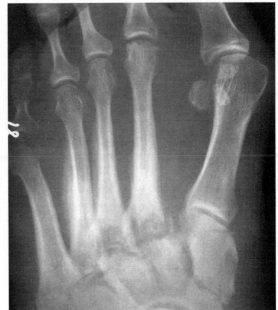

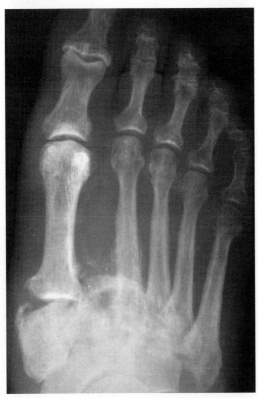

FIG. 5-37. Neuropathic arthropathy of the TMT joints. **A:** Fracture-dislocation of Lisfranc's joint, classic for neuropathic arthropathy. Also observe the irregular joint space narrowing and osteophytes involving the naviculomedial cuneiform joint. **B:** Fracture-dislocation of Lisfranc's joint, sclerosis and new bone formation of the metatarsals, and fracture deformity of the second metatarsal head. Findings can all be seen in neuropathic arthropathy. Incidentally noted is hallux valgus deformity. **C:** Diabetic neuropathic arthropathy of the foot is associated with extensive vascular calcifications.

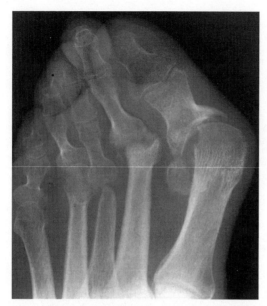

FIG. 5-38. Neuropathic arthropathy of the MTP joints. Dissolution of the joints, osteophyte formation, subluxation and dislocations, and resorptive changes most marked in the third metatarsal.

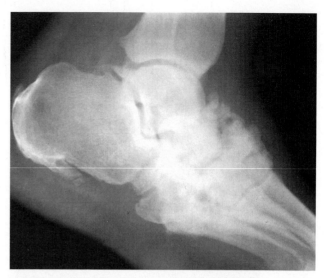

FIG. 5-40. Hypertrophic reparative or sclerotic phase of neuropathic arthropathy. Lateral view of the foot demonstrates dissolution of the joints, sclerosis with osteophyte formation, dislocations and subluxations, fractures with debris, and joint distension.

berg's infraction (Fig. 5-41A).[21] If the foot is imaged in the acute phase when extensive bone resorption can be present, it may be difficult to exclude infection.[7] Radiographic findings that would favor a neuropathic joint over osteomyelitis include (1) location in the midfoot, (2) polyarticular impairment, (3) absence of localized cortical lesions, and (4) some distance between a known soft tissue infection and bone changes; conversely, (1) abnormalities involving the toes or metatarsal heads and (2) cortical lesions that are better circumscribed and located close to a known soft tissue infection favor osteomyelitis over a neuropathic joint.[14] Patients with acutely evolving neuropathic osteoarthropathy or recent fractures (see Fig. 5-41B) related to the disease can have MRI signal-intensity changes within the bone marrow and contiguous soft tissues similar to those seen in osteomyelitis.[14] Abnormal areas have low signal intensity on T1-weighted sequences and high signal intensity on T2-

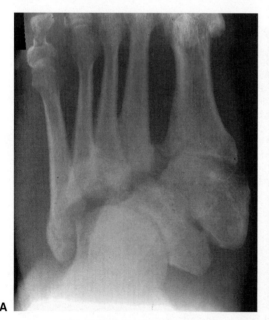

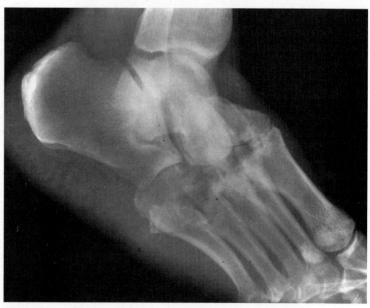

A   **B**

FIG. 5-39. Acute resorptive or hyperemic phase of neuropathic arthropathy. AP (**A**) and oblique (**B**) images of the midfoot demonstrate extensive bone resorption at Lisfranc's joint that could be confused with infection.

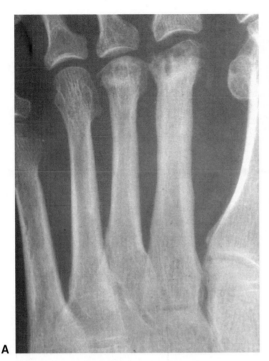 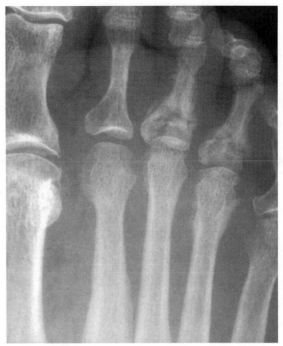

FIG. 5-41. Fractures associated with neuropathic arthropathy. **A:** Fracture deformities of the third and fourth metatarsal heads, resembling Freiberg's infraction. There is also sclerosis and cortical thickening of the metatarsals. **B:** Fractures of the third and fourth proximal phalanges and resorptive changes in the metatarsal heads.

weighted sequences, leading to potential diagnostic pitfalls. To avoid misdiagnosing acutely evolving neuropathic osteoarthropathy as osteomyelitis, one must carefully consider the patient's clinical history, the correlating radiograph, and possibly the bone scan before making a final interpretation of the MRI.[14] Often, biopsy is required to make the definitive diagnosis.

Initial management of acute neuropathic osteoarthropathy includes open reduction and arthrodesis, total-contact cast or brace, and amputation. Patients with chronic neuropathic joints are initially treated in a total-contact cast or molded orthotic insert, with or without bracing.[16]

METABOLIC ARTHRITIDES

Gouty Arthritis

Gout is a common, episodic, and self-limited inflammatory arthropathy[17] caused by biochemical derangement leading to the development of hyperuricemia. Only a few with elevated urate, however, ever develop an acute attack of gouty arthritis.[29] The radiologic hallmarks of gouty arthritis are asymmetric soft tissue swelling, tophi, and cortical erosions with overhanging margins. The distribution of gout tends to be asymmetric, and it usually involves fewer joints than in rheumatoid arthritis. There is a predilection for the lower extremities, especially the feet, which are involved in approximately 85% of the cases.

Tophaceous gout is the chronic phase of the disease char-

acterized by the deposition of monosodium urate crystals in the synovial fluid and the articular and periarticular structures, resulting in irritation and inflammation of the involved structures. Monosodium urate crystals are strongly birefringent needle-shaped crystals. Tophi are generally located close to joints in the subarticular bones, bursae, tendon sheaths, and articular cartilage[27], but they most commonly involve the first MTP joint (Fig. 5-42). Tophi may eventually erode the underlying bone, producing eccentric punched-out lytic lesions with overhanging edges of bone and well-defined, sharply marginated sclerotic borders (Fig. 5-43A to C).[27] These erosions may be intraarticular or extraarticular and can result in significant bony destruction, even the disappearance of phalanges (see Fig. 5-43D), or pathologic fractures. Intraosseous urate deposits are rare, but when they do occur, they are located in the metaphyseal ends of tubular bones within the periosteal covering or in the subchondral spongy bone.[29] The bones then slowly expand and undergo cystic change. Rarely, tophi calcify (see Fig. 5-43E), thus distinguishing them from rheumatoid nodules. Intraosseous calcifications, if present, are punctate and circular.

Involved digits exhibit eccentric and asymmetric joint swelling. Joint space loss is often absent, but there can be asymmetric joint space loss late in the disease process.[21] Bone mineralization is generally normal, but occasionally be mild osteopenia is present. Although bony proliferation resulting in overhanging edges is typical of gout, osteophytes are not characteristic of gout. Chronic gout often results in

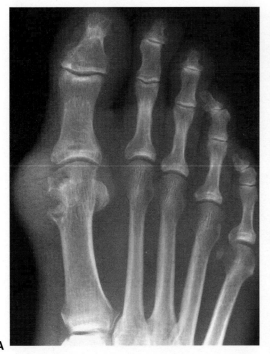

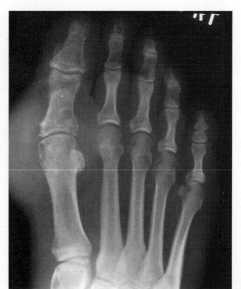

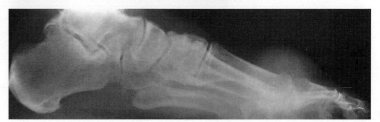

FIG. 5-42. Gouty arthritis of the first MTP joint. **A:** Extensive erosive changes of the medial aspect of the first MTP joint, primarily involving the head of the metatarsal. Note the extensive tophaceous soft tissue mass involving the medial, more than the lateral, aspect of the joint. **B** and **C:** Larger tophus in a different patient, with relatively less erosive changes of the first MTP joint.

FIG. 5-43. Gouty tophi. **A** to **C:** Tophi are associated with varying degrees of characteristic bone erosion in the first IP joints. The tophi can eventually erode the underlying bone, producing punched-out lytic lesion with overhanging edges of bone and well-defined, sharply marginated sclerotic borders[25]. *(continued)*

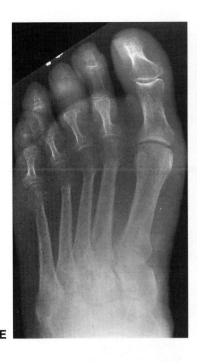
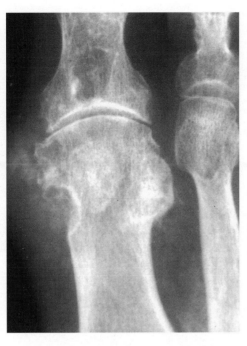

E

FIG. 5-43. *Continued.* **D:** Erosions due to tophi can result in significant bony destruction, even the disappearance of phalanges, as in this case involving the third toe. **E:** Rarely, tophi calcify, distinguishing it from a rheumatoid nodule.

an enlarged, irregular first metatarsal head. Malalignment and subluxations are rare in gout, but hallux valgus deformity is observed frequently. Gout can involve both the first IP joint and the first MTP joint in association with first MTP joint changes. IP erosions can be medial or lateral and marginal or central (Fig. 5-44). Involvement of the remainder of the foot is less common (Fig. 5-45).

The ankle joint is rarely afflicted with gout, but posterior calcaneal erosions are common (Fig. 5-46). Retrocalcaneal bursitis is associated with soft tissue swelling, Achilles tendon thickening, and erosions of the posterior tendon secondary to tophi. In addition, the Achilles tendon can undergo fusiform or nodular enlargement[20] and may eventually rupture. TMT joint erosions may be marked. The monosodium urate crystals can inflict an intense inflammatory reaction, resulting in enhancement of tendon sheaths, ligaments, mus-

FIG. 5-44. Gouty arthritis of the fifth DIP joint. Large cysts and erosions occur on either side of the joint. A large tophus is present medially.

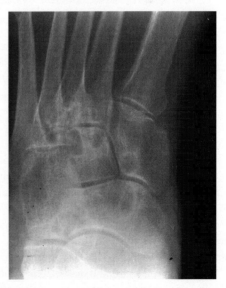

FIG. 5-45. Gouty arthritis of the midfoot. Prominent subchondral cysts throughout the midfoot, which is an uncommon site for gout.

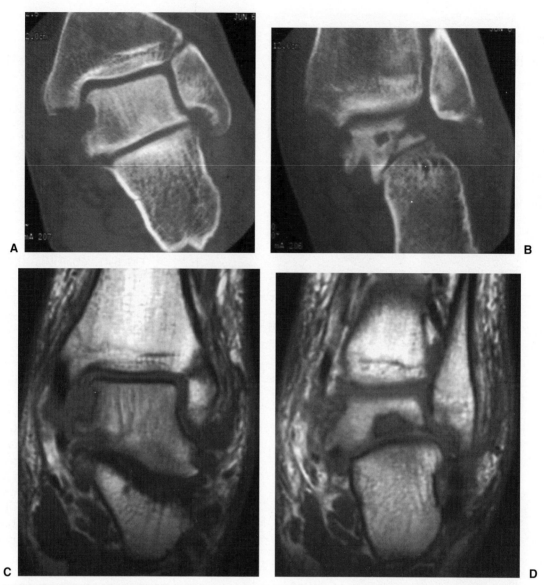

FIG. 5-46. Gouty arthritis of the ankle. Coronal CT images displayed in bone windows through the (**A**) medial and (**B**) posterior ankle joint display the extensive erosions involving the medial and lateral malleoli and the medial and posterior talus. **C** and **D**: Coronal T1-weighted images through the corresponding regions demonstrate low signal intensity soft tissue foci associated with the erosive changes. These abnormalities proved to be gouty tophi at arthroscopy. *(continued)*

cles, and bone marrow; these changes can be easily appreciated on MRI.

MRI reflects the changes caused by the proliferative synovitis. Tophi are almost universally isointense to muscle on T1-weighted imaging, but they can have variable T2-weighted characteristics depending on the degree of calcification (Fig. 5-47).[29] The T2-weighted signal is most commonly heterogeneously low to intermediate, but it can range from homogeneously increased to near-homogeneously decreased.[29] Although it is unusual to have tophi without prior episodes of gouty arthritis, soft tissue inflammation or masses without articular disease can be a diagnostic dilemma; tophi could be mistaken for neoplasm. Tophaceous gout should be considered when there is a heterogeneous low-to-intermediate signal mass associated with adjacent osseous erosive changes in the right clinical setting.

Calcium Pyrophosphate Dihydrate Deposition or Pseudogout

The radiologic hallmarks of pseudogout are as follows: joint pain; calcification of fibrocartilage and hyaline cartilage, articular and periarticular structures, ligaments, and tendons; and atypical degenerative arthritis with atypical joints involved in atypical areas, prominent subchondral cysts, and destruction sometimes resembling neuropathic arthropathy. It infrequently affects the foot and ankle.

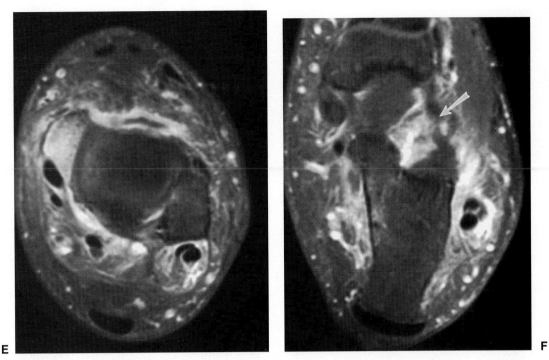

FIG. 5-46. *Continued.* Axial T1-weighted, fat-suppressed, gadolinium-enhanced images at the levels of the (**E**) ankle joint and (**F**) sinus tarsi demonstrate marked enhancement of the tophi throughout the ankle, with associated synovial enhancement of the extensor and peroneal tendon sheaths. Also notice the marked enhancement within the sinus tarsi (*arrows*).

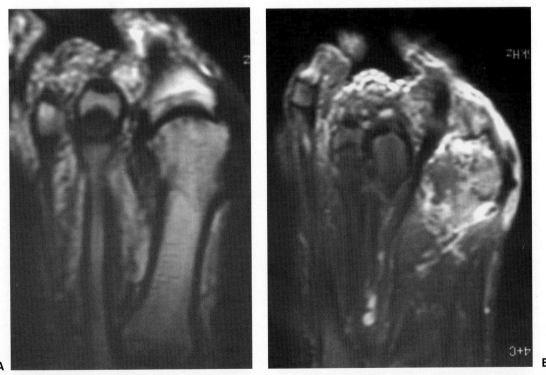

FIG. 5-47. Gouty tophi on MRI. T1-weighted (**A**) and T1-weighted fat-suppressed (**B**), gadolinium-enhanced images through the first MTP joint demonstrate marginal erosive changes and enhancement of the tophus and adjacent synovium. T2-weighted (not shown) characteristics are variable, depending on the degree of calcification; however, the signal is most commonly heterogeneously low to intermediate.

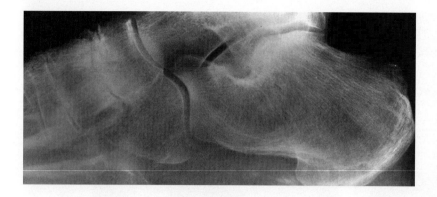

FIG. 5-48. Calcium pyrophosphate dihydrate deposition (CPPD). Lateral image of the foot demonstrates calcification of the plantar aponeurosis and arthropathy involving the naviculocuneiform joint.

Pseudogout is a disorder that results from the excessive buildup or impaired degradation of pyrophosphate, leading to crystal deposition, synovitis, and arthritis. It usually manifests in the sixth and seventh decades by chondrocalcinosis and associated secondary osteoarthritis.[22] The frequency of calcium pyrophosphate dihydrate deposition is 1 in 1,000 and increases with age.[22] This disorder can occur sporadically or in association with such metabolic disorders as hemochromatosis, phosphate and magnesium imbalances, hyperparathyroidism, and hypothyroidism.[22] Patients can present with (1) acute episodes of arthritis in large and medium sized joints, (2) chronically with degenerative changes and mild inflammatory episodes, (3) symmetric polyarthritis mimicking rheumatoid arthritis, or (4) destructive arthropathy.[17] The weakly birefringent, variably shaped crystals can be recovered from synovial fluid, even in uninflamed joints, and intracellularly. Calcification (Fig. 5-48) of cartilage, ligaments, and tendons is also common, particularly in the Achilles tendon. Pseuodogout can present with sclerosis, osteophytosis, cartilage loss, and subchondral cysts, similar to osteoarthritis. However, it differs from osteoarthritis in that it involves unusual joints, involves unusual sites within the affected joint, and exhibits prominent subchondral cysts, bone destruction, and variable osteophyte formation.[21] The arthropathy most commonly affects the tarsal and MTP joints, and the MTP joints may demonstrate capsular calcification.

Hemochromatosis

The radiologic hallmarks of hemochromatosis are osteoporosis, chondrocalcinosis, and atypical degenerative-type arthritis with more symmetric joint-space narrowing and predilection for the metacarpophalangeal and wrist joints. Foot and ankle involvement occurs occasionally and does not differ in appearance from involvement elsewhere in the body (Fig. 5-49).

Hemochromatosis is a chronic disease in which iron is excessively deposited in various tissues, resulting in parenchymal fibrosis, damage, and dysfunction. Hemochromatosis may arise as a primary idiopathic disorder, or it may occur secondarily to cirrhosis, multiple transfusions, or excessive iron ingestion. This disorder is more common in men and arises after the age of 40 years.

Approximately half of the patients with idiopathic hemochromatosis have arthritis similar to degenerative arthritis or calcium pyrophosphate dihydrate deposition disease.[11] The arthritis consists of osteoporosis, subchondral cysts, bony eburnation, sclerosis, and loss of joint space.[21] Cystic lesions are subchondral and can become quite large. Sclerosis is due to subchondral trabecular thickening beneath eroded cartilage surfaces. The joint space narrowing is typically uniform. Chondrocalcinosis is often present and is prominent.

COLLAGEN VASCULAR DISEASE

Systemic Lupus Erythematosus

Systemic lupus erythematosus is a deforming, nonerosive (Jaccoud-like) arthropathy that can involve the foot and ankle. The articular deformities of lupus arthropathy are due

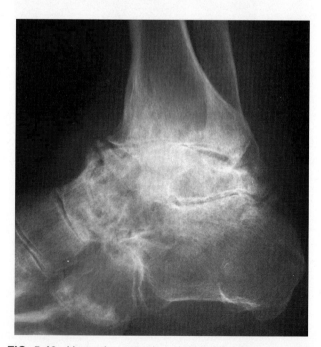

FIG. 5-49. Hemochromatosis arthritis of the foot and ankle. There is fairly uniform loss of articular cartilage throughout the foot and ankle, resulting in sclerosis and hypertrophic changes.

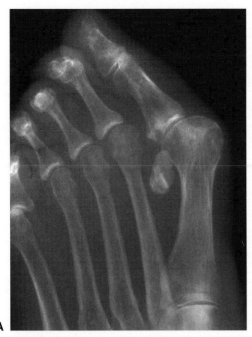
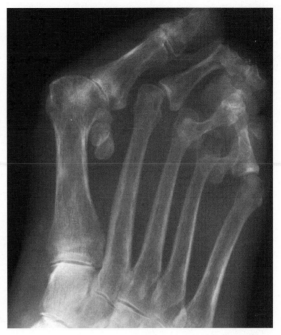

A   B

FIG. 5-50. Systemic lupus erythematosus (SLE) of the foot. AP views of the (**A**) right and (**B**) left feet demonstrate bilateral hallux valgus deformities, fibular deviation and subluxations of the left second through fifth MTP joints, and osteoporosis.

to capsular and ligamentous laxity, contracture, and muscle imbalance as a result of intraarticular and periarticular inflammation and eventual fibrosis.[21] The arthropathy often is evident early in the disease, although it is more common and severe in patients with chronic disease.[21] Typical findings include soft tissue swelling, regional osteoporosis, hallux valgus deformity (Fig. 5-50), subluxation of the MTP joints (see Fig. 5-50B), and widening of the forefoot.[21] Joint space narrowing, rare hook erosions of the metatarsal heads, subchondral cysts of the metatarsal heads, and osteonecrosis of the small bones of the foot can also be observed. Systemically or locally injected steroids can lead to tendon weakening and rupture, most commonly involving the Achilles tendon. Soft tissue calcifications can be diffuse, linear, streaky, or nodular in the subcutaneous and deeper soft tissues, plaque-like periarticular, or arterial. Patients with systemic lupus erythematosus are more prone to osteomyelitis and septic arthritis of the ankle resulting from steroid use.[1]

REFERENCES

1. Ansell BM. Juvenile rheumatoid arthritis, juvenile chronic arthritis, and juvenile spondyloarthropathies. Curr. Opin. Rheumatol. 1992; 4: 706–712.
2. Avila R, Pugh DG, Slocumb CH, Winkelmann RK. Psoriatic arthritis. A roentgenologic study. Radiology 1960; 75:691–701.
3. Azouz EM, Duffy CM. Juvenile spondyloarthropathies. Clinical manifestations and medical imaging. Skeletal Radiol. 1995; 24:399–408.
4. Bouysset M, Tavernier T, Tebib J, Noel E, Tillmann K, Bonnin M, Eulry F, Bouvier M. CT and MRI evaluation of tenosynovitis of the rheumatoid hindfoot. Clin. Rheumatol. 1995; 14:303–307.
5. Cofield RH, Morrison MJ, Beabout JW. Diabetic neuropathy in the foot. Patient characteristics and patterns of radiographic change. Foot Ankle 1983; 4:15–22.
6. El-Khoury GY, Kathol MH, Brandser EA. Seronegative spondyloarthropathies. Radiol. Clin. North Am. 1996; 34:343–357.
7. Flemming D. Approach to the foot. pp 69–104. In Brower A, ed. Arthritis in Black and White. 2nd Ed. Philadelphia, W.B. Saunders, 1997; pp. 69–104.
8. Greenfield GB. Radiology of Bone Dysplasias. 4th ed. Philadelphia, J.B. Lippincott, 1986.
9. Greenspan A. Orthopaedic Radiology. A Practical Approach. 2nd Ed. Philadelphia, Lippincott–Raven. 1997.
10. Holmes GB, Hill N. Fractures and dislocations of the foot and ankle in diabetics associated with Charcot joint changes. Foot Ankle Int. 1994; 15:182–185.
11. Jensen PS. Hemochromatosis. A disease often silent but not invisible. AJR Am. J. Roentgenol. 1976; 126:343–351.
12. Kettering JM, Towers JD, Rubin DA. The seronegative spondyloarthropathies. Semin. Roentgenol. 1996; 3:220–228
13. Kucukdeveci AA, Kutlay S, Seckin B, Aarasil T. Tarsal tunnel syndrome in ankylosing spondylitis. Br. J. Rheumatol. 1995; 34(5):488–9.
14. Marcus CD, Ladam-Marcus VJ, Leone J, Malgrange D, Bonnet-Gausserand FM, Menanteau BP. MR imaging of osteomyelitis and neuropathic osteoarthropathy in the feet of diabetics. Radiographics 1996; 16:1337–1348.
15. Martel W, Stuck KJ, Dworin AM, Hylland RG. Erosive osteoarthritis and psoriatic arthritis. A radiologic comparison in the hand, wrist, and foot. AJR Am. J. Roentgenol. 1980; 134:125–135.
16. Myerson MS, Henderson MR, Saxby T, Short KW. Management of midfoot diabetic neuroarthropathy. Foot Ankle Int. 1994; 15:233–241.
17. Pascual E. The diagnosis of gout and CPPD crystal arthropathy. Br. J. Rheumatol. 1996; 35(4):306–308.
18. Peterson CC, Silbiger ML. Reiter's syndrome and psoriatic arthritis. Their roentgen spectra and some interesting similarities. AJR Am. J. Roentgenol. 1967; 101:860–971.
19. Prieur AM. Chronic arthritis in children. Curr. Opin. Rheumatol. 1994; 6:513–517.
20. Reber P, Crevoisier Z, Noesberger B. Unusual localization of tophaceous gout. A report of four cases and review of the literature. Arch. Orthop. Trauma Surg. 1996; 115:297–299.
21. Resnick D. Diagnosis of Bone and Joint Disorders. 3rd Ed. Philadelphia, J.B. Lippincott, 1995.
22. Rivera-Sanfeliz G, Resnick D, Haghighi P, Wong W, Lanier T. Tophaceous pseudogout. Skeletal Radiol. 1996; 25:699–701.
23. Roberton DM, Cabral DA, Malleson PN, Petly RE. Juvenile psoriatic

arthritis. Follow-up and evaluation of diagnostic criteria. J. Rheumatol. 1996; 23:166–170.

24. Sanders TG, Linares R, Su A. Rheumatoid nodules of the foot. MRI appearances mimicking an indeterminate soft tissue mass. Skeletal Radiol. 1998; 27:457–460.

25. Sequeira W. The neuropathic joint. Clin. Exp. Rheumatol. 1994; 12: 325–337.

26. Sugimoto H, Takeda A, Masuyama J, Furuse M. Early-stage rheuma-toid arthritis. Diagnostic accuracy of MR imaging. Radiology 1996; 198:185–192.

27. Surprenant MS, Levy AI, Hanft JR. Intraosseous gout of the foot. An unusual case report. J. Foot Ankle Surg. 1996; 35:237–243.

28. Tucker LB. Juvenile rheumatoid arthritis. Curr. Opin. Rheumatol. 1993; 5:619–628.

29. Yu JS, Chung C, Recht M, Dailiana T, Jurdi R. MR imaging of topha-ceous gout. AJR Am. J. Roentgenol. 1997; 168:523–527.

Radiology of the Foot and Ankle, Second Edition,
edited by Thomas H. Berquist.
© 2000 by Mayo Foundation.
Published by Lippincott Williams & Wilkins, Philadelphia.

CHAPTER 6

Bone and Soft Tissue Tumors and Tumor-like Conditions

Thomas H. Berquist and Richard A. McLeod

The World Health Organization has classified bone and soft tissue tumors.[35] The current list consists of 82 soft tissue lesions and 50 bone tumors or tumor-like conditions.[24,57]

Skeletal neoplasms of the foot and ankle do not constitute a major part of orthopedic oncology.[16] They comprise only about 1 to 2% of primary skeletal neoplasms.[16,35] The foot and ankle are exceedingly rare sites for skeletal metastasis (0.007 to 0.3%).[4,16,41,81] The prevalence of foot and ankle lesions is somewhat greater if one also considers lesions that may simulate skeletal neoplasms, such as fibrous dysplasia, Paget's disease, cysts, osteomyelitis, aneurysmal bone cyst, giant cell reaction, stress fractures, intraosseous ganglia, and bizarre periosteal osteochondromatosis proliferation (Fig. 6-1).[62]

Of the 8,542 primary bone tumors studied by Dahlin and Unni,[16] only 286 (3.4%) occurred in the foot and ankle. Malignant lesions slightly outnumbered the benign lesions by 157 to 129. Both malignant and benign bone tumors were more frequent in the distal tibia and fibula than in the bones of the foot. If one considers only the foot, benign lesions outnumber malignant lesions by 4 to 1. Which lesions are most common varies by series, and the data are more confusing if one considers the foot alone or the foot and ankle together. In some series, giant cell tumors are most common, and in others, osteoid osteomas lead the list. Chondrosarcoma and Ewing's sarcomas appear to be the most common malignant bone tumors (Table 6-1).[16,35]

Soft tissue lesions are more common than skeletal tumors in the foot and ankle. Benign soft tissue lesions are much more common than malignant lesions.[24,83] Table 6-2 summarizes common soft tissue lesions in the foot and ankle.[24,83]

T. H. Berquist: Mayo Medical School, Mayo Clinic Jacksonville, Jacksonville, Florida 32224; Mayo Foundation, Mayo Clinic, Rochester, Minnesota 55905.

R. A. McLeod: Mayo Medical School (Emeritus), Rochester, Minnesota 55905.

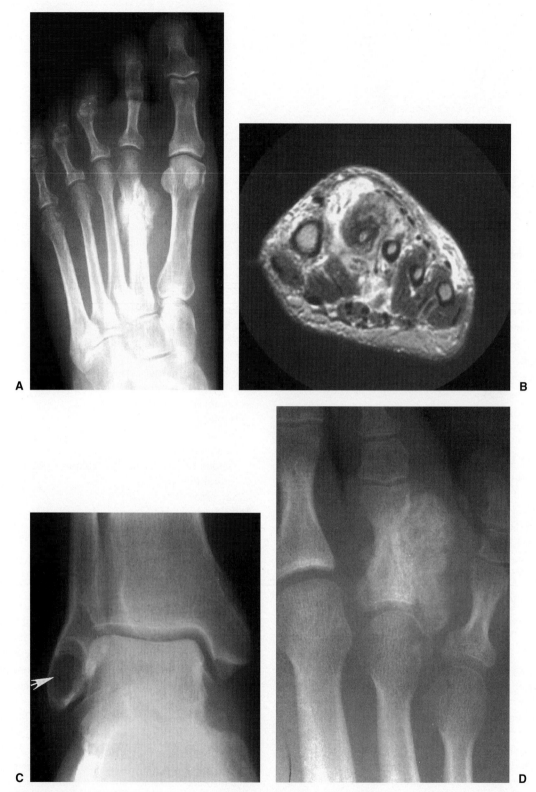

FIG. 6-1. A and **B:** Lesions that may be confused with tumors. A healing fracture of the second metatarsal (**A**), which can be confused with osteogenic sarcoma. MRI (**B**) demonstrates a large ossifying hematoma surrounding the fracture site, which could be confused with soft tissue extension of bone (**C**). Intraosseous ganglion of the lateral malleolus (*arrow*). Sharp margin with a thin sclerotic rim. The lesion abuts the articular cortex (**D**). Periosteal osteochondromatous proliferation. This benign reactive lesion may mimic osteochondroma or osteogenicsarcoma. Although attached to bone, the bone is normal, and there is no continuity of cortical and cancellous bone, nor is there the flaring usually seen with osteochondroma.

TABLE 6-1. *Bone lesions (tumors and tumor-like) of the foot and ankle[a,b]*

Malignant
  Osteosarcoma
  Chondrosarcoma
  Ewing's Sarcoma
  Hemangioendothelial sarcoma
  Fibrosarcoma
  Lymphoma
  Adamantinoma
  Plasmacytoma
  Multiple myeloma
  Metastases
Benign
  Osteochondroma
  Nonossifying fibroma
  Giant cell tumor
  Osteoid osteoma
  Exostosis
  Aneurysmal bone cyst
  Simple bone cyst
  Enchondroma
  Chondromyxoid fibroma
  Chondroblastoma
  Fibrousdysplasia
  Osteoblastoma
  Fibrous histiocytoma

[a] Data from references 16 and 35.
[b] In order of decreasing frequency, order may vary with specific series.

TABLE 6-2. *Soft tissue lesions of the foot and ankle[a,b]*

Ganglion cysts
Fibrohistiocytic tumors
Glomus tumor
Synovial sarcoma
Clear cell sarcoma
Lipoma
Liposarcoma
Angioscarcoma
Rhabdomyosarcoma
Hemangiopericytoma
Fibromatosis
Giant cell tumor tendon sheath

[a] Data from references 6, 24, 35, and 83.
[b] In order of decreasing frequency.

TABLE 6-4. *Enneking staging of benign lesions[a]*

Stage	Lesion characteristics
1	Static or healing spontaneously
2	More aggressive, evidence of slow growth, less mature histologically
3	Aggressive, may invade adjacent structures, histologically immature

[a] Data from references 23 and 83.

These lesions, specifically bone lesions, pose a challenging problem for the diagnostician. Because such lesions are rare, the index of suspicion usually is low. The clinical diagnosis is further complicated because, at presentation, most patients have vague symptoms, such as pain or a pressure sensation, and the physical examination usually reveals either a mass or no abnormality.

The primary roles of imaging are detection and classification or staging.[6,10] Proper staging of bone and soft tissue lesions is essential for treatment planning. This requires a thorough knowledge of the soft tissue compartments of the foot and ankle. Staging of bone and soft tissue lesions is based on tumor extent (intracompartmental or extracompartmental), histologic grade, and whether metastasis are present (Table 6-3).[24,83] Benign soft tissue lesions are graded based on their aggressiveness and histologic appearance (Table 6-4).[83] Staging systems, although modified by some authors, are based on Enneking's system.[23]

Conventional radiographs constitute the initial study of choice. Most bone lesions are detected on roentgenograms, which also provide information that allows estimation of the aggressiveness of a tumor and its probable histologic diagnosis. When malignancy is suspected, or resection is required, additional studies are usually required.[10,11,13,33] The accurate determination of tumor location and extent, as well as its effect on adjacent structures, is required before treatment can begin. For this, computed tomography (CT) and magnetic resonance imaging (MRI) have generally been most valuable and are used routinely.[15,51] Each technique is useful for the detection or the exclusion of recurrences and for follow-up after chemotherapy or radiation therapy.[2,34,44,53,89] In most cases, MRI is preferred over CT.[2,6,8] Specific lesions are reviewed separately, with emphasis on significant clinical and image features.

TABLE 6-3. *Enneking staging system[a]*

Stage	Grade	Site	MRI/CT features
IA	Low	Intracompartmental	Tumor confined to bone or soft tissue compartment
IB	Low	Extracompartmental	Lesion extends beyond compartment
IIA	High	Intracompartmental	Same as IA, may be more inhomogeneous
IIB	High or low	Intracompartmental	Same as IIA, poorly defined
IIIA	High or low	Intracompartmental	Same as IA or IIA with metastasis
IIIB	High or low	Extracompartmental	Same as IB or IIB with metastasis

[a] From Enneking, ref. 23, with permission.

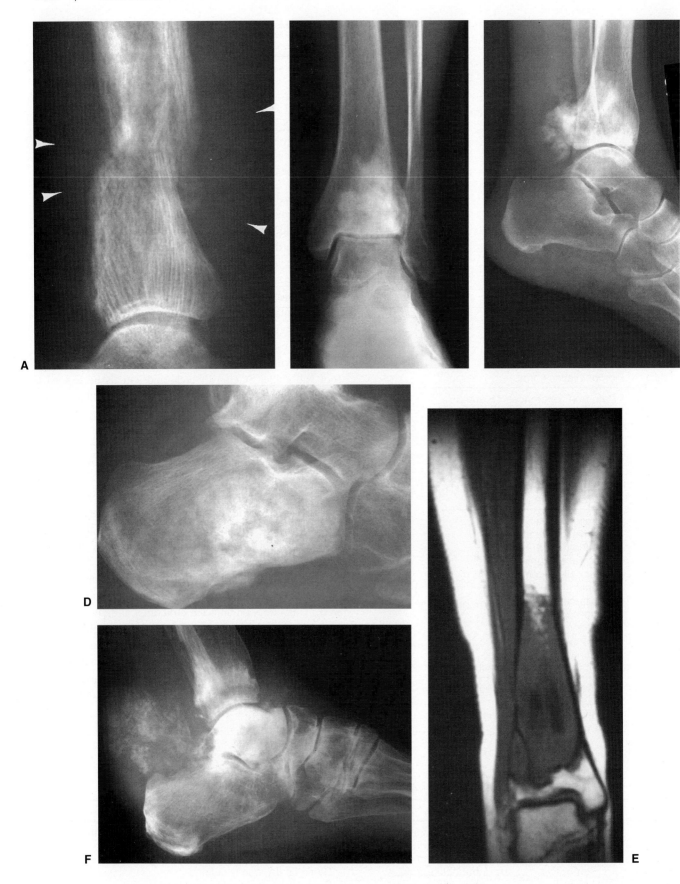

A

B,C

D

E

F

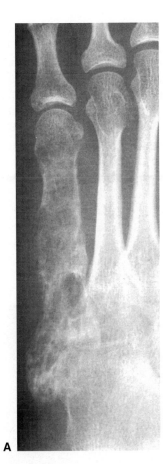

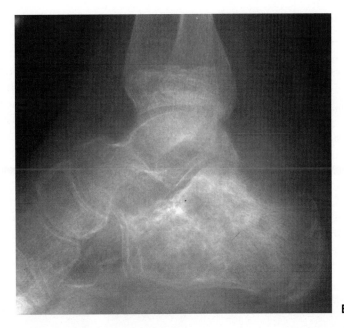

FIG. 6-3. A: Ewing's sarcoma of the fifth metatarsal. One sees a long extensive lesion with poor margination and a mixture of reactive sclerosis and lytic destruction. **B:** Ewing's sarcoma of the calcaneus. The irregular admixture of lucency and sclerosis and the soft tissue mass are usual.

MALIGNANT BONE TUMORS

Osteosarcoma

Osteogenic sarcoma (Fig. 6-2) has a highly variable appearance but consists of a sarcomatous stroma with cells that produce osteoid.[7,17] It is slightly more common in males than in females, and its peak incidence is seen in the second decade of life. Most osteogenic sarcomas occur around the knee. Osteosarcoma in the foot is rare in some series (1% of 2,525 cases).[7,35] Of the osteogenic sarcomas studied by Dahlin and Unni,[16] only 2.8% arose in the foot and ankle. However, the tumor is still the most common malignancy of this region, especially in childhood.[68] Of the 38 osteogenic sarcomas in the series of Dahlin and Unni, 27 occurred in the distal tibia and fibula, 10 in the tarsal bone, and 1 in a metatarsal joint. The appearance of osteogenic sarcoma is variable (see Fig. 6-2).[7,40] It may be osteolytic or osteosclerotic, but it is most often a combination of the two. Cortical and medullary destruction and poor margination are usually present, indicative of the malignant nature. Periosteal new bone formation is usually found and often takes the form of Codman's triangles or "sunburst" spiculation. Matrix ossification and soft tissue extension are frequent and are useful diagnostic clues (see Fig. 6-2F). Matrix ossification may be recognized as such because of its fluffy, cloud-like, amorphous appearance. CT or MRI is helpful for pretreatment staging when limb-salvage surgery is considered (see Fig. 6-2F). Surgery is the primary treatment modality, although preoperative chemotherapy is given.[6,16,75] Osteogenic sarcoma may complicate Paget's disease (see Fig. 6-2A), it may arise in bone that has been previously radiated, and it is rarely seen in association with bone infarcts.[56]

FIG. 6-2. A: Osteogenic sarcoma arising in Paget's disease of the lower tibia. Note the thickened cortex and coarsened trabecula, indicative of Paget's disease. Note the soft tissue mass (*arrowheads*), cortical destruction, and pathologic fracture resulting from sarcoma. **B and C:** Osteogenic sarcoma of the lower end of tibia. Note larger soft tissue extension posteriorly. Matrix ossification combined with evidence of malignancy strongly favors this diagnosis. **D:** Osteogenic sarcoma of calcaneus. Poor margin and matrix ossification favor this diagnosis. Ewing's sarcoma may have a similar appearance. **E:** MRI of central low-grade osteogenic sarcoma of lower tibia. Coronal SE 500/20 image gives an accurate depiction of the longitudinal extent. Note cortical breakthrough laterally. T2-weighted or gadolinium enhanced images would demonstrate soft tissue changes and cortical breakthrough more clearly. **F:** Osteogenic sarcoma of the tibia, talus, and calcaneus arising in a former World War II radium dial painter.

Ewing's Sarcoma

Ewing's sarcoma (Fig. 6-3) is a highly malignant tumor consisting of small, round cells with little intercellular stroma. Most of the tumors occur in children between the ages of 5 and 15 years. The tumors are most commonly located in the pelvis and lower extremity. Of the Ewing's sarcomas studied by Dahlin and Unni,[16] and by Mirra[57], 8.7% and 5%, respectively, occurred in the foot and ankle. The incidence of foot and ankle lesions was higher in younger patients.[16,68] This may be related to the central shift in marrow elements with skeletal maturation. Of the 35 tumors in the series of Dahlin and Unni,[16] 15 occurred in the distal tibia and fibula, 10 in the tarsal bones, 7 in the metatarsals, and 3 in the phalanges. Others also report the highest incidence in the calcaneus and metatarsals.[35,86]

Ewing's sarcoma tends to present as a diaphyseal lesion extensively involving the bone of origin.[71] The matrix may be lytic or sclerotic, or it may have an irregular mixture of both.[68,70] Generally, there is an irregular permeative type of bone destruction, along with poor margination. Periosteal reaction is often prominent and frequently takes a multilaminal form. Most lesions have an associated soft tissue mass, which may be large. Occasionally, little or no alteration of the bone is seen on the radiograph (Fig. 6-4), in which case CT or MRI may be required for demonstration.[6,38,43] MRI is superior for evaluating soft tissue extension and therefore is more commonly used in our practice (Fig. 6-5).[6]

Combination chemotherapy has shown promising results. Surgical resection or amputation for foot and ankle lesions has many proponents. Ewing's sarcoma is relatively radio-

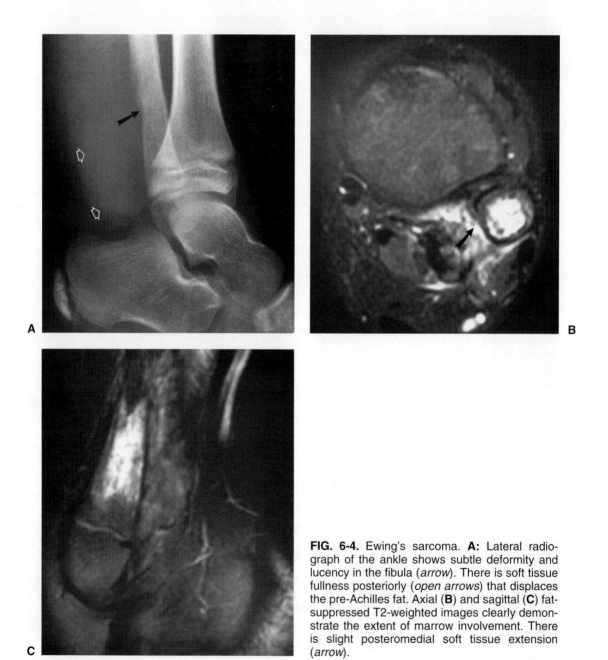

FIG. 6-4. Ewing's sarcoma. **A:** Lateral radiograph of the ankle shows subtle deformity and lucency in the fibula (*arrow*). There is soft tissue fullness posteriorly (*open arrows*) that displaces the pre-Achilles fat. Axial (**B**) and sagittal (**C**) fat-suppressed T2-weighted images clearly demonstrate the extent of marrow involvement. There is slight posteromedial soft tissue extension (*arrow*).

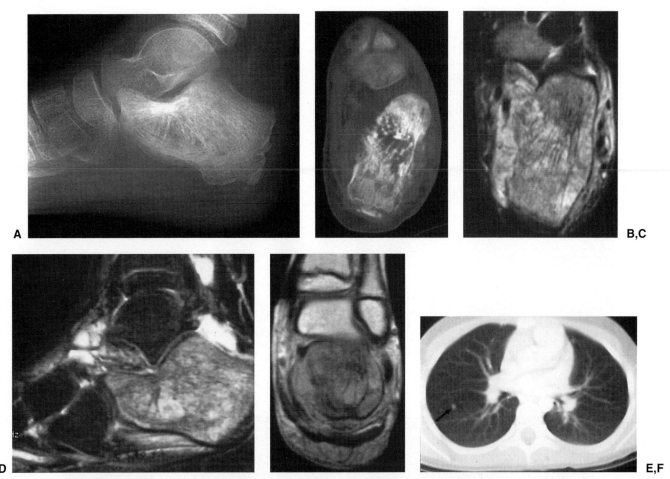

FIG. 6-5. Ewing's sarcoma **A:** Lateral view of the calcaneus shows increased sclerosis. **B:** CT scan demonstrates medial and lateral cortical destruction. Axial (**C**) and sagittal (**D**) fat-suppressed T2-weighted and coronal (**E**) proton-density MRI show that the entire calcaneus is involved with soft tissue extension. Note the expansion on the coronal image (**E**). CT scan of the chest (**F**) performed as part of staging shows a lung metastasis on the right (*arrow*).

sensitive, and some clinicians still consider it the prime treatment modality. Reports indicate that the classic 5-year survival rate of approximately 15% has increased and at the present time is between 40% and 56%, or even higher.[6,16,70]

Chondrosarcoma

Chondrosarcoma (Figs. 6-6 and 6-7) is usually a low-grade sarcoma composed predominantly of hyaline cartilage. It is most common in the fourth through the sixth decades of life. More than three-fourths of the tumors arise centrally from the axial skeleton or the proximal humeri or femurs. This tumor accounts for 3.5% of all primary osseous malignancies.[35] Of the chondrosarcomas studied by Dahlin and Unni,[16] 3.5% were seen in the foot and ankle. Of the 22 tumors, 13 occurred in the distal tibia and fibula, 5 in the tarsals, 3 in the metatarsals, and 1 in the phalanges. In the review by Walling and Gasser,[83] chondrosarcoma was the most common primary osseous malignancy in the foot. The hindfoot was the most common location for this neoplasm.

Other investigators reported the highest incidence in the metatarsals (Fig. 6-8), followed by the calcaneus.[35,61,74] Rarely, chondrosarcoma can arise in existing synovial chondromatosis.[66]

Lytic destruction, poor margin, and soft tissue extension are usually present and indicate a malignant process.[49] About two-thirds of the tumors contain punctate calcification—a finding highly suggestive of the diagnosis. Periosteal new bone is usually scant or absent.[16,49]

About 10% of chondrosarcomas arise in a preexisting benign lesion, which is usually a solitary osteochondroma or one of multiple lesions in a patient with multiple hereditary exostosis. Rarely, chondrosarcoma may complicate a solitary enchondroma or one lesion of many in a patient with Ollier's disease or Maffucci's syndrome. Radical surgery is the best treatment and, in this location, is usually curative.[49,86]

Routine radiographs (see Figs. 6-6 and 6-8) and CT are useful to characterize the matrix and histology of chondrosarcoma. Although MRI is also valuable (see Fig. 6-8), if scans are not compared with radiographs, the diagnosis of a cartilaginous lesion may be difficult.[6]

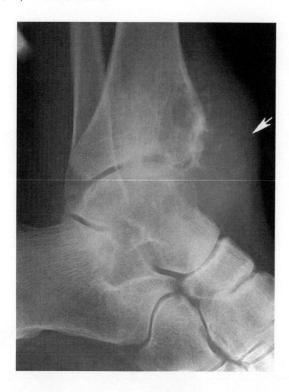

FIG. 6-6. Chondrosarcoma of the lower tibia. Cortical destruction and soft tissue mass (*arrow*) indicate malignancy. Subtle punctate calcification suggests chondrosarcoma.

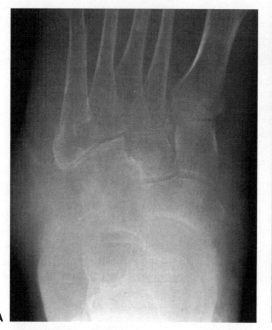

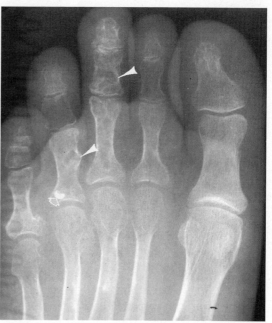

A   B

FIG. 6-7. Chondrosarcoma of the cuboid arising in a patient with enchondromatosis and soft tissue hemangiomas (Maffucci's syndrome). Note the malignant-appearing lesion of the cuboid (**A**), with bone destruction and a large soft tissue mass. **B:** Note the multiple enchondromas of phalanges (*arrowheads*). A phlebolith, indicative of soft tissue hemangioma, is projected over the base of the fourth proximal phalanx (*open arrow*).

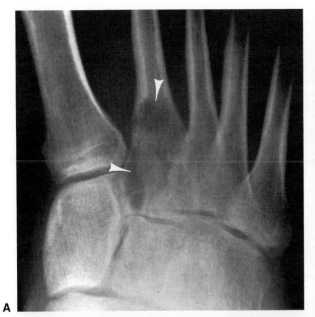

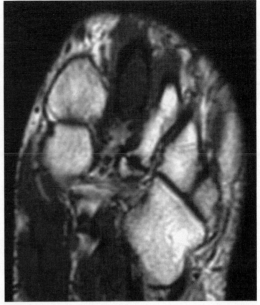

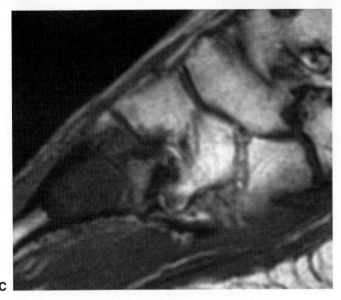

FIG. 6-8. Chondrosarcoma of the second metatarsal. **A:** AP radiograph demonstrates a poorly defined lytic lesion in the proximal second metatarsal (*arrowheads*). Coronal (**B**) and sagittal (**C**) SE 500/11 images demonstrate a low-intensity lesion that expands the cortex. *(continued)*

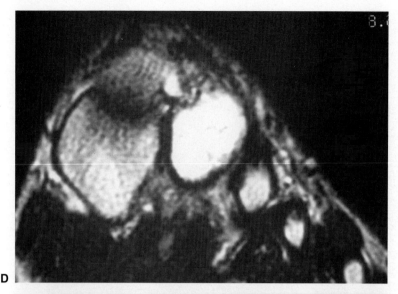

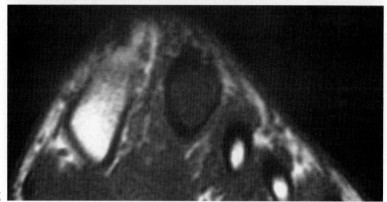

FIG. 6-8. *Continued.* Axial SE 2000/80 (**D**) and SE 500/11 (**E**) images show fairly homogeneous signal intensity with no low-intensity foci to suggest cartilage or calcified areas in the lesion.

Hemangioendothelial Sarcoma

Hemangioendothelial sarcoma (Figs. 6-9 and 6-10) is a vasoformative sarcoma that varies from a borderline to high-grade malignancy.[85] The lesion occurs in patients of all ages (20 to 80 years), having no definite age predilection. Males are affected in 63% of cases.[35] It occurs throughout the skeleton and, unlike the other malignant bone tumors, has a predilection for the foot and ankle. In the compilation by Dahlin and Unni,[16] 16.7% of these lesions occurred in the foot and ankle region. In another series of 93 patients, 7% involved the foot.[57] Of the 10 patients who had biopsies of the lesions, 4 had the lesion in the distal tibia, 1 in the tarsal bones, 2 in the metatarsals, and 3 in the phalanges. There were more lesions than this, because multifocal lesions were counted as only a single lesion with localization based on the biopsy site. The radiographic appearance is nonspecific. The most common presentation is one showing an area of lytic destruction without matrix mineralization, reactive sclerosis, or periosteal new bone (see Figs. 6-9 and 6-10). The radiographic appearance correlates approximately with the histologic grade. High-grade lesions appear more permeative and destructive than low-grade lesions. About one-third of hemangioendothelial sarcomas are multifocal. Low-grade lesions are well marginated and tend to have sclerotic borders. Nine of the 10 patients had multifocal lesions that were limited to the involved lower extremity.[16,85]

Routine radiographs (see Figs. 6-9 and 6-10) demonstrate multiple lucent or lytic areas. This feature should suggest the lesion. On occasion, CT or MRI may add information concerning the aggressiveness or histology of these multifocal lesions.[16,35]

Fibrosarcoma

Fibrosarcoma (Fig. 6-11) is a spindle cell sarcoma with a "herringbone" pattern of growth. The tumors occur with equal distribution in patients who are in the second through the sixth decade of life and arise most commonly from the lower femur or the proximal tibia.[16,35,80] Of the fibrosarcomas studied by Dahlin and Unni,[16] 4.4% arose in the foot and ankle. Like osteogenic sarcoma, fibrosarcomas arise almost exclusively in the ankle and hindfoot. None of our patients had tumor in the forefoot.

The tumor tends to be large, diaphyseal or metaphyseal, and eccentrically located. Generally, the tumor is purely lytic with sclerosis either absent or scant (see Fig. 6-11). Poor margination, bone destruction, and soft tissue extension are frequent (Fig. 6-12). Periosteal reaction is occasionally seen, but it is usually not a prominent feature.[16,35,68]

Nearly one-third of fibrosarcomas arise in preexisting lesions, such as Paget's disease, radiated bone, infarcts, or low-grade chondrosarcoma.[16,56] Treatment generally consists of aggressive surgical resection.[16,84]

Lymphoma

Lymphoma (Figs. 6-13 and 6-14) consists of a diffuse proliferation of mixed cells without matrix production. About half of patients with skeletal lymphoma have soft tissue disease elsewhere in the body. Any age group may be affected, although lymphoma is rarely seen in patients less than 10 years old. Any bone may be involved, and multicentric lesions (see Fig. 6-13) are common. The femur is the most common site. Lymphoma is rare in the foot and ankle, with only 1.7% occurring in this region.[16,86]

The appearance of lymphoma is so similar to that of Ewing's sarcoma that the radiologist may be left with the patient's age as the most reliable clue to the diagnosis (compare Figs. 6-3 and 6-14). Because of this overlap in appearance, the term "small round cell tumor" is sometimes used. Despite the similarities between lymphoma and Ewing's sarcoma, distinguishing them is worthwhile because of the better prognosis and the likelihood of disease elsewhere in patients with lymphoma.[16]

Lymphomas are frequently extensive, and although they

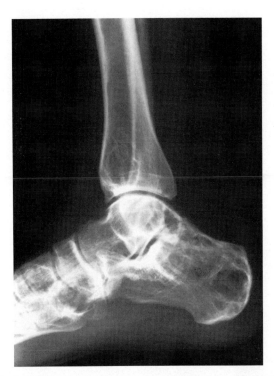

FIG. 6-9. Multicentric hemangioendothelial sarcoma of the foot and ankle. Note the lesions in the tibia, talus, calcaneus, cuboid, and cuneiform bones. Clustering of lesions in one geographic region is typical, and there is a predilection for this site.

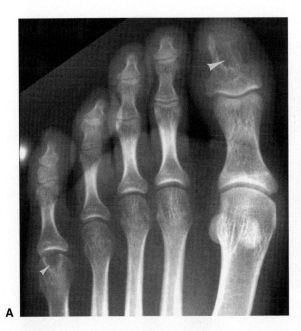

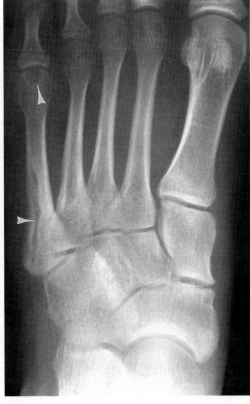

FIG. 6-10. AP views of the forefoot (A) and midfoot (B) show a multicentric hemangioendothelial sarcoma of foot. Note the lesions in the first distal phalanx, fifth metatarsal head, and fifth metatarsal base (*arrowheads*). Multiple lesions in a single foot and ankle are highly suggestive of this diagnosis.

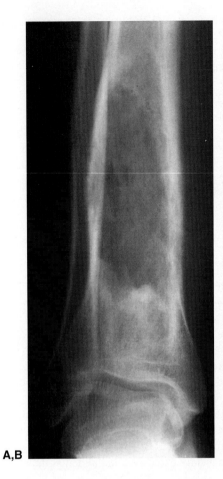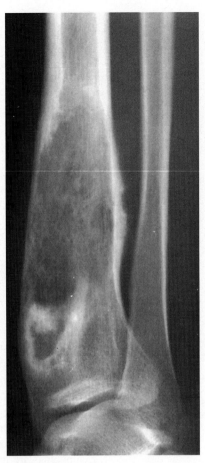

A,B

FIG. 6-11. Fibrosarcoma of the lower tibia. AP (**A**) and lateral (**B**) radiographs demonstrate poor margination and cortical destruction favoring malignancy. This tumor is usually purely lytic, although a small amount of sclerosis (as seen here) occasionally occurs.

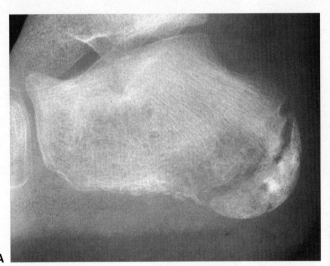

A

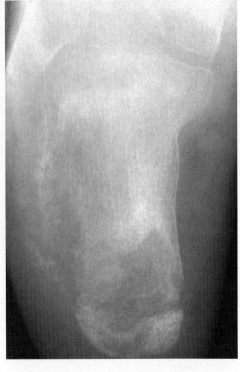

B

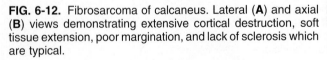

FIG. 6-12. Fibrosarcoma of calcaneus. Lateral (**A**) and axial (**B**) views demonstrating extensive cortical destruction, soft tissue extension, poor margination, and lack of sclerosis which are typical.

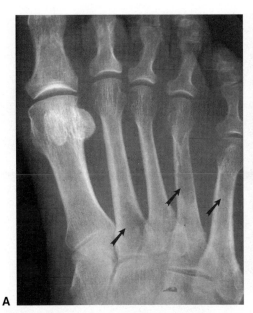 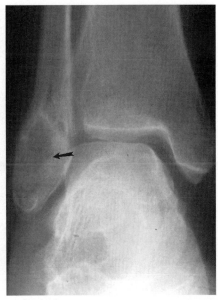

FIG. 6-13. Multiple lesions of lymphoma of the foot and ankle. AP radiographs of the foot (**A**) and ankle (**B**) show nonspecific lytic lesions of the lateral malleolus and the second, fourth, and fifth metatarsals (*arrows*). This is an unusual site.

may be either lytic (see Fig. 6-13) or sclerotic (see Fig. 6-14), most consist of a mixture of the two. Periosteal new bone is less common and less striking than that seen with Ewing's sarcoma. Generally, the appearance of lymphoma is one of poor margination and soft tissue mass. MRI is useful for detection of soft tissue involvement. Though this finding is useful and may cause lymphoma to be added to

the differential diagnosis, MRI adds little specificity to radiographic features.[6,38] The primary treatment is radiation therapy, with or without chemotherapy, depending on the extent of the disease.[16,84]

Adamantinoma

Adamantinoma (Fig. 6-15) is an extremely rare tumor, having a peak incidence in patients who are in the third decade of life. More than 90% of adamantinomas arise in the tibia. Of the adamantinomas studied by Dahlin and Unni,[16] 17.4% occurred in the ankle region, in either the tibia or the fibula.

This tumor is generally centered in the tibial diaphysis.[82] Eccentric lucency, surrounded and connected by sclerosis, is the usual appearance. Larger lesions often demonstrate a dominant central lesion. Expansion is common. Multicentricity occurs, and the fibula is the most common secondary site. Routine radiographs and CT (see Fig. 6-15) are most useful for evaluating subtle osseous changes and cortical expansion.[6]

Metastasis/Myeloma

Metastasis involve the skeletal much more commonly than primary bone tumors (25:1).[35] However, metastasis and myeloma rarely involve the hands and feet.[3,4,83,86] From 20 to 30% of patients with malignancy develop skeletal metastasis.[41] However, only 0.3% or fewer have lesions involving the foot and ankle.[41,83] About one-half of lesions involve the tarsal bones, especially the calcaneus. The metatarsals are second in order of frequency.[35] As a rule, primary lesions

FIG. 6-14. Lymphoma of the calcaneus. Lateral view of the calcaneus demonstrates considerable sclerosis involving the entire calcaneus.

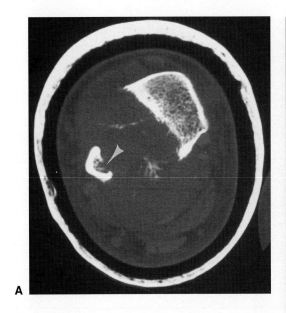
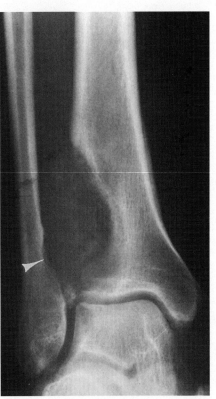

FIG. 6-15. Axial CT (**A**) and AP radiograph (**B**) of adamantinoma of lower tibia. There is direct extension into the fibula (*arrowhead*). This presentation does not permit radiographic diagnosis.

above the diaphragm more frequently involve the hands, and tumors below the diaphragm involve the foot.[35] However, statistically most metastatic lesions to the foot arise from the colon (17%), kidney (17%), lung (15%), bladder (10%), and breast (10%).[35,83,86] Melanoma can also involve the foot. The primary tumor is usually a subungual lesion.[81]

Clinically, patients present with pain and swelling. A palpable mass is not uncommon. The clinical findings may be difficult to differentiate from infection.[4,41] However, the extent of bone destruction and more profound soft tissue mass point to metastasis.[4]

Radiographs may be negative initially. However, bone destruction and soft tissue mass usually develop within 3 to 4 weeks after the onset of symptoms. Bone destruction that does not cross the joint space with prominent soft tissue mass help to differentiate metastasis from infection. Radionuclide bone scans or MRI are positive before radiographic changes occur.[6]

BENIGN BONE TUMORS AND CYSTS

Osteochondroma

Osteochondroma (Fig. 6-16) is a benign growth having a thin cartilage cap reminiscent of an epiphyseal plate with maturation occurring by endochondral ossification to bone trabeculae. Osteochondromas are most commonly discovered in the second decade of life, and the lower femur is the most common site. The lesion is the most common of the benign tumors (50%), and its true incidence is even higher,

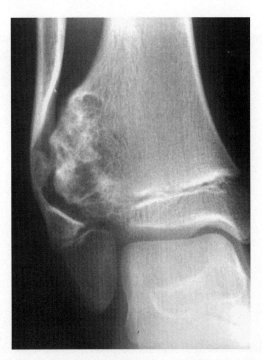

FIG. 6-16. Osteochondroma of the lower tibia. Continuity of cortical and cancellous bone is almost diagnostic. Note pressure erosion and deformity of the adjacent fibula.

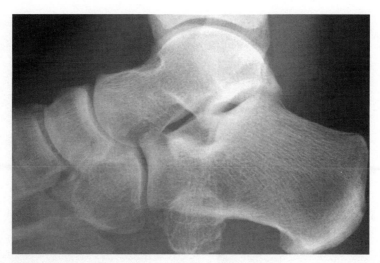

FIG. 6-17. Osteochondroma of the calcaneus. The bone projection or growth consisting of benign trabecular bone with smooth surface is characteristic. This location is unusual, except in patients with multiple hereditary exostoses.

because biopsy is often not necessary.[16,35,76] Of the 34 foot and ankle lesions, 28 occurred in the distal tibia and fibula, 5 in the tarsal bones, and 1 in a metatarsal. Calcaneal lesions (Fig. 6-17) are rare.[76] Of the osteochondromas studied by Dahlin and Unni,[16] 4.7% occurred in the foot and ankle. An osteochondroma arising in the foot is rare and generally occurs as one of the lesions in a patient with multiple hereditary exostoses.[16,76]

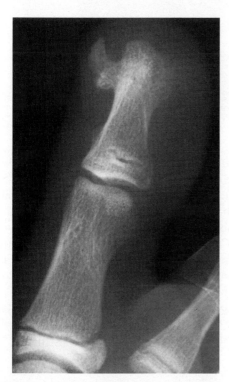

FIG. 6-18. Subungual exostosis of the great toe. The appearance is similar to an osteochondroma.

The lesion presents as a peripheral bone projection or growth with flaring or a lack of tubulation of the affected bone. It is composed of benign regular trabecular bone and has a smooth cortical surface. The finding of cortical and cancellous bone extending from the osteochondroma to the bone of origin is essentially diagnostic.[16]

Subungual exostoses are radiologically similar to osteochondromas.[19] They are not true tumors, probably representing reactive lesions secondary to trauma or pressure or both. They arise dorsal from distal phalanges beneath the nail bed. They have a pronounced predilection for the great toe. Forty-three of the 50 lesions studied by Dahlin and Unni[17] arose at that site (Fig. 6-18).

Osteochondromas have a characteristic radiographic appearance (see Figs. 6-16 and 6-17). Additional studies are rarely indicated, except for operative planning or when adjacent neurovascular structures are involved by the lesion (Figs. 6-19 and 6-20). In this setting, CT or MRI may be required.[6]

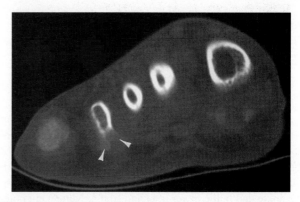

FIG. 6-19. Patient with plantar forefoot pain and normal radiographs. Axial CT image demonstrates a fourth metatarsal osteochondroma (*arrowheads*) compressing the plantar nerve.

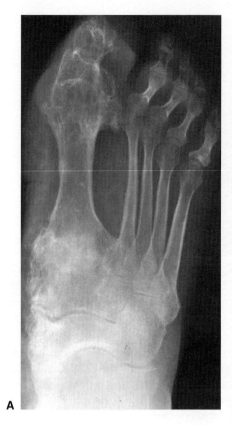

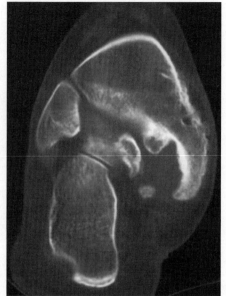

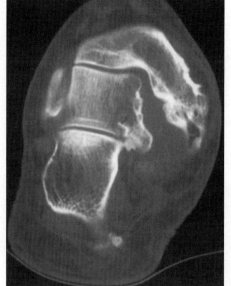

FIG. 6-20. Patient with foot and ankle pain and deformity. The AP radiograph (**A**) demonstrates midfoot and distal great toe deformities. Coronal CT images (**B** and **C**) demonstrate multiple osteochondromas medially involving the malleolus, talus, and calcaneus. The tarsal tunnel was compressed.

No treatment is required unless the lesion becomes symptomatic or unless significant cosmetic deformity occurs. Simple excision is curative. Malignant transformation is extremely rare.

Nonossifying Fibroma

Nonossifying fibromas (Fig. 6-21) are fibrous tumors that are most commonly seen in patients who are in the second decade of life.[16,30] The tumors are most commonly seen in the lower femur and the lower tibia. Of the nonossifying fibromas studied by Dahlin and Unni,[16] 32.3% occurred in the ankle and in the lower tibia and fibula. None were noted in the foot.

These lesions arise eccentrically in the metaphyseal cortical bone.[60] Expansion is common, and nearly all the lesions are sharply marginated (see Fig. 6-21). The margin is often scalloped, having a thin rim of sclerosis. Some of the lesions are multilocular, and multiple lesions are occasionally observed (Fig. 6-22). The bony axis of the lesion parallels that of the bone of origin.[16,60]

Treatment is not required when the lesion is small and typical. Curettage with bone grafting is required when pathologic fracture is imminent. Pathologic fracture (Fig. 6-23) is considered imminent when both the anteroposterior and lateral views of the ankle show that more than 50% of the cortical bone is involved.[16] Routine radiographs (see Figs. 6-21 and 6-23) are usually diagnostic. MRI, especially if not compared with radiographs, can be misleading.[6]

Osteoid Osteoma

Osteoid osteoma (Fig. 6-24) is a small tumor with a peculiarly limited growth potential and consists of an interlacing

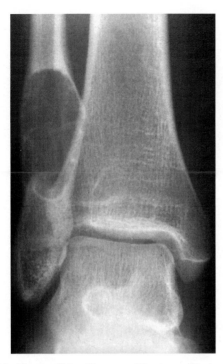

FIG. 6-21. Nonossifying fibroma of the lower fibular diametaphysis. Note the sharp margin, thin sclerotic rim, and expansion.

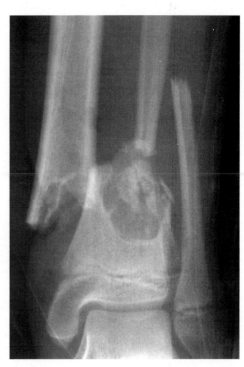

FIG. 6-23. Large nonossifying fibroma of the lower tibia, with pathologic fracture.

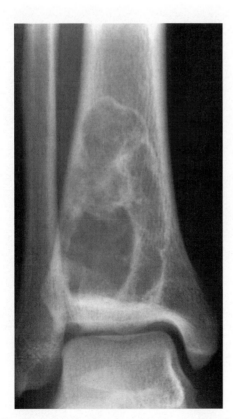

FIG. 6-22. Nonossifying fibroma of the lower tibia. The sharp, scalloped, and sclerotic margin is typical, as is the eccentric metaphyseal location.

network of osteoid trabeculae with a less fibrovascular connective tissue in between. Lesions may be cortical, intraosseous, or intraarticular. Cortical lesions are most common. Intraarticular lesions are less common and are more difficult to diagnose.[72] About 80% of osteoid osteomas are found in males, and most of the tumors arise in patients between 5 and 25 years of age. The femur and tibia are the most common sites.[72] Up to 5 to 8% arise in the talus.[72] Of the osteoid osteomas studied by Dahlin and Unni,[16] 10.6% occurred in the foot and ankle. Of these 26 tumors, 15 arose in the lower end of the tibia, 8 in the tarsals, and 3 in the phalanges.

The typical appearance is that of a small lucent nidus usually surrounded by sclerosis.[12,79,83] The tumor is rarely larger than 1 cm, and it most commonly lies in the cortex. The nidus may be ossified centrally (see Fig. 6-24; Fig. 6-25) or throughout. About one-fourth of the tumors are not seen on the roentgenogram, and therefore, an isotope bone scan (see Fig. 6-24B), tomograms (see Fig. 6-24A), or CT may be required for identification.[6,77] Tumors that arise in cancellous bone or in a subperiosteal or intracapsular location often provoke little or no reactive sclerosis. However, on MRI, one may see extensive marrow edema and synovial inflammation.[6]

Conservative surgical removal is curative. This may be accomplished surgically, arthroscopically, by percutaneous bone biopsy, or by using radiofrequency ablation.[72,78,84]

Giant Cell Tumor

Giant cell tumor (Figs. 6-26 and 6-27) is a benign tumor with multinucleated giant cells scattered in a field of similar

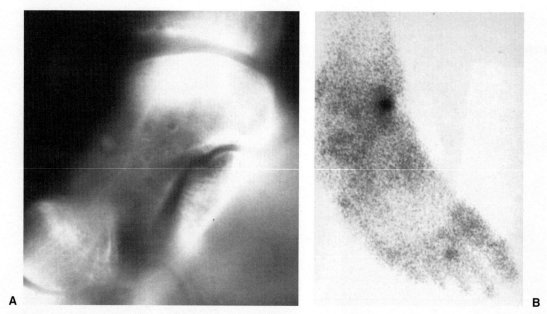

FIG. 6-24. Osteoid osteoma of the talus. The lesion was not seen on routine roentgenograms but is well demonstrated by tomogram (**A**) and isotope bone scan (**B**).

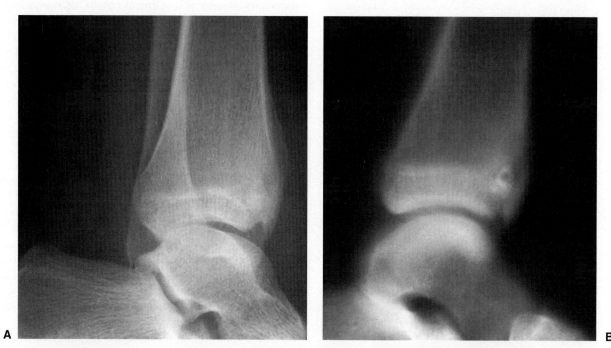

FIG. 6-25. Osteoid osteoma of the anterior lower tibia. A small, round sclerotic tumor near physis with benign periosteal new bone is demonstrated on the routine radiograph (**A**) and tomogram (**B**).

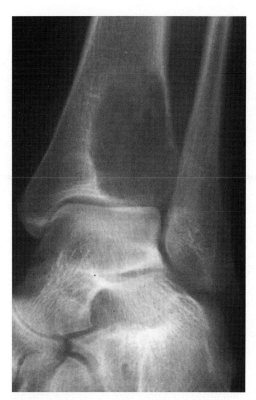

FIG. 6-26. Giant cell tumor abutting the end of the lower tibia. The eccentric location and lack of matrix or reactive mineral are characteristic.

but mononuclear cells. This lesion accounts for 5% of biopsied bone lesions.[60] This tumor is more common in females, and most of the tumors occur in patients between the ages of 20 and 40 years. The most common sites are the ends of the long bones (especially the distal femur and radius and the proximal tibia) and the sacrum.[15] About 70% of these tumors occur about the knee.[60] Of the giant cell tumors studied by Dahlin and Unni,[16] 6.1% occurred in the foot and ankle. O'Keefe and associates[65] reported an incidence of 4% in the foot and ankle. Of the 26 tumors, 21 arose in the distal tibia, 4 in the tarsals, and 1 in a metatarsal. Compared with giant cell tumors found elsewhere in the skeleton, lesions of the small bones of the foot are seen in younger patients, recur at a higher rate, and may be multifocal.[16,65]

Radiographically, the lesion location and geographic pattern with a nonsclerotic margin (see Fig. 6-26) usually suggest the diagnosis. Additional studies such as MRI and CT may not be necessary. However, MRI using T1- and T2-weighted sequences may assist in predicting the histologic features of the lesion. The lesion is of intermediate to low intensity on T1-weighted sequences (see Fig. 6-27) and may be of low intensity on T2-weighted sequences because of hemosiderin in giant cells.[6] Giant cell tumors enhance with intravenous gadolinium, but the pattern is nonspecific. Fluid-fluid levels have also been reported in giant cell tumors.[36]

Treatment is curettage and bone packing using graft material or methyl methacrylate.[60,83] Some clinicians prefer

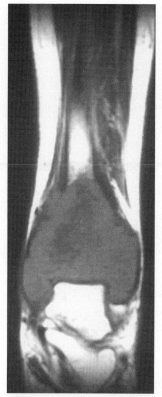

A

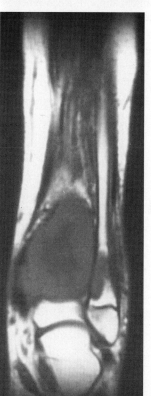

B

FIG. 6-27. MRI of a giant cell tumor of the lower tibia. Coronal SE 500/20 images (**A** and **B**) demonstrating the location, signal intensity and appearance are typical. There is unsuspected extension of the tumor into the fibula (**B**).

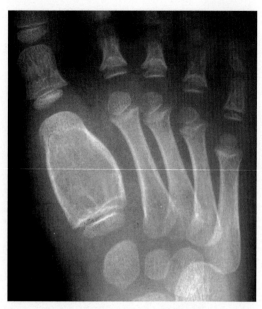

FIG. 6-28. Aneurysmal bone cyst of the first metatarsal characterized by pronounced expansion and metaphyseal location.

Aneurysmal Bone Cyst

An aneurysmal bone cyst (Figs. 6-28 and 6-29) is composed of cavernous blood-filled spaces with thin fibrous walls.[16,29] These lesions are probably not true neoplasms but rather a reactive process. Most occur in patients younger than 20 years of age. Aneurysmal bone cysts arise throughout the skeleton but most commonly occur in the metaphyses of large bones (especially femur and tibia) and the dorsal elements of the spine.[16,83] Of the aneurysmal bone cysts studied by Dahlin and Unni,[16] 11% occurred in the foot and ankle. Of the 24 lesions, 15 occurred in the tibia and fibula, 4 in the tarsals, 3 in the metatarsals, and 2 in the phalanges (Fig. 6-30).

Aneurysmal bone cysts often show pronounced expansion or ballooning of the affected bone (see Figs. 6-28 to 6-30). Significant matrix mineralization is not seen. A surrounding rim of sclerosis and periosteal new bone formation are common. Usually, a thin shell of bone contains the expansile process. This lesion can be aggressive, with cortical destruction and soft tissue extension. When this occurs, confusion with malignancy is possible.

Radiographically, the foregoing features are easily observed. However, differentiation from other expanding lesions is not always possible (see Fig. 6-30). MRI may demonstrate increased signal intensity on T1-weighted images resulting from blood. In addition, fluid-fluid levels are commonly seen with aneurysmal bone cysts on both CT and MRI.[6] This finding is not specific. Fluid-fluid levels have been described in benign and malignant bone lesions.[6,36]

methyl methacrylate because of thermal extension and immediate mechanical support. Recurrence is not unusual and is reported in 10 to 30% of patients whose lesions are treated with curettage.[60,83] En bloc resection or wide excision results in fewer recurrences, but more extensive reconstruction is required to preserve joint function.[83]

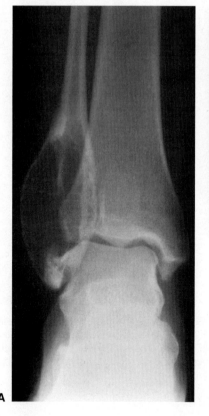

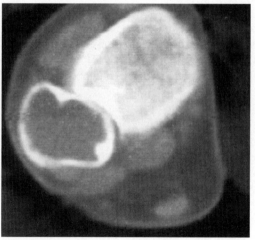

FIG. 6-29. AP view (**A**) and CT scan (**B**) show marked fibular expansion. There are no fluid-fluid levels noted on CT. This aneurysmal bone cyst of the lower fibula exhibits pronounced expansion.

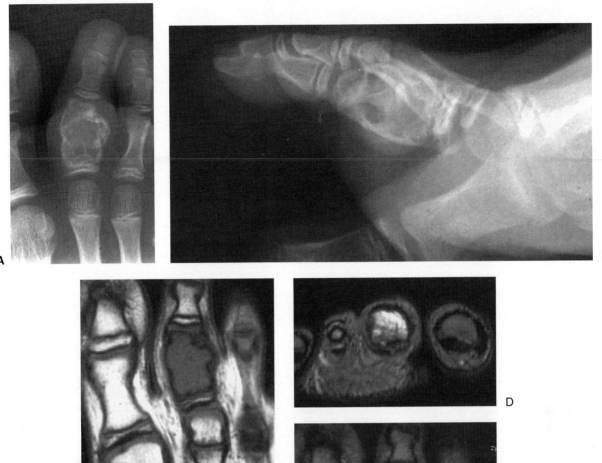

FIG. 6-30. Aneurysmal bone cyst of the second proximal phalanx. The growth plates are still open, effectively excluding giant cell tumor from the differential diagnosis. AP (**A**) and lateral (**B**) radiographs show the expanded septated appearance. Coronal SE 500/11 MRI (**C**) demonstrates a lesion with signal intensity slightly higher than muscle. Axial (**D**) and coronal (**E**) SE 2000/80 images show high signal intensity with septation and small fluid-fluid levels.

Surgical removal with bone grafting is the recommended treatment and is usually curative, although recurrence is possible. Cellular tissue should be removed to be certain the aneurysmal bone cyst did not arise from a more aggressive lesion.[83]

Simple Bone Cyst

Simple bone cysts (Fig. 6-31), like aneurysmal bone cysts, are probably not true neoplasms. This lesion consists of a cystic cavity filled with straw-colored fluid. Bone cysts are detected most commonly in patients who are in the first 2 decades of life.[16,83] The most common sites are the metaphyses of the upper humerus and femur. Of the 13 foot and ankle cysts reported by Walling and Gasser, 11 arose in the calcaneus, thus making it the most common calcaneal lesion.[16,83]

Radiographically, location in the anterior calcaneus near the junction of the atrium and middle third is characteristic. A well-marginated and purely lytic process is seen. The cysts

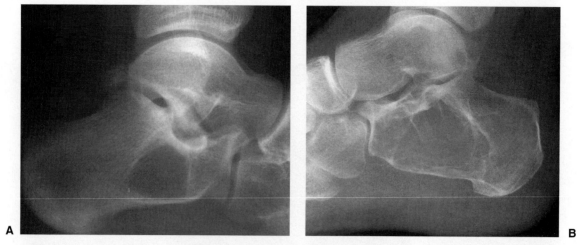

FIG. 6-31. A: Simple cyst of the anterior calcaneus. Location, sharp margin, and lack of matrix mineral are typical. **B:** Simple cyst of the calcaneus. The cyst is larger than usual, but the appearance and location are otherwise typical.

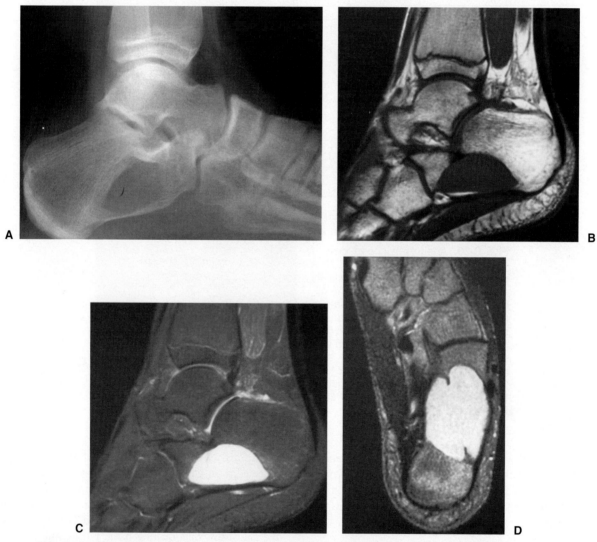

FIG. 6-32. Simple cyst. **A:** Lateral view of the calcaneus shows a lucent lesion anteriorly. The margins are not as sharp as the cysts in Fig. 6-31. **B:** Sagittal SE 500/22 MRI shows a homogeneous low-intensity lesion that is not fat. Sagittal (**C**) and axial (**D**) T2-weighted images show a uniformly high-intensity lesion consistent with a cyst. Note that fat suppression was used on image **C.**

are variable in size and often show mild expansion. They are round to oval, and light trabeculation (see Fig. 6-31B) may be seen. The cysts may be bilateral. On occasion, it may be difficult to differentiate a simple cyst from a pseudocyst or an intraosseous lipoma.[6,28] CT or MRI may solve this problem because fat is easily differentiated from fluid (Fig. 6-32).[6,45]

Observation, curettage, and steroid injection are possible approaches to treatment.[83] Compared with large bone lesions, these cysts do not respond as well to steroid injection. They may, in fact, be a different entity.[74]

Enchondroma

Enchondroma (Figs. 6-33 and 6-34) is a benign hypocellular neoplasm of cartilage found in patients of any age, but more commonly it is seen in the second decade of life.[35,83,86] About 60% of these lesions occur in the hand. The foot is the second most common site (8%).[35] Of 16 enchondromas in the foot, 13 occurred in the forefoot, with 11 of these located in the phalanges.[16] The incidence in men and women is equal.[16,35]

These intramedullary lesions have benign radiographic features consisting of sharp margination and expansion (see Figs. 6-33 and 6-34). Punctate cartilage-type calcification is seen in most cases and is a useful diagnostic clue (see Figs. 6-33 and 6-34). The enchondroma may be solitary or multiple.[15] CT and MRI (Fig. 6-35) are rarely indicated.[6]

If the roentgenogram shows a characteristic lesion, treatment is not necessary. Simple curettage may be done when

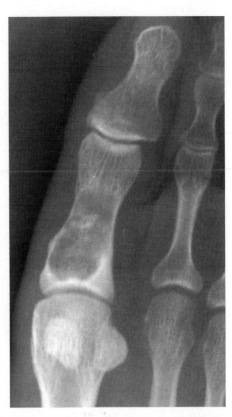

FIG. 6-34. Enchondroma of the first proximal phalanx. Punctate calcification, benign features, and location are essentially diagnostic.

there is pain, pathologic fracture, or equivocal radiographic findings.[16,84]

Chondromyxoid Fibroma

Chondromyxoid fibroma (Fig. 6-36) is a rare benign lesion of cartilage, arising most commonly in patients who are in the second and third decades and more often in males.[69] This lesion accounts for less than 1% of primary bone tumors.[64] The lesion is most common in the knee region and has a predilection for the tibia. Involvement of the foot and ankle is common.[5] Of the chondromyxoid fibromas studied by Dahlin and Unni,[16] 28.2% occurred in the foot and ankle. Baron and colleagues reported 56 cases with 21 in the tarsal bones, 21 in the metatarsals, and 14 involving the phalanges. Despite the rarity of this lesion, it was the most common benign metatarsal lesion.[16]

Radiologically, the tumor is usually seen in an eccentric metaphyseal location.[27,64] The margins are typically sharp, sclerotic, and scalloped. Matrix calcification only rarely occurs (see Fig. 6-36).[16,64] Additional imaging studies do not improve the ability to characterize this lesion histologically.[6]

Conservative resection may be curative. However, recurrences have been reported. Recurrences are especially common in the foot and in younger patients. Baron and associates[5] reported recurrence rates of 25 to 30% in young

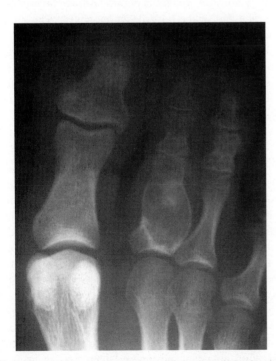

FIG. 6-33. Benign enchondroma of the second proximal phalanx. There is a sharp sclerotic margin, expansion, and punctate calcification, which are characteristic of this tumor.

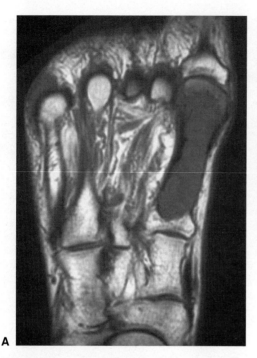

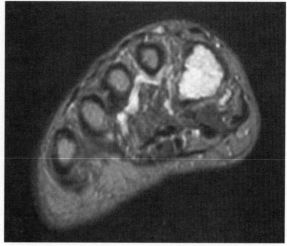

FIG. 6-35. Enchondroma. Coronal SE 500/20 (**A**) and axial SE 2000/80 (**B**) images demonstrate a large lesion without soft tissue involvement. Without the radiograph, it is difficult to predict the histology of this lesion.

children. O'Connor and colleagues[64] reported recurrence in 3 of 4 forefoot chondromyxoid fibromas.

Chondroblastoma

Chondroblastoma (Fig. 6-37), like chondromyxoid fibroma, is a rare benign tumor of cartilage derivation. Like

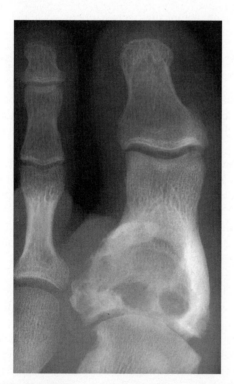

FIG. 6-36. Chondromyxoid fibroma of the proximal phalanx. Expansion, lobulation, surrounding sclerosis, and lack of matrix calcification are usual findings.

chondromyxoid fibroma, this lesion represents only about 1% of primary bone tumors.[35,86] It is more common in males, and 80% of patients are in the second and third decades of life.[16,27] The most common sites are the knee, shoulder, and hip region. Of the chondroblastomas studied by Dahlin and Unni,[16] 7.6% occurred in the foot and ankle, with the talus and calcaneus the preferred sites. Fink and associates[27] reported that 42 of 322 cases (13%) involved the foot.

Like giant cell tumor, chondroblastoma invariably involves the end of the bone or an apophysis. The tumor is characterized by sharp margination, often with a sclerotic rim. Expansion is present in more than half the patients, and matrix calcification occurs in about one-fourth (Fig. 6-38).[50] CT is particularly useful to evaluate the margins and matrix calcifications. Conservative surgery is the usual treatment, with curettage and bone grafting.[16,27]

Osteoblastoma

Osteoblastoma (Figs. 6-39 and 6-40) is a rare benign osseous neoplasm that is closely related to osteoid osteoma, but it has the capability for greater growth.[16,35] Common locations include the dorsal elements of the spine, mandible, and long bones. Of the osteoblastomas studied by Dahlin and Unni,[16] 75% occurred in males, and most patients are in the second and third decades of life. Six percent of these tumors occurred in the foot and ankle.[16]

The radiographic appearance is variable and is often nonspecific.[52] The lesion may resemble osteoid osteoma, except for its increased size. Other helpful clues include matrix ossification, abundant surrounding sclerosis, expansion, and benign-appearing new bone formation. As with osteoid osteoma, ossification of the central tumor nidus occurs and is

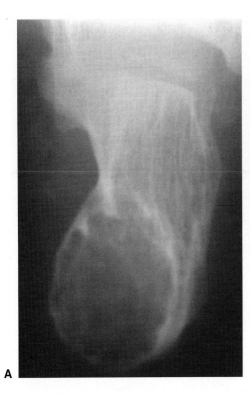

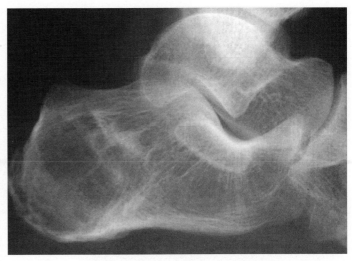

FIG. 6-37. Chondroblastoma of the calcaneus. Axial (**A**) and lateral (**B**) radiographs showing a lesion with a sharp, sclerotic margin and location at bone end are usual.

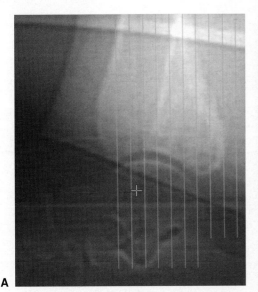

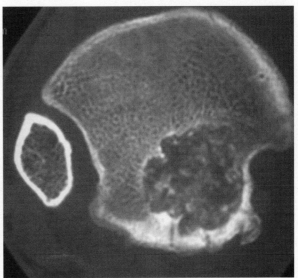

FIG. 6-38. Scout sagittal (**A**) and axial (**B**) CT images demonstrated a large distal tibial lesion with calcified matrix consistent with chondroblastoma.

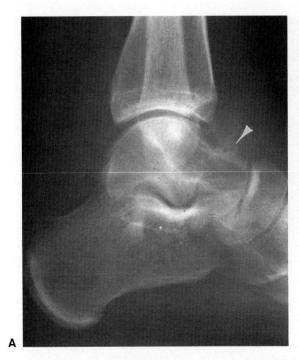

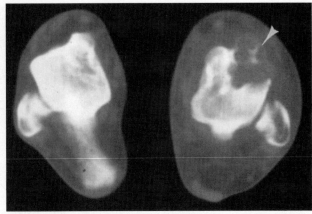

FIG. 6-39. Osteoblastoma of the talus. Lateral radiograph (**A**) and CT scan (**B**) show a markedly expansile lesion of the superior aspect of the talus (*arrowhead*).

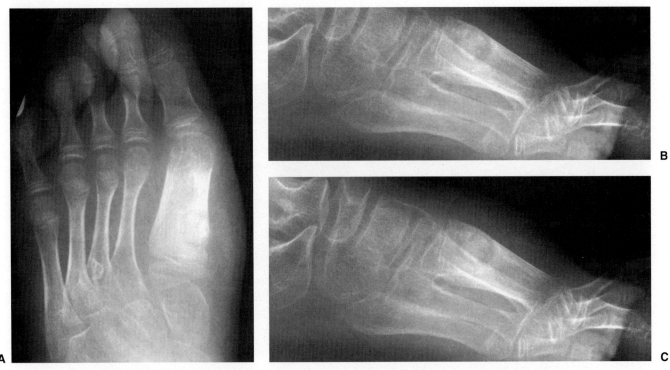

FIG. 6-40. Osteoblastoma of the first metatarsal. AP (**A**) and lateral (**B**) radiographs demonstrate an oval ossified tumor with a lucent halo and surrounding sclerosis. Tumor has prevented tubulation of the metatarsal.

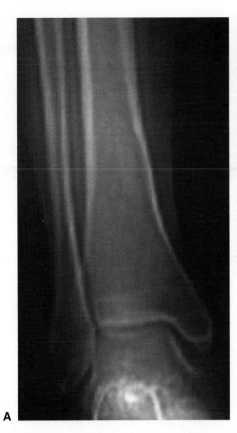
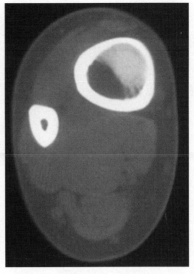

FIG. 6-41. Fibrous dysplasia. CT scout image (**A**) and axial image (**B**) demonstrate a ground-glass lesion with slight cortical thinning.

strongly suggestive of the diagnosis. The radiographic appearances may simulate that of sarcoma in about one-fourth of the cases.[16,35] As with osteoid osteoma, CT is most useful to demonstrate the characteristic radiographic features.[52] Conservative surgery is the treatment of choice.[16,84]

Fibrous Dysplasia

Fibrous dysplasia is a metaplastic process that uncommonly involves the foot. Only 2% of 334 cases reported by Johnston[35] involved the foot. Most cases occur in patients less than 30 years of age. Males and females are affected equally.[16,35]

Radiographically, fibrous dysplasia may present as isolated or multiple lesions. Lesions may be round lobulated, expansile, or lytic, or they have a ground-glass appearance (Fig. 6-41).[16,86] Radiographic features are usually characteristic. However, other benign lesions such as enchondroma, bone cyst, and nonossifying fibroma may have a similar appearance. When the histologic pattern is not clear, we prefer CT (see Fig. 6-41). MRI, especially with gadolinium, may cause this benign process to appear aggressive.[6]

No treatment is necessary unless the lesion is large enough to predispose to fracture. In this setting, curettage and packing with bone or methyl methacrylate are indicated.[84]

SOFT TISSUE TUMORS AND CYSTS

Like their counterparts arising from the skeleton, soft tissue tumors of the foot and ankle are uncommon (see Table 6-2).[6,18,20,24,37,39,46,48,67] Kirby and associates[39] reviewed 83 cases; 87% were benign and 13% malignant. Radiographs have significant limitation as a method to study the soft tissues and thus are less useful in soft tissue tumors than in skeletal tumors. Although valuable information may be present on the radiograph (Fig. 6-42), the information is seldom definitive, and negative findings on examination do not exclude a soft tissue mass. Currently, CT and MRI are the modalities of choice for evaluation of known or suspected soft tissue lesions (see Fig. 6-42; Fig. 6-43).

Although CT is a valuable imaging technique for all parts of the body, it has limitations in the foot and ankle region. The small size of the various structures, the paucity of fat, and the beam-hardening artifact from the cortical bone all combine to diminish potentially the quality of CT images. The intravenous infusion of contrast medium is sometimes useful to image isodense intramuscular tumors or arteriovenous malformation, to demonstrate tumor vessels or enhancement, or to show the relationship of the tumor with adjacent vessels.[51,53]

The foot and ankle region is an ideal area for MRI study. Chapter 2 describes MRI techniques, but a review of certain techniques is warranted here. The small dimensions allow the use of circumferential coils or small partial volume extremity coils.[6,37,38] Coil size, slice thickness, and field of view should be selected to achieve optimal image quality, but also to ensure that the entire area is well demonstrated on MRI.[6,42,43] Imaging should be performed in at least two planes selected to demonstrate the extent and compartment

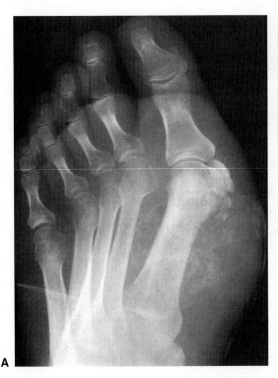

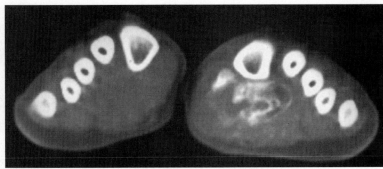

FIG. 6-42. Soft tissue chondroma of the foot seen on an AP view of the foot (**A**) and axial CT image (**B**). Note the partially calcified mass. Separation from bone is well demonstrated by CT.

involvement of the lesion.[6,23] Conventional spin-echo (SE) sequences using T1- and T2-weighting are usually adequate to detect and characterize the lesion (see Fig. 6-43). Additional sequences such as short TI inversion recovery (STIR) (subtle marrow and soft tissue masses) or intravenous gadolinium are useful in selected cases.[6,25]

In general, neither CT nor MRI provides histologic speci-

ficity, but certain MRI features are useful in predicting the nature of the lesion.[6,38] Several useful, although imperfect, criteria are available for distinguishing benign from malignant lesions. These include signal intensity, signal homogeneity or inhomogeneity, border definition, and neurovascular or bone involvement.[6,51]

Benign lesions tend to have sharp margins with a homoge-

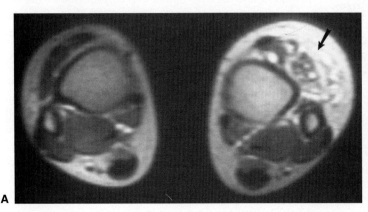

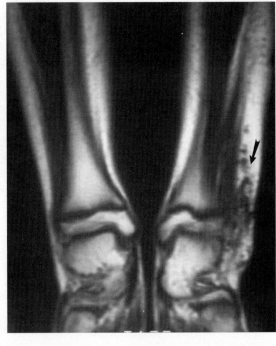

FIG. 6-43. Axial T2-weighted (**A**) and coronal T1-weighted (**B**) images demonstrating the characteristic features of a benign hemangioma. Serpiginous vessels (*arrow* in **B**) and multiple punctate vessels (*arrow* in **A**) are typically demonstrated.

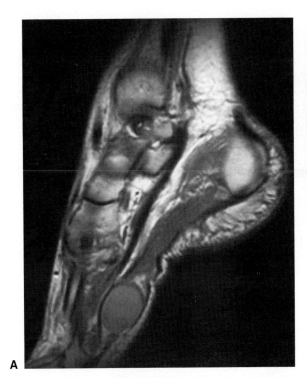

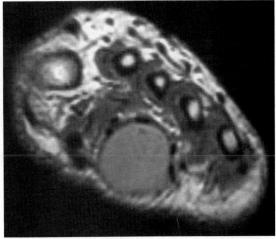

FIG. 6-44. Sagittal (A) and axial (B) proton-density images of a large, well-defined schwannoma.

neous signal intensity (Figs. 6-44 and 6-45). Malignant tumors are poorly marginated, and they are frequently inhomogeneous (Fig. 6-46).[6]

The inhomogeneity in malignant lesions is due to intralesional necrosis or hemorrhage or both. Involvement of multiple muscle groups or compartments is more commonly asso-

ciated with malignancy (see Fig. 6-46).[6,23,51] When there is altered density or signal in the adjacent fat or muscle beyond the confines of the mass, a malignant process is favored. Invasion or destruction of adjacent bone is uncommon in all soft tissue tumors, but when seen, the invasion or destruction is more frequently associated with a malignant tumor.[6,51,89]

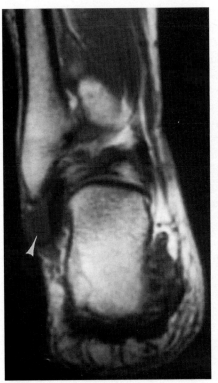

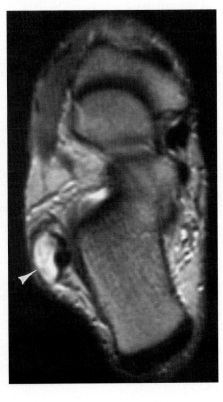

FIG. 6-45. Coronal SE 500/11 (A) and axial SE 2000/80 (B) images of a ganglion cyst of the peroneal tendon sheath (arrowhead).

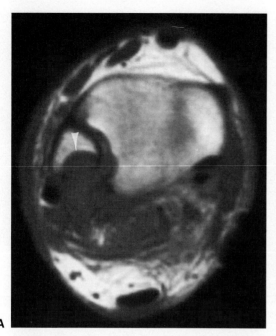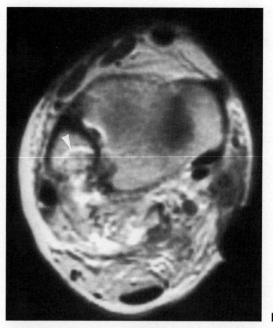

FIG. 6-46. Malignant fibrous histiocytoma. Axial SE 500/20 (**A**) and SE 2000/80 (**B**) images demonstrate an inhomogeneous ankle mass with fibular involvement (*arrowheads*). The inhomogeneity and irregularity of the lesion margins are most easily appreciated on the T2-weighted sequence (**B**).

Tumor calcification has diagnostic significance. Such mineral is best detected by CT or radiography. Subtle calcifications may be difficult to detect on MRI. Phlebolith-type calcification identifies a soft tissue mass as either a hemangioma or an arteriovenous malformation. Small, scattered flecks of calcification favor a malignant sarcoma. When large chunks of calcification are noted in a soft tissue mass, the usual diagnosis is either soft tissue osteogenic sarcoma or synovial sarcoma.[51]

Most soft tissue masses that are imaged by MRI demonstrate low signal intensity in T1-weighted pulse sequences and high signal intensity on T2 sequences. Caution must be exercised when predicting the benign or malignant nature of a soft tissue tumor based on image appearance alone. All the previously mentioned findings are occasionally identified in both benign and malignant tumors. However, if these criteria are carefully applied, more than 80% of the tumors can be correctly identified as being either benign or malignant. In addition, over time, significant experience has been gained concerning a significant number of lesions. Most data have been generated for the more common benign lesions.[6,39]

Lipomas/Liposarcomas

Fatty tissue has high signal intensity on T1-weighted MRI. The signal intensity is suppressed with T2-weighting or by using fat suppression techniques.[6] Fat-containing tumors generally follow the signal intensity of subcutaneous fat. Multiple benign and malignant lesions have been described

that vary in signal intensity and morphology.[6,21,61] The MRI appearance of these lesions is summarized as follows:

Lipoma: Lipomas are benign tumors with fat signal intensity and homogeneous signal, except for occasional well-defined fibrous septa. Subcutaneous lipomas are smaller and better defined than deep or intermuscular lesions. From 5 to 7% are multiple.[6,61]

Heterotopic lipomas: These fatty tumors occur in association with nonadipose tissue and may be intramuscular, intermuscular in tendon sheaths, or intraarticular.

Variants: Mixed lesions including adipose and other tissues. This list includes angiolipoma, lipoblastoma, and neurofibroma. These lesions have mixed signal intensity on MRI and may be difficult to differentiate from liposarcomas.

Liposarcomas: Liposarcomas are the second most common malignant soft tissue tumor and account for 16 to 18% of soft tissue malignancies.[6,24,61] Low-grade liposarcomas look like lipomas with focal areas of low intensity on T1-weighted sequences.[6] High-grade lesions may contain little fat, and therefore a fatty tumor may not be considered on MRI.

Fatty tumors in the foot are uncommon in our experience.[6] Kirby and associates[39] found that the majority occurred in the ankle and dorsum of the foot.

Hemangiomas

Hemangiomas (see Fig. 6-43) and vascular malformations closely resemble normal blood vessels.[6,14] There are fre-

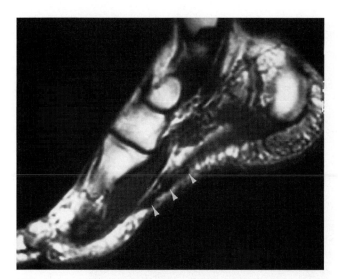

FIG. 6-47. Plantar fibromatosis. Sagittal SE 500/11 image demonstrates low-intensity thickening and nodularity (*arrowheads*) of the plantar fascia.

quently associated nonvascular tissues such as fat (angiolipoma).[6,35,86] Hemangiomas are among the most common benign soft tissue tumors (7%).[35] The incidence of this lesion in the foot and ankle varies from 26 to 30%.

MRI features (see Fig. 6-43) are usually characteristic with numerous vascular channels in soft tissue. In selected cases, gadolinium with fat suppressed T1-weighted sequences or MRI angiographic techniques, improve the accuracy of diagnosis.[6]

Fibromatosis

Fibromatosis relates to various proliferating fibroses tissue lesions that include benign fibromatosis, aggressive fibromatosis (desmoid tumors), and fibrosarcoma.[6,24,26,32,58]

Anatomically, fibromatoses may be classified as superficial or deep.[6,24] Superficial fibromatoses generally involve the fascia such as plantar fibromatosis (Fig. 6-47).[35,83] Lesions usually present as irregular low-intensity areas of nodularity or thickening on MRI. The lesions are obvious on sagittal and coronal MRI (see Fig. 6-47).[24,35] Symptomatic patients may be treated conservatively with footwear modification and antiinflammatory medication. Surgery should be avoided.[83]

Deep fibromatosis usually presents between adolescence and 40 years of age. Two-thirds of lesions involve the lower extremity. Lesions are almost always isolated, although multiple lesions have been reported in up to 15% of patients.[6,24] Younger patients have a more guarded prognosis and a higher recurrence rate. Recurrence rates in all patients may be as high as 77%. These tumors are often large and malignant-appearing on MRI. Neurovascular encasement and bone involvement are common (Fig. 6-48). MRI features are useful in suggesting the diagnosis in these patients. Typically, significant portions of the lesion are low to intermediate in signal intensity on both T1- and T2-weighted sequences.[32] One may see areas of high signal intensity or enhancement with gadolinium, depending on cellularity of the lesion.[6,32] Fibrosarcomas also occur more commonly in the lower extremity, but they do not frequently involve the foot. Only about 3% of fibrosarcomas involve the foot. Most patients are in the 40- to 70-year age range. Image features do not differ significantly from those of other aggressive fibrous lesions.[6,35]

Ganglion Cysts

Ganglion cysts are among the most common benign lesions in the foot and ankle. In our experience, most involve the tendon sheaths about the ankle and the dorsum of the foot. Lesions are most common in adults. Some series note

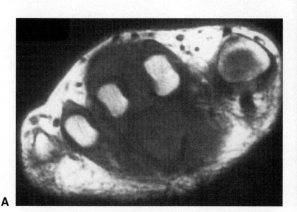
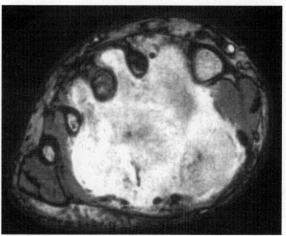

FIG. 6-48. Desmoid tumor. Axial SE 500/20 (**A**) and SE 2000/80 (**B**) images demonstrate a large lesion involving multiple plantar and dorsal compartments. There are areas of low intensity on the T2-weighted sequence (**B**).

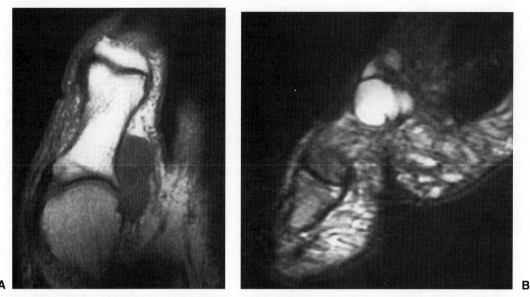

A   B

FIG. 6-49. Ganglion cyst. Coronal SE 500/11 (**A**) and sagittal SE 2000/80 (**B**) images demonstrate a lobulated ganglion adjacent to the metatarsophalangeal joint.

a prevalence of 3:1 for women over men.[35] The origin of these lesions is unclear. However, synovial herniation and repetitive trauma have been implicated.[6,24] Lesions are usually filled with viscous or gelatinous fluid that is difficult to aspirate. Lesions may be simple, septated, or lobulated.

MRI features are characteristic in uncomplicated (no hemorrhage or infection) ganglion cysts. Lesions are well defined with low signal intensity on T1-weighted sequences and uniformly high signal intensity on T2-weighted sequences (Fig. 6-49).[6] Gadolinium is usually not indicated.

However, the cyst wall enhances, and the fluid does not (Fig. 6-50).[6]

Tendon Sheath Giant Cell Tumors

Giant cell tumors of the tendon sheath have histologic features resembling those of pigmented villonodular synovitis. Location is the main differentiating feature.[6,35] These lesions are most common in the 30- to 50-year age groups. Giant cell tumors of the tendon sheath occur most commonly

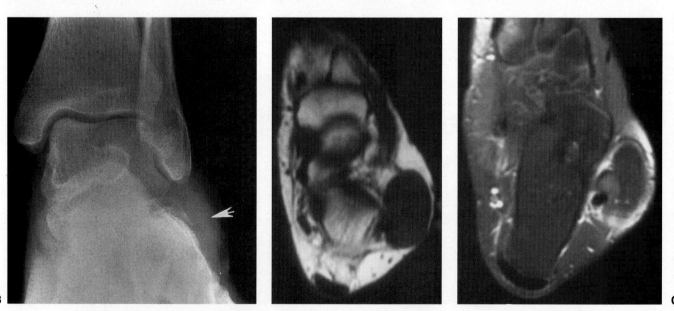

A,B   C

FIG. 6-50. Ganglion cyst. AP radiograph (**A**) of the ankle demonstrates focal swelling below the lateral malleolus (*arrow*). Axial SE 500/11 (**B**) and postgadolinium fat-suppressed SE 500/11 (**C**) images show a low-intensity lesion with no central enhancement.

in the hands and feet. About 17% of lesions occur in the foot and ankle.[6,35,83]

Radiographs may demonstrate a focal soft tissue mass, and bone erosion may be evident, especially with phalangeal lesions.[35] MRI is most specific for diagnoses of giant cell tumors. Image features are similar to pigmented villonodular synovitis.[6] Therefore, when soft tissue lesions along the tendon have low signal intensity on T1-weighted images and significant areas of low signal on T2-weighted sequences, a giant cell tumor of the tendon sheath is the likely diagnosis.[22,31] Gadolinium is usually not useful. However, lesions do enhance (Fig. 6-51).[6]

Lesions are treated with surgical resection. Recurrence is not uncommon.

Neural Lesions

Neuroma, neurofibroma, schwannoma (neurilemoma), and Morton's neuroma may be noted in the foot and an-

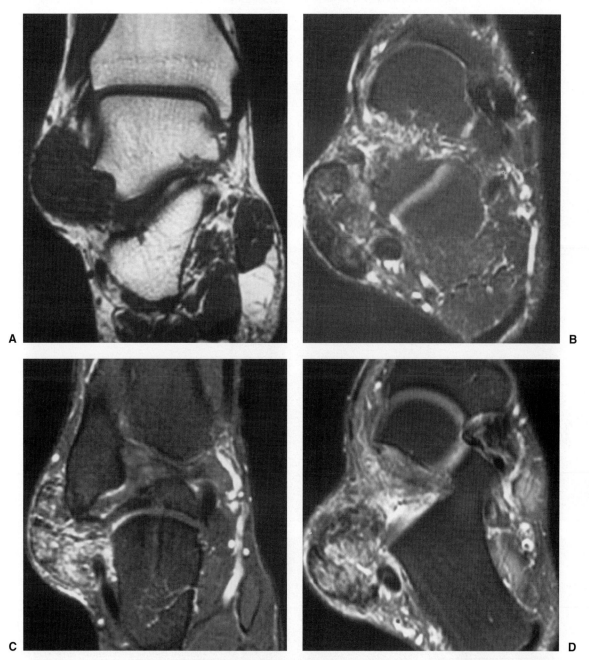

FIG. 6-51. Giant cell tumor of the tendon sheath. Coronal T1-weighted (**A**) and axial fat-suppressed T2-weighted (**B**) images demonstrate a large, low-intensity mass along the peroneal tendons. A significant portion of the mass remains low intensity on the T2-weighted image (**B**). Gadolinium was given intravenously, and postinjection coronal (**C**) and axial (**D**) T1-weighted fat-suppressed images demonstrate irregular enhancement of the lesion.

kle.[35,83] Neurofibromas are most often seen in patients between 20 and 40 years of age. Cutaneous nerves are most commonly affected. Multiple lesions are seen with cutaneous syndromes such as von Recklinghausen's disease (neurofibromatosis).[35,83] In the foot, most of these lesions occur in the heel and great toe.[35]

Patients with schwannomas fall into the same age range as neurofibromas. Lesions are most common in the flexor regions of the extremities (see Fig. 6-44).[6,24] Lesions are usually well defined and oval. Schwannomas are encapsulated and displace nerve fibers, so they can be shelled out surgically, thus preserving the neural tissue.[35] Neurofibromas extend between nerve fibers, so removal without including a portion of the involved nerve is difficult.[83]

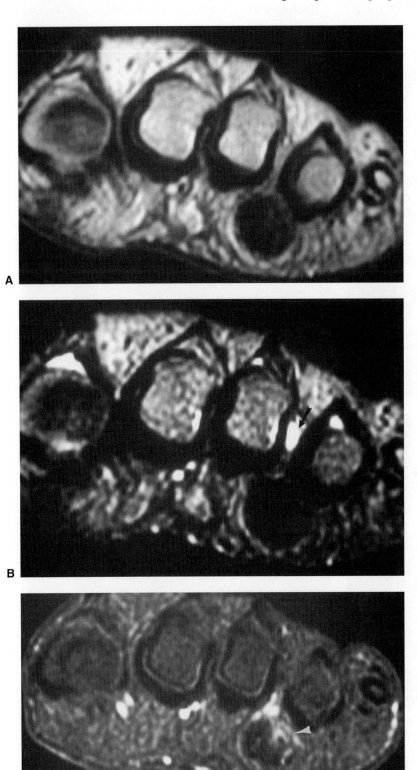

FIG. 6-52. Morton's neuroma. Axial SE 500/11 (**A**) and SE 2000/80 (**B**) images show a large plantar mass. The bursa (*arrow*) is clearly different in location and appearance compared with the neuroma. Fat-suppressed T1-weighted postgadolinium image (**C**) demonstrates irregular peripheral enhancement of the lesion (*arrowhead*).

Malignant nerve sheath tumors are rare and are usually associated with neurofibromatosis. Although malignant lesions are reported in 10 to 25% of patients with neurofibromatosis, the lesion is rare in the foot.[24,35]

Morton's neuroma is a pseudotumor of the interdigital nerve.[59,87,88] The lesion is considered traumatic and is believed to be related to repetitive traumic compressing of the nerve against the transverse intermetatarsal ligament.[6,87,88] Patients usually complain of pain and numbness in the forefoot that is increased with walking or standing and is relieved by rest.[55,87,88] Differential diagnosis clinically includes avascular necrosis, ischemic disease, capsulitis, bursitis, and foreign body.[54]

MRI is the technique of choice when imaging of these neural lesions is required.[6] Schwannomas are generally round or oval with low intensity on T1-weighted images and high intensity on T2-weighted images (see Fig. 6-44).[6] Neurofibromas may have a similar appearance or may have mixed signal intensity because of the fibrous tissue intermixed with neural tissue. Morton's neuromas are located on the plantar aspect of the transverse ligament. These lesions are often small, but they can be identified on T1-weighted images because of the adjacent high-signal-intensity fat. Signal intensity on T2-weighted images may also be low. Gadolinium enhancement patterns are not uniform. Morton's neuromas are easily differentiated from fluid-filled bursae, which are located dorsal to the ligament. Fluid-filled bursae

have high signal intensity on T2-weighted sequences (Fig. 6-52).[6,87,88]

Sarcomas

Soft tissue malignancies are uncommon in the foot. In addition, MRI features are less histologically specific. Therefore, we can discuss these lesions as a group.[6,24,39] Certain lesions, such as liposarcoma, fibrosarcoma, and malignant schwannoma, were noted earlier.[24] Other soft tissue sarcomas in the foot and ankle include rhabdomyosarcoma, leiomyosarcoma, malignant fibrous histiocytoma, and synovial sarcoma. Synovial sarcoma deserves further discussion because of its MRI appearance.[6,9] This lesion accounts for 10% of all malignant primary soft tissue tumors.[24] Most occur in the lower extremity, and most are extraarticular occurring along fascial planes near joints. Most lesions are slow growing and therefore may be mistaken for a benign process.[24,47,59,73]

Routine radiographs may be normal, or a soft tissue mass may be visible. Soft tissue calcification may be present in up to 33% and adjacent bone involvement in 11 to 20%.[24,47,59,73] MRI is useful to evaluate the extent of involvement and to stage the lesion.[6] However, in some cases, the lesion may mimic a benign cyst or ganglion because of its cystic appearance (see Fig. 6-31; Figs. 6-53 and 6-54). Therefore, small lesions could be confused with a benign process.[6,59]

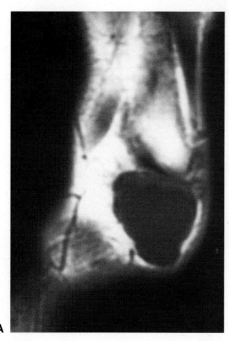

A

FIG. 6-53. Benign ganglion cyst. Sagittal T1-weighted (**A**) and axial proton-density (**B**) and T2-weighted SE (**C**) images demonstrate a well-defined homogeneous lesion consistent with a cyst.

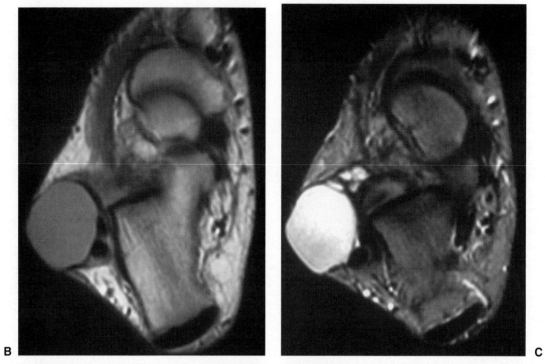

FIG. 6-53. Continued.

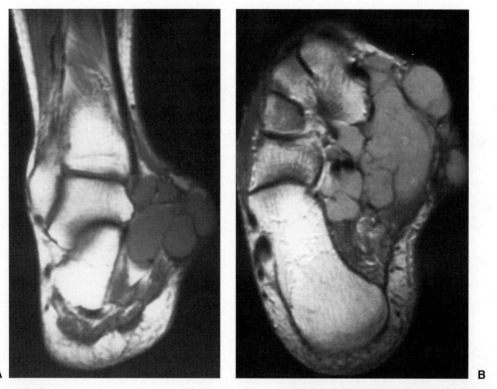

FIG. 6-54. Synovial sarcoma. Coronal SE 500/11 (A) and axial SE 2000/20 (B) images demonstrate a large multicystic or septated lesion. (Note the similarity in signal intensity compared with Fig. 6-53B.)

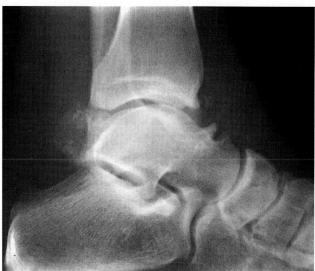

FIG. 6-55. Synovial osteochondromatosis. Lateral view of the ankle demonstrates numerous small calcific densities within the joint capsule in the absence of osteoarthritis.

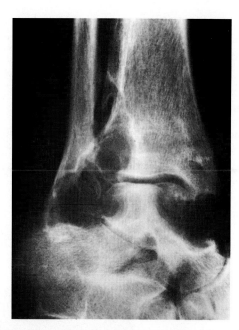

FIG. 6-57. Pigmented villonodular synovitis of the ankle. AP view of the ankle shows multiple bone erosions on both sides of the joint and all within the joint capsule.

JOINT LESIONS

Synovial Chondromatosis

Synovial chondromatosis (Figs. 6-55 and 6-56) is a rare condition in which cartilaginous bodies are produced via metaplasia of the synovium.[55] This monoarticular process may affect any joint, but it is especially common in the knee, elbow, hip, and shoulder. Usually, the diagnosis is readily

suggested from the radiographic appearance, which shows from one to innumerable round calcific densities within the joint capsule. If the cartilage bodies are uncalcified, the radiograph may be normal. If this is the case, arthrography (conventional or CT) may be useful. Subtle changes may be

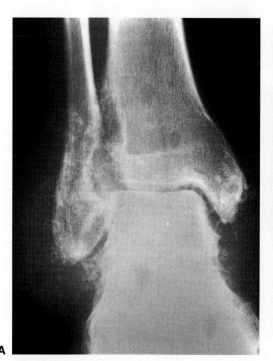
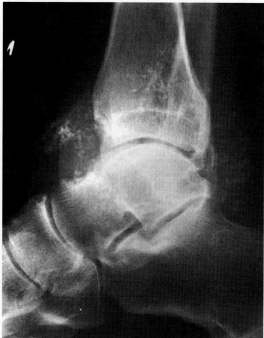

FIG. 6-56. Synovial osteochondromatosis of ankle. In addition to typical numerous intracapsular densities, multiple erosions of the tibia, fibula, and talus are seen on the AP (A) and lateral (B) radiographs.

difficult to detect with MRI unless intraarticular contrast is used. Erosion of adjacent bone may occur.[63] Surgical removal is the preferred treatment.

Pigmented Villonodular Synovitis

Pigmented villonodular synovitis is a benign inflammatory process of unknown cause. It is a monoarticular process that may be seen in any joint, although 80% of cases involve the knee. The fingers, ankle, hip, wrist, and shoulder may also be involved. Radiographically, one sees localized erosive changes of bone on either side of the joint (Fig. 6-57).[22,31] In more advanced change, there is loss of articular cartilage, along with bone destruction and cysts.[1] In some cases, the only finding is that of fluid or synovitis of the joint. The synovial masses do not calcify, but hemosiderin deposition is common and is practically diagnostic. Such deposition may be seen as areas of hazy, high density on CT (Fig. 6-58).

MRI features of pigmented villonodular synovitis are often distinctive. On T1-weighted images, one sees areas of low or intermediate signal intensity. Areas of intermediate and low intensity are also seen on T2-weighted images (Fig. 6-59). Image changes, similar to those seen in giant cell tumors of the tendon sheath, are believed to be related to hemosiderin deposition with preferential shortening of T2 relaxation times.[6]

Surgery is the treatment of choice. Recurrence rates are high (50%) (Fig. 6-60).

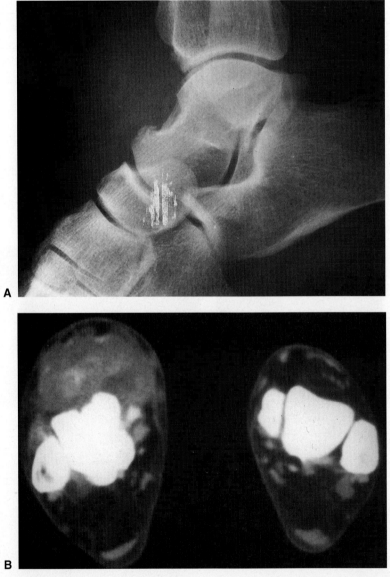

FIG. 6-58. Pigmented villonodular synovitis of the ankle seen on the lateral radiograph (**A**) and CT (**B**). Note erosion of the dorsal aspect of the talus, with a soft tissue mass containing faintly radiodense deposits of hemosiderin. These deposits are common, but actual calcification does not occur.

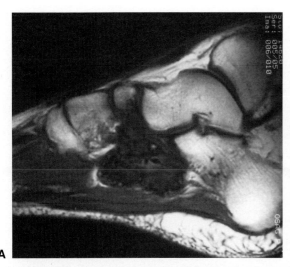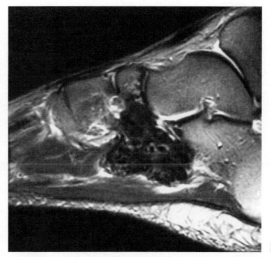

FIG. 6-59. Pigmented villonodular synovitis of the midfoot. Sagittal SE 500/11 (**A**) and SE 2000/60 (**B**) images show a large, irregular low-intensity mass.

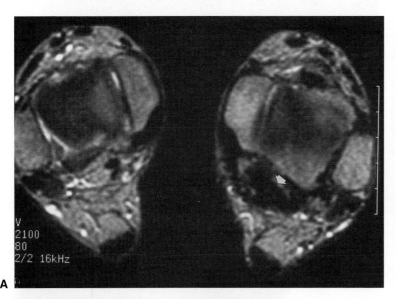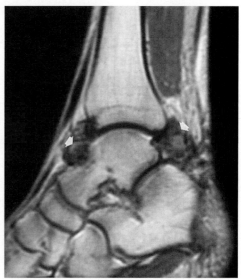

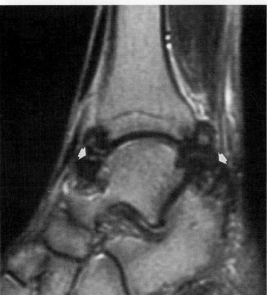

FIG. 6-60. Recurrent pigmented villonodular synovitis (PVNS). Axial SE 2000/60 (**A**) and sagittal SE 2000/20 (**B**) and 2000/80 (**C**) images preoperatively show PVNS involving the ankle (*arrows*). *(continued)*

354 / CHAPTER 6

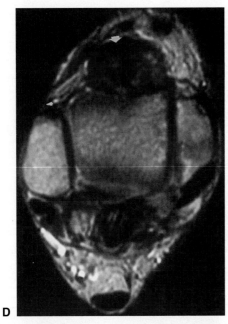
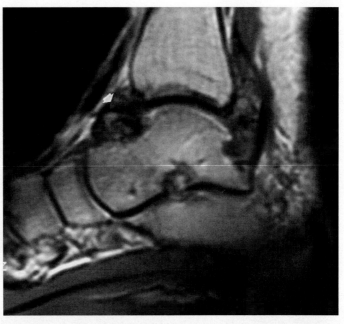

FIG. 6-60. *Continued.* One year later, there is recurrent tumor with more prominent anterior involvement (*arrow*) shown on axial (**D**) and sagittal (**E**) SE 2000/80 images.

REFERENCES

1. Abrahams TG, Pavlov H, Bansal M, Bullough P. Concentric joint space narrowing of the hip associated with hemosiderotic synovitis (HS) including pigmented villonodular synovitis (PVNS). Skeletal Radiol. 1988; 17:37–45.
2. Aisen AM, Martel W, Braunstein EM, McMillin KI, Phillips WA, Kling TF. MRI and CT evaluation of primary bone and soft-tissue tumors. AJR Am. J. Roentgenol. 1986; 146:749–756.
3. Antonijevic N, Radosevic-Radohovic N, Colovic M, Joronovick V, Rolovic Z. Multifocal plasmacytoma of hand and foot bones. Leuk Lymphoma 1996; 21:505–507.
4. Baran R, Tosti A. Metastatic carcinoma of the terminal phalanx of the big toe. Report of 2 cases and review of the literature. J. Am. Acad. Dermatol. 1994; 31:259–263.
5. Baron RL, Galinski AW, Vlahos M, Heiring M. Chondromyxoid fibroma. J. Am. Podiatr. Med. Assoc. 1996; 86(5):212–216.
6. Berquist TH. MRI of the Musculoskeletal System. 3rd Ed. Philadelphia, Lippincott–Raven, 1996.
7. Biscaglia R, Gasbarrini A, Böhling T, Bacchini P, Bertoni F, Picci P. Osteosarcoma of the bones of the foot. An easily misdiagnosed malignant tumor. Mayo Clin. Proc. 1998; 73:842–847.
8. Bloem JL, Falke THM, Taminiau AHM, Doornbos J, Van Oosterom AT, Steinerj RM, Overbosch EEH, Ziedses des Plantes BG Jr. Magnetic resonance imaging of primary malignant bone tumors. Radiographics 1985; 5:853–886.
9. Borg AA, Wynn-Jones C, Dawes PT. Synovial sarcoma manifesting as a single joint flair of rheumatoid arthritis. Clin. Rheumatol. 1993; 12:89–92.
10. Brien EW, Mirra JM, Kerr R. Benign and malignant cartilage tumors of bone and joint. Their anatomic and theoretical basis with emphasis on radiology, pathology, and clinical biology. The intramedullary cartilage tumors. Skeletal Radiol. 1997; 26:325–353.
11. Casadei R, Ruggieri P, Guseppe T, Biagini R, Mercuri M. Ankle resection arthrodesis in patients with bone tumors. Foot Ankle Int. 1994; 15(5):242–249.
12. Chang JL, Ireland ML. Osteoid osteoma of the os calcis in a teenage athlete. Med. Sci. Sports Exer. 1993; 25(1):2–8.
13. Chore LB, Malawer MM. Analysis of surgical treatment of 33 foot and ankle tumors. Foot Ankle Int. 1994; 15(4):175–181.
14. Cohen EK, Kressel HY, Perosio T, Burk DL, Dalinka MK, Kanal E, Schieber ML, Fallon MD. MR imaging of soft tissue hemangiomas. Correlation with pathologic findings. AJR Am. J. Roentgenol. 1988; 150:1079–1081.
15. Dahlin DC. Giant cell tumor of bone. Highlights of 407 cases. AJR Am. J. Roentgenol. 1985; 144:955–960.
16. Dahlin DC, Unni KK. Bone Tumors: General Aspects and Data on 8,542 Cases. Springfield, IL, Charles C Thomas, 1986.
17. Dahlin DC, Unni KK. Osteosarcoma of bone and its important recognizable varieties. Am. J. Surg. Pathol. 1977; 1:6172.
18. Delsmann BM, Pfahler M, Nerlick A, Refior HJ. Primary leiomyosarcoma affecting the ankle joint. Foot Ankle Int. 1996; 17(7):420–424.
19. dePalma L, Gigante A, Specchia N. Subungual exostosis of the foot. Foot Ankle Int. 1996; 17(12):758–763.
20. Dokter G, Linclau LA. The accessory soleus muscle. Symptomatic soft tissue tumor or accidental finding. Neth. J. Surg. 1981; 33(3):146–149.
21. Dooms GC, Hricak H, Sollitto RA, Higgins CB. Lipomatous tumors and tumors with fatty component. MR imaging potential and comparison of MR and CT results. Radiology 1985; 157:479–483.
22. Dorwart RH, Genant HK, Johnston WH, Morris JM. Pigmented villonodular synovitis of synovial joints. Clinical, pathologic, and radiologic features. AJR Am. J. Roentgenol. 1984; 143:877–885.
23. Enneking WF. Musculoskeletal Tumor Surgery. New York, Churchill Livingstone, 1983.
24. Enzinger FM, Weiss SW. Soft Tissue Tumors. St. Louis, C.V. Mosby, 1983.
25. Erlermann R, Reiser WF, Peters PF, Vasallo P, Nommensen B, Kusnierz-Glaz CR, Ritter J, Roessner A. Musculoskeletal neoplasms. Static and dynamic Gd-DTPA–enhanced MR imaging. Radiology 1989; 171:767–773.
26. Feld R, Burg DL, McCue P, Mitchell DG, Lackman R, Rifkin MD. MRI of aggressive fibromatosis. Frequent appearance of high signal on T2-weighted images. Magn. Reson. Imaging 1990; 8:583–588.
27. Fink BR, Temple T, Chiricosta FM, Mizel MS, Murphey MD. Chondroblastoma of the foot. Foot Ankle Int. 1997; 18(4):236–242.
28. Fox IM. Intraosseous lipoma of the 5th metatarsal. J. Foot Ankle Surg. 1994; 33(2):138–140.
29. Fraipont MJ, Thordarson DB. Aneurysmal bone cyst of the navicular. A case report and review of the literature. Foot Ankle Int. 1996; 17(11):709–711.
30. Glochenberg A, Sobel E, Noel JF. Nonossifying fibroma. Four cases

and a review of the literature. J. Am. Podiatr. Med. Assoc. 1997; 87(2): 66–69.

31. Goldberg RP, Weissman BN, Naimark A, Braunstein E. Femoral neck erosions. Sign of hip joint synovial disease. AJR Am. J. Roentgenol. 1983; 141:107–111.

32. Hartman TE, Berquist TH, Fetsch JF. MR imaging of extra-abdominal desmoids. Differentiation from other neoplasms. AJR Am. J. Roentgenol. 1992; 158:581–585.

33. Hudson J, Cobby M, Yates P, Watt I. Extensive infiltration of bone with marrow necrosis in a case of hairy cell leukemia. Skeletal Radiol. 1995; 24:228–231.

34. Hudson TM, Hamlin DJ, Enneking WF, Pettersson H. Magnetic resonance imaging of bone and soft tissue tumors. Early experience in 31 patients compared with computed tomography. Skeletal Radiol. 1985; 13:134–146.

35. Johnston MR. Epidemiology of soft-tissue and bone tumors of the foot. Clin. Podiatr. Med. Surg. 1993; 10(4):581–607.

36. Kaplan PA, Murphe M, Greenway G, Resnick D, Sartoris DJ, Harms S. Fluid levels in giant cell tumors of bone. A report of 2 cases. J. Comput. Tomogr. 1987; 11:151–155.

37. Kiegley BA, Haggar AM, Gaba A, Ellis BI, Froelich JW, Wei KK. Primary tumors of the foot. MR imaging. Radiology 1989; 171: 755–759.

38. Kier R. MR imaging of foot and ankle tumors. Magn. Reson. Imaging 1993; 11:149–162.

39. Kirby EJ, Shereff MJ, Lewis MM. Soft-tissue tumors and tumor-like lesions of the foot. Analysis of eighty-three cases. J. Bone Joint Surg. Am. 1989; 71:621–626.

40. Kumar R, David R, Madewell JE, Lindell MM Jr. Radiographic spectrum of osteogenic sarcoma. AJR Am. J. Roentgenol. 1987; 148: 767–772.

41. Leonheart EE, DiStazio J. Acrometastasis. J. Am. Podiatr. Med. Assoc. 1994; 84(12):625–627.

42. Levey DS, Park Y-H, Sartoris DJ, Resnick D. Imaging methods for assessment of pedal soft-tissue neoplasms. Clin. Podiatr. Med. Surg. 1993; 10(4):617–632.

43. Levey DS, Sartoris DJ, Resnick D. Advanced diagnostic imaging techniques for pedal osseous neoplasms. Clin. Podiatr. Med. Surg. 1993; 10(4):655–682.

44. Lukens JA, McLeod RA, Sim FH. Computed tomographic evaluation of primary osseous malignant neoplasms. AJR Am. J. Roentgenol. 1982; 139:45–48.

45. Mald, McCarthy EF, Bluemke DA, Frassica FJ. Differentiation of benign from malignant musculoskeletal lesions using MR imaging. Pitfalls in MR evaluation of lesions with cystic appearance. AJR Am. J. Roentgenol. 1998; 170:1251–1258.

46. Mahajan H, Kern EE, Waleace S, Abello R, Benjamin R, Evans HL. Magnetic resonance imaging of malignant fibrous histiocytoma. Magn. Reson. Imaging 1989; 7:283–288.

47. Mahajan H, Lorigan JG, Shuklauda A. Synovial sarcoma, MR imaging. Magn. Reson. Imaging 1989; 7:211–216.

48. Math KR, Pavlov H, DiCarlo E, Bohne WAO. Spindle cell lipoma of the foot. A case report and review of the literature. Foot Ankle Int. 1995; 16(4):220–226.

49. McLeod RA. Chondrosarcoma. In Taveras JM, Ferucci JT, eds. Radiology. Diagnosis, Imaging, Intervention. Vol. 5. Philadelphia, J.B. Lippincott, 1986; pp. 1–12.

50. McLeod RA, Beabout JW. The roentgenographic features of chondroblastoma. AJR Am. J. Roentgenol. 1973; 118:464–471.

51. McLeod RA, Berquist TH. Bone tumor imaging: contribution of CT and MRI. In Unni KK, ed. Bone Tumors. New York, Churchill Livingstone, 1988; pp. 1–34.

52. McLeod RA, Dahlin DC, Beabout JW. The spectrum of osteoblastoma. AJR Am. J. Roentgenol. 1976; 126:321–335.

53. McLeod RA, Stephens DH, Beabout JW, Sheedy PF III, Hattery RR. Computed tomography of the skeletal system. Semin. Roentgenol. 1978; 13:235–247.

54. Mendicino SS, Rochett MS. Morton's neuroma. Update and imaging. Clin. Podiatr. Med. Surg. 1997; 14:303–311.

55. Milgram JW. Synovial osteochondromatosis. A histopathological study of thirty cases. J. Bone Joint Surg. Am. 1977; 59:792–801.

56. Mirra JM, Bullough PG, Marcove RC, Jacobs B, Havos AG. Malignant fibrous histiocytoma and osteosarcoma in association with bone infarcts. J.Bone Joint Surg. Am. 1979; 56:932–940.

57. Mirra J, Picci P, Gold R. Bone Tumors. Clinical, Radiological, Pathological Correlation. Philadelphia, Lea & Febiger, 1989.

58. Morrison WB, Schweitzer ME, Wapner KL, Lackman RD. Plantar fibromatosis: a benign aggressive neoplasm with characteristic appearance on MR images. Radiology 1994; 193:841–845.

59. Morton MJ, Berquist TH, McLeod RA, Unni KK, Sim FH. MR imaging of synovial sarcoma. AJR Am. J. Roentgenol. 1991; 156: 337–340.

60. Moser RP Jr, Sweet DE, Haseman DB, Madewell JE. Multiple skeletal fibroxanthomas. Radiologic–pathologic correlation of 72 cases. Skeletal Radiol. 1987; 16:353–359.

61. Munk PL, Lee MJ, Janzen DL, Connell DG, Logan RM, Poon PY, Bainbridge TC. Lipoma and liposarcoma. Evaluation using CT and MR imaging. AJR Am. J. Roentgenol. 1997; 169:589–594.

62. Nora FE, Dahlin DC, Beabout JW. Bizarre parosteal osteochondromatous proliferations of the hands and feet. Am. J. Surg. Pathol. 1983; 7:245250.

63. Norman A, Steiner GC. Bone erosion in synovial chondromatosis. Radiology 1986; 161:749–752.

64. O'Connor PJ, Gibson WW, Hardy G, Butt WP. Chondromyxoid fibroma of the foot. Skeletal Radiol. 1996; 25:143–148.

65. O'Keefe RJ, O'Donnell RJ, Temple T, Scully SP, Mankin HJ. Giant cell tumor of bone in the foot and ankle. Foot Ankle Int. 1995; 16(10): 617–623.

66. Ontell F, Greenopan A. Chondrosarcoma complicating synovial chondromatosis. Findings with magnetic resonance imaging. Can. Assoc. Radiol. J. 1994; 45(4):318–323.

67. Panicek DM, Go SD, Healey JH, Leung DHY, Brennan MF, Lewis JJ. Soft-tissue sarcoma involving bone or neurovascular structures. MR imaging prognostic factors. Radiology 1997; 205:871–875.

68. Posteraro RH. Radiographic evaluation of pedal osseous tumors. Clin. Podiatr. Med. Surg. 1993; 10(4):633–653.

69. Rahimi A, Beabout JW, Ivins JC, Dahlin DC. Chondromyxoid fibroma. A clinicopathologic study of 76 cases. Cancer 1972; 30:726–736.

70. Reinus WR, Gilula LA. IESS Committee. Radiology of Ewing's sarcoma. Intergroup Ewing's sarcoma study (IESS). Radiographics 1984; 4:929–944.

71. Reinus WR, Gilula LA, Shirley SK, Askin FB, Siegal GP. Radiographic appearance of Ewing sarcoma of the hands and feet. Report from the intergroup Ewing sarcoma study. AJR Am. J. Roentgenol. 1985; 144: 331–336.

72. Resnick RB, Jarolem KL, Sheskier SC, Desai P, Cisa J. Arthroscopic removal of osteoidosteoma of the talus. A case report. Foot Ankle Int. 1995; 16(4):212–215.

73. Sanchez-Reyes JM, Mexia MA, Tapia DQ, Arambru JA. Extensively calcified synovial sarcoma. Skeletal Radiol. 1997; 26:671–673.

74. Sans M, Nubiola D, Alejo M, Diaz F, Anglada A, Antonell J, Bragues J. Mesenchymal chondrosarcoma of the foot, an unusual location. Case report and review of the literature. Med. Pediatr. Oncol. 1996; 26: 139–142.

75. Scarborough MT, Helmstedter CS. Arthrodesis after resection of bone tumors. Semin. Surg. Oncol. 1997; 13:25–33.

76. Sella EJ, Chrostowski JH. Calcaneal osteochondromas. Orthopedics 1995; 18(6):573–574.

77. Shereff MJ, Cullivan OPA, Johnson KA. Osteoid-osteoma of the foot. J. Bone Joint Surg. Am. 1983; 65:638–641.

78. Snow SW, Sobel M, DiCarlo EF, Thompson FM, Deland JT. Chronic ankle pain caused by osteoid osteoma of the neck of the talus. Foot Ankle Int. 1997; 18(2):98–106.

79. Swee RG, McLeod RA, Beabout JW. Osteoid osteoma. Detection, diagnosis, and localization. Radiology 1979; 130:117–123.

80. Taconis WK, Mulder JD. Fibrosarcoma and malignant fibrous histiocytoma of long bones. Radiographic features and grading. Skeletal Radiol. 1984; 11:237–245.

81. Tamburri SA, Boberg JS. Skeletally metastatic malignant melanoma of the foot. J. Foot Ankle Surg. 1994; 33(4):368–372.

82. Unni KK, Dahlin DC, Beabout JW, Ivins JC. Adamantinomas of long bones. Cancer 1974; 34:1796–1805.

83. Walling AK, Gasser SI. Soft-tissue and bone tumors about the foot and ankle. Clin. Sports Med. 1994; 13(4):909–938.

84. Williams RP, Pechero G. Management of soft-tissue and bone tumors of the foot. Clin. Podiatr. Med. Surg. 1993; 10(4):717–725.

85. Wold LE, Unni KK, Beabout JW, Ivins JC, Bruckman JE, Dahlin DC. Hemangioendothelial sarcoma of bone. Am. J. Surg. Pathol. 1982; 6: 59–70.

86. Wu KK. Differential diagnosis of pedal osseous neoplasms. Clin. Podiatr. Med. Surg. 1993; 10(4):683–715.

87. Zanetti M, Ledermann T, Zollinger H, Hodler J. Efficacy of MR imaging in patients suspected of having Morton's neuroma. AJR Am. J. Roentgenol. 1997; 168:529–532.

88. Zanetti M, Strehle JK, Hollinger H, Hodler J. Morton neuroma and fluid in the intermetatarsal bursae on MR images of 70 asymptomatic volunteers. Radiology 1997; 203:516–520.

89. Zimmer WD, Berquist TH, McLeod RA, Sim FH, Pritchard DJ, Shives TC, Wold LE, May GR. Bone tumors. Magnetic resonance imaging versus computed tomography. Radiology 1985; 155:709–718.

Radiology of the Foot and Ankle, Second Edition,
edited by Thomas H. Berquist.
© 2000 by Mayo Foundation.
Published by Lippincott Williams & Wilkins, Philadelphia.

CHAPTER 7

Infection

Thomas H. Berquist

Infections of the foot and ankle can occur at any age. Clinical presentation varies with the patient's age, clinical status (i.e., diabetes mellitus, immunosuppression, debilitating disease, postoperative status), location of infection, and type of organism.[1,28,31,171,172] Symptoms may have an abrupt onset or a more chronic or subacute course leading to diagnostic and therapeutic challenges for clinicians and radiologists.

Infections are usually bacterial, but fungal, viral, and parasitic infections may also occur. Infections are usually categorized by site. Osteomyelitis involves the bone, septic arthritis the joints, infectious tendinitis the tendon and tendon sheath, and cellulitis the subcutaneous tissues.[27] Deep soft tissue infection may be severe, resulting in necrotizing fasciitis.[154,160,179] Bursae may also become infected (septic bursitis).[27]

Infections occur by three routes: (1) direct implantation, such as a puncture wound or surgery; (2) hematogenous spread; and (3) spread from a contiguous source such as a diabetic ulcer.[27,36,97,145] Imaging techniques provide valuable information regarding the extent of involvement (e.g., bone, soft tissue, tendon sheath). The value of each technique differs, depending on the type of infection suspected. Table 7-1 provides examples of advantages of common imaging procedures used to evaluate infection.

This discussion considers each category of infection separately. Bone, soft tissue, and joint involvement are discussed separately. The final section of this chapter is devoted to infections in the diabetic foot.

OSTEOMYELITIS

The term "osteomyelitis" is reserved for infections involving bone. This term is generally applied to infections whether cortex, marrow, or periosteum is involved. Resnick and Niwayama[145] further categorized infection describing cortical infection as suppurative periostitis. Sclerosing

T. H. Berquist: Mayo Medical School, Mayo Clinic Jacksonville, Jacksonville, Florida 32224; Mayo Foundation, Mayo Clinic, Rochester, Minnesota 55905.

TABLE 7-1. *Imaging of foot and ankle infections*[a]

Technique	Applications
Computed tomography	Subtle cortical bone destruction Cloacae Sequestra Gas in soft tissues
MRI	Early/subtle changes in marrow, soft tissue, tendon sheaths, bursae, and fascia
Ultrasound	Fluid collections or abscesses in soft tissue Joint fluid
Radionuclide scans (^{99m}Tc, ^{67}Ga, ^{111}In WBC)	Early bone involvement Subtle postoperative infections

[a] Data from references 3, 19, 41, 56, 86, 116, and 145.

(Garré's sclerosing osteomyelitis) osteomyelitis is a term applied to infections that lead to extensive periosteal new bone formation with minimal suppuration.[129,145] Brodie's abscess is a localized nidus of infection surrounded by dense bony reaction.[25,73,119]

Osteomyelitis may develop by several routes of contamination. These mechanisms include (1) trauma or penetrating wounds leading to direct contamination, (2) direct bone involvement resulting from spread from a local soft tissue infection, (3) hematogenous osteomyelitis from organisms reaching bone via the circulation, or (4) contamination from surgical procedures.[27,145] In the foot, the most common mechanism is trauma, which may lead to direct bone involvement or soft tissue infection and subsequent osteomyelitis.[25,27,36,97]

Hematogenous Osteomyelitis

The calcaneus is the most commonly affected bone in the foot. The other tarsal bones and metatarsals are involved less frequently.[50,132,138,145,148] Hematogenous osteomyelitis is most common in children and older adults. Traditionally, hematogenous osteomyelitis has been categorized according to age group (infants, children, and adults) because of differences in clinical and radiographic features.[19,21,35,39,42,50,52,135,145,163] The degree of periosteal attachment, vascular anatomy, and variations in the growth plate have a significant impact on the nature of osteomyelitis in these different age groups.[27,50,111,117,157,162,163]

In infants (less than 1 year of age), vessels in the long bones extend beyond the undeveloped growth plate into the epiphysis. The vessels terminate in the venous lakes similar to the sinusoids in the metaphyseal region of children[145,157,163,168] (Fig. 7-1). This vascular pattern accounts, in part, for the higher evidence of epiphyseal and joint space infections in infants with osteomyelitis. If the diagnosis is not established, abnormalities in the growth plate can lead to deformity or cessation of growth.[145] The periosteum is also more loosely attached in infants. Therefore, infections easily elevate and penetrate the periosteum leading to more frequent soft tissue infection and striking periosteal changes on radiographs.[27,145,162]

Metaphyseal and diaphyseal vascular patterns change with development and evolution of the physis (1 to 16 or more years). During this period, the growth plate separates the metaphyseal and epiphyseal blood supply. The metaphyseal vessels in the child are tortuous and form venous lakes in the medullary portion of the metaphysis. Flow rates are reduced in the metaphysis, thus making this region of bone most susceptible to infection.[19,33,124,168] Similar metaphyseal equivalent infections occur near the cartilage in flat and nontubular bones (scapula, ilium, clavicle, calcaneus) in children.[132] Vascular anatomy in these regions is similar to the metaphysis of long bones. Nearly 25% of childhood infections occur in metaphyseal equivalent sites of nontubular bones.[27,72,145]

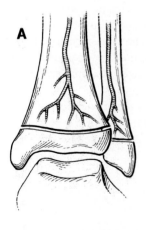
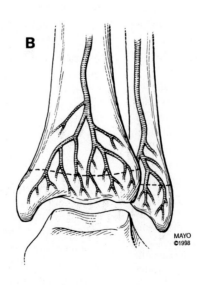

FIG. 7-1. Illustrations demonstrating vascular patterns at the metaphyseal epiphyseal junction in a child (**A**) and adult (**B**).

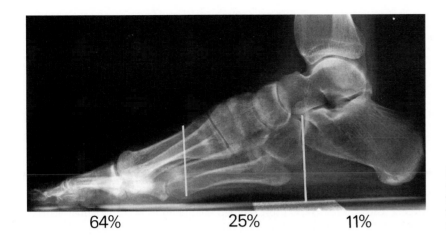

64%   25%   11%

FIG. 7-2. Lateral radiograph of the foot demonstrating the zones of the foot where puncture wounds occur: forefoot (metatarsal necks to toes), midfoot (calcaneal joint to metatarsal necks), and heel (subcalcaneal region).

The adult vascular pattern evolves with closure of the growth plate (see Fig. 7-1B). The metaphyseal vessels enter the epiphysis, thereby allowing infection to involve this region of bone and, more frequently, to enter the adjacent joint space. Periosteum in the adult is more firmly attached, so elevation is more subtle than in children. Infection is more likely to spread along the medullary space. In adults, the spine and bones of the feet are common sites of osteomyelitis.[145,163,168] Clinically, hematogenous osteomyelitis tends to present with a more abrupt onset (fever, local swelling, limp or reduced motion in the involved joint) in children.[24,25,117,122,124] Involvement of multiple sites is more common in infants. In adults, symptoms are often more subtle and only affect one site. Bacteria, mycobacteria, fungi, and viral organisms can all be involved. *Staphylococcus aureus* is commonly implicated in children and adults, and group B streptococcal organisms are found in infants.[8,9]

Osteomyelitis Secondary to Local Extension

Direct extension of soft tissue infection into adjacent bone or joint structures occurs most commonly in the skull, facial bones, and peripheral extremities.[92,163,165] Initial soft tissue infections may be secondary to burns, penetrating trauma, or soft tissue ulceration and necrosis from diabetes mellitus and ischemic disease.[53,63,92]

Infections resulting from puncture wounds in the plantar aspect of the foot are particularly common.[98,99,163,173] Most injuries occur in the barefoot child.[97,120] About 1% of emergency room visits are related to puncture wounds. Up to 15% of these injuries result in infection. Most puncture wounds involve the forefoot (64%), with 25% occurring in the midfoot and 11% in the heel or hindfoot (Fig. 7-2).[97] Punctures are usually due to nails (80%), needles (7%), wood slivers (4%), and glass (2%).[86,97] Organisms common in the soil, such as *Pseudomonas aeruginosa,* are commonly isolated.[163,167] Soft tissue infection is due to *S. aureus* or *S. epidermidis* in 75% of cases. *P. aerginosa* accounts for only 16% of soft tissue infections but most commonly involves bone.[97] These wounds lead to soft tissue infection with os-

teomyelitis or joint space infections occurring because of direct extension of the soft tissue process. Osteomyelitis in the calcaneus from heel puncture (blood tests) in infants has been reported.[26]

Frostbite, burns, and other forms of ischemic disease can also affect the soft tissues. Necrotic tissue easily becomes infected. Extension to bone can occur if the condition is not properly treated.[145,163]

Spread of infection in the soft tissues tends to follow the medial, intermediate, or lateral tissue compartments (Fig. 7-3). These divisions are created by fibrous septa arising from the plantar aponeurosis.[75,152] The greatest potential space exists in the intermediate or central compartment (see Fig. 7-3). Direct contamination to the medial compartment or

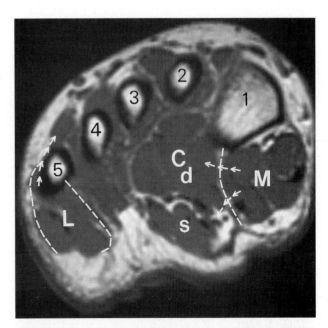

FIG. 7-3. Axial SE 500/11 MRI of the foot demonstrating the compartments and direction infections spread (*arrows*). *1–5,* metatarsals; *M,* medial compartment; *C,* central (intermediate) compartment with deep (*d*) and superficial (*s*) sections; *L,* lateral compartment.

TABLE 7-2. *Plantar compartments of the foot*[a]

Compartment	Anatomic Contents
Medial	Adductor hallucis, flexor hallucis brevis and flexor hallucis longus tendon
Lateral	Flexor digiti minimi, abductor digiti minimi
Central	Flexor digitorum brevis, flexor digitorum longus tendons, quadradus plantae, lumbrical muscles, adductor hallucis

[a] Data from references 75 and 152.

the lower leg via the flexor hallucis longus can occur.[145] Extension from an infection in the lateral compartment usually enters the dorsal soft tissues of the foot (see Fig. 7-3). Medial compartment extension tends to decompress into the intermediate compartment.[75,145] Table 7-2 summarizes the contents and anatomy of the plantar compartments of the foot. The central (intermediate) compartment (see Fig. 7-3) is divided by transverse fascia into deep (adductor hallucis muscle) and superficial compartments.

Osteomyelitis resulting from local soft tissue infection in diabetic patients presents a more complex problem.[171,172] Waldvogel and Popageogion[172] noted that 33% of their patients with osteomyelitis had diabetes. Osteomyelitis was most frequently noted in the phalanges and peripheral joints of the foot. Most patients were 50 to 70 years old. Greenwood[79] noted histories of infection in 25% of diabetic patientss, with 10% of diabetic patients presenting with active infection at any given time. Infections tended to develop at pressure points (metatarsal heads and heel), where ischemic changes are more advanced.

Osteomyelitis in Violated Bone

Osteomyelitis may develop following surgical procedures, deep puncture wounds that directly involve bone, or open fractures. Diagnoses in these settings may be particularly difficult because of soft tissue injury and the presence of distorted bony anatomy.[32] The latter may result from fracture or orthopedic manipulation and the presence of orthopedic fixation devices or prosthesis. This mechanism of contamination is not unlike that of direct puncture or infection from an adjacent source.

Diagnosis

Early detection of osteomyelitis can be difficult. The patient's age, mechanism of contamination, offending organism, previous or current medications, and other factors may affect the clinical and radiographic features of the disease process.[159,162,163,168]

Clinical features of osteomyelitis differ in infants, children, and adults. Infants generally present with swelling and may be unwilling to move the involved extremity. Children (1 to 16 years old) usually present with a more aggressive clinical picture including high fever, localized pain, swell-

ing, and redness over the site of involvement. In adults, symptoms can be subtle. Laboratory studies may reveal an elevated erythrocyte sedimentation rate and leukocytosis, but blood cultures may be negative in up to 50% of patients.[33,79,145]

Radiographic features of osteomyelitis vary with age, clinical setting, and type of technique used. Early diagnosis and treatment are essential to avoid chronic infection and potential complications.

Routine Radiography

The earliest radiographic features of acute hematogenous osteomyelitis are due to soft tissue changes.[32,33] These changes are subtle and may only be evident if comparison views of the uninvolved extremity are obtained. Computed radiographic images are easily manipulated on the imaging work station. Therefore, soft tissues can be more easily evaluated. Swelling of the deep soft tissues adjacent to the involved bone develops 2 to 3 days after the onset of acute hematogenous osteomyelitis. This swelling results in irregularity or displacement of the deep fat planes. Diagnosis at this stage may lead to complete resolution before bone changes develop. As soft tissue involvement progresses, the deep tissue involvement becomes more superficial. This feature is useful in differentiating osteomyelitis from cellulitis. Cellulitis involves the superficial tissues initially and is more commonly noted in infections resulting from puncture wounds. If the infection is not treated, the process progresses to involve the deep tissues, periosteum, cortex, and finally the medullary bone. This is a reversal of the pattern seen with hematogenous osteomyelitis (Fig. 7-4).[145]

Bone changes are not usually evident for 10 to 14 days or until 35 to 50% of the bone has been destroyed.[47,49,145] Bone and periosteal abnormalities vary with patient's age, the type of bone involved, and the organism. There are also subtle differences depending on the clinical presentation (acute, subacute, or chronic). The most common bacterial organism identified in hematogenous osteomyelitis is *S. aureus* (81 to 92% of cases).[145] Beta-hemolytic streptococcal infections are not uncommon in infants.[39,82,113,145] Other organisms are identified less frequently, although pneumococcal, gonococcal, and meningiococcal infections do occur. These organisms and certain of the gram-negative bacteria (*Escherichia coli, P. aeruginosa, Klebsiella,* and *Aerobacter*) are more common in debilitated patients, such as those with alcoholism, diabetes, or hypogammaglobulinemia.[47,53,60,70,82,90,92,103,115,145]

Generally, the radiographic changes resulting from acute osteomyelitis do not allow the causative organism to be identified.[23,29,145] In infants (less than 1 year old), lytic areas appear in the metaphysis of the tubular bones or calcaneus near the tuberosity. Impressive periosteal reaction and soft tissue abscess formation may develop along tubular bones. The latter are due to the loosely attached periosteum in this age group. Joint space involvement is also common because

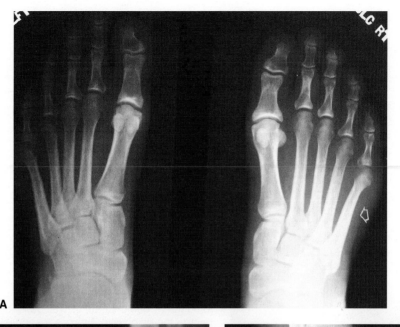

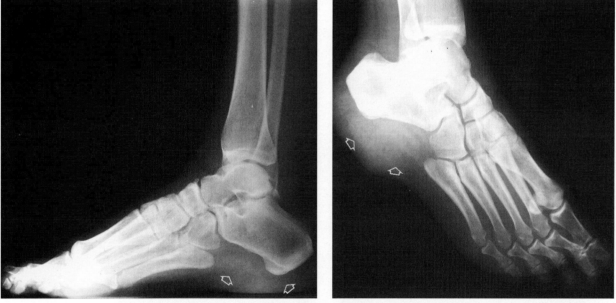

FIG. 7-4. Soft tissue changes due to infected puncture wound. AP (**A**), lateral (**B**), and oblique (**C**) radiographs show soft tissue swelling and increased soft tissue density (*open arrows*). No bone involvement is evident.

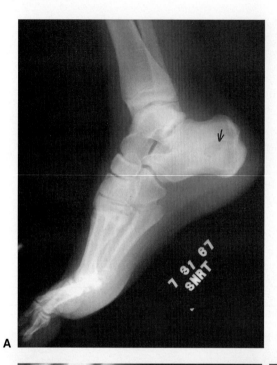

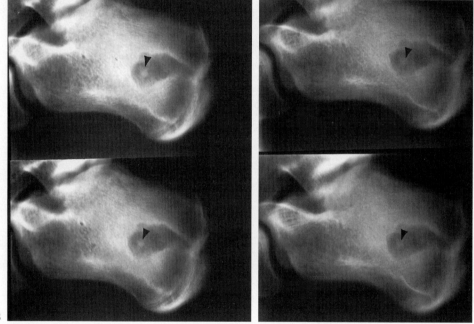

FIG. 7-5. A: Lateral radiograph of the foot demonstrating a lytic area in the posterior calcaneus (*arrow*). **B:** Lateral tomograms demonstrate a well-defined lytic area with a tract to the epiphysis. There is a sequestrum (*arrowhead*) anteriorly.

of the vascular communication between the metaphysis and epiphysis. Sequestra may also be evident. These features are often better demonstrated with conventional computed tomography (Fig. 7-5). Children have similar radiographic features, except the growth plate and vascular anatomy reduce the incidence of epiphyseal and joint space involvement in the foot and ankle (Figs. 7-6 through 7-8).[116,117,119,121–123]

Acute hematogenous osteomyelitis in adults may involve the epiphysis, metaphysis, or diaphysis.[23,27,33,145] Epiphyseal involvement results in more frequent extension into the joint space (Fig. 7-9). Periosteal changes are less obvious because the periosteum is more firmly attached to bone in adults than in infants and children. Progression into cortical and periosteal tissues can lead to soft tissue abscess and fistula formation.[145]

Subacute or chronic osteomyelitis may develop when diagnosis is delayed or the infection is improperly treated. There is no distinct method of separating these categories of infection, although chronic infection is the term applied to infections of more than 6 weeks' duration.[27] Again, radiographic features vary depending on the organism, type of therapy, and presence of other underlying diseases (Figs. 7-

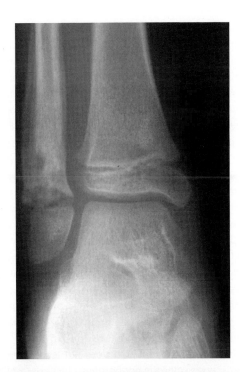

FIG. 7-6. AP view of the ankle in a child with classic osteomyelitis. There are lytic areas in the fibular metaphysis with periosteal new bone formation. The epiphysis is normal.

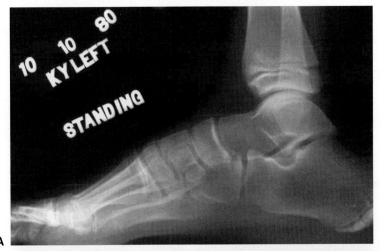

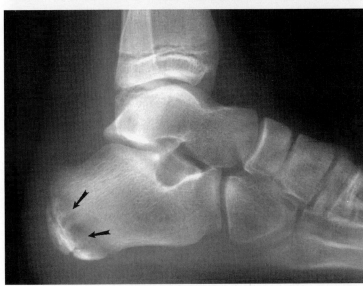

FIG. 7-7. A: Lateral view of the left foot is normal. **B:** Lytic changes (*arrows*) adjacent to the calcaneal growth plate due to osteomyelitis.

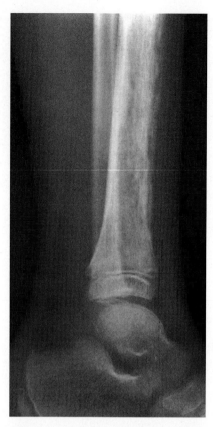

FIG. 7-8. Lateral radiograph of the lower leg demonstrates a permeative pattern in the anterior cortex and marrow from osteomyelitis.

10 through 7-12). The periosteal changes may be extensive, forming a dense involucrum (sclerotic layer of bone usually around sequestra) that surrounds the shaft of tubular bones (see Fig. 7-12). Small perpendicular cortical tunnels or cloacae may be present that result when necrosis extends through the bone. When this occurs, radiographs may demonstrate adjacent abscesses in the soft issues.[28,33] Areas of necrotic or dead bone may also be evident. Radiographically, these sequestra are often more dense than the surrounding osteoporotic or hyperemic bone that surrounds them in the medullary or cortical regions (see Fig. 7-5). This appearance results from devascularization of sequestra, which prevents these islands of bone from participating in the usual hyperemic changes responsible for osteoporosis or lucency in the vascularized bone.[24,33,140] Granulation tissue and suppuration also surround sequestra.[28,145,158] Sequestra are usually not evident for at least 3 weeks, and size variation may make them difficult to identify using conventional radiographs. Conventional tomography and computed tomography (CT) are useful in identification of subtle sequestra (see Fig. 7-5).[20,27,31]

In certain cases, infection does not lead to necrosis, but instead causes sclerotic nonpurulent changes.[145,158] The term Garré's sclerosing osteomyelitis should be used in this setting.[163,169] This type of response is more common in the mandible and long bones of the lower extremity than in the foot (Fig. 7-13).

Localized abscesses (Brodie's abscess) also occur. Patients are usually not systemically ill and often have symptoms for weeks or months. The distal tibia is a common site of involvement. These abscesses are usually due to *S. aureus,*

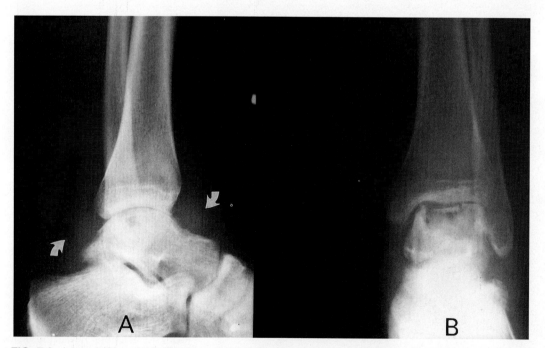

FIG. 7-9. Lateral (**A**) and AP (**B**) views of the ankle demonstrate a large effusion (*curved arrows*) with destructive changes in the talus due to osteomyelitis extending into the joint space.

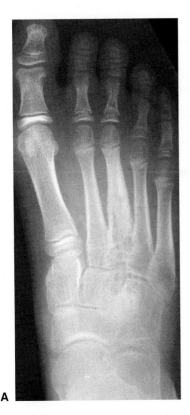

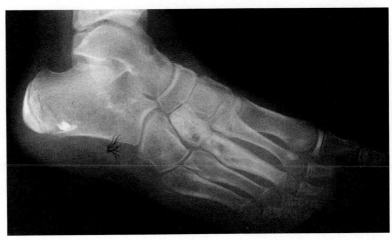

FIG. 7-10. AP (**A**) and oblique (**B**) radiographs demonstrate scleroses and thickening of the cortex and trabeculae of the lateral cuneiform and third metatarsal with loss of joint space due to chronic osteomyelitis and joint space infection.

A

but in up to 50%, no organism can be identified.[32,119] Abscesses are usually metaphyseal (60%), well marginated with dense surrounding sclerosis, and range from 4 mm to 4 cm in size (Fig. 7-14). Central sequestra have been identified in up to 20% of patients.[32,119] When cortical involvement occurs, these lesions present radiographically as a small, lucent nidus surrounded by dense cortical reaction, a feature not

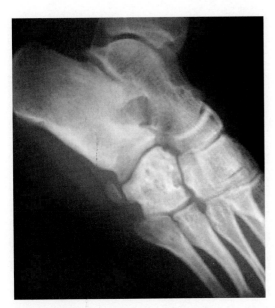

FIG. 7-11. Mixed lytic and sclerotic changes in the cuboid due to chronic osteomyelitis.

unlike osteoid osteoma. Diaphyseal involvement may also occur, especially in adults (Fig. 7-15).[32,158] Abscesses may have a serpiginous tract that communicates with the growth plate (see Fig. 7-5).[73]

As mentioned earlier, most pyogenic bacterial infections have similar radiographic features. However, certain organisms (e.g., mycobacteria, fungi) have different radiographic and clinical features.

Salmonellosis

Salmonella (*S. typhi, S. paratyphi, S. choleraesuis, S. typhimurium,* and *S. arizonae*) can involve bone (approximately 1%).[145,162] Osteomyelitis with *Salmonella* occurs more commonly in patients with sickle cell disease or other hemoglobinopathies, leukemia, lymphoma, and systemic lupus erythematosus.[47,145] The exact mechanism of contamination in *Salmonella* osteomyelitis is uncertain. Patients with sickle cell disease probably develop hematogenous osteomyelitis resulting from bowel infarcts that allow organisms to enter the circulation. Osteomyelitis due to *Salmonella* has a predilection for the medullary region of the diaphysis and areas of bone infarction.[31,60,134,135,145]

Tuberculosis

Tuberculosis osteomyelitis can involve patients in all age ranges, but it is rare in infants.[80,129,133] Bone and joint involvement occurs in 3 to 5% of patients with tuberculosis

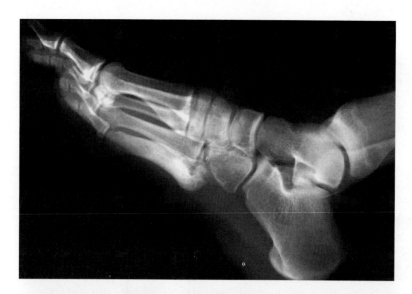

FIG. 7-12. Lateral view of the foot shows chronic osteomyelitis of the fifth metatarsal. Changes are secondary to a previous nail puncture with *Pseudomonas* infection.

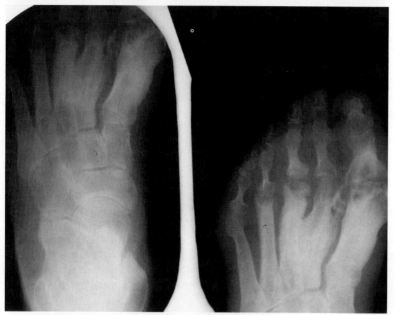

FIG. 7-13. AP views of the foot demonstrate sclerosing osteomyelitis in the first through third metatarsals. There are also chronic destructive changes in the first metatarsophalangeal joint and collapse of the third and fourth metatarsal necks.

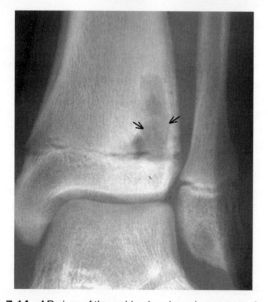

FIG. 7-14. AP view of the ankle showing a large metaphyseal Brodie's abscess (*arrows*).

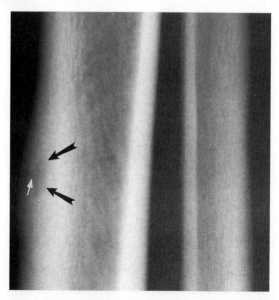

FIG. 7-15. Small oval Brodie's abscess (*black arrows*) with cortical thickening. There is also a sinus tract (*white arrow*).

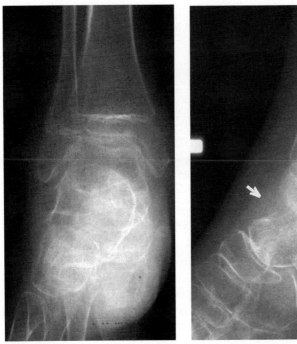 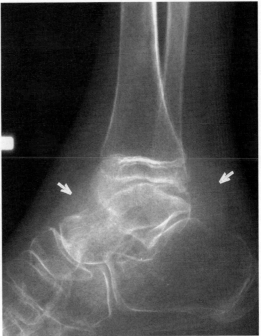

FIG. 7-16. A 12-year-old child with osteopenia, joint space narrowing, and a large effusion (*arrows*) resulting from tuberculosis seen on AP (**A**) and lateral (**B**) radiographs.

(Fig. 7-16).[133,145] The infection is more common in the presence of debilitating disease and drug addiction and in certain groups of immigrants.[145] *Mycobacterium tuberculosis* is contracted via inhalation, whereas *M. bovis* was common following ingestion of contaminated milk products.[59,129] The latter accounted for up to 20% of musculoskeletal tuberculosis in the past, but it has been largely eradicated. *M. tuberculosis* still accounts for some cases of infectious arthropathy (spine, hip, knee), but less frequently it causes primary osteomyelitis. When present, the disease usually presents with hematogenous dissemination to the metaphyseal region of long bones in children and the epiphysis in adults. Pulmonary involvement is evident in 50% of patients. The shafts of the metatarsals (tuberculous dactylitis) may show obvious layered periostitis (Fig. 7-17). This type of osteomyelitis is most common in children but has been described in adults.[59, 64,145] Multiple metatarsals may be involved in up to 33% of patients. Congenital syphilis can produce a similar radiographic appearance, but it typically involves both feet and ankles and there is less soft tissue swelling than with tuberculous dactylitis.[64,145]

Circumscribed lytic lesions (cystic tuberculosis) may also

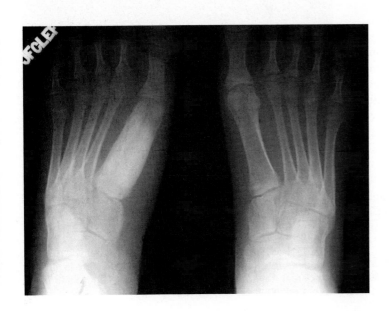

FIG. 7-17. AP radiographs of the feet demonstrate periosteal thickening and sclerosis due to tuberculosis. The laminated appearance of the periosteum is common with tuberculosis.

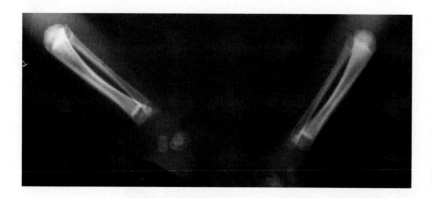

FIG. 7-18. Leg and ankle radiographs in a neonate with congenital syphilis. Note the symmetric periosteal new bone.

be evident, although these changes are more common in the large long bones of the lower extremity than the foot. These lesions may be difficult to differentiate from eosinophilic granuloma, sarcoidosis, cystic angiomatosis, and plasmacytomas.[145]

Tuberculous osteomyelitis can be difficult to differentiate from acute pyogenic osteomyelitis and fungal infection. However, tuberculosis and fungal disease tend to have a more subtle course requiring more time for bone and joint changes to occur. With pyogenic infection, the course is much more rapid and joint involvement is less common than with tuberculosis (see Fig. 7-16).[32,145]

Syphilis

The organism of syphilis, *Treponema pallidum,* is a spirochete that may be transmitted transplacentally or by sexual contact in adults. The organism reaches the musculoskeletal system via the circulation. Bone involvement in the neonate may include the diaphysis and metaphysis. The process is usually symmetric (Fig. 7-18).[45,141]

Spirochetes inhibit bone formation, thereby resulting in osteoblastic degeneration. If the infant survives, bone manifestations include widening of the zone of provisional calcification, lucent bands similar to those seen with leukemia or neuroblastoma, and periosteal new bone formation (see Fig. 7-18). These changes are usually symmetric and involve multiple long bones compared with osteomyelitis resulting from more common organisms, which is generally local and asymmetric (see Fig. 7-18).[46] Syphilitic lesions may regress only to reappear in 5 to 20 years. At this time, the changes resemble the adult form of the disease. The adult or acquired form of syphilis affects the skeleton in 0.5 to 20% of patients. This hematogenous involvement leads to periosteal new bone formation that is generally laminar and evolves into cortical thickening with areas of lytic necrosis (Fig. 7-19). The skull is involved in up to 9% of patients.[145] The tibia and foot are also frequently involved (see Figs. 7-18 and 7-19). These lytic areas or gummas do not appear for several years. Histologically, one sees caseating necrosis and giant cells resembling a tubercle. Less commonly, dactylitis, similar to that seen in tuberculosis, develops in the tubular bones of the hands and feet.[145,146]

Fungal Infections

Osteomyelitis of fungal origin should be considered in debilitated patients, diabetic patients, patients taking steroids, and patients with osteomyelitis who reside in certain geographic regions. Actinomycosis (*Actinomyces israelii* or *A. bovis*) is present in the oral cavity. Osseous involvement generally results from local extension, but hematogenous spread can also occur.[145,147] Obviously, local extension most commonly involves the facial bones. Involvement of the foot and ankle is uncommon.

Cryptococcosis (*Crytococcus neoformans*) can be ac-

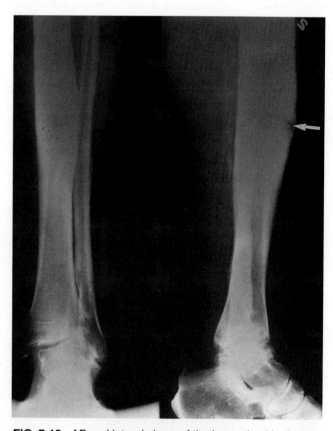

FIG. 7-19. AP and lateral views of the leg and ankle demonstrate neurotrophic arthropathy with talar tilt. There is marked periosteal new bone formation on the tibia and distal fibula with a midtibial gumma (*arrow*).

quired by direct implantation into open wounds in the foot because the organism is present in the soil. Skeletal involvement is reported in 5 to 10% of patients.[104] Destructive bone lesions are commonly associated with draining sinuses.[174]

Blastomycosis (*Blastomyces dermatiditis*) is prevalent in the Ohio and Mississippi River valleys. Contamination can occur via the skin or by inhalation, which leads to pulmonary involvement. Thus, osteomyelitis may follow direct or hematogenous contamination. Skeletal involvement occurs in up to one-half of patients with pulmonary involvement. The tibia and tarsal bones are commonly affected.[38] Radiographically, there are patchy destructive lesions and draining sinuses. Whitehouse and Smith[174] suggested that lytic bone lesions, soft tissue infection, and pulmonary disease should suggest the diagnosis of blastomycosis.

Coccidioidomycosis (*Coccidioides immitis*) is an inhalation disease endemic in the southwestern portion of the United States.[22,29,44,140] Bone involvement occurs frequently (10 to 20%).[174] About one-third of cases initially present with transient polyarthritis.[22,44] Areas of bony prominence, such as the calcaneal tuberosity, and the diaphysis of the metatarsals are common sites of involvement (Fig. 7-20). Involvement is often symmetric with aggressive periostitis, unlike osteomyelitis resulting from more typical organisms.[44,145,174] Associated pulmonary involvement is common.[174]

Histoplasma capsulatum and *H. duboisii* are present in the soil, contaminating the lungs (histoplasmosis) initially. The axial skeleton is more commonly involved than the foot

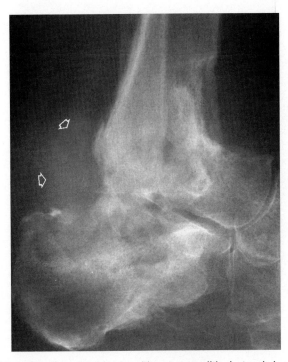

FIG. 7-20. *Coccidioides immitis* osteomyelitis. Lateral view of the calcaneus shows marked soft tissue swelling posteriorly (*open arrows*) with lytic destructive changes on the calcaneus, talus, and tibia.

and ankle. Children are affected more frequently than adults.[93,140]

Other fungal infections that may affect the foot and ankle include sporotricosis, candidiasis, mucormycosis, and aspergillosis.[145] Multiple lytic lesions, usually eccentric and well marginated, are typical. Radiographic changes do not vary significantly from those described earlier.

Miscellaneous Infections

Leprosy may also cause osteomyelitis in the foot.[61] Osteomyelitis develops in 3 to 5% of patients following a long (3- to 6-year) incubation period. The process usually follows soft tissue involvement, so bone involvement begins in the periosteum.[61,145] The phalanges are most commonly involved. Differentiation of the neurotrophic changes from chronic infection is difficult radiographically.[61]

Rubella and cytomegalic inclusion disease can present with similar radiographic findings in neonates who are infected during the first trimester of pregnancy.[145,150] Periosteal changes, if present, are not usually as dramatic as in congenital syphilis (Fig. 7-21). The long bones are most commonly affected. Mixed lucent and sclerotic changes in the metaphysis result in a "celery stalk" appearance (see Fig. 7-21). With healing, a prominent line often forms at the metaphyseal margin.[145,150] Adults and older children rarely have radiographic findings, even though clinical arthropathy has been described.[145]

Parasitic infections rarely affect the skeleton. Soft tissue involvement with subsequent cystic calcification can develop. This feature is more common with cysticerosis (*Taenia solium*) and trichinosis (*Trichinella spiralis*). Ecchinococcus granulosis may involve the adult skeleton in 1 to 2% of patients. Radiographically, areas of involvement are cystic with central trabeculation. Cortical expansion can also develop.[145]

Radiographic features of osteomyelitis differ if the source is a contiguous infection rather than an infection acquired by the hematogenous route (see Figs. 7-2 and 7-5). Bone involvement following contiguous infection generally follows local trauma, vascular insufficiency, or other devitalizing mechanisms that allow soft tissues to become infected (see Fig. 7-3). The plantar surface of the foot is frequently involved.[63,145,158] Anatomic studies have demonstrated that the deep layers of the midplantar intermuscular planes are most commonly involved in spread of these infections.[145,152] *P. aeruginosa* is present in the soil and is frequently implicated. The earliest radiographic findings are swelling and distortion of the plantar fat and septa (see Fig. 7-4). As with hematogenous infection, the radiographic features are not usually evident for 10 to 21 days. Bone involvement begins in the periosteum and outer cortex, unlike hematogenous osteomyelitis, which typically involves the metaphyseal marrow. Periosteal changes are more common in children because of the loose periosteal attachment. Cortical and

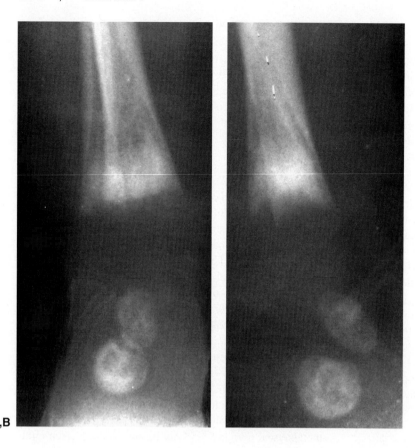

FIG. 7-21. AP (**A**) and lateral (**B**) radiographs demonstrate sclerotic changes with celery stalk appearance due to rubella infection in a neonate.

A,B

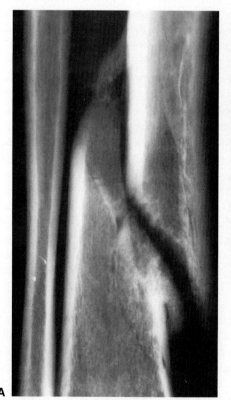

A

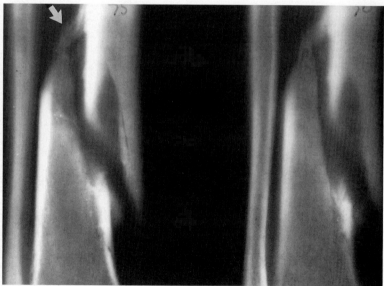

B

FIG. 7-22. Routine AP radiograph (**A**) and tomograms (**B**) of a distal tibial fracture. The cortex is normal, fracture margins are sharp and there are no lytic areas in the bone. No infection is present.

medullary involvement follows the reverse order of hematogenous osteomyelitis.[141,145]

Osteomyelitis After Surgery or Fracture

Routine radiographic findings in osteomyelitis following surgical intervention or fracture may be especially subtle. After acute fracture, necrosis of osteocytes occurs at the fracture line extending to the area of closest vascular supply. This causes widening and some irregularity of the fracture line (Fig. 7-22). Complex or comminuted fractures may have multiple fragments at the fracture site. Some of these fragments may lose their blood supply and resemble sequestra. Additional confusion may occur because of the osteoporosis that occurs with immobilization. The degree of periosteal callus is variable depending on the extent of injury and size of the hematoma adjacent to the fracture site. In the foot and ankle, hematomas are generally smaller than in the thigh or calf, so callus is generally less exuberant.[19,32]

Sequential radiographs are useful in following the progress of normal fracture healing. Any variation in the normal sequence of radiographic or clinical findings such as delay in union, local pain, erythema, or swelling may suggest infection.[32] Radiographic features (see Fig. 7-22; Fig. 7-23) are similar to those mentioned earlier, but they may be obscured by architectural changes near the fracture. This can reduce the confidence in radiographic findings and delay diagnosis. Conventional tomography or CT, magnetic resonance imaging (MRI), and isotope studies (see next sections) may be most useful in this setting (Figs. 7-24 and 7-25).

Following surgical treatment, such as internal fixation of fracture, joint replacement, or arthrodesis, detection of infection may also be difficult. Clinical signs are often subtle. Certain radiographic findings (irregularity of the fracture [see Fig. 7-23], new soft tissue swelling, lucent areas in sclerotic or reinforced bone) may be helpful (Fig. 7-26). When traction pins or screws have been used, well-marginated lucent tracts are usually easily demonstrated on routine radiographs (Fig. 7-27).[76,127] It is important to view these areas en face, so infections are not overlooked. This is most easily accomplished if the tracts are fluoroscopically positioned. If a sequestrum can be identified (Fig. 7-28), infection is likely.[77,131]

Radioisotope Imaging in Osteomyelitis

The importance of early diagnosis of osteomyelitis cannot be overstated. Radiographic findings do not appear for 10 to 21 days.[2,25,32,95,145,156] Radioisotope imaging has evolved as a highly sensitive tool for early diagnosis of osteomyelitis.[7,11,17,54,55,67,78,84] Currently, technetium-99m methylene diphosphate (MDP), gallium-67, and indium-111– or technetium-99m nexamethyl propylenamine oxine–labeled leukocytes are the most commonly used isotopes for bone scintigraphy.[27,32,54]

Technique (see Chapter 2) is important regardless of the radioisotope selected. Technetium-99m MDP studies may detect osteomyelitis within 24 to 48 hours of onset.[32] Three-phase studies are normally obtained providing an early angiographic phase, a blood pool phase, and delayed images.

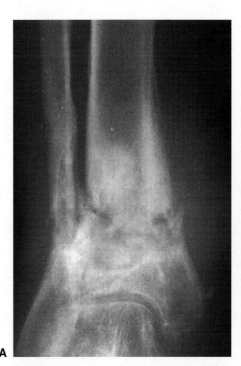
A

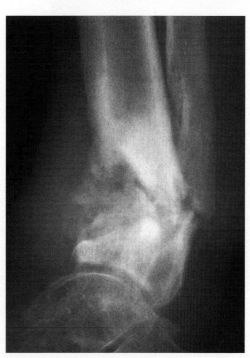
B

FIG. 7-23. AP (**A**) and lateral (**B**) views of the ankle show an old fracture with periosteal new bone along the tibia and fibula. There is soft tissue swelling, sclerosis, and scattered lytic areas with an irregular fracture margin due to osteomyelitis.

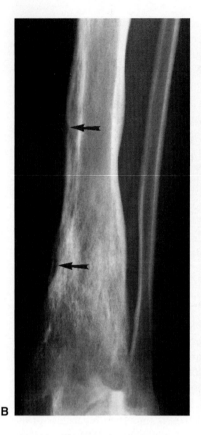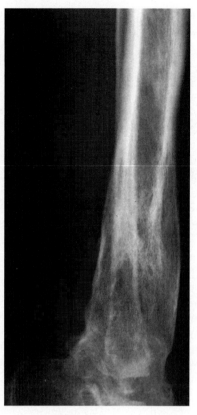

A,B

FIG. 7-24. AP (**A**) and lateral (**B**) views demonstrate prominent trabeculae, cortical thickening, and areas as sclerosis due to chronic osteomyelitis after fracture and tibiotalar arthrodesis. There are two cloacae medially (*arrows*) on the AP view (**A**).

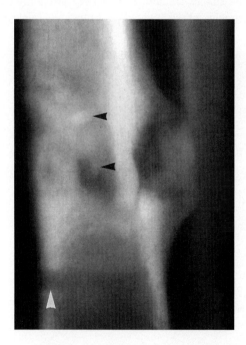

FIG. 7-25. Tomogram of the distal tibia shows sclerosis at the old fracture site with central lucency and several sequestra (*arrowheads*). There is callus laterally and a pin tract inferiorly (*white arrowhead*).

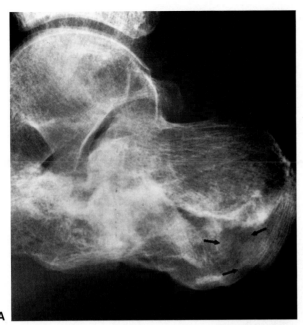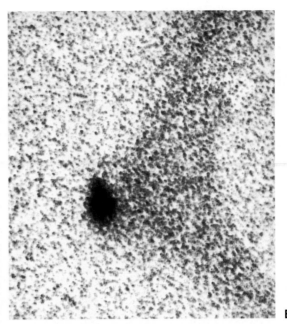

A B

FIG. 7-26. A: Lateral view of the calcaneus shows an old fracture with scleroses along the anterior aspect of the fracture line below the subtalar joint. There is a lucent area posteriorly (*arrows*). **B:** Indium-111–labeled white blood cell scan demonstrates a focal area of increased tracer in the posterior calcaneus due to osteomyelitis.

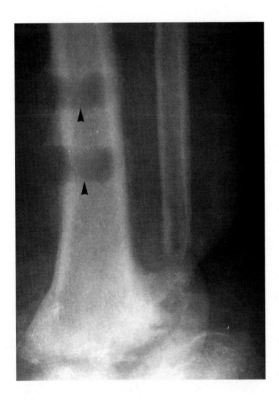

FIG. 7-27. Ankle arthrodesis that was fixed with an external fixation device. The fusion site is irregular. The pin tracts (*arrowheads*) are wide and irregular with periosteal reaction because of osteomyelitis.

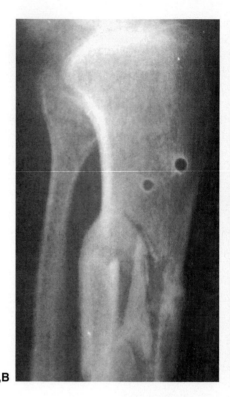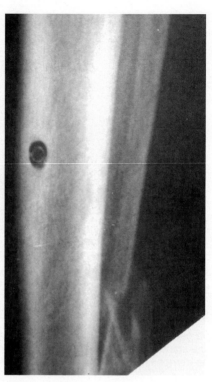

A,B

FIG. 7-28. A: Lateral view of the upper tibia showing normal well-marginated pin tracts. B: Fluoroscopically positioned image showing a ring sequestrum due to osteomyelitis. (From Nguyen, ref. 131, with permission.)

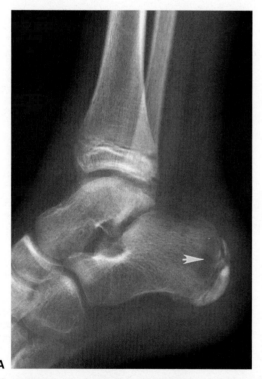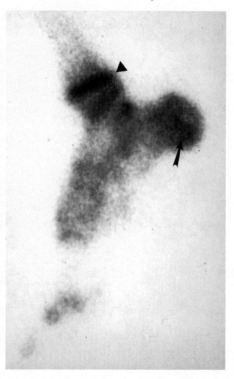

A

B

FIG. 7-29. A 13-year-old patient with heel pain and osteomyelitis. A: Routine radiograph shows a focal lucent area near the growth plate (*arrow*). B: Delayed image on a technetium-99m bone scan demonstrates diffuse uptake in the posterior calcaneus (*arrow*). There is also increased uptake of tracer in the distal tibial epiphyses (*arrowhead*), a normal finding in children.

This approach is useful in differentiating cellulitis from osteomyelitis. Patients with cellulitis demonstrate increased tracer activity during the early phases with near-normal activity on the delayed images. Osteomyelitis causes abnormal tracer accumulation on all three phases.[27,32,54] Gilday[70] and Howie and colleagues[83] studied a large series of patients using early (blood pool) and delayed images. Osteomyelitis was demonstrated as a focal area of increased uptake in bone on both early and late images (Fig. 7-29). Patients with cellulitis have diffuse increased uptake in soft tissue areas on both early and delayed studies without definite focal bone uptake. Maurer and associates[108] believed that this technique did not increase the sensitivity, but, in their experience, the false-positive rate was reduced from 25 to 6 percent.

A large review series by Howie and colleagues[83] studied 280 patients. Patients were divided into two groups: definitely positive for osteomyelitis and definitely negative. Using the three-phase bone scan with technetium-99m pyrophosphate, all patients with cellulitis or soft tissue abscess were correctly separated from those with osteomyelitis. However, 8 of 39 patients diagnosed as osteomyelitis had septic arthritis. The accuracy of this technique was equal in all age groups, all skeletal sites, and throughout the course of the disease process.

O'Mara and associates[136] reported that technetium-99m studies were 76% sensitive and 99% specific with an overall accuracy of 93%, compared with a sensitivity of 24%, specificity of 99%, and overall accuracy of 79% for routine radiographs. Isreal and colleagues,[84] using a quantitative technique, compared lesion with nonlesion tracer uptake ratios at 4 and 24 hours. Using a ratio of 1.18 ± 0.18 for osteomyelitis and 0.98 ± 0.05 for soft tissue infection, sensitivity was 82%, specificity was 92%, and accuracy was 95%. A 24/4 hour ratio of greater than or equal to 1.06 was the most reliable indicator of osteomyelitis. Other reports present sensitivities ranging from 69 to 100% and specificity ranges of 38 to 82% (Table 7-3).[27]

Although areas of osteomyelitis are almost always hot on bone scintigraphy, reports have noted photopenic areas in early osteomyelitis,[87,88,127,155] probably because infection is localized in the marrow space, with increased pressure causing reduced flow. Because this is now well recognized, the photopenic area can be equally diagnostic of early osteomyelitis or septic arthritis.[127] Although bone scanning is useful in adults and children, its utility for neonatal osteomyelitis is controversial. Ash and Gilday[7] reported that isotope scans detected just over 25% of sites with proven osteomyelitis. Some authors have reported that isotope scans in suspected neonatal osteomyelitis should be reserved for patients who have equivocal clinical and radiographic findings.[121] Bessler and colleagues[21] showed that with proper technique all sites of osteomyelitis could be detected in the neonatal age group. This included 10 sites that were radiographically normal.

Additional differential diagnostic problems with bone scintigraphy occur in patients with bone infarction. Majd and Frankel[106] demonstrated normal "blood pool" images with focal increased uptake on delayed images in patients with bone infarcts resulting from sickle cell disease.

Further isotope studies are useful to improve specificity of technetium-99m scans (Figs. 7-30 and 7-31). Gallium-67 and indium-111– or technetium-99m hexamethyl propyleneamine oxine–labeled leukocyte scans are most commonly used.[3,4,51,54,55,109,115,116,143,169]

Gallium-67 accumulates in sites of infection in bone or soft tissues. Abnormal uptake may also occur in certain neoplasms, hematomas, and areas of increased bone turnover such as healing fractures, surgical sites, and neurotrophic arthropathy.[27,32,54,149,169] Gallium-67 studies are usually combined with technetium bone scans to improve accuracy.[27,32,149] Studies are considered positive for infection when uptake of gallium-67 is greater than that of technetium in the expected site of abnormality. Rosenthall and colleagues[149] reported osteomyelitis, joint space infection, or cellulitis in patients with the foregoing incongruent radiotracer pattern. Sensitivities and specificities vary from 69 to 70% and 83 to 93%, respectively, using combined technetium-99m and gallium-67 citrate[2,27,51,54,149] (see Table 7-3).

Indium-111–labeled leukocytes have been used for detection of infection for years. More recently, technetium-99m hexamethyl propyleneamine oxine–labeled leukocytes have also been used to detect early infection.[27,32] Labeled leukocytes studies are generally considered more specific than gallium-67 studies.[27,32,115,116] In addition, both leukocyte techniques have isotopes that are more ideally suited for gamma camera imaging.[32,115,116]

Indium-111–labeled leukocytes are most useful in the postoperative setting.[91,105,115,116] Mauer and colleagues[109] found that combined technetium bone scans and indium-111–labeled leukocyte studies improved the specificity of diagnosing infection in diabetics (see Fig. 7-31). Disadvantages are also reported with radioisotope-labeled leukocyte studies. Because lymphocytes are not labeled, there is reduced sensitivity for detection of chronic infections.[27] Spatial resolution may also make it difficult to differentiate bone and soft tissue involvement.[32,115,116]

Both gallium-67 citrate and indium-111–labeled leukocyte studies are combined with technetium-99m MDP scans.

TABLE 7-3. *Imaging of osteomyelitis[a]*

Technique	Sensitivity (%)	Specificity (%)
Routine radiographs	43–75	75–83
Three-phase bone scan (^{99m}Tc MDP)	69–100	38–99
Gallium-67 (combined with ^{99m}Tc MDP)	69–70	83–93
Indium-111–labeled white blood cells	82–96	73–90
MRI	82–100	53–94

[a] Data from references 27, 32, 83, 110, and 136.

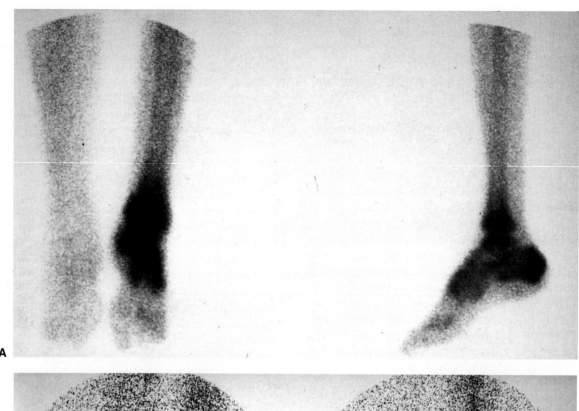

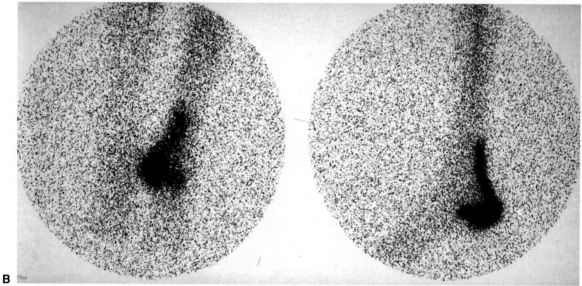

FIG. 7-30. Adult with suspected osteomyelitis. **A:** Technetium-99m MDP scans show increased uptake in the ankle, midfoot, and hindfoot. **B:** Indium-111–labeled leukocyte images demonstrate intense uptake in the posterior calcaneus and Achilles tendon due to infection.

Therefore, the study requires up to 3 days to complete.[27] In some cases, the cost is greater than that of MRI.[54]

Magnetic Resonance Imaging

MRI is a sensitive technique that provides excellent tissue contrast, and images can be obtained in multiple planes. MRI has a proven impact on diagnoses and clinical decision making.[5,12–16,43,56,128]

Technique is important to optimize image quality and to characterize lesions accurately. General MRI techniques for the foot and ankle are reviewed in Chapter 2. However, certain approaches specific to osteomyelitis are reviewed in this section.

Screening examinations for infection can be accomplished with conventional spin-echo (SE) sequences. Both T1- and T2-weighted sequences should be performed. Osteomyelitis is seen as low signal intensity in marrow on T1-weighted (SE 500/10) sequences. Contrast compared with the normal high signal intensity of marrow makes lesions easy to

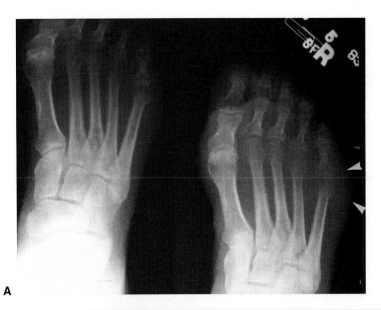

FIG. 7-31. Diabetic with suspected osteomyelitis in the lateral foot. **A:** Radiographs demonstrate swelling (*white arrowheads*) and loss of joint space in the fifth metatarsophalangeal joint. **B:** Technetium-99m MDP study demonstrates uptake in the fifth metatarsal, more evident near the joint. **C:** Indium-111–labeled leukocyte images show focal uptake due to infection.

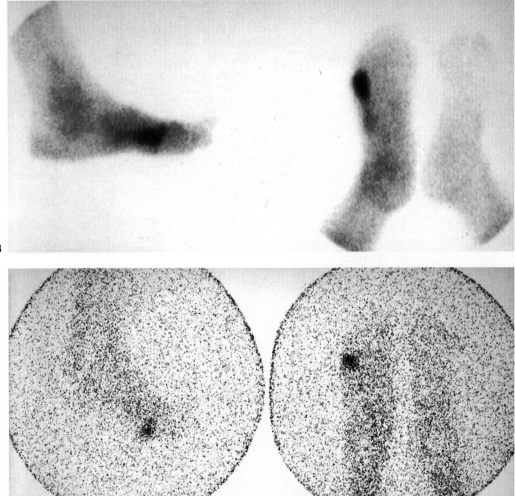

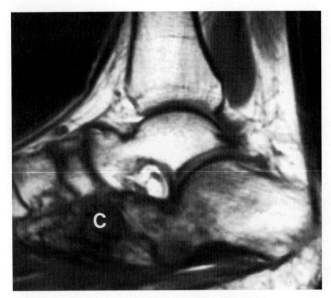

FIG. 7-32. Sagittal SE 500/10 image of the foot shows low signal intensity in the cuboid (*C*) and anterior calcaneus due to osteomyelitis.

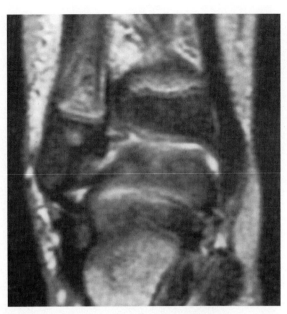

FIG. 7-34. Child with osteomyelitis of the distal fibula. Coronal T2-weighted image demonstrates high signal intensity in the periosteum and soft tissues and focal epiphyseal increased signal intensity due to osteomyelitis.

identify (Fig. 7-32). T1-weighted sequences are less useful for demonstrating cortical and soft tissue involvement except fatty tissues. Osteomyelitis is seen as high signal intensity in marrow on T2-weighted sequences. With T2-weighted sequences, the fat signal in marrow is suppressed (Fig. 7-33). T2-weighted sequences are more useful for evaluating the cortex and adjacent soft tissues (see Fig. 7-33 and Fig. 7-34).[19,62,112]

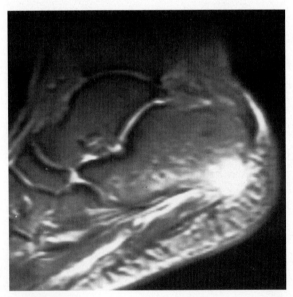

FIG. 7-33. Sagittal SE 2000/80 image of the calcaneus shows bright signal intensity in the posterior calcaneus and adjacent soft tissues due to infection from a puncture wound. Radiographs were normal.

Additional sequences or gadolinium may be useful in some situations. Short TI inversion recovery (STIR) sequences provide excellent contrast because of the high signal intensity of water (e.g., edema, infection) and suppression of fat signal intensity. However, anatomic detail is inferior to that of SE sequences in our experience. Despite this disadvantage, a negative STIR image has a negative predictive value of about 100% for osteomyelitis.

Gadolinium can be given intravenously and combined with fat-suppressed T1-weighted images. Advantages of this approach include differentiation of inflammation or cellulitis from abscesses. The fluid in an abscess does not enhance, whereas cellulitis and the abscess wall do enhance.[37,118] Granulation tissue also enhances, but sequestra do not.[27] The utility of gadolinium is diminished in patients with significant vascular disease. Morrison and associates[126] reported sensitivity of 88% and specificity of 93% with gadolinium studies compared with 79 and 53% for nongadolinium images. Multiple series report sensitivities of 82 to 100% and specificities of 53 to 94% for diagnoses of osteomyelitis with conventional MRI techniques.[14,27,37,62,126,166,179]

The role of MRI is more limited in patients with previous surgery, fracture, or orthopedic implants. Most orthopedic appliances are nonferromagnetic, but local image distortion may make evaluation of bone and adjacent soft tissues difficult. In patients with previous surgery or chronic infection, interpretation of MRI may be more difficult. The diagnoses of osteomyelititis should be made with caution unless sequestra (low signal intensity on T1- and T2-weighted sequences), fluid collections, abscesses, or sinus tracts are identified.[19]

Computed Tomography

CT has been replaced by MRI in most patients. However, CT still offers an option to MRI and may be useful in certain situations.[10,27,152,158] Both CT and MRI demonstrate subtle changes earlier, and lesions are more conspicuous compared with routine radiographs (Fig. 7-35).[10,27,158] CT can detect subtle marrow and cortical abnormalities and small gas collections. Findings more specific to infection including sequestra (see Fig. 7-35), cloacae, and involucra.[27,32] Sequestra and cloacae may also be defined using conventional tomography (see Fig. 7-5).

Treatment

Treatment of osteomyelitis depends on multiple factors. Osteomyelitis is considered acute when symptoms are less than 1 month in duration. If symptoms and signs are present for longer than 1 month, the condition is considered chronic.[69]

Medical and surgical management of osteomyelitis can be difficult, especially if early diagnosis is not achieved. The site or sites of involvement must be identified and the organism isolated so proper antimicrobial therapy can be instituted. Blood cultures are only positive in about 50% of patients. Therefore, open or image-guided biopsies may be required. Management is particularly difficult in patients with diabetes mellitus, debilitating disease, or ischemic disease and devitalized tissues. This setting can result in amputation of the involved bone or a more proximal amputation in the case of vascular disease.[53,69,79]

Patients with chronic infection may be treated with debridement and vascularized muscle, bone, or omental

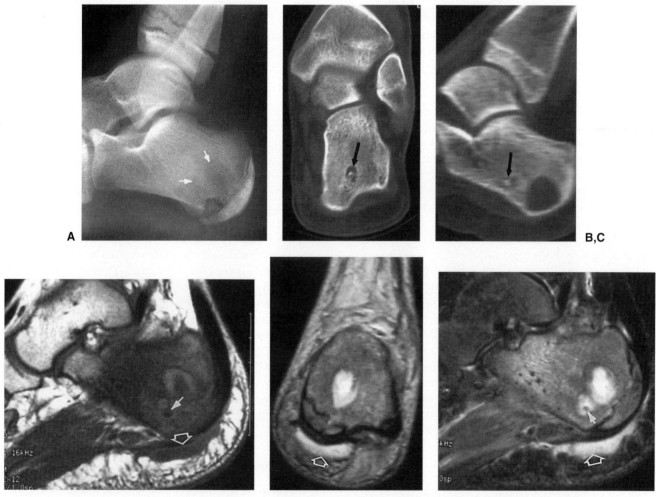

FIG. 7-35. Chronic osteomyelitis with sequestrum. **A:** Routine radiograph of the calcaneus demonstrates a focal lucent area near the physis with a less distinct area of decreased bone density posteriorly (*arrows*). Coronal (**B**) and reconstructed sagittal (**C**) CT images show a large area of low attenuation in the posterior calcaneus and a sequestrum (*arrow*) not evident on the radiograph. Sagittal SE 500/11 (**D**) and coronal (**E**) and sagittal (**F**) T2-weighted images demonstrate soft tissue fluid (*open arrows*) and the posterior calcaneal infection. The sequestrum is seen as a small focus of low signal intensity (*small arrows*).

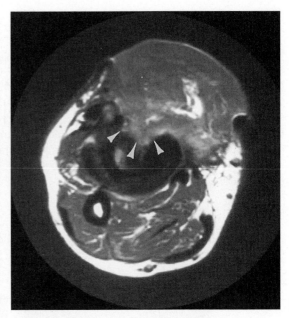

FIG. 7-36. Chronic osteomyelitis treated with debridement and vascularized muscle flap. **A:** Radiographs demonstrate bone sclerosis and the operative site (*arrow*). **B:** Axial SE 500/10 MRI shows the normal signal intensity of the muscle filling the dead space (*arrowheads*) left by surgery.

grafts.[6,177] The role of this treatment is to obliterate necrotic and infected tissue, to fill the resulting dead space in bone, and to provide a vascular supply to aid in healing.[6,19,65,69] Imaging of these patients plays an important role preoperatively and postoperatively. It is essential to define the area of involvement and to exclude skip lesions before surgery. Postoperatively, imaging is useful, to be certain the dead space is completely filled and the graft is viable. Routine radiographs and tomography are not optimal for preoperative or postoperative evaluation. CT could be used preoperatively, but the multiplanar imaging of MRI is superior for defining the extent of involvement and for excluding skip lesions.[19] Postoperative MRI clearly demonstrates the muscle or omental graft (Fig. 7-36). The position and viability can also be assessed. In the early postoperative period, the muscle may have high signal because of edema, and later fatty replacement is not uncommon. Images should be obtained in two planes (axial and either coronal or sagittal) to confirm that graft material fills the dead space.[19] Vascular integrity of the graft can be evaluated with static or dynamic gadolinium studies using fat-suppressed T1-weighted sequences.[19,170]

Complications

Patients who are not properly diagnosed or treated may develop extensive osteolysis leading to destruction of large segments of the involved bone or bones. When this stage is evident, proper therapy may have little effect, leading to the need for amputation of portions of the foot or ankle.[69,145]

Osteomyelitis can affect the growth plates in infants and children and may lead to asymmetric growth or cessation of growth.[26,145] Involvement of the distal tibial physis is most important in the foot and ankle. Weight bearing and foot function can be significantly affected if the growth plate is not parallel to the ground. This can lead to early degenerative arthritis and the need for corrective osteotomy. Leg-lengthening procedures or epiphysiodesis of the opposite extremity may be needed in patients with leg-length discrepancy.

Patients with chronic osteomyelitis and chronic draining sinuses can develop epidermoid or squamous cell carcinomas. This complication has been reported in 0.5% of patients with chronic foci of osteomyelitis.[66] These changes are not usually evident for 20 to 30 years. Other histologic forms of malignancy, such as fibrosarcoma, have also been reported. Patients with malignant degeneration may have increased pain or a soft tissue mass in a previously quiescent infected area, but these symptoms are not specific.[145] MRI may be most sensitive in detecting an active process (either inflammation or tumor), but findings are not specific. Therefore, open or percutaneous biopsy is usually necessary to establish the diagnosis.

Differential Diagnosis

A complete discussion of the list of potential differential diagnostic entities is beyond the scope of this chapter. However, certain conditions do require mention. The mixed lytic and sclerotic changes may be noted, especially in the calcaneus and tarsal bones, with infection and Ewing's sarcoma (see Chapter 6). The patient's age (children) is not always helpful because both conditions are seen in this age group. When sclerotic changes or prominent trabeculae are noted

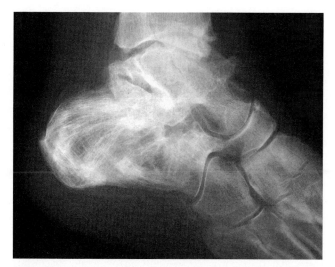

FIG. 7-37. Lateral view of the calcaneus on a patient with Paget's disease. There is no soft tissue swelling or focal lytic areas in this patient. Compare with Figures 7-4, 7-5, and 7-26.

in the adult, Paget's disease should be included in the differential diagnosis (Fig. 7-37).[145,174]

Cystic lesions can be seen with fungal infections and tuberculosis. This finding can also be seen with other conditions including eosinophilic granuloma, sarcoid, and cystic angiomatosis.[145,174] A small cortical Brodie's abscess can be confused with an osteoid osteoma. The patient's age and symptoms (night pain relieved by aspirin) may be helpful, but in either case surgery is usually required.

Foreign body reactions and stress fractures, especially in the tarsal bones and sesamoids, can also cause confusion.[50,76,148,168] Chapter 6 addresses other entities that may be confused with infection.

Diagnosis of osteomyelitis, staging of the extent of bone involvement, and differentiation of infection from other conditions can be challenging. Clinical data can be extremely useful. However, the index of clinical suspicion is not always high, a factor that makes the role of imaging more significant. Appropriate use of imaging is more critical in today's cost-conscious environment. Table 7-4 provides a suggested algorithm for imaging osteomyelitis. Some controversy exists regarding MRI (limited to STIR or fat-suppressed T2-weighted sequences versus complete study) compared with radionuclide scans because of cost and time required for the latter. I prefer MRI (see Table 7-4) in many situations. A more specific approach for infection in diabetics is reviewed in the last section of this chapter.

JOINT SPACE INFECTIONS

Joint space infections may be due to any of the previously mentioned organisms, although *S. aureus* is by far the most common.[18,33,89,145] Infections may develop at any age but are more frequent in children.[71,138] Patients taking steroids and those with debilitating illnesses also have a higher incidence of septic arthritis. Like osteomyelitis, contamination of joint spaces can occur via the hematogenous route, by direct extension from soft tissue or adjacent bone, and following surgery. In the foot, direct extension is a much more common mechanism of contamination than in more proximal joints. Hematogenous involvement in the ankle occurs more commonly in children.[50,138,145]

TABLE 7-4. *Imaging approaches for osteomyelitis*[a]

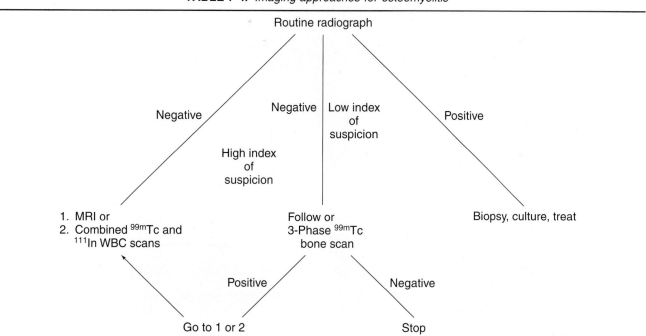

[a] Data from references 12, 27, 32, 74, 110, and 136.

Hematogenous spread indicates that infection follows vascular involvement of the synovium from a distant source. The synovial membrane becomes infected before contamination of synovial fluid.[8,176] The joint reaction (articular cartilage, synovial proliferation, and fluid changes) varies depending on the type of organism involved. Destructive changes are more rapid with pyogenic infection compared with a more subtle and prolonged course with organisms such as *Mycobacterium* and *Brucella*.[18,32,50]

Infants (less than 1 year of age) and adults more frequently develop septic arthritis because of direct extension of osteomyelitis from adjacent bones. This occurs because the vascular supply crosses the growth plate region into the epiphysis (see Fig. 7-1). In children (age 1 until the time of growth plate fusion), the growth plate serves as a barrier to the longitudinal spread of infection.[145,168,171,172] Direct involvement of the joint resulting from local soft tissue infection is particularly common in the foot.[40,174] This is especially true in diabetic patients and in those with vascular disease in whom soft tissues are frequently devitalized.[57,58,63,103] Patients undergoing surgical procedures in joints of the foot and ankle may also develop joint space infections (Fig. 7-38).[32,145]

Radiographic Features

Infectious arthritis most commonly involves the larger joints (hip and knee), but the articulations of the foot and ankle may also be affected. Monoarticular involvement is common, a finding that is useful in differentiating this entity from other arthropathies that are more commonly polyarticular or bilateral (e.g., rheumatoid arthritis).[49,89] Occasionally, patients with rheumatoid arthritis being treated with steroids develop infections in multiple joints. In this setting, or in other patients taking systemic steroids, a rapidly enlarging effusion with new erosive changes suggests superimposed infection.[144,145]

The earliest radiographic findings involve the soft tissues. Periarticular swelling and effusions are most easily detected in the ankle (Fig. 7-39).[30] This finding is most easily detected on the lateral view. The smaller joints are more difficult to evaluate. Subtle increased density around the joints or displacement of the muscle planes may be the only radiographic features initially. Local hyperemia may lead to juxtaarticular osteoporosis, especially in pyogenic (bacterial) infections.[30,32] Aspirations may be negative in the early stages of disease because the synovium is usually involved before the fluid. Sympathetic sterile effusions may also be evident in adjacent joints, thus adding to the diagnostic dilemma early in the course of the disease.[11] Involvement of multiple joints in the lower extremity can occur with certain infections, namely gonococcal arthritis (see Fig. 7-39).[145]

Destructive changes in articular cartilage begin early (2 to 3 days) with pyogenic infections. Cartilage destruction may involve the articular margins or central joint surfaces (Fig. 7-40). In weight-bearing joints, such as the ankle, the weight-bearing cartilage is usually affected first. Tuberculo-

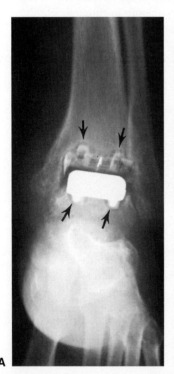
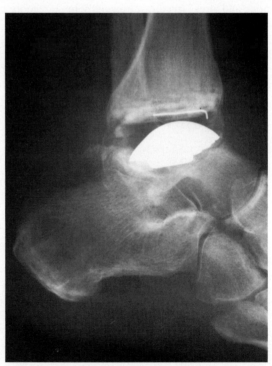

FIG. 7-38. Loose, infected ankle arthroplasty. AP (**A**) and lateral (**B**) radiographs demonstrate lucency (*arrows*) about the components. Joint aspiration obtained cloudy fluid resulting from infection with *S. aureus*.

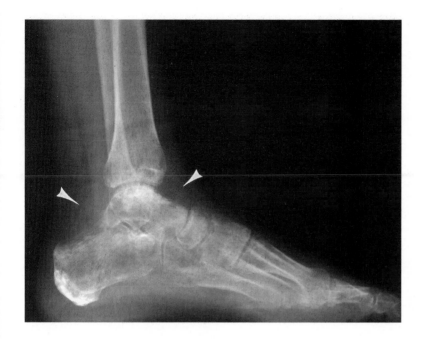

FIG. 7-39. Lateral view of the foot and ankle demonstrating aggressive osteopenia with an ankle effusion (*arrowheads*) from gonococcal arthritis.

sis and certain fungal infections not only evolve much more slowly (weeks to months), but also erosive changes from cartilage destruction are more common at the periphery of the joint.[30] These changes are less clear cut in the smaller joints of the foot. This is due in part to the problem of over-penetration seen in the distal foot radiographically.[32]

The pathogenesis of cartilage lysis is not completely clear, but several factors are probably responsible. Fibrin deposits on the articular cartilage can reduce the normal flow of nutrients to articular cartilage.[48] Leukocytes are prevalent in pyogenic infections. Lysozymes in leukocytes release enzymes that destroy cartilage rapidly (over a period of days). Articular cartilage is also destroyed more rapidly in patients with debilitating illnesses or in patients receiving immunosuppressive therapy.[30,145] Changes progress much more

slowly (weeks to months) in patients with tuberculosis or fungal infections. In this setting, one sees an associated lymphocytic response in synovial fluid. Similar enzymatic effects do not occur, a finding that may explain the slower progression of the joint changes. Moreover, the peripheral pannous formation seen in more indolent forms of infection may explain the preservation of the joint space and the frequency of marginal joint erosions. Serial radiographs and the location of the erosive changes can be helpful in differentiating bacterial (rapid aggressive changes) from tuberculous or fungal infections, which progress more slowly.[30,32]

Occasionally, air can be identified in the joint or adjacent soft tissues. Air-forming organisms such as *Clostridium perfringens* (formerly known as *C. welchii*), *E. coli*, and certain anaerobic streptococci may cause this appearance. Air may

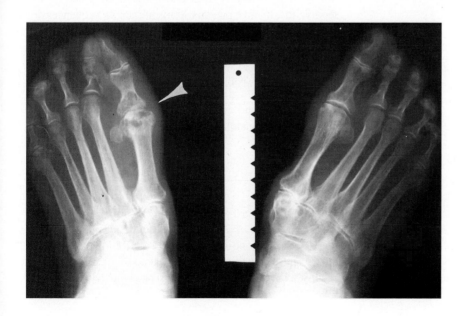

FIG. 7-40. Standing AP view of the feet demonstrates swelling and erosive changes (*arrowhead*) in the left great toe due to joint space infection secondary to *S.* aureus.

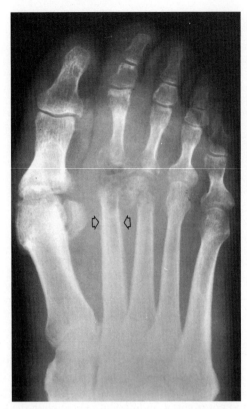

FIG. 7-41. *E. coli* septic arthritis. AP radiograph of the foot demonstrating joint space destruction involving the first through third metatarsophalangeal joints with air in the soft tissues. Associated osteomyelitis and periosteal reaction are present along the second metatarsal (*open arrows*).

also enter the joint and soft tissues when an open wound is present or following aspiration of the joint (Fig. 7-41).[23,153]

If diagnosis is delayed, joint infections can progress to involve the bones on either side of the joint (see Fig. 7-41). Further progression may result in fibrous or bony ankylosis and growth disturbances in children.[30,145]

Radionuclide Imaging

As with osteomyelitis, technetium-99m MDP scans may be performed using the three-phase technique. Increased uptake of isotope in the synovium is seen during the angiographic and blood pool phases. On the delayed images, the uptake is increased in the articular regions of the joints involved with infectious arthritis.[30,54,94]

In some patients, early images may demonstrate a photopenic area surrounding the joint space. This is most often seen in larger joints such as the hip or ankle. This finding is likely due to the tense effusion present in early infection. Kloiber and colleagues[94] examined this feature in hips and found that it correlated with effusions but was not evident after aspiration of the joint. The effusion is postulated to comprise local vessels leading to decreased tracer. As the

infection progresses, the uptake in the joint increases.[30,94] Technetium-99m MDP studies are sensitive but not specific for infection.

When technetium bone scans are equivocal but clinical suspicion is high, further studies are indicated.[17,101] Gallium-67 or indium-111–labeled leukocytes should be considered in this setting.[20,159] Lisbona and Rosenthal[101] noted that both gallium-67 citrate and technetium-99m MDP bone scans were positive in just over 50% of patients with septic arthritis. In the remaining cases, the technetium bone scan was negative but gallium scans were positive. The focus of infection was evident in these patients, and it was possible to differentiate osteomyelitis from joint space infection or cellulitis in adults and older children, but not in infants.

Indium-111– or technetium-99m hexamethyl propyleneamine oxine–labeled leukocytes can also be used to detect septic arthritis.[27,32] Leukocyte labeling makes these techniques more useful in acute than chronic infections. For the latter, lymphocyte labeling may be more useful.[27,30,105]

Magnetic Resonance Imaging

CT is used infrequently for diagnosis of patients with suspected acute joint space infections. Subtle articular changes and fluid can be identified. However, I most often rely on MRI for diagnostic studies and reserve CT for selected situations or biopsy guidance.[10,158,175]

MRI can detect subtle bone and cartilage erosions earlier than routine radiographs.[19,20] Synovial inflammatory changes can also be evaluated. Intravenous gadolinium provides additional data in patients with early synovial inflammation.[19] Conventional MRI clearly demonstrates joint fluid (Fig. 7-42).[86] However, signal intensity of fluid is not particularly useful for differentiating infection from other causes of joint effusion.[19,30,85]

MRI techniques used when joint space is suspected do not differ significantly from the approach suggested for osteomyelitis. In most patients, conventional SE sequences detect joint fluid (see Fig. 7-42), soft tissue inflammation, and early cartilage or marrow changes (Fig. 7-43). Early cartilage abnormalities may be more easily detected using T2-weighted fast SE sequences with fat suppression or gradient-echo sequences with thin-section volume acquisition.[19] Early synovial and marrow changes can be seen using fat-suppressed postgadolinium T1-weighted sequences (Fig. 7-44).[19,125]

Ultrasound

The musculoskeletal applications of ultrasound continue to expand.[27,85,86,130] Although ultrasound is not of value for characterizing bone changes, fluid collections, joint effusions, and periostitis can be evaluated.[27,85] Ultrasound is readily available and is inexpensive compared with MRI.

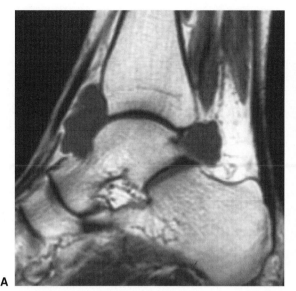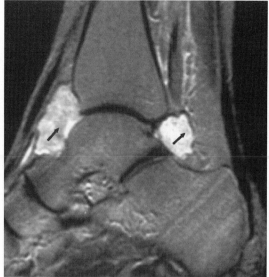

FIG. 7-42. Sagittal SE 500/11 (**A**) and SE 2000/80 (**B**) MRI demonstrates a large effusion with joint space narrowing. The fluid is low intensity on the T1-weighted image (**A**) and *not* uniformly high intensity on the T2-weighted sequence (**B**). The areas of inhomogeneity (*arrows*) suggest that this is not a simple effusion.

However, I generally reserve ultrasound for guidance of aspiration or biopsy techniques.

Interventional Techniques

Usually, the involved joint is clinically obvious, but in the midfoot, evaluation of more than one joint may be re-

quired. In this setting, available imaging studies should be reviewed to select the aspiration and biopsy site. Moreover, the technique selected for guidance is based on available image studies. Fluoroscopy, CT, or ultrasound can be selected depending on bone and soft tissue changes as well as examiner preference. Using image guidance and sterile preparation techniques (see Chapter 2), the joints of the foot

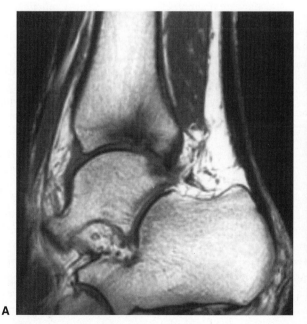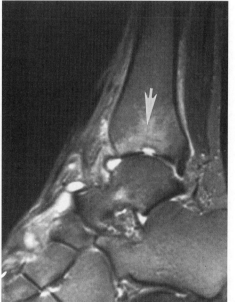

FIG. 7-43. Joint space infections in two patients. **A:** Sagittal T1-weighted image demonstrates tibial marrow abnormality due to bone involvement. **B:** Sagittal T2-weighted image demonstrates effusions with marrow edema (*arrow*) and a central articular defect.

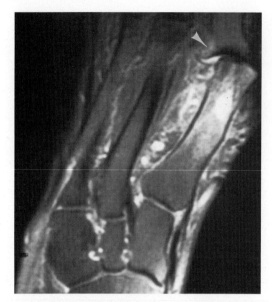

FIG. 7-44. Coronal postgadolinium image using an SE 500/11 sequence with fat suppression shows joint incongruency with marrow enhancement in the first metatarsal and at the margin of the proximal phalanx (*arrowhead*). There is also a joint effusion and soft tissue involvement.

can be easily entered and aspirated. If no fluid is obtained, a small amount of contrast (0.5 ml) can be injected to confirm needle position. If the needle is intraarticularly placed and no fluid is obtained, the joint should be flushed with nonbacterostatic sterile saline and reaspirated. Typically, a 22-gauge needle is adequate for aspiration of the small joints of the foot. If thick, purulent material is present, a larger needle (18 gauge) may be needed.[19,32]

The fluid can be sent for Gram stain, culture, sensitivity, and any other indicated laboratory studies. Aerobic and anaerobic bacterial studies are routinely ordered along with mycobacteria and fungal cultures. If indicated, an arthrogram can be performed after the aspiration is completed. Generally, other than confirming needle position, arthrography does not add significant new information. In granulomatous or chronic infection, synovial biopsy may be required. This can also be easily accomplished using imaging techniques for guidance.[19]

Treatment

Most joint space infections are treated with appropriate antibiotics after the organism has been isolated. When appropriate therapy is instituted early, joint damage can be kept in check. In the case of previous surgery or metallic implants, the devices may need to be removed and reoperation considered following appropriate therapy.[151,160]

Diabetic patients and patients with ischemic disease may be particularly difficult to treat. In this setting, amputations may be indicated. Whether a local or more proximal amputation is performed, it is essential to obtain postoperative radio-

graphs to serve as a baseline. This method allows further infections to be more easily detected (Fig. 7-45).

Differential Diagnosis

Monoarticular arthropathies should be considered infectious until proven otherwise. Occasionally, other conditions that may be monoarticular can be confused with infection. Juvenile rheumatoid arthritis, pigmented villonodular synovitis, and even adult-onset rheumatoid arthritis can present with monoarticular involvement initially. When this occurs, the foot and ankle are not usually involved initially.[145] MRI may be useful in differentiating pigmented villonodular synovitis from other arthropathies. On T2-weighted images, the paramagnetic effect of hemosiderin shortens the T2 relaxation phenomenon, so dark areas are seen instead of the usual high intensity seen with inflammation.

It becomes more difficult when infection is superimposed on existing arthropathy or when more than one joint is involved, such as in gonococcal arthritis. In this setting, serial radiographic change or an asymmetric increase in joint symptoms should increase the suspicion that superimposed infection may be present.[144]

Neurotrophic arthropathy can be difficult to differentiate from infection. Similarly developing infection in patients with neurotrophic arthropathy can be difficult to detect. Radiographic features are often subtle. A more complete discussion of the diabetic foot is included later in this chapter.

Complications

Complications of joint space infection can be avoided if they are diagnosed and treated early. Complications include articular destruction, which can lead to ankylosis or degenerative arthritis.[30] Osteomyelitis can develop in adjacent bones, leading to chronic or recurrent infections. Certain adjacent soft tissue structures such as the periarticular ligaments and tendons can also be involved, leading to chronic instability that will exaggerate arthropathy of the involved and adjacent joints.

SOFT TISSUE INFECTIONS

Soft tissue infections in the foot and ankle may involve distinct regions such as tendon sheaths or fascia or may involve multiple tissues that can extend to the bone and joints.[154,161] Soft tissue infections of the foot and ankle are particularly common in children with exposed bare feet.[86,87,97,99,120,167] Trauma can be related to puncture wounds and lawn mower accidents, for example. Elderly persons, diabetic patients, and patients with vascular disease also frequently develop chronic ulcerations and infections in the foot and ankle.[100]

Diffuse soft tissue inflammation, usually superficial, is termed cellulitis. This category of soft tissue infection is often obvious clinically. Patients present with pain, swelling,

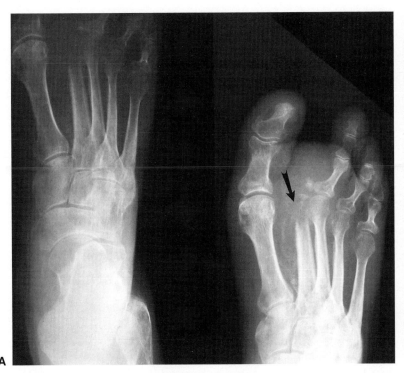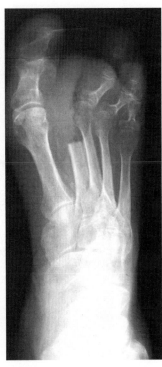

FIG. 7-45. Diabetic joint space infection. The second digit had been amputated previously. **A:** AP radiographs demonstrates destruction of the second metatarsal head (*arrow*). **B:** A second operation with resection of the distal second metatarsal was required. Note the sharp, well-defined surgical images that serve as a baseline for follow-up imaging.

and erythema of the involved region. Offending organisms include streptococci, staphylococci, and, with puncture wounds, *Pseudomonas*.[97,98,120] Imaging of patients with cellulitis is indicated to exclude bone and joint involvement and to detect foreign bodies. Tables 7-3 and 7-4 summarize the effectiveness of imaging techniques and approaches previously described to evaluate patients with suspected osteomyelitis. Detection of foreign bodies that may require excision can be difficult. Routine radiographs may suffice for opaque foreign bodies (e.g., metal, certain types of glass). However, nonopaque objects such as wood are more difficult to localize. MRI (Fig. 7-46) can be used, but more recently ultrasound has been advocated. Jacobson and associates[85] reported a 95% sensitivity for detecting wood slivers using ultrasound. On ultrasound, foreign bodies are hyperechoic with posterior acoustic shadowing (Fig. 7-47). This finding is important because up to 38% of foreign bodies go undetected, resulting in increased difficulty in clearing the infection.[85]

Fasciitis, specifically necrotizing fasciitis, is an uncommon but serious soft tissue infection.[154,178] The condition most often affects older patients (50 to 70 years old) with preexisting conditions such as cancer, alcoholism, drug abuse, and inadequate nutrition.[178] Early symptoms may be subtle. Clinically, the disorder may resemble cellulitis involving the subcutaneous tissues.[27] Cellulitis can be treated with antibiotics, but necrotizing fasciitis requires surgical intervention with debridement and fasciotomy.[154]

Multiple organisms are common in this disease process. Up to 75% of patients have mixed infections. Staphylococci and streptococci are most common. *C. perfringens* is isolated in 5 to 15% of patients.[178]

Because clinical diagnosis is difficult, imaging plays a significant role to early diagnosis of necrotizing fasciitis. The main role of imaging should be to differentiate cellulitis from necrotizing fasciitis or bone and joint involvement.[154,178] Both CT and MRI play a role in this regard.[142,154,178] Facial thickening, deep inflammatory changes involving the muscles, abscesses, and gas in the deep soft tissues are the typical finding describe with necrotizing fasciitis.[178] CT can be performed less expressively than MRI. Fascial thickening and gas in the soft tissues are easily identified. For these reasons, some authors prefer CT in patients with suspected fasciitis.[178]

MRI using conventional SE or fast SE T2-weighted sequences can clearly demonstrate inflammatory changes in muscle fascia and subcutaneous tissues. Fluid collections or abscesses are also easily demonstrated.[154] I prefer to add postgadolinium fat-suppressed T1-weighted sequences in patients with suspected infection regardless of the type (e.g., cellulitis, fasciitis, osteomyelitis). Subtle gas collections may be less obvious with MRI compared with CT.[27,178]

Bursae and tendon sheaths may also become infected.[27,31,98] Tendon sheaths are lined with synovium and may become inflamed by chronic trauma, rheumatoid arthritis, or infection. Infections of bursae and tendon sheaths are most

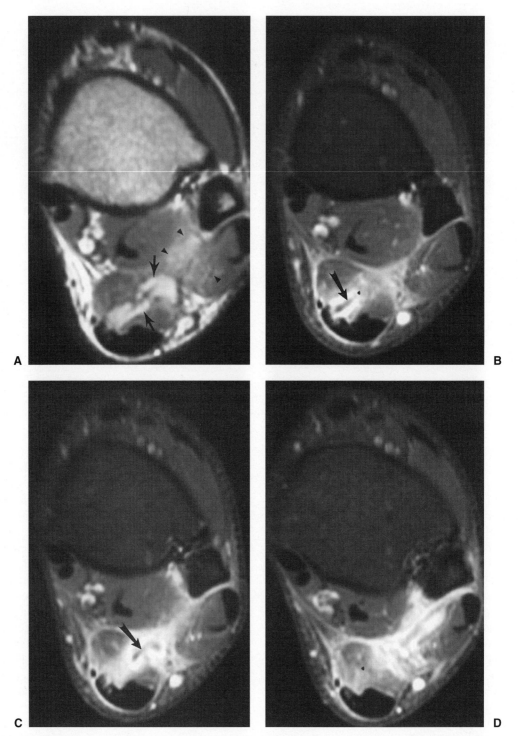

FIG. 7-46. Posterior puncture wound with a thorn imbedded in the Achilles tendon **(A)**. Axial proton density MRI shows an abscess anterior to the Achilles tendon (*arrows*) and soft tissue inflammation (*arrowheads*). Fat-suppressed T2-weighted fast SE images **(B–D)** demonstrate the thorn (*arrow*) and soft tissue infection to better advantage. There is no bone involvement. Treatment is foreign body removal and soft tissue debridement.

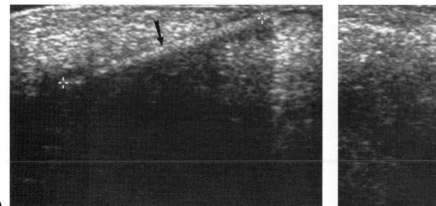
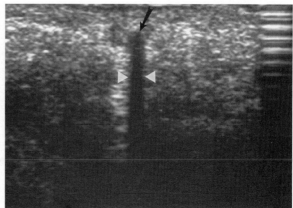

FIG. 7-47. A: Longitudinal sonogram shows a hyperechoic wooden foreign body (*arrow*) with posterior acoustic shadowing. **B:** Transverse sonogram shows a hyperechoic wooden foreign body (*arrow*) with posterior acoustic shadowing (*arrowheads*).

often related to direct puncture wound or adjacent soft tissue cellulitis.[27] Most bursal infections occur in the knee and elbow. The foot is not commonly involved.

Image features of infected bursae or tendon sheaths are not specific. Fluid in the bursa or tendon sheath can occur with multiple inflammatory and traumatic disorders. The degree of distension may be useful (Figs. 7-48 and 7-49). However, demonstration of fluid is primarily useful to provide a site for aspiration and culture. Fluid can be detected with MRI, CT, and ultrasound. I prefer MRI for diagnostic studies because adjacent soft tissue and bone can also be effectively evaluated. Aspiration may be most easily accomplished with ultrasound guidance.

DIABETIC FOOT

Foot disorders account for more hospitalizations than other conditions associated with diabetes mellitus.[27,34,36] Arthropathies are discussed in Chapter 5, and ischemic disorders are emphasized in Chapter 8. However, because of the complexity of diabetic foot infection, more specific data on this aspect of pedal diabetic foot disease are warranted here.

Ischemic and neuropathic (lack of sensation) disease in the diabetic cause confusion clinically and on images when trying to define the presence and extent of infection.[27,36,56,74,100,107] Diabetic foot infections result in health bills of more than $200,000,000 per year in the United States.[100] Up to

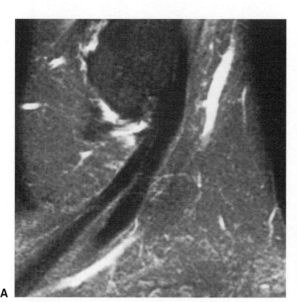
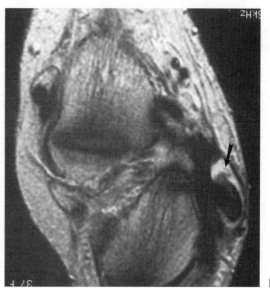

FIG. 7-48. Tenosynovitis due to tendon microtrauma. **A:** Sagittal fat-suppressed fast SE T2-weighted image of the peroneal tendons with minimal fluid in the tendon sheaths. **B:** Axial T2-weighted image shows fluid about the tendon (*arrow*) with slightly increased signal in the tendon.

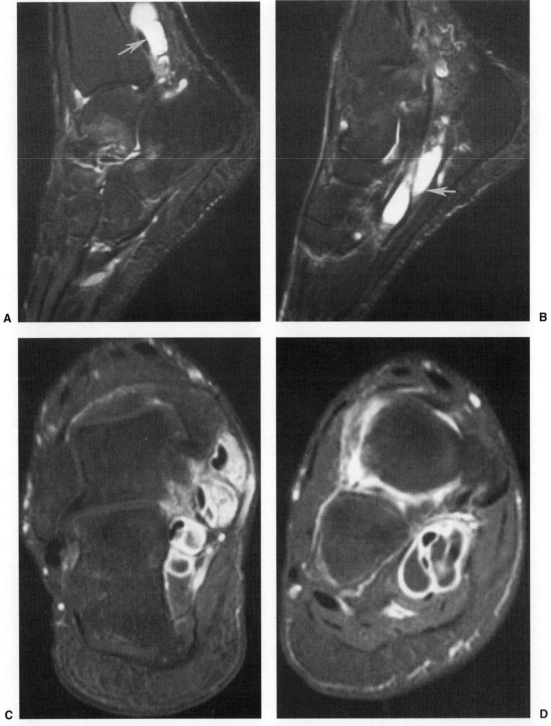

A

B

C

D

FIG. 7-49. Advanced fluid distension of the tendon sheaths. **A and B:** Sagittal fat-suppressed fast SE T2-weighted images demonstrate marked tendon sheath distension (*arrows*). **C:** Axial fat-suppressed fast SE T2-weighted sequence demonstrates inhomogeneous signal intensity and distension of the tendon sheaths. **D:** Axial fat-suppressed T1-weighted sequence after gadolinium shows synovial enhancement with low intensity fluid.

6% of diabetic patients undergo lower extremity amputations because of infection and ischemic disease.[27]

Detection and differentiation of soft tissue infection from osteomyelitis is a common problem in diabetics. Cellulitis and soft tissue swelling are common. Foot ulcerations are on pressure areas from footwear and in weight-bearing areas of the foot.[36,56,100,164] Ulcerations occur most commonly below the metatarsal heads, at the tips of the toes, over digital foot deformities (hammer toe, claw toe), beneath the calcaneus, and over the malleoli.[74] Puncture wounds and foreign bodies may go unnoticed because of senory defects.[36]

Foot ulcerations are particularly important to evaluate. Not all ischemic ulcers become infected or lead to eventual osteomyelitis.[36] However, more than 90% of cases of osteomyelitis result from contiguous spread of infection from foot ulcers.[41,74] Therefore, ulcerations are debrided and cultured, and images are obtained to exclude foreign bodies and early bone involvement.[36,74] Clinically, infection or ulceration is suggested when the patient has local erythema, purulent material, a sinus tract, or crepitation in the adjacent soft tissues.[36]

Detection of osteomyelitis is difficult because of the lack of significant clinical symptoms and altered bone response from ischemic disease. Bone healing and reactive changes such as periostitis are reduced in the diabetic. Clinical symptoms and signs such as fever, septicemia, and laboratory data including leukocytosis, erythrocyte sedimentation rate elevation, and bacteremia may be absent.[74] The most common organisms are S. aureus and S. epidermidis. Other organisms may be isolated from puncture wounds.[36,75,99,120]

Routine Radiography

Routine radiographs remain the initial screening examination in diabetic patients with suspected osteomyelitis. Although sensitivity is less than more expressive techniques, radiographs, specifically serial studies, can be valuable (Fig. 7-50). Differentiation of neurotrophic arthropathy from infection can cause confusion.[114] Neurotrophic arthropathy is typically hypertrophic (bone sclerosis, osteophytes) (Fig. 7-51 and 7-52) in the midfoot and hindfoot but may be atrophic (osteopenia, no bone production), especially in the forefoot (Fig. 7-53).[27,74] Diminished bone density and subtle lytic areas (see Fig. 7-53) or erosions are more suggestive of in-

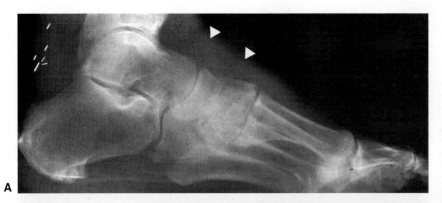
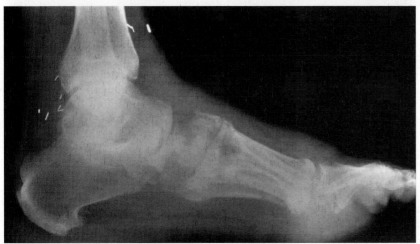
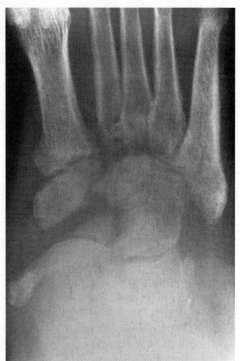

FIG. 7-50. Diabetic foot with S. aureus osteomyelitis and joint space infection. **A:** Initial lateral view demonstrates dorsal soft tissue swelling (*arrowheads*) with no bone destruction. Lateral (**B**) and AP (**C**) views 3 weeks later demonstrate obvious bone destruction with poorly defined margins.

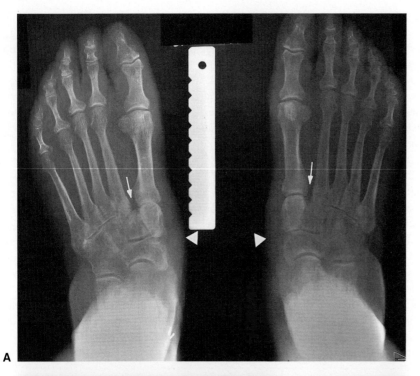

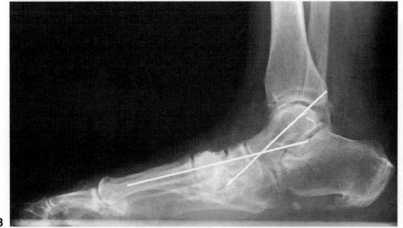

FIG. 7-51. Early diabetic foot deformity due to neurotrophic disease. **A:** Standing AP views demonstrate medial swelling (*arrowheads*) and diastases of the first to second metatarsal bases (*arrows*). **B:** Lateral radiograph demonstrates increased bone density due to arch collapse and bone overlap on the midfoot. Note the negative talar–first metatarsal angle (*white lines*).

fection. Most authors report sensitivities of 43 to 75% and specificities of 69 to 83% for radiographic diagnosis of osteomyelitis in the diabetic foot.[27,96,179]

Radionuclide Imaging

Sensitivity and specificity of radionuclide imaging vary with the technique employed. Three-phase bone scans are highly sensitive but nonspecific. A normal technetium-99m MDP study effectively excludes osteomyelitis. However, this assumes adequate flow to deliver the isotope.[56] False-negative studies can occur in the presence of significant ischemic disease.[74] Abnormal uptake can occur with infection and neurotrophic arthropathy.[96,102,137,179]

Combined technetium-99m and gallium-67 citrate studies have improved accuracy, but significant problems still exist with false-positive studies because of neurotrophic arthropathy. Therefore, many clinicians prefer indium-111–labeled leukocytes in diabetic patients, especially in the presence of neurotrophic arthropathy.[27,74,96] Sensitivity of indium-111–labeled leukocyte studies is reported to approach 96% compared with 80 to 86% for technetium-99m MDP studies.[55] However, false-positive rates result in lower specificity. Disadvantages of indium-111 studies include cost (usually combined with technetium study), time (24 hours or more), low count rates, and poor resolution that results in difficulty in separating soft tissue from bone involvement.[56,74,96]

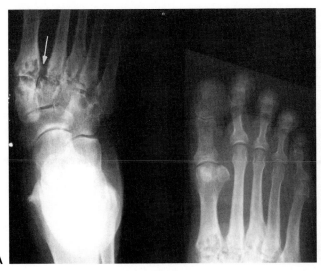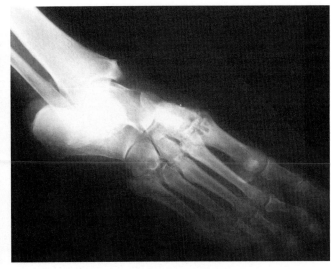

A   **B**

FIG. 7-52. Neurotrophic arthropathy. **A:** AP views demonstrate widened first-to-second metatarsal space (*arrow*) with well-defined erosions and increased bone density. **B:** Oblique radiograph shows well-defined erosions with increased bone density and hypertrophy at the first metatarsal base.

Magnetic Resonance Imaging

CT was used before the development of MRI for evaluating marrow, soft tissue, cortical, or periosteal changes and to detect gas in the soft tissues.[74] MRI has replaced CT in most situations. MRI features of soft tissue or bone involve-

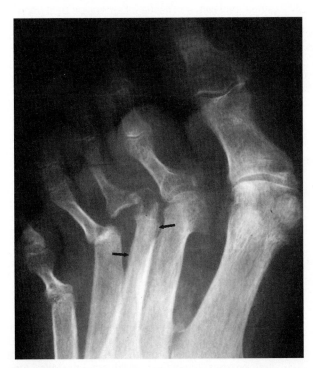

FIG. 7-53. AP radiograph of the forefoot demonstrates bone resorption without new bone formation in the distal fourth and fifth metatarsals. There is dislocation of the third metatarsophalangeal joint with lytic changes in the metatarsal head and subtle (*arrows*) periosteal new bone. This area was infected.

ment have been clearly described.[12,45,56,107,118,125,180] Soft tissue abnormalities are easily appreciated because of the superior tissue contrast of MRI.[19] Ulcerations, sinus tracts (Fig 7-54), fluid collections or abscesses, and cellulitis are easily identified using conventional T1- and T2-weighted sequences. These soft tissue changes are valuable secondary signs that can be used to improve accuracy of diagnosing osteomyelitis. Morrison and associates[125] reviewed these secondary signs as they affect diagnoses of osteomyelitis. Sensitivities and specificities for sinus tracts were 32% and 85%, cellulitis 84% and 30%, soft tissue abscess 26% and 74%, ulcers 41% and 81%, and cortical tract or disruption 86% and 78%, respectively.[125]

The MRI features of osteomyelitis have been described using conventional SE and STIR sequences.[12,45,55,81,107,118] Infection is low intensity on T1-weighted sequences and high intensity on T2-weighted and STIR sequences (Fig. 7-55). These MRI features are 90 to 100% sensitive and are 71% specific for diagnosis of osteomyelitis.[81,107] Marrow edema may also have this appearance (Figs. 7-56 and 7-57).[45,118] Sensitivities and specificities for diagnoses in diabetics are lower, 82% and 80%, respectively.[126] Neurotrophic arthropathy accounts for a significant portion of this problem. Usually, hypertrophic neuroarthropathy is seen as low intensity on both T1- and T2-weighted sequences.[12,107] Gadolinium studies are useful for evaluating abscesses and soft tissue masses (Fig. 7-58). However, enhancement occurs with infection and edema. In addition, poor perfusion, especially in the forefoot, may reduce the usefulness of gadolinium.[45,118]

Comparison with radiographs is especially important when interpreting MRI in patients with diabetic foot infections (Figs. 7-57 to 7-59). Clinical (e.g., cellulitis, ulcera-

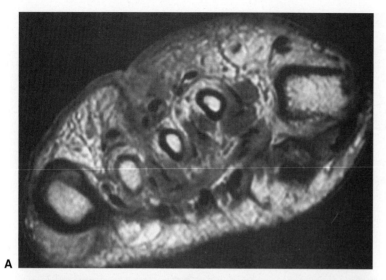

A

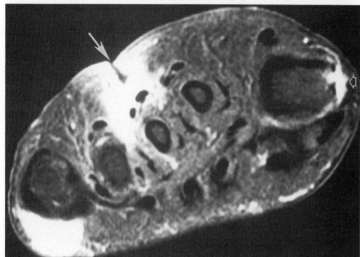

B

FIG. 7-54. Proton density (**A**) and fat-suppressed T2-weighted (**B**) images of the foot demonstrate a dorsal sinus tract with soft tissue inflammation best seen on the T2-weighted image (**B**) (*arrow*). There is an enlarged plantar bursa beneath the fifth metatarsal and fluid with a degenerative erosion (*open arrow*) in the first metatarsal. There is cortical thickening in the fifth metatarsal but no increased signal to suggest infection.

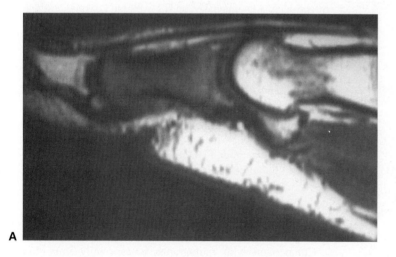

A

FIG. 7-55. Diabetic patient with osteomyelitis of the great toe. Sagittal SE 500/11 (**A**) and SE 2000/80 (**B**) images demonstrate abnormal signal intensity in the first proximal phalanx due to osteomyelitis. *(continued)*

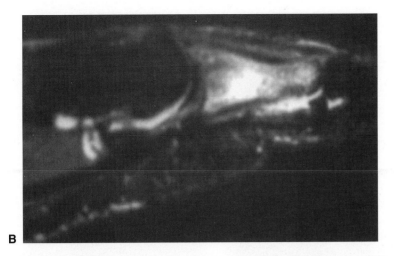

B

FIG. 7-55. *Continued.*

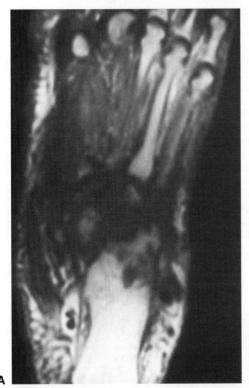

A

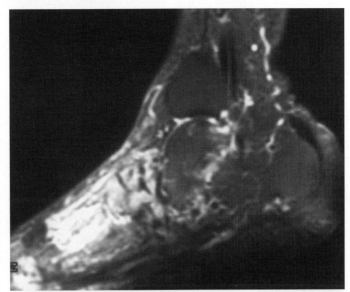

B

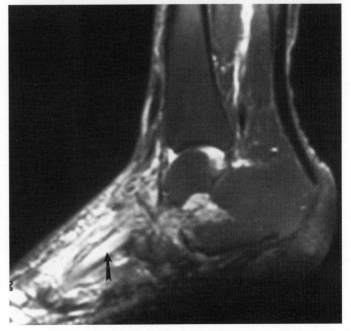

C

FIG. 7-56. Diabetic patient with neurotrophic arthropathy and osteomyelitis. Coronal SE 500/11 image (**A**) demonstrates normal marrow in the fourth metatarsal. Signal intensity in the adjacent metatarsals is difficult to evaluate because of partial volume effect. Sagittal fat-suppressed T2-weighted fast SE sequences images (**B** and **C**) demonstrate normal marrow in the hindfoot with high intensity in the soft tissues and metatarsal (*arrow* in **C**) resulting from infection.

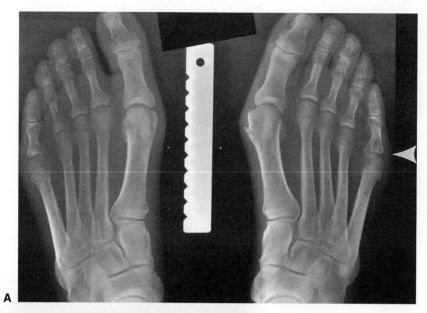

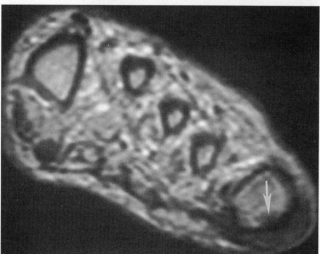

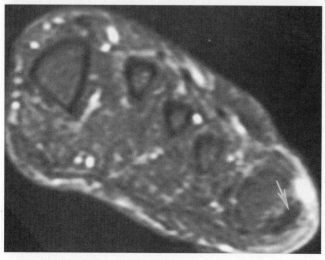

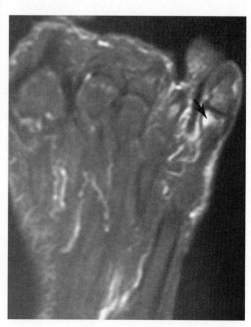

FIG. 7-57. Diabetic patient with swelling over the fifth metatarsophalangeal joint. **A:** Standing AP radiograph of the feet is normal. The *arrowhead* points to site of clinical swelling and erythema. Axial T1-weighted image (**B**) shows low intensity along the fifth metatarsal head with no definite marrow abnormality except at the lateral margin (*arrow*). Postgadolinium axial (**C**) and coronal (**D**) images using T1-weighted fat-suppressed sequences demonstrate soft tissue enhancement from inflammation. The questionable area on **B** (*white arrow*) does not enhance. Coronal image (**D**) shows phalangeal enhancement (*arrow*). Biopsy was positive for osteomyelitis.

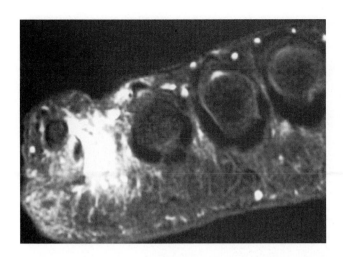

FIG. 7-58. Axial postgadolinium fat-suppressed image demonstrates a large area of soft tissue enhancement between the metatarsals resulting from infection. No abscess is present.

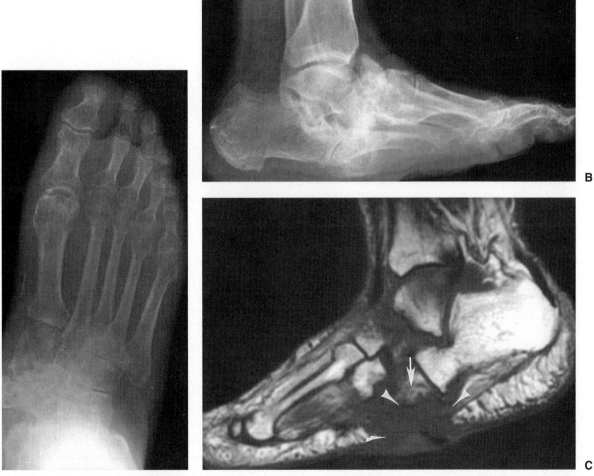

FIG. 7-59. Diabetic patient with neurotrophic arthropathy and plantar draining ulcer. AP (**A**) and lateral (**B**) radiographs demonstrate midfoot fragmentation with increased bone density and rocker bottom deformity. No destructive lesions or erosions are present. Sagittal SE 500/11 T1-weighted images (**C** and **D**) demonstrate normal marrow, except for areas of avascular necroses in the talus and abnormal cuboid (*arrow*). The soft tissue inflammation with the ulceration are of low intensity (*arrowheads*). The talus is vertically oriented (*white lines*). *(continued)*

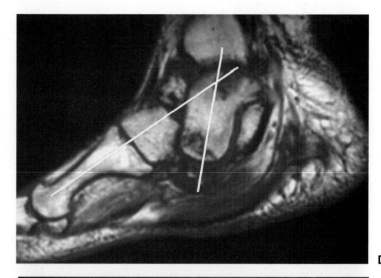

D

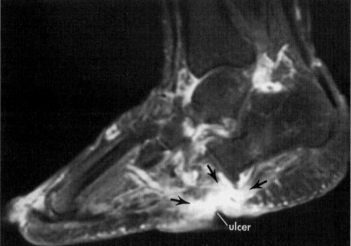

ulcer

E

FIG. 7-59. *Continued.* **E:** Sagittal fat-suppressed T2-weighted fast SE sequence demonstrates high-signal-intensity soft tissue near the ulcer (*arrows*) with an absent cuboid. The signal intensity in the other visualized osseous structures is normal.

tions) and routine radiographic features are essential in planning a cost-effective approach to diagnoses of infection in diabetic foot disease. Table 7-5 summarizes three approaches to diabetic foot infection in common clinical and radiographic settings.

Treatment

Up to 25% of diabetic patients develop foot problems resulting in hospitalization and eventual amputation in 6 to 7%.[100] Multiple factors must be considered in planning therapy for diabetic infections. Glycemic control is an important factor. Chronic hyperglycemia reduces cellular and humoral response to infection. Ischemic disease retards healing and reduces effectiveness of antibiotic therapy.[36,100] About 80% of patients with foot lesions also have neuropathy that leads to recurrent cutaneous injury and joint destruction.[100]

Infections may be superficial, or they may involve the deep soft tissues or bone and joints. Usually, superficial infections result from ulceration, puncture wounds, or poor foot and nail hygiene. If left unattended, superficial infec-

tions can lead to more extensive cellulitis, fasciitis, deep muscle and tendon involvement, and eventual osteomyelitis or septic arthritis (Fig. 7-60).[36,69] Superficial infections are most often caused by staphylococci (*S. aureus* or *S. epidermidis*) and streptococci. Surgical debridement of infected and necrotic tissue is essential. This should be followed by elevation of the involved extremity, careful wound care, and intravenous antibiotics for 6 to 10 weeks.[36,56,69,100] Non-weight bearing and control of blood sugar levels are also important.[36,100]

Deep soft tissue and bone and joint involvement must be treated more aggressively. Deep infections may be caused by the organisms noted earlier. However, multiple organisms, including anaerobic organisms, are more often cultured in deep infection (60% of cases).[56,100] Surgical intervention is often extensive in these patients. Unfortunately, culture material from sinus tracts and superficial ulcers is often inaccurate. Accuracy rates may be as low as 49%.[68] Therefore, examination of deep tissue specimens or bone biopsy is usually necessary to isolate the organism or organisms.[69] Before surgical planning, it is also important to be certain the blood

TABLE 7-5. *Diabetic foot infections: imaging approaches*[a]

Soft Tissue Swelling and/or Erythema with No Ulceration (See Fig. 7–56)

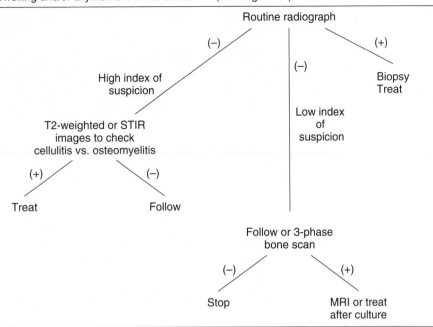

Soft Tissue Ulceration (see Fig. 7–57)

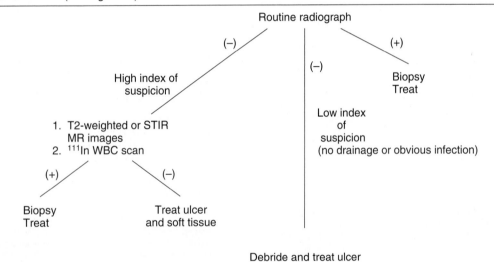

Neurotrophic Arthropathy with or without Ulceration (see Figs. 7–49 and 7–57)

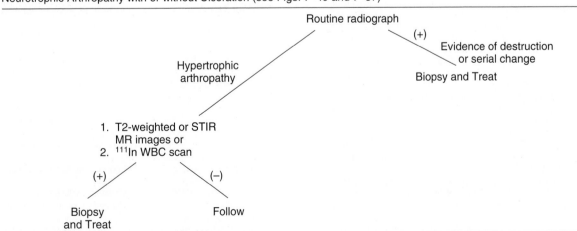

[a] Data from references 19, 25, 45, 56, 73, 100, 125, and 126.

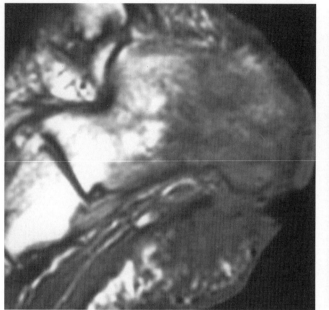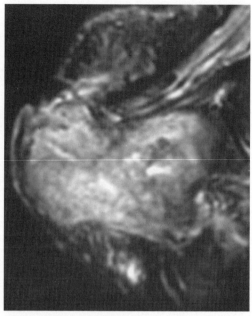

FIG. 7-60. Diabetic patient with calcaneal ulceration and osteomyelitis. Sagittal SE 500/11 (**A**) and T2-weighted images (**B**) demonstrate a heel ulcer and abnormal calcaneal signal abnormality resulting from clinical osteomyelitis.

supply is adequate. This may be accomplished with noninvasive techniques, MR angiography, or conventional angiographic techniques. Tissue debridement, amputation of specific digits or forefoot segments, or more proximal amputation can be planned appropriately with accurate vascular mapping.

REFERENCES

1. Alldred AJ, Nesbit NW. Hydatid disease of bone in Australia. J. Bone Joint Surg. Br. 1964; 46:260–267.
2. Alazvaki N, Fierer J, Resnick D. Chronic osteomyelitis. Monitoring by 99m-Tc–phosphate and 57-Ca citrate imaging. AJR Am. J. Roentgenol. 1985; 145:767–771.
3. Al-Sheikh W, Sfakianakis GN, Mnaymneh W, Houroni Z, Heal H, Duncan, RC, Burnett A, Ashlear FS, Serafui AN. Subacute and chronic bone infection. Diagnosis using In-111, Ga-67, Tc-99m MDP bone scintigraphy and radiography. Radiology 1985; 155:501–506.
4. Ang JGP, Gelfand MJ. Decreased gallium uptake in acute hematogenous osteomyelitis. Clin. Nucl. Med. 1983; 8:301–303.
5. Anzilotti K, Schweitzer ME, Hecht P, Wapner K, Kahn M, Ross M. Effect of foot and ankle MR imaging on clinical decision making. Radiology 1996; 201:515–517.
6. Arnold PG, Irons GB. Lower extremity muscle flaps. Orthop. Clin. North Am. 1984; 15:441–449.
7. Ash JM, Gilday DL. The futility of bone scanning in neonatal osteomyelitis. J. Nucl. Med. 1980; 21:417–420.
8. Atcheson SG, Ward JR. Acute hematogenous osteomyelitis progressing to septic synovitis and eventual pyarthrosis. Arthritis Rheum. 1978; 21:968–971.
9. Autto JH, Ayoub EM. Streptococcal osteomyelitis and arthritis in the neonate. Am. J. Dis. Child. 1978; 129:1449–1451.
10. Azouz EM. Computed tomography in bone and joint infections. Can. Assoc. Radiol. 1981; 3:102–106.
11. Baker SB, Robinson DR. Sympathetic joint effusion in septic arthritis. JAMA 1979; 240:1989.
12. Batte WG, Schweitzer ME, Morrison WB, Johnson PA, Juneja V, Deely DM. Accuracy of MR imaging for diagnosis of acute osteomyelitis. Prospective clinical study at 550 sites. Presented RSNA, Chicago, 1998.
13. Beltran J, Campanini S, Knight C, McCalla M. The diabetic foot. Magnetic resonance imaging evaluation. Skeletal Radiol. 1990; 19: 37–41.
14. Beltran J, McGhee RB, Shaffer PB, Olsen JO, Bennett WF, Foster TR, McCalla MS, Iskra LA, Blagg RL, Biller DS. Experimental infections of the musculoskeletal system evaluation with MR imaging and Tc-99m MDP and Ga-67 scintigraphy. Radiology 1988; 167: 167–172.
15. Beltran J, Noto AM, Herman LT, Mosure JC, Burk JM, Christoforidis AJ. Joint effusions. MR imaging. Radiology 1986; 158;133–137.
16. Beltran J, Noto AM, McGhee RB, Freedy RM, McCalla MS. Infections in the musculoskeletal system. High-field strength MR imaging. Radiology 1987; 164:449–454.
17. Berkowitz ID, Wenzel W. ''Normal'' technetium bone scans in patients with acute osteomyelitis. Am. J. Dis. Child. 1980;134;828–830.
18. Berney S, Goldstein M, Bishko F. Clinical and diagnostic features of tuberculous arthritis. Am. J. Med. 1972; 53:36–42.
19. Berquist TH. MRI of the Musculoskeletal System. 3rd Ed. Philadelphia, Lippincott-Raven, 1996.
20. Berquist TH, Brown ML, Fitzgerald RH, Jr., May GR. Magnetic resonance imaging. Applications in musculoskeletal injection. Magn. Reson. Imaging 1985; 3:219–230.
21. Bessler EL, Conway JJ, Weiss SC. Neonatal osteomyelitis examined by bone scintigraphy. Radiology 1984; 152:685–688.
22. Bisla RS, Taher TH. Coccidiomycosis of bone and joints. Clin. Orthop. 1976; 121:196–204.
23. Bliznak J, Ramsey J. Emphysematous septic arthritis due to E. coli. J. Bone Joint Surg. Am. 1976; 59:145–145.
24. Blockney NJ, Watson JT. Acute osteomyelitis in children. J. Bone Joint Surg. Br. 1970; 52:77–87.
25. Bonakdapour A, Gaine VD. Radiology of osteomyelitis. Orthop. Clin. North Am. 1983; 14:21–37.
26. Borris LC, Helleland H. Growth disturbance in the hind foot following osteomyelitis of the calcaneus in the new born. J. Bone Joint Surg. Am. 1986; 68:32–35.
27. Boutin RD, Joachim B, Sartoris DJ, Reilly D, Resnick D. Update of imaging of orthopedic infections. Orthop. Clin. North Am. 1998; 29: 41–66.

28. Brayton RG, Stokes PE, Schwartz MS. The effect of alcohol and various diseases on leukocyte mobilization, phagocytosis and intracellular bacterial killing. N. Engl. J. Med. 1970; 282:123–132.

29. Bried JM, Speer DP, Shehah ZM. *Coccidiodes immitis* osteomyelitis in a 12 month old child. J. Pediatr. Orthop. 1987; 7:328–330.

30. Brower AC. Septic Arthritis. Radiol. Clin. North Am. 1996; 34:293–310.

31. Brown JT, Miller A. Peroneal tenosynovitis following acute gonnoccal infection. Am. J. Orthop. 1996; 25:445–447.

32. Brown ML, Kamida CB, Berquist TH, Fitzgerald RH. An imaging approach to musculoskeletal infections. In Berquist TH, ed. Imaging of Orthopedic Trauma and Surgery. Philadelphia, WB Saunders, 1986; pp. 731–753.

33. Butt WP. The radiology of infection. Clin. Orthop. 1973; 96:20–30.

34. Bybee JD, Rogers DE. Phagocytic activity of polymorphonuclear leukocytes obtained from patients with diabetes mellitus. J. Lab. Clin. Med. 1964; 64:1–13.

35. Capitano MA, Kirkpatrick JA. Early roentgen observations in acute osteomyelitis. AJR Am. J. Roentgenol. 1970; 188:488–496.

36. Caputo GM, Cavanaugh PR, Ulbrecht JS, Gibbons GW, Karchmer AW. Assessment and management of foot disease in patients with diabetes. N. Engl. J. Med. 1994; 331:854–860.

37. Chandnani VP, Beltran J, Morris CS, Dhalil SN, Mueller CF, Burk JM, Bennett WF, Shaffer PB, Vasila MS, Reese J, Ridgeway JA. Acute experimental osteomyelitis and abscesses. Detection with MR imaging versus CT. Radiology 1990; 174:223–226.

38. Cherniss, EI, Waisbren, BA. Blastomycosis osteomyelitis. A clinical study of 40 cases. Ann. Intern. Med. 1956:44;105–123.

39. Chilton SJ, Aftimos SF, White PR. Diffuse skeletal involvement of streptococcus osteomyelitis in the neonate. Radiology 1988; 134:390.

40. Chused MJ, Jacobs WM, Sty JR. *Pseudomonas* arthritis following puncture wounds of the foot. J. Pediatr. 1979; 94:429–431.

41. Cicchinelli LD, Corey SV. Imaging of the infected foot. Fact or fancy? J. Am. Podiatr. Med. Assoc. 1993; 83:576–594.

42. Clarke AM. Neonatal osteomyelitis. A disease different from osteomyelitis in older children. Med. J. Aust. 1958; 1:237–239.

43. Cohen MD, Klatte ER, Baekner R, Smith JA, Mortin-Simmerman P, Carr BR, Provisor AJ, Weetman RM, Coates T, Siddiqui A, Weisman SJ, Berkow R, McKenna S, McGuire WA. Magnetic resonance imaging of marrow disease in children. Radiology 1984; 151:715–718.

44. Conaty JP, Biddle M, McKeever FM. Osseous coccidiodal granuloma. J. Bone Joint Surg. Am. 1959; 41:1109–1122.

45. Craig JG, Amin MB, Wu K, Eyler WR, van Holsbeeck MT, Bouffard JA, Shirazi K. Osteomyelitis of the diabetic foot: MR imaging-pathologic correlation. Radiology 1997; 203:849–855.

46. Cremin BJ, Fisher RM. The lesions of congenital syphilis. Br. J. Radiol. 1970; 43:333–341.

47. Curtiss PH. Some uncommon forms of osteomyelitis. Clin. Orthop. 1973; 96:84–87.

48. Curtiss PH. The pathophysiology of joint infection. Clin. Orthop. 1973; 96:129–135.

49. Dalinka MK, Lally JF, Konwer G. The radiology of osseous and articular infection. CRC Radiol. Nuc. Med. 1975; 7:1–64.

50. D'Amato CR, Pitchon HE. Hematogenous osteomyelitis of the tarsal navicular. J. Med. Soc. N. J. 1985; 82:644–647.

51. Deysine M, Rofkin H, Tucker I. Diagnosis of chronic and postoperative osteomyelitis with gallium-67 citrate scans. Am. J. Surg. 1975; 129:632–635.

52. Dick VQ, Nelson JD, Hatalin KC. Osteomyelitis in infants and children. Am. J. Dis. Child. 1975; 129:1273–1278.

53. Dillon DS. Successful treatment of osteomyelitis and soft tissue infections in ischemic diabetic legs by local antibiotic injections and end diastolic pneumatic pressure boot. Ann. Surg. 1986; 204:643–649.

54. Donohoe KJ. Selected topics in orthopedic nuclear medicine. Orthop. Clin. North Am. 1998; 29:85–101.

55. Duzynsky DO, Kuhn JF, Afshani E. Early radioisotope diagnosis of acute osteomyelitis. Radiology 1975; 117:337–340.

56. Eckman MH, Greenfield S, Mackey WC, Wong JE, Kaplan S, Sullivan L, Dukes K, Pauher SG. Foot infections in diabetic patients. JAMA 1995; 273:712–720.

57. Edmonds ME. The diabetic foot. Pathophysiology and treatment. Clin. Endocrinol. Metab. 1986; 15:889–916.

58. Ellenberg M. Diabetic foot. N. Y. State J. Med. 1973; 73:2778–2781.

59. Enarson DA, Fuji M, Nakielna EM, Grzybowski S. Bone and joint tuberculosis. A continuous problem. Can. Med. Assoc. J. 1979; 120:139–145.

60. Engh CA, Hughes JL, Abrous RC, Bowerman JW. Osteomyelitis in the patient with sickle cell disease. Diagnosis and management. J. Bone Joint Surg. Am. 1971; 53:1–15.

61. Enna CD, Jacobson RR, Rausch RO. Bone changes in leprosy. A correlation of clinical and radiographic features. Radiology 1971; 100:295–306.

62. Erdman WA, Tomburro F, Jayson HT, Weatherall PT, Ferry KB, Peshock RM. Osteomyelitis. Characteristics and pitfalls of MR imaging. Radiology 1991; 180:533–539.

63. Feingold ML, Resnick D, Niwayama G, Garrett L. The plantar compartment of the foot. A roentgen approach. Invest. Radiol. 1977; 12:281–288.

64. Feldman F, Auerback R, Johnston A. Tuberculosis dactylitis in the adult. AJR Am. J. Roentgenol. 1971; 112:460–479.

65. Fitzgerald RH, Ruttle PE, Arnold PG, Kelly PJ, Irons GB. Local muscle flaps in treatment of chronic osteomyelitis. J. Bone Joint Surg. Am. 1985; 67:175–185.

66. Fitzgerald RH, Brewer NS, Dohlin DS. Squamous cell carcinoma complicating chronic osteomyelitis. J. Bone Joint Surg. Am. 1976; 58:1146–1148.

67. Fleisher GR, Paradise JE, Plotkin SA. Falsely normal radionuclide scans for osteomyelitis. Am. J. Dis. Child 1980; 134:499–502.

68. Fletcher DB, Scales PV, Nelson AD. Osteomyelitis in children. Detection by magnetic resonance. Radiology 1984; 150:57–60.

69. Gentry LO. Osteomyelitis: options for diagnosis and management. J. Antimicrob. Chemother. 1988; 21:115–128.

70. Gilday DL. Problems of scintigraphic detection of osteomyelitis. Radiology 1980; 135:791.

71. Gillespie R. Septic arthritis of childhood. Clin. Orthop. 1973; 96:152–159.

72. Gilmour WN. Acute hematogenous osteomyelitis. J. Bone Joint Surg. Br. 1962; 44:841–853.

73. Gohil VK, Dalinka MK, Edeiken J. The serpiginous tract. A sign of subacute osteomyelitis. J. Can. Assoc. Radiol. 1973; 24:337–339.

74. Gold RH, Tong DJF, Crim JR, Seeger LL. Imaging of the diabetic foot. Skeletal Radiol. 1995; 24:563–571.

75. Goodwin DW, Salonen DC, Yu JS, Brossman J, Trudell DJ, Resneck DL. Plantar compartments of the foot. MR appearance in cadavers and diabetic patients. Radiology 1995; 196:623–630.

76. Gray PF. Osteomyelitis of the metatarsal sesamoid. Am. Fam. Physician 1981; 24:131–133.

77. Green SA, Ripley MJ. Chronic osteomyelitis in pin tracts. J. Bone Joint Surg. Am. 1984; 66:1092–1098.

78. Greene G, Mauer AH, Malmud LS, Clorkes ND. "Cold spot" imaging with gas gangrene in three phase skeletal scintigraphy. Clin. Nucl. Med. 1983; 8:410–412.

79. Greenwood AM. A study of the skin in 500 cases of diabetes mellitus. JAMA 1927; 89:714–781.

80. Haygood TM, Williamson SL. Radiographic findings of extremity tuberculosis in childhood. Back to the future. Radiographics 1994; 14:561–570.

81. Horowitz SD, Durham JR, Nease B, Lukens ML, Wright JG, Smead WL. Prospective evaluation of magnetic resonance imaging in the management of acute diabetic foot infections. Ann. Vasc. Sug. 1993; 7:44–50.

82. Howard JB, McCracken GH Jr. The spectrum of group B streptococcal infections in infancy. Am. J. Dis. Child 1974; 129:1449–1451.

83. Howie DW, Savage JB, Wilson TG. Technetium phosphate bone scan in diagnosis of osteomyelitis in children. J. Bone Joint Surg. Am. 1983; 65:431–437.

84. Isreal O, Gips S, Jerushalmi J, Frenkel A, Front D. Osteomyelitis and soft tissue infection. Differential diagnosis with 24 hr/4 hr ratio of Tc-99m MDP uptake. Radiology 1987; 163:725–726.

85. Jacobson JA, Andresen R, Jaovisidha S, DeMalseneer S, Foldes K, Trudell DR, Resnick D. Detection of ankle effusion. Comparison study in cadavers using radiography, sonography and MR imaging. AJR Am. J. Roentgenol. 1998; 170:1231–1238.

86. Jacobson JA, Powell A, Craig JG, Bouffard JA, van Holsbeeck MT. Wooden foreign bodies in soft tissue. Detection at US. Radiology 1998; 206:45–48.

87. Johnson PH. *Pseudomonas* infection of the foot after puncture wounds. JAMA 1968; 204:262–266.

88. Jones DC, Cady RB. Cold bone scans in acute osteomyelitis. J. Bone Joint Surg. Br. 1981; 63: 376–378.

89. Kelly PJ. Bacterial arthritis in adults. Orthop. Clin. North Am. 1975; 6:973–982.

90. Kelly PJ. Osteomyelitis in the adult. Orthop. Clin. North Am. 1975; 6:983–987.

91. Kim EE, Pjara EA, Lowry PA, Gobuty AH, Traina JF. Osteomyelitis complicating fracture. Pitfalls in 111-In leukocyte scintigraphy. AJR Am. J. Roentgenol. 1987; 148:927–930.

92. Kirchenbaum SE, Minenberg ML. Pedal and lower extremity complications of substance abuse. Am. J. Podiatr. 1982; 72:380–387.

93. Klingberg WG. Generalized histoplasmosis in infants and children. J Pediatr. 1950; 36:728–741.

94. Kloiber R, Pavlosky W, Portner O, Gortke K. Bone scintigraphy of hip joint effusions in children. AJR Am. J. Roentgenol. 1983; 140: 995–999.

95. Kolyvas E, Rosenthall L, Ahronheim GA. Serial 67-Ga citrate imaging during acute osteomyelitis in childhood. J. Clin. Nucl. Med. 1978; 3:461–466.

96. Larcos G, Brown ML, Sutton RL. Diagnosis of osteomyelitis of the foot in diabetic patients. Value of 111-In leukocyte scintigraphy. AJR Am. J. Roentgenol. 1991; 157:527–531.

97. Laughlin TJ, Armstrong DG, Caporusso J, Lavery LA. Soft tissue and bone infections from puncture wounds in children. West. J. Med. 1997; 166:126–128.

98. Lavery LA, Harkless LB, Ashry HR, Felter-Johnson K. Infected puncture wounds in adults with diabetes. Risk factors for osteomyelitis. J. Foot Ankle Surg. 1994; 33:561–566.

99. Lavery LA, Walker SC, Hackless LB, Felder-Johnson K. Infected puncture wounds in diabetic and non-diabetic adults. Diabetes Care 1995; 18:1588–1591.

100. Lipsky BA, Pecosaro RE, Wheat LJ. The diabetic foot. Soft tissue and bone infection. Infect. Dis. Clin. North Am. 1990; 4:409–432.

101. Lisbona R, Rosenthal L. Radionuclide imaging of septic joints and their differentiation from periarticular osteomyelitis and cellulitis in pediatrics. Clin. Nucl. Med. 1997; 2:337–343.

102. Littenberg B, Mushlin AL. Technetium bone scanning in the diagnosis of osteomyelitis: A meta-analysis of test performance. J. Gen. Intern. Med. 1992; 7:158–164.

103. Little JR, Kobyaski GS, Sonnenwirth AC. Infection in the diabetic foot. In Levin ME, O'Neil LW, eds. The Diabetic Foot. 3rd Ed. St. Louis, CV Mosby, 1983; pp. 113–147.

104. Littman MC. Cryptococcosis (torulosis). Am. J. Med. 1959; 27: 976–999.

105. Magnuson JE, Brown ML, Hauser MF, Berquist TH, Fitzgerald RH. Indium-111 white blood cell scintigraphy versus other imaging tests in suspected orthopedic prosthesis infection. A comparison. Radiology 1988; 168:235–239.

106. Majd M, Frankel RS. Radionuclide imaging in skeletal inflammatory and ischemic disease in children. AJR Am. J. Roentgenol. 1976; 126: 832–841.

107. Marcus CD, Ladam-Marcus VJ, Leone J, Malgrange D, Bonnet-Gausserand FM, Menanteau BP. MR imaging of osteomyelitis and neuropathic osteoarthropathy in the feet of diabetics. Radiographics 1996; 16:1337–1348.

108. Mauer AH, Chen DCP, Camargo EE. Utility of three phase skeletal scintigraphy in suspected osteomyelitis. J. Nucl. Med. 1981; 22: 941–949.

109. Mauer AH, Millmond SH, Knight LC, Mesgerzehdeh M, Siegel JAM, Shuman CR, Adler LP, Green GS, Malmud LS. Infection in diabetic osteoarthropathy. Use of Indium-labeled leukocytes for diagnosis. Radiology 1986; 161:221–225.

110. Mazua JM, Ross G, Cummings RJ. Usefulness of magnetic resonance imaging for diagnosis of acute musculoskeletal infections in children. J. Pediatr. Orthop. 1995; 15:144–147.

111. McClatchey WM. Pseudopodia from hemophilus influenza in the adult. Arthritis Rheum. 1979; 22:681–683.

112. McKenna S, McGuire WA. Magnetic resonance imaging of bone marrow disease in children. Radiology 1984; 151:715–718.

113. Meinen IA, Jacobs NM, Yeh TF, Libern LD. Group B streptococcal osteomyelitis and septic arthritis. Am. J. Dis. Child. 1979; 133: 291–296.

114. Mendelson EB, Fisher MR, Deschler TW. Osteomyelitis in the dia-

115. Merkel KD, Brown ML, Dewanjee MR, Fitzgerald RH. Comparison of indium labeled leukocyte imaging with sequential technetium-gallium scanning in diagnosis of low grade musculoskeletal sepsis. A prospective study. J. Bone Joint Surg. Am. 1985; 67:465–476.

116. Merkel KD, Fitzgerald RH, Brown ML. Scintigraphic evaluation of musculoskeletal sepsis. Orthop. Clin. North Am. 1984; 15:401–416.

117. Miller EH, Semian DW. Gram negative osteomyelitis following puncture wounds of the foot. J. Bone Joint Surg. Am. 1975; 57:535–537.

118. Miller TT, Randolph DA Jr, Staron RB, Feldman F, Cushin S. Fat-suppressed MRI of musculoskeletal infection. Fast T2-weighted techniques versus gadolinium enhanced T1-weighted images. Skeletal Radiol. 1997; 26:654–658.

119. Miller WB, Murphy WA, Gilula LA. Brodie's abscess. Reappraisal. Radiology 1979; 132:15–23.

120. Miron D, Raz R, Kaufman B, Fridus B. Infections following nail puncture wounds of the foot. Case reports and review of the literature. Isr. J. Med. Sci. 1993; 29:194–197.

121. Mok PM, Reilly BJ, Ash JM. Osteomyelitis in the neonate. Clinical aspects and the role of radiography and scintigraphy in diagnosis and management. Radiology 1982; 145:677–682.

122. Mollan RA, Piggot J. Acute osteomyelitis in children. J. Bone Joint Surg. Br. 1977; 59:2–7.

123. Moore TE, Yuh WTC, Kathol MH, El-Khoury GY, Corson JD. Abnormalities of the foot on patients with diabetes mellitus. Findings on MR imaging. AJR Am. J. Roentgenol. 1991; 157:813–816.

124. Morrey BF, Bianco AJ, Rhodes KA. Hematogenous osteomyelitis in uncommon sites in children. Mayo Clin. Proc. 1978; 53:707–713.

125. Morrison WB, Schweitzer ME, Ganville-Batte W, Radack DP, Russel KM. Osteomyelitis of the foot. Relative importance of primary and secondary MR imaging signs. Radiology 1998; 207:625–632.

126. Morrison WB, Schweitzer ME, Wapner KL, Hecht PJ, Gonnon FH, Behm WR. Osteomyelitis in feet of diabetics. Clinical accuracy, surgical utility and cost effectiveness of MR imaging. Radiology 1995; 196:557–564.

127. Murray IPC. Photopenia in skeletal scintigraphy of suspected bone and joint infection. Clin. Nucl. Med. 1982; 7:13–20.

128. Mushlin AI, Littenberg B. Diagnosing pedal osteomyelitis. Testing choices and their consequences. J. Gen. Intern. Med. 1994; 9:1–7.

129. Myers JA. Tuberculosis among adults and children. 3rd Ed. Springfield, IL, Charles C Thomas.

130. Nazarian LN, Rowool NM, Martin CE, Schweitzer ME. Synovial fluid in the hind foot and ankle. Detection of amount and distribution with US. Radiology 1995; 197:275–278.

131. Nguyen VD, London J, Cone RO III. Ring sequestrum. Radiographic characteristics of skeletal fixation pin tract osteomyelitis. Radiology 1986; 158:129–131.

132. Nixon GW. Hematogenous osteomyelitis of metaphyseal equivalent locations. AJR Am. J. Roentgenol. 1978; 130:123–129.

133. O'Connor B, Steel WM, Saunders R.: Disseminated bone tuberculosis. J. Bone Joint Surg. Am. 1970; 52:537–542.

134. Ogden JA, Light TR. Pediatric osteomyelitis. Arizona hinshavii osteomyelitis. Clin. Orthop. 1979; 139:110–113.

135. Ogden JA, Lister G. The pathology of neonatal osteomyelitis. Pediatrics 1975; 55:474–478.

136. O'Mara RE, Wilson GA, Burke AM. Skeletal Imaging in Osteomyelitis. J. Nucl. Med. 1983; 24:71.

137. Park HM, Wheat J, Siddiqui A. Scintigraphic evaluation of diabetic osteomyelitis. J. Nucl. Med. 1982; 23:569–573.

138. Paterson DC. Acute suppurative arthritis in infancy and childhood. J. Bone Joint Surg. Br. 1970; 52:474–482.

139. Peh WCG, Brockwell J, Chau MT, Ng MMT. Imaging features of dissecting neuropathic joints. Aust. Radiol. 1995; 39:249–253.

140. Pritchard DJ. Granulomatous infections of bones and joints. Orthop. Clin. North Am. 1975; 6:1029–1047.

141. Rafii M, Firooznia H, Galimbu C, McCawley DI. Hematogenous osteomyelitis with fat-fluid level shown by CT. Radiology 1984; 153: 493–494.

142. Rahmouni A, Chosedow O, Mathieu D, Gulorquieva E, Jazaerb N, Radier C, Faivre JM, Rogeau JC, Vasile N. MR imaging of acute infectious cellulitis. Radiology 1994; 192:493–496.

143. Raptopoulos V, Doherty PW, Gross TP. Acute osteomyelitis. Advan-

tage of white cell scans for early detection. AJR Am. J. Roentgenol. 1982; 139:1077–1082.

144. Resnick D. Pyarthrosis complicating rheumatoid arthritis. Roentgenographic evaluation of 5 patients and a review of the literature. Radiology 1975; 114:581–586.

145. Resnick D, Niwayama G. Diagnosis of Bone and Joint Disorders. 3rd Ed. Philadelphia, WB Saunders, 1995.

146. Reynolds FW, Wasserman H. Destructive osseous lesions in early syphilis. Arch. Intern. Med. 1942; 69:263–276.

147. Rhangos WC, Check EW. Mycotic infections in bone. South. Med. J. 1964; 57:664–674.

148. Robb JE. Primary acute hematogenous osteomyelitis of an isolated metatarsal in children. Acta Orthop. Scand. 1984; 55:334–338.

149. Rosenthall L, Lisbona R, Hernandez M. ^{99m}Tc-PP and ^{67}Ga citrate imaging following insertion of orthopedic appliances. Radiology 1979; 133:717–721.

150. Rudolph AJ, Singleton EB, Rosenberg HS, Suger DB, Phillips CA. Osseous manifestations of congenital rubella syndrome. Am. J. Dis. Child. 1965; 110:428–433.

151. Sarto LA. The infected implant. Clin. Podiatr. 1984; 1:199–209.

152. Sartoris DJ, Devine S, Resnick D, Gallranson F, Fierer J, Witztun K, Vasquez T, Kerr R, Pineda C. Plantar compartmental infection in the diabetic foot. The role of computed tomography. Invest. Radiol. 1985; 20:772–784.

153. Schiller M, Donnelly PJ, Melo JC, Riff MJ. *Clostridium perfringens* septic arthritis. Clin. Orthop. 1979; 139:92–95.

154. Schmid MR, Kossmann T, Duewell S. Differentiation of necrotizing fasciitis and cellulitis using MR imaging. AJR Am. J. Roentgenol. 1998; 170:615–620.

155. Scoles PV, Hilty MD, Sfakianadeis GN. Bone scan patterns in acute osteomyelitis. Clin. Orthop. 1980; 153:210–217.

156. Segall GM, Nino-Murcia M, Jacobs T, Chang K. The role of bone scan and radiography in the diagnostic evaluation of suspected pedal osteomyelitis. Clin. Nucl. Med. 1989; 14:255–260.

157. Seldin DW, Heiken JP, Feldman F, Alderson PO. Effect of soft tissue pathology on detection of pedal osteomyelitis. J. Nucl. Med. 1985; 26:988–993.

158. Seltzer SE. Value of computed tomography in planning medical and surgical treatment of chronic osteomyelitis. J. Comput. Assist. Tomogr. 1984; 8:482–487.

159. Sfakianakis G, Al-sherkh W, Spolecinsky E. Correlation of In-111–WBC, gallium-67 scintigraphy, computed tomography, ultrasonography and plain radiography in diagnosis of focal infection. J. Nucl. Med. 1983; 24:P38.

160. Shapiro SE, Spurling DC, Cavaliere R. Infections following implant arthroplasties of the forefoot. Clin. Podiatr. Med. Surg. 1996; 13: 767–791.

161. Shukla PC. Plantar cellulitis. Pediatr. Emerg. Care 1994; 10:23–25.

162. Specht EE. Hemoglobinopathies with salmonella osteomyelitis: Orthopedic aspects. Clin. Orthop. 1971; 79:110–118.

163. Steinback HL. Infection in bone. Semin. Roentgenol. 1966; 1: 337–369.

164. Sugarman B, Hawes S, Musher DM, Klima M, Young EI, Pircher F. Osteomyelitis beneath pressure sores. Arch. Intern. Med. 1983; 143: 683–688.

165. Swischuk LE, Jorgenson F, Jorgenson A, Caper D. Wooden splinter induced pseudotumors and osteomyelitis-like lesions or bone and soft tissues. AJR Am. J. Roentgenol. 1974; 122:176–179.

166. Tang JSH, Gold RH, Bassett LW, Weeger LL. Musculoskeletal infections of the extremities. Evaluation with MR imaging. Radiology 1988; 166:205–209.

167. Toohey JS. Pseudomonas osteomyelitis following puncture wounds of the foot. Kans. Med. 1993; 94:325–326.

168. Trueta J. Three types of acute hematogenous osteomyelitis. A clinical and vascular study. J. Bone Joint Surg. Br. 1959; 41:671–680.

169. Tumeh SS, Aliabadi P, Weissman BN, McNeil BJ. Chronic osteomyelitis. Bone and gallium scan patterns associated with active disease. Radiology 1959; 158:685–688.

170. Varnell RM, Flint DW, Dalley KW, Moravelle KR, Cummings CW, Shuman WP. Myocutaneous flap failure. Early detection with Gd-DTPA-enhanced MR imaging. Radiology 1989; 173:755–758.

171. Waldvogel FA, Medoff G, Schwartz MN. Osteomyelitis. A review of the clinical features, therapeutic conditions, and unusual aspects. N. Engl. J. Med. 1978; 282:198–206.

172. Waldvogel FA, Popageogion PS. Osteomyelitis. The past decade. N. Engl. J. Med. 1980; 303:306–370.

173. Weber EJ. Plantar puncture wounds. A survey to determine the incidence of infection. J. Accid. Emerg. Med. 1996; 13:274–277.

174. Whitehouse WM, Smith WS. Osteomyelitis of the feet. Semin. Roentgenol. 1970; 5:367–377.

175. Wing VW, Jeffrey RB, Federle MP, Helms CA, Trafton P. Chronic osteomyelitis examined by CT. Radiology 1985; 154:171–174.

176. Wofsy D. Culture negative septic arthritis and bacterial endocarditis. Arthritis Rheum. 1980; 23:605–607.

177. Wood MB, Cooney WP III. Vascularized bone segment transfers for management of chronic osteomyelitis. Orthop. Clin. North Am. 1984; 15:401–472.

178. Wysoki MG, Santora TA, Shah RM, Friedman AC. Necrotizing fasciitis: CT characteristics. Radiology 1997; 203:859–863.

179. Yuh WTC, Sato Y, El-Khoury GY, Hawes DR, Platz CE, Cooper RR, Corvy RJ. Osteomyelitis of the foot in diabetics: evaluation with plain film, ^{99m}Tc-MDP bone scintigraphy and MR imaging. AJR Am. J. Roentgenol. 1989; 152:795–800.

180. Zlatkin MB, Pathria M, Sartoris DJ, Resnick D. The diabetic foot. Radiol. Clin. North Am. 1987; 25:1095–1105.

Radiology of the Foot and Ankle, Second Edition,
edited by Thomas H. Berquist.
© 2000 by Mayo Foundation.
Published by Lippincott Williams & Wilkins, Philadelphia.

CHAPTER 8

Bone and Soft Tissue Ischemia

Thomas H. Berquist, Hugh J. Williams, Jr., and W. Andrew Oldenburg

Ischemic necrosis is a common problem in the foot, particularly in diabetic patients and in patients with other vascular diseases. Necrosis of bone and that of soft tissues are considered separately because their underlying causes and imaging evaluation differ considerably.

OSTEONECROSIS

The terms applied to ischemic bone disease can be confusing. Osteonecrosis is used to describe death of bone and

T. H. Berquist: Mayo Medical School, Mayo Clinic Jacksonville, Jacksonville, Florida 32224; Mayo Foundation, Mayo Clinic, Rochester, Minnesota 55905.

H. J. Williams, Jr. and W. A. Oldenburg: Mayo Medical School, Mayo Clinic Jacksonville, Jacksonville, Florida 32224.

marrow cell components.[222] Although originally (in the 19th century), the cause was considered to be infectious, no organisms could be cultured. The lack of evidence for infection coupled with the loss of blood supply as identified histologically led to the terms ischemic necrosis and aseptic necrosis to describe this condition.[190,222] Today, two distinct terms are applied to osteonecrosis based on the area of bone involved. Avascular necrosis is the term applied to ischemic necrosis involving the epiphyseal region. Osteonecrosis in the diaphysometaphyseal portion of bone is termed a bone infarct.[222]

Osteochondrosis is a loosely used term that generally applies to ischemic disease in the apophysis of the immature skeleton. Osteochondritis and apophysitis or epiphysitis are also frequently used interchangeably to describe clinical symptoms involving these sites in children.[180] Certain of these conditions are most likely ischemic, whereas others simply represent normal variations in ossification.[22,178,179]

For purposes of this section, the pathogenesis of osteonecrosis and its associated radiographic features are reviewed. Other common conditions in the foot and ankle considered in the "osteochondroses" category are also discussed.

Etiology of Ischemic Necrosis in Bone

The etiology of osteonecrosis is not always clear (Table 8-1). However, several mechanisms are implicated in reduced blood flow. Vascular supply to a region may be reduced by traumatic disruption of the blood supply, vascular occlusion (thrombosis or sludging), vascular compression, or prolonged vasospasm.[19,92,126,222] The type of vessels involved and the anatomic site (epiphysis, metaphysis, or diaphysis) are important. Arterial collateral vessels serve a protective function, whereas sinusoids are more susceptible to occlusion, especially in patients with sickle cell disease or other hemoglobinopathies. The epiphyses have fewer collaterals, especially before growth plate closure. The surface area of articular cartilage is a significant factor in the tarsal bones because this reduces the available penetration area for vessels. The talus, for example, has an extensive articular surface reducing entrance points for blood supply resulting in increased susceptibility to osteonecrosis.[172,174] The articular cartilage receives much of its nutrients from synovial fluid, a feature that excludes this area from the ischemic process.[26,79,241]

Certain clinical conditions and mechanisms are well ac-

TABLE 8-1. *Osteonecrosis conditions and mechanisms*

Conditions	Suggested origin
Trauma	Disruption of blood supply[79,172,174,179,222]
Hemoglobinopathies (sickle cell disease)	Sinusoidal sludging[179,222]
Vasculitis	Vascular occlusion[179,222]
Steroids (Cushing's disease, exogenous)	Fat cell hypertrophy Fatty liver, fat emboli[55,179,243]
Alcohol	Fatty liver, fat emboli[55,179,243] Toxic effect on osteocytes
Gaucher's disease	Sinusoidal packing with lipid-laden histiocytes[179,243]
Histiocytosis	Increased extravascular pressure[179]
Dysbaric disorders	Air embolism Nitrogen in fat cells, increased pressure Fat emboli[28,51,54]
Pancreatitis	Probably alcohol related[179]
Infection	Increased extravascular pressure[179]
Radiation	Primarily hemopoeitic necrosis[21,179]
Idiopathic	Unknown[179,222]
Hereditary	Unknown[179,222]

cepted as causes of osteonecrosis (see Table 8-1). Traumatic transsection of vessels and intraluminal thrombosis are well documented. In certain situations, the pathogenesis is more controversial. Dysbaric osteonecrosis has increased because of space exploration, expansion of off-shore oil exploration, and deep sea exploration. Osteonecrosis occurs because of rapid changes in pressure resulting in release of gases, primarily nitrogen (nitrogen narcosis) into the blood and soft tissues. Microgas emboli result in ischemic changes in the affected area, including bone. Nitrogen appears to have a propensity for accumulation in fat and marrow. Thus vascular insult may be direct (gas emboli) or indirect (accumulation in fat cells). Disruption of fat cells with associated fat emboli has also been implicated.[28,51,54,223] The incidence of dysbaric osteonecrosis is higher in obese patients, in patients with repeated exposures to pressure changes, and in patients with rapid, high-pressure exposures. The incidence in deep sea divers maybe as high as 10 to 20%.[33] The most common sites of necrosis are the humerus and femur. Foot and ankle involvement is rare.[28,33,51,54,174]

Marrow cell packing and other extravascular diseases (see Table 8-1) increase pressure in the marrow compartment causing extrinsic vascular compromise. These conditions affect the femoral head much more frequently than the bones of the foot and ankle.[38,41,55,179,222,243]

Cushing's disease and iatrogenic steroid administration are commonly associated with avascular necrosis. The exact cause is unclear. However, fat cell hypertrophy and fatty liver with fat embolization (see Table 8-1) have been implicated.[55,179,243] Steroid-induced osteonecrosis is most common in the hips, shoulders, and knees. The foot and ankle are involved less frequently.

Certain diseases affect the vessel walls, leading to ischemic changes. These conditions include lupus erythematosus, arteriosclerosis, and rheumatoid arthritis.[41,174,180,222] Resnick and associates[180] reported widespread osteonecrosis of the foot in systemic lupus erythematosus. Soft tissue ischemia is more common in the foot and ankle in patients with arteriosclerosis and other vascular diseases. Other potential causes and mechanisms of osteonecrosis are summarized in Table 8-1.

Histologic and Imaging Features of Bone Necrosis

A predictable histologic response occurs regardless of the underlying cause of bone necrosis. The stages are progressive, but overlap is considerable, so a clear definition between each phase may not be distinguishable. Most data, including those presented later, are based on histologic studies of the hip (Table 8-2); however, similar changes occur in other areas of the skeleton. Image features vary with location, stage of necrosis, and the imaging modality applied.[15,19,89]

TABLE 8-2. *Stages and imaging features of osteonecrosis based on changes in the hip*[a]

Histologic stage	Radiographic stage (Ficat classification)	Routine radiograph	Imaging features	
			Radionuclide scans	MRI features
I	0	Normal	± (May have "cold spot" after acute trauma)	Diffuse signal abnormality ↑ signal T2WI, ↓ signal T1WI (see Fig. 8-1)
II	I	Usually normal	Photopenic region or increased uptake	Necrotic zone normal intensity, surrounding zone of ↑ intensity T2WI, ↓ intensity T1WI (see Fig. 8-5)
III and IV	II	Subchondral lucent or sclerotic changes	Increased uptake, occasionally may look normal (see Fig. 8-4)	Necrotic zone normal to mixed intensity, new bone ↓ intensity on T1WI and T2WI, hyperemic area ↑ T2WI, ↓ T1WI
V	III	Crescent sign, mixed lucent and sclerotic changes (see Fig. 8-7)	Increased uptake	Same as II with subchondral fracture
—	IV	Articular collapse and degenerative changes (see Fig. 8-8)	Increased uptake	Similar to radiographic findings

T1WI, T1-weighted image; T2WI, T2-weighted image
[a] Data from references 14, 19, 55, 90, 222, and 226.

Stage I

Cell death occurs in stages, beginning with alterations in cellular enzyme systems.[19,92,222] If ischemic changes persist, the enzymatic abnormalities lead to cessation of metabolic processes resulting in cell necrosis. These effects occur at different times depending on the cell type. Hematopoietic cells undergo necrotic change 6 to 12 hours after blood supply is interrupted. Necrosis takes 12 to 48 hours to develop in osteocytes, osteoblasts, and osteoclasts and 2 to 5 days in fat cells.[92,222,223,243]

Histologic changes of cell necrosis are not evident for 48 to 72 hours using conventional light microscopy. Therefore, it is not surprising that radiographs are entirely normal during the earliest phases of osteonecrosis (see Table 8-2).[14,55,90] Radionuclide scans may be positive early. Both increased uptake of radiotracer and photopenic regions ("cold spots") have been described with avascular necrosis.[14,72,73] Magnetic resonance imaging (MRI) has become the technique of choice for detection of early bone necrosis and to differentiate avascular necrosis from other causes of hip pain.[14,17,92,141,227] Theoretically, MRI can detect abnormalities as early as 2 to 5 days after insult resulting from fat necrosis and edema.[141,153,154,226] Imaging changes are primarily due to inflammatory or hyperemic changes that lead to decreased signal on T1-weighted images and increased signal on T2-weighted images (Fig. 8-1).[14] Spectroscopic studies may be particularly useful during the early stages of osteonecrosis.[76] However, spectroscopy has not been commonly used clinically for this purpose to date.

Stage II

Progression to the second stage requires viable tissue and adequate blood supply at the margin of the necrotic bone.[179,222] In this setting, the necrotic cellular debris evokes a local inflammatory response in the viable surrounding bone. This stimulus leads to vasodilatation, fluid accumulation in the adjacent tissue, and an influx of inflammatory cells at the necrotic margin.[179,222] Histologically, the involved region demonstrates a necrotic zone surrounded by ischemic and hyperemic zones.[179]

At this stage (histologic stage II; see Table 8-2), subtle radiographic abnormalities may be present. Radiographs may reveal an area of increased density that is more apparent than real. The dense area is really normal bone density and represents the necrotic area that is surrounded by the osteopenic bone (Fig. 8-2). The osteopenic appearance is due to the hyperemic response (Hawkins' sign).[79,222] Early changes of avascular necrosis may be more easily appreciated with computed tomography (CT) or conventional tomography (Fig. 8-3). Radionuclide scans generally demonstrate increased uptake in the involved bone (Fig. 8-4). On occasion, a photopenic region may be noted in the necrotic area if this zone of necrosis is large enough.[14–17,19,71,72,92,168]

MRI often demonstrates an area of normal signal intensity surrounded by a low-intensity zone on T1-weighted images (Fig. 8-5) (see Table 8-2).[14,16,19,92,227] On T2-weighted images, the area adjacent to the necrotic zone typically has increased signal intensity because of reactive hyperemia and

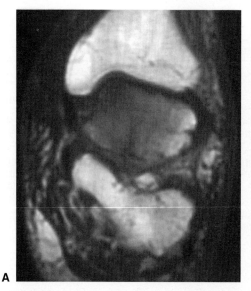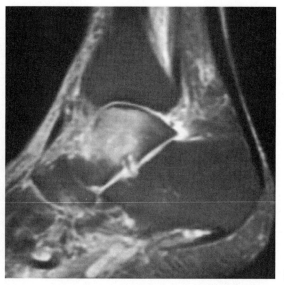

FIG. 8-1. Coronal T1-weighted (SE 500/11) (**A**) and sagittal fat suppressed T2-weighted fast SE (**B**) images demonstrate signal abnormality in the talus due to edema or early avascular necrosis.

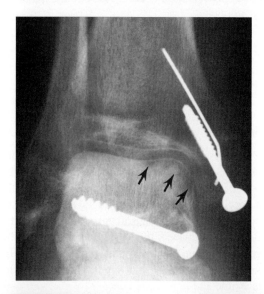

FIG. 8-2. Complex ankle injury with internal fixation of the medial malleolus and talar fracture. AP view taken 6 weeks after injury shows subchondral osteopenia due to hyperemia in the medial aspect of the talus (*arrows*). Bone density of the lateral portion is normal. Avascular necrosis developed in the lateral segment.

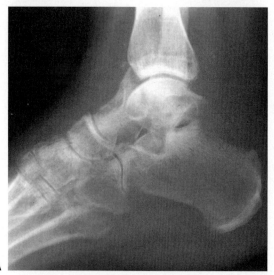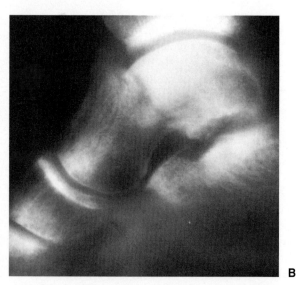

FIG. 8-3. Three months after closed reduction of a Hawkins type III talar neck fracture. (**A**) Lateral view does not show evidence of abnormal bone density. Lateral tomogram (**B**) clearly demonstrates the fracture and sclerosis of the talus due to avascular necrosis.

408

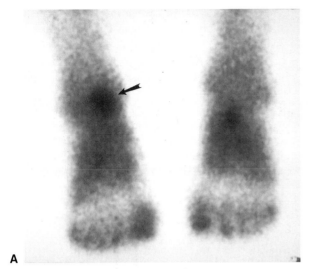 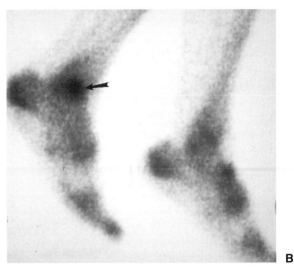

A   B

FIG. 8-4. AP and lateral technetium-99m MDP scans of the ankle after trauma. Increased radiotracer uptake in the medial body of the talus (*arrow*) is due to avascular necrosis.

inflammation (Fig. 8-6).[14,16,19,153,154,227] Changes appear more advanced than suspected from reviewing the routine radiographs.[14]

Stages III and IV

With progression of stage II into stage III, a reactive zone develops around the necrotic tissue.[179] New bone begins to form at the margin of the ischemic and viable cells. Remodeling of the reactive zone results in trabecular resorption, which, in turn, causes trabecular reinforcement along the resorptive margin.[179,222]

These histologic changes (stages III and IV; see Table 8-2) correspond to Ficat stage II radiographically.[54,90] Radiographically, the necrotic zone has a normal to dense appearance. This zone is surrounded by mixed lucent and sclerotic zones. The sclerotic area is caused by new bone reinforce-

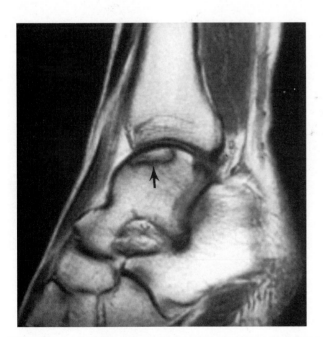

FIG. 8-5. Sagittal SE 500/11 image demonstrates avascular necrosis of the talus. The necrotic zone has signal intensity similar to fat surrounded by a low-intensity margin (*arrow*).

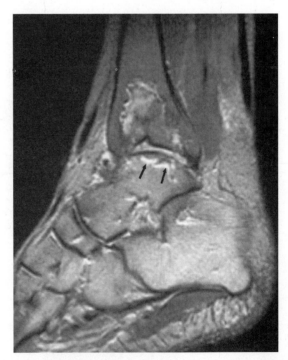

FIG. 8-6. Sagittal T2-weighted (SE 2000/80) image in a patient receiving steroid therapy. Noted are a distal tibial infarct and talar avascular necrosis surrounded by a margin of increased signal intensity (*arrows*).

TABLE 8-3. *MRI signal intensity in osteonecrosis*[a]

Tissue	Signal intensity	
	T2WI	T1WI
Fat	Low	High
Fibrous, fiber bone	Low	Low
Inflammatory	High	Low
Blood	High (> fat)	High (≅ fat)

T1WI, T1-weighted image; T2WI, T2-weighted image.
[a] Data from references 14, 15, 92, 140, 153, 154, and 226.

ment (see Table 8-2). Radionuclide scans generally show increased uptake at this stage. MRI has a more varied appearance, with low intensity in the area of new bone formation on both T1-weighted sequences.[14,16,92,153,154] Hyperemic zones are similar to earlier stages with intensity higher than marrow on T2-weighted sequences and lower intensity than marrow on T1-weighted sequences (Table 8-3).[14,15,19,92,141,154,226]

Stage V

Progressive trabecular resorption leads to subchondral collapse and fracture. This is accompanied by flattening of the articular surface. These changes eventually lead to degenerative arthritis.[14,55,90,179,222]

In the hip, a linear fracture (crescent sign) is seen in the subchondral area. Similar features can be seen in the talus and metatarsal heads, but irregular fragmentation is more common (Fig. 8-7). Flattening or step-off of the articular cortex is often observed simultaneously. Joint space narrowing and degenerative changes follow (Fig. 8-8) (see Table 8-2). At this stage, MRI features are similar to the radiographic findings. Before stage IV (Ficat), MRI features appear more advanced.[14,15,19]

The radiographic stages of osteonecrosis are not pure but overlap, as do histologic changes. Early diagnosis with MRI appears to be more specific and sensitive than with radionuclide scans in the hip. Sensitivity and the typical segmental patterns are particularly useful and can also be applied in early diagnosis of avascular necrosis in the talus and metatarsal heads.[14,15,226,251]

Specific Sites and Problems in the Foot and Ankle

It is not unusual for osteonecrosis to develop in other bones in the foot and ankle. Infarcts do occur in the distal tibia, but avascular necrosis is uncommon.[222] The cause of these infarcts is variable (see Table 8-1). In the next sections, osteonecroses in specific sites is reviewed.

Tarsal Bones

Avascular necrosis in the tarsal bones, particularly the talus, is not uncommon and generally follows significant trauma.[15,26,79,168,170] Necrosis results from the tenuous vascular supply of the talus and certain other tarsal bones that have extensive articular surface area and fewer entrance sites

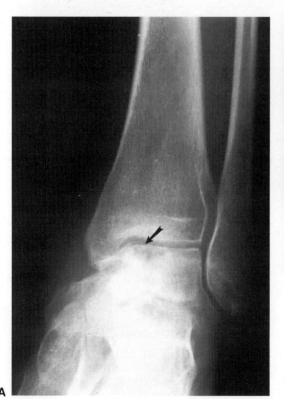

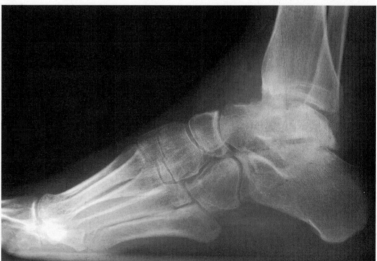

FIG. 8-7. Mortise (**A**) and lateral (**B**) views of the ankle demonstrate talar density changes and articular collapse (*arrow*).

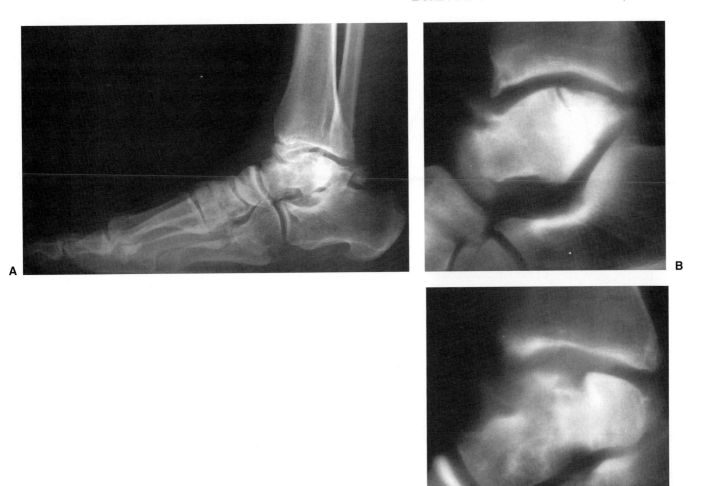

FIG. 8-8. Lateral radiograph (**A**) demonstrates increased talar density, flattening, and degenerative arthritis. Lateral tomograms (**B** and **C**) demonstrate bone sclerosis and fragmentation.

for vascular supply.[15,26,222] The blood supply of the talus is primarily via the posterior tibial, peroneal, and dorsalis pedis arteries (Fig. 8-9). The arteries of the tarsal canal and tarsal sinus are the most important branches.[178,222] Fractures of the talar neck place the body of the talus at risk for avascular necrosis.[26,79] Avascular necrosis following talar neck injury is most common after complex fracture dislocations (Hawkins' type III to IV).[79] As noted in Chapter 4, the earliest radiographic findings may not be evident for 6 to 8 weeks. Hawkins' sign (see Fig. 8-2) is useful in predicting the viability of the talus following injury. When the vascular supply is intact, subchondral osteopenia can be identified by 6 weeks. Absence of this sign suggests that avascular necrosis will occur (see Fig. 8-3).[26,79]

Early treatment of patients with talar avascular necrosis is essential to prevent articular collapse. Isotope studies may be positive 72 hours after fracture (see Fig. 8-4). However, in the presence of talar neck fractures. increased uptake may be seen at the fracture site. A cold spot, in the presence of a fracture, is a more useful sign of early avascular necrosis. Later, increased uptake near the fracture or in the absence

of fracture is a useful sign of avascular necrosis (see Fig. 8-3). MRI of the tarsal bones (see Fig. 8-1) is the most effective technique for early detection of avascular necrosis.[14,15,153,226,251] MRI also provides a method for following this process. With revascularization, signal intensity gradually returns to normal.[14] Revascularization usually begins medially and may require 3 years to complete.[79,222]

Detection of posttraumatic avascular necrosis of the other tarsal bones may be imaged using a similar approach. Radiographically, changes in bone density may be the only finding (Fig. 8-10). This finding may be more difficult to detect in the cuneiforms because of bony overlap (Fig. 8-11). In this setting, subtle changes may be more easily appreciated using technetium-99m methylene diphosphonate (MDP) scans or conventional tomography or CT. Again, MRI may be more sensitive, in many cases allowing detection before radiographic changes are present.[14,153,251] However, the MRI appearance of avascular necrosis in the cuneiforms and navicular is not as well established. Therefore, findings are less specific than in other areas of the skeleton (e.g., talus, hip).[14,15,18]

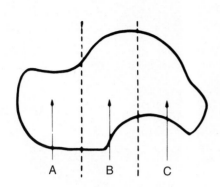

MEDIAL VIEW OF THE TALUS
SHOWING THE AREAS COVERED
BY THE FOLLOWING SECTIONS

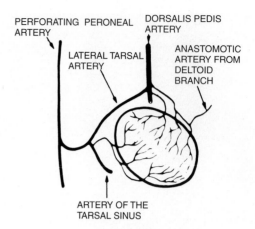

A   BLOOD SUPPLY TO THE
     HEAD OF THE TALUS

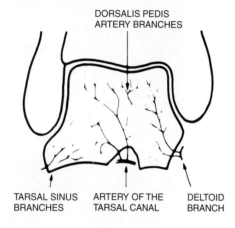

B   BLOOD SUPPLY TO THE
     MIDDLE ONE - THIRD
     OF THE TALUS

A

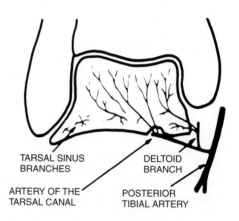

C   BLOOD SUPPLY TO THE
     POSTERIOR ONE - THIRD
     OF THE TALUS

FIG. 8-9. Illustrations of the blood supply of the talus seen in the coronal (**A**) and sagittal (**B**) planes. (From Mulfinger and Trueta, ref. 163, with permission.) *(continued)*

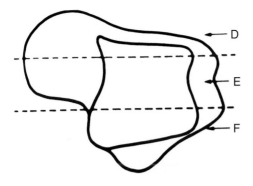

DORSAL VIEW OF THE TALUS
SHOWING THE AREAS COVERED
BY THE FOLLOWING SECTIONS

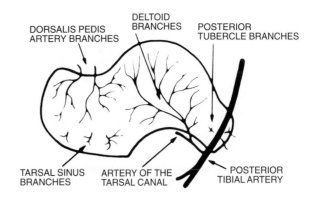

A   BLOOD SUPPLY TO THE
     MEDIAL ONE-THIRD
     OF THE TALUS

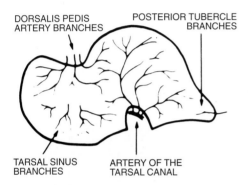

B   BLOOD SUPPLY TO THE
     MIDDLE ONE-THIRD
     OF THE TALUS

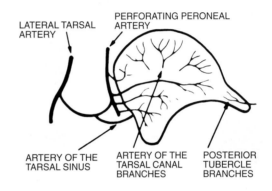

C   BLOOD SUPPLY TO THE
     LATERAL ONE-THIRD
     OF THE TALUS   B

FIG. 8-9. *Continued.*

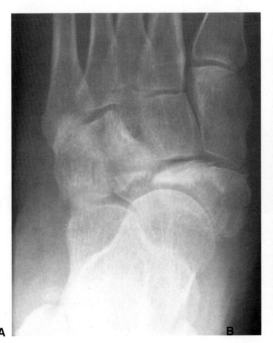

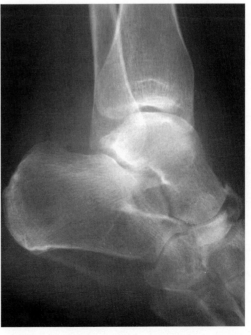

FIG. 8-10. AP (**A**) and lateral (**B**) radiographs demonstrate a navicular fracture with lateral sclerosis due to avascular necrosis.

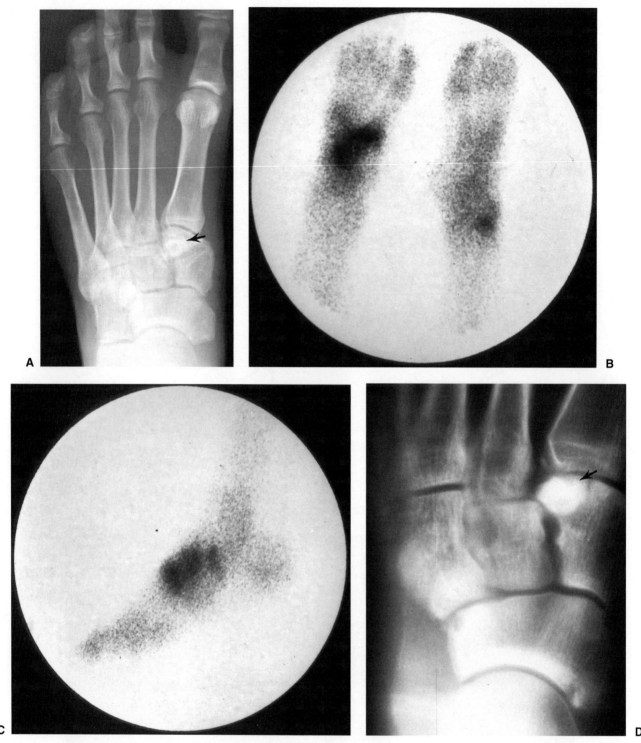

FIG. 8-11. Old Lisfranc's injury with persistent foot pain. The AP radiograph (**A**) shows a suspicious area of increased density in the medial cuneiform (*arrow*). Radionuclide scans (technetium-99m MDP) in the AP (**B**) and lateral (**C**) projections show increased tracer in the midfoot. Tomogram (**D**) demonstrates an old fracture distally with sclerosis resulting from avascular necrosis of the distal fragment (*arrow*).

Metatarsals and Sesamoids

Freiberg[57] first described collapse of the metatarsal heads in 1914 (Fig. 8-12). The original description was based on a group of patients with metatarsalgia and collapse of the metatarsal head. The abnormality was attributed to avascular necrosis. To date, most clinicians still believe that this condition is due to ischemic necrosis secondary to repetitive trauma.[179,210,222] As originally described, the second metatarsal (68% of cases) is most commonly involved (Fig. 8-13).[57,179,210] This may be due to its length and firmer proximal fixation in the mortise formed by the cuneiforms.[138,139,170,179] The third (27%), fourth (4%), and, less commonly, the fifth (1%) metatarsal heads may also be affected (Fig. 8-14).[179] The condition is more commonly reported in women (female-to-male ratio, 4:1), a finding that may be at least partially due to footwear (high heels).[170,179] Symptoms most commonly occur between 13 and 18 years of age (Table 8-4). Avascular necrosis of the first metatarsal head has also been reported following bunionectomies.[138]

Radiographic features of Freiberg's disease are similar to avascular necrosis in other articular areas. Unlike in Köhler's disease, the changes are not self-limited, and deformities usually persist, especially once articular collapse has taken place (see Figs. 8-3 and 8-4).

Osteonecrosis of the first metatarsal sesamoids has also been reported.[91,94,97,180] The condition is more common in women. Although the cause is not always clear, the changes are most likely related to repeated trauma. Ogata and colleagues[165] did report four cases in patients with no significant history of trauma. This group was also free of any other foot deformities. Radiographically, one usually sees sclerosis and irregularity of the involved sesamoid (generally the medial sesamoid). Radionuclide scans may be useful in the early stages (Fig. 8-15). However, usually by the time physician assistance is sought, changes are sufficient to

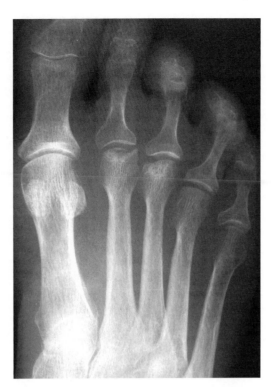

FIG. 8-13. AP view of the forefoot demonstrating avascular necrosis of the second and third metatarsal heads with articular collapse. Joint spaces are preserved.

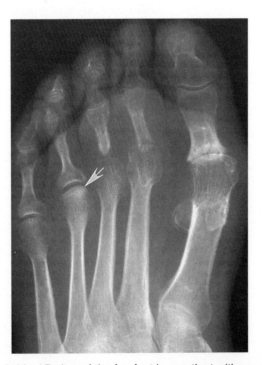

FIG. 8-14. AP view of the forefoot in a patient with previous resection arthroplasties of the first and third metatarsophalangeal joints. Sclerosis and flattening of the fourth metatarsal head (*arrow*) are due to avascular necrosis.

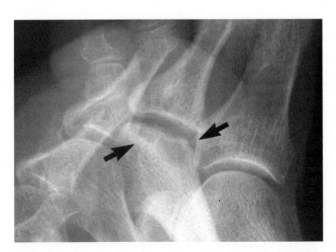

FIG. 8-12. Localized oblique view of the second metatarsal head demonstrating flattening and deformity (*arrows*) from Freiberg's disease.

TABLE 8-4. *"Osteochondrosis" of the foot and ankle*[a]

Disease/Reporting author(s)	Site	Radiographic appearance	Age (yr)	Mechanism
Freiberg's	Metatarsal head (usually second, third, or fourth)	Progressing through stages of AVN leading to flattening of the metatarsal head	13–18	AVN due to trauma
Köhler's	Navicular	Flattening and sclerosis	3–7	AVN due to trauma or normal variant
Sever's	Calcaneal apophysis	Sclerotic and fragmented	9–11	Normal variant
Siffert and Arkin	Distal tibial epiphysis	Sclerosis and flattening	≤11	AVN due to trauma
Leeson and Weiner (Buschke's disease)	Cuneiforms	Flattening and sclerosis	4–7	Disorder of endochondral ossification

AVN, avascular necrosis.

[a] Data from references 22, 57, 114, 143, 161, 179, 180, 197, and 222.

detect the abnormality with sesamoid views (see Chapter 2) or conventional tomography or CT (Fig. 8-16).

Osteochondrosis is a term frequently used interchangeably or confused with osteonecrosis (see Table 8-4).[179,197,198] Osteochondrosis is a term more appropriately used to describe a group of conditions that tend to involve the immature skeleton affecting the epiphyses or apophyses.[22] Siffert and Arkin[207] divided this condition into three categories. Articular forms present with deformity of the evolving epiphysis with potential for joint deformity. Freiberg's disease and Köhler's disease (Fig. 8-17) are included in this category in the foot. The nonarticular form of this condition involves areas of ligament or tendon attachment to the apophysis. Sever's disease is an example of this category in the foot. The third category, physeal, is most commonly seen in the spine (Scheuermann's disease) and proximal tibia (Blount's disease).[206,207]

Although it is a useful concept, this classification excludes normal variants or growth variations that constitute a large percentage of patients diagnosed with osteochondroses.[22,222] Brower[22] believed that most osteochondroses are due to normal growth variations, growth disturbances without osteonecrosis, or osteonecrosis. Most patients are diagnosed before their teenage years, and white male patients are most commonly affected. Osteochondroses are rare in black children. A history of trauma is common.[22,197,222] The radiographic features of these conditions are similar, presenting with fragmentation, sclerosis, and, not uncommonly, reossification with bone remodeling to nearly normal osseous contour.[22,179]

The origin of conditions described as osteochondroses is not always clear. Therefore, commonly used eponyms will most likely continue to be used. Köhler's disease is a commonly used term to describe osteochondroses of the navicular (see Fig. 8-17).[114,115] The cause is controversial, but histologically the disease was believed to be due to ischemia.[114,170,179,194] Most patients are 3 to 7 years old (see Table 8-4). The condition is six times more common in males, and it is

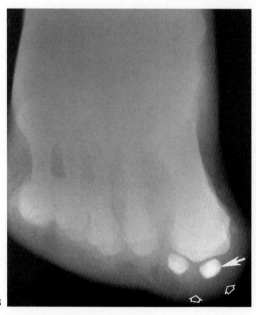
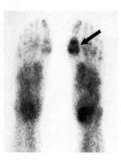

FIG. 8-15. Sesamoid view demonstrates soft tissue swelling (*open arrows*) with sclerosis of the medial sesamoid (*arrow*). Plantar technetium-99m MDP scan shows marked increased uptake in the sesamoids (*arrow*).

A,B

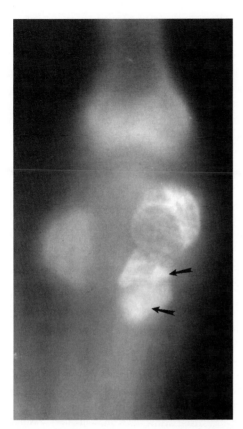

FIG. 8-16. AP tomogram of the sesamoids demonstrates a bipartite medial sesamoid with sclerosis and fragmentation of the proximal medial segment (*arrows*) resulting from avascular necrosis.

unilateral in 75 to 80% of patients.[170] Patients often present with localized pain and tenderness. Up to 35% of patients have a history of trauma.[179] Bone changes have an appearance similar to normal irregular ossification of the navicular (see Fig. 8-17). Therefore, the diagnosis cannot be made

unless symptoms of local pain, swelling, and reduced motion are present.[139,170] Certain authors believe that the diagnosis of Köhler's disease cannot be made unless a normal navicular becomes sclerotic and fragmented.[22]

Because most symptoms are unilateral, it may be helpful to obtain radiographs of both feet for comparison. Serial radiographs may be useful because a normal bone may become abnormal, or the typical changes of avascular necrosis may evolve.[170,179,194] Isotope studies may be confusing in the maturing skeleton, but decreased uptake has been described early. Later increased uptake occurs during the revascularization phases.[165] In the majority of cases, the condition is self-limiting and the bone returns to normal. Therefore, aggressive use of imaging procedures is generally not indicated.[19,194]

Sclerosis and fragmentation of the calcaneal ossification center (Fig. 8-18) were described by Sever.[197] As originally described, the condition was believed to be due to ischemic necrosis. The finding was most common in 9- to 11-year-old children and was originally believed to fit into the ischemic necrosis category. This condition is now considered a normal variant.[22,179,203]

Other less commonly known osteochondroses have also been reported. The distal tibia, talus, fifth metatarsal base, and cuneiforms can be involved.[22,138,143,149,206]

Siffert and Arkin[207] described osteonecrosis of the distal tibial epiphysis in 1950. Ischemic changes in the distal epiphyses were reported after crush injuries. Histologic evaluation of the injured epiphyses confirmed avascular necrosis. This condition is rare in our experience.

Leeson and Weiner[128] reviewed osteochondrosis of the cuneiforms (Buschke's disease). This is a rare osteochondrosis believed to be due to a disorder of endochondral ossification. Patients present with pain and local tenderness over the cuneiform.[162,181] Radiographically, there may be swelling and the typical fragmented sclerotic appearance of the

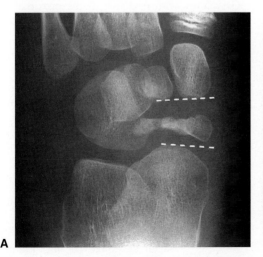
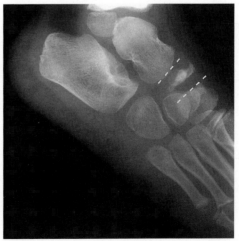

FIG. 8-17. AP (**A**) and lateral (**B**) radiographs demonstrate a compressed navicular. The space (*dotted lines*) occupied by the navicular is normal indicating an intact cartilage model (Köhler's disease).

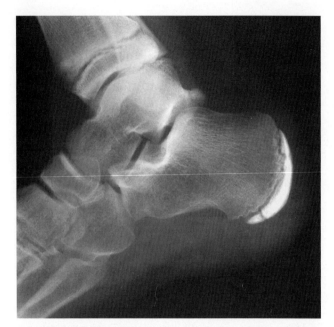

FIG. 8-18. Lateral view of the calcaneus showing sclerosis of the posterior ossification center ("Sever's disease"). This is a normal variant.

cuneiform, similar to the navicular in Figure 8-17. The condition is usually self-limited and resolves in 6 to 24 months.[128,162]

Treatment

Treatment of avascular necrosis depends on the anatomic site, the severity of symptoms, and the patient's age and condition. The potential for poor results and sequelae is increased in children.[170] When possible, regardless of the age group, conservative therapy is preferred, to maintain normal function and to preserve normal weight distribution in the foot.[138]

Talus and Tarsal Bones

Treatment of patients with avascular necrosis of the talus and other tarsal bones is controversial. In most cases, avascular necrosis follows fracture or fracture/dislocation. The extent of necrosis depends on the degree of fracture displacement and the individual variations in vascular supply.[26,79,172,174] Most clinicians agree that non-weight bearing should be maintained only until union has been established, because complete revascularization can take 2 to 3 years.[26,79,138] In certain cases, a patellar tendon-bearing brace can be used at this point to provide further protection until revascularization is complete.[80,139] More recently, core decompression has been advocated for patients when talar collapse has not occurred. Mont and associates[157] reviewed 17 core decompressions and reported good to excellent results in 82% 7 years after the procedure. The remaining 3 patients had early failure and required tibiotalar fusion.

Generally, patients with avascular necrosis of a tarsal bone can be pain-free even if some collapse occurs.[138] When symptoms are present and other joints, such as the subtalar joint, are involved, operative therapy may be indicated. There are numerous procedures for resolving this problem. However, it is important to include all painful tarsal joints. For example, ankle arthrodesis will provide little benefit if the subtalar joint is also involved. Often the patient's symptoms and data obtained from routine radiographs provide the necessary information. Occasionally, CT or tomography is useful to delineate the extent of joint involvement more clearly. In some patients, it is useful to perform diagnostic anesthetic injections to define the exact site or sites of pain. This can be easily accomplished using routine arthrographic approaches with fluoroscopic guidance (see Chapter 2). A small amount of contrast should be injected prior to anesthetic injection to confirm needle position.[15]

Once the involved areas have been clearly defined, the proper surgical therapy can be instituted. Tibiotalar joint involvement can be treated with ankle arthrodesis. However, involvement of both the tibiotalar and subtalar joints is more common in patients who remain symptomatic. In this setting, triple arthrodesis, talectomy, and other techniques may be indicated. Although talectomy may be effective, it results in loss of length (approximately 1.5 inches) on the involved side.[18,131,138] Joint arthrodesis may also be applied to treating avascular necrosis in other tarsal bones that do not respond to conservative therapy (Fig. 8-19).

Metatarsals

Treatment of avascular necrosis in the metatarsals and sesamoids can also be difficult. Generally, decreasing activity or walking cast immobilization is successful. In patients with persistent symptoms, surgical therapy may be required. Reshaping the second metatarsal head may be all that is required. Because of the length and weight-bearing function, resection of the second metatarsal head should be avoided.[138] Osteotomy with resection of the proximal portions of the third or fourth proximal phalanges can be effective when these metatarsals are involved. Arthrodesis may be the best method of resolving problems secondary to first metatarsal head involvement.[138]

Avascular necrosis of the sesamoids may also require surgical intervention. Resection of a single sesamoid is reasonable. However, the muscle insertion of the flexor hallucis longus is affected if both medial and lateral sesamoids of the great toe are removed. This can result in a "cock-up" deformity of the great toe.[91,94,138,165,177]

Complications of Avascular Necrosis

The most common complications of avascular necrosis are persistent pain and degenerative arthritis. The latter can lead to functional and anatomic deformity of the foot. When surgical therapy is required (see Chapter 10), the clinician

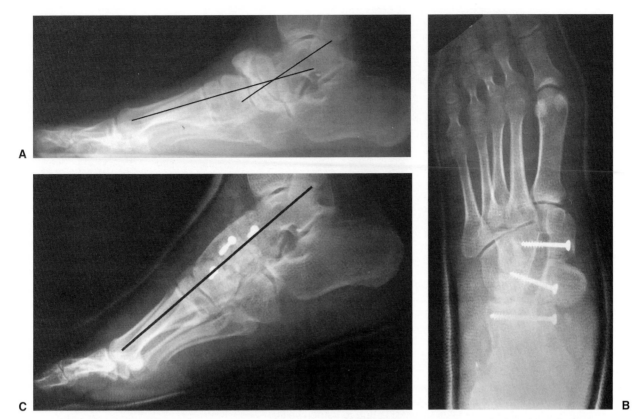

FIG. 8-19. Standing lateral view (**A**) of the foot shows avascular necrosis of the navicular with collapse of the navicular and longitudinal arch (*lines*). The patient responded to dorsal arthrodesis with bone graft and screw fixation. The postoperative AP (**B**) and lateral (**C**) radiographs demonstrate improved tarsal alignment (*black lines*).

must carefully follow results with appropriate imaging techniques to be certain that complications related to surgery (fusion failure or infection) do not occur (Fig. 8-20). Conventional or tomography or CT, MRI, and radionuclide studies may be useful in this setting. Selection of the most appropriate technique depends on the suspected complication (nonunion, infection, or both) and the amount of metal (see Fig. 8-20) used for fusion.

Indium-111–labeled white blood cells are useful depending on the clinical setting. Indium-111–labeled white blood cells are most specific for detection of infection, especially in the presence of metal implants and postoperative changes.[15] MRI is an excellent technique for evaluating union after arthrodesis. When fusion is solid, contiguous bone contact is seen. With nonunion, there is high signal intensity at the fusion site on T2-weighted (TE 60 or more, TR 2000) sequences. Fibrous union has low intensity on both T1- and T2-weighted sequences.[15,19]

Malignant degeneration is a rare complication of bone infarcts in the distal tibia. Fibrosarcomas, osteosarcomas, and malignant fibrous histiocytomas have been reported in association with bone infarcts.[37,61,152] CT and MRI are useful in detecting this often subtle malignant degeneration.[15,19]

SOFT TISSUE ISCHEMIA

Numerous vascular and systemic diseases have been implicated as causes of soft tissue ischemia.[1–3,34,36,39,46,49,53,150] In certain cases, the ischemic changes may also involve bone, but as a rule soft tissue involvement predominates.

Vascular diseases can be divided into several categories. In some cases, vascular response to cold, chemicals, or other stimuli leads to vasospasm.[46, 48] Actual vascular occlusion and abnormal arteriovenous communications may also lead to soft tissue ischemia.[34]

Vasospastic Disorders

The exact cause of most vasoconstrictive conditions is unknown.[53,98,101,104,113,144] Occlusive vascular disorders involve larger vessels. Vasospastic disorders involve the smaller arteries or arterioles and venioles. These small vessels have highly concentrated spirally oriented smooth muscles. The muscle pattern is at least partially responsible for the vasospasm that occurs in this group of disorders[101,135,144] Both the hands and feet may be affected in these conditions. However, erythromelalgia more commonly involves the feet, as compared with Raynaud's disease, in which the hands are more commonly symptomatic.[53]

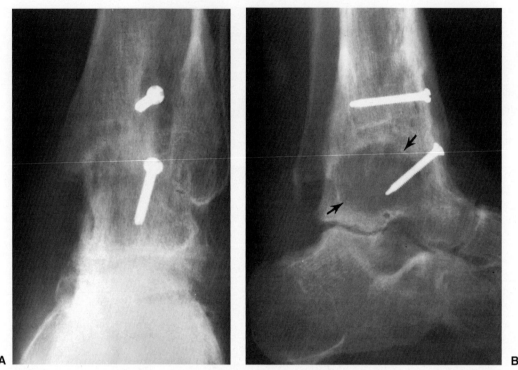

FIG. 8-20. **A:** and lateral (**B**) views of the ankle following tibiotalar arthrodesis. Noted are advanced arthrosis with loss of the subtalar joint and ankylosis of the calcaneocuboid articulation. In addition, a large lucent area in the talus (*arrows*) is due to osteomyelitis.

Erythromelalgia

This condition may be primary (as in Raynaud's disease) or associated with other diseases such as hypertension, polycythemia, or vascular occlusive diseases.[9,98,101,113,144] There is no age or sex predilection. Patients present with episodes of erythema, warmth, and pain in the involved extremities. The feet are more commonly involved than the hands. This feature is useful in differentiating this condition from other vasospastic disorders. The pain, which may be disabling, is usually confined to the toes and balls of the feet. Pain is increased when the feet are in a dependent position and when they are exposed to increased temperature. Pain is similar to that described with frostbite, peripheral neuropathy, and thromboangiitis obliterans. However, the typical history (pain increased with heat, decreased with cold, feet affected more than the hands) allows one to establish the diagnosis.[9,144,150]

Raynaud's Disease and Phenomenon

Raynaud's phenomenon is manifested by repeated episodes of pallor, cyanosis, and erythema in the extremities. Symptoms are usually associated with cold exposure or emotional stimuli.[53] This symptom complex is referred to as Raynaud's disease when the patient has no associated systemic diseases. When associated with a systemic disease, the condition is referred to as Raynaud's syndrome or phenomenon.[101,144,150] Raynaud's phenomenon may be associated with occlusive vascular disease, repetitive trauma (usually occupational), neurogenic conditions (syringomyelia, thoracic outlet syndrome), certain medications (specifically beta blockers) or chemical exposure (ergotamines, polyvinyl chloride), and commonly, connective tissue diseases. For example, 90% of patients with scleroderma have Raynaud's phenomenon.[101,113,120]

The exact cause of Raynaud's disease is unclear. However, it has been postulated that increased sympathetic nerve activity and hyperactive muscle response in vessel walls are responsible for the vasoconstrictive changes. The changes noted clinically are due to initial vasoconstriction (pallor), followed by cyanosis (deoxygenated hemoglobin from stasis in arterioles), and finally redness in the involved extremities from reactive hyperemia. Although the foregoing pattern is classically described, clinical evidence suggests that cyanosis often precedes pallor. The onset of symptoms is generally gradual, and prognosis is excellent, except when associated with severe systemic diseases such as scleroderma. In severe long-standing cases, the media may hypertrophy, leading to thrombosis and gangrene.[53,101,120]

Acrocyanosis

Acrocyanosis is a rare condition that results in persistent cyanosis of the hands and less commonly the feet. The disorder is more common in females and usually presents in young or middle-aged women.[53,101,113,120]

The cause is unknown, but changes are presumed to follow arteriolar constriction, which leads to slow flow and cyanosis from desaturated hemoglobin in the cutaneous vessels. Arteriole constriction is precipitated by cold stimuli. The bluish discoloration of the extremities is also more obvious when the extremities are in the dependent position. Cyanosis typically clears when the extremities are elevated. Unlike in Raynaud's phenomenon, the extremities are cool, wet, and clammy. There is generally no pain, and ulceration and gangrene are unusual.[53,101,113,120,144]

Livedo Reticularis

Livedo reticularis is a condition seen in young adults. Males and females are affected with equal frequency. The exact cause is unknown.[52,101,113,120,144] Cholesterol embolization affecting the dermal arteries may result in livedo reticularis affecting the trunk and the lower extremities in patients with atheromatous disease of the aorta.

Proliferative changes are seen in the arterioles of the skin histologically. These changes result in constriction, slow flow, and desaturation of hemoglobin, which, when entering the dilated capillaries and veins, gives a localized, lace-like cyanotic appearance. There are normal areas of skin color among the areas of involvement, giving the skin its reticular or lace-like appearance.[52,101] Vasospasticity is reduced with warming, which may return the skin to normal color.[101,120]

Most patients seek medical attention because of concern over the appearance of their skin. Ulceration and other ischemic complications are rare.[52,101,120,144]

Vascular Disease due to Cold Exposure

The three basic conditions in this category are trenchfoot, frostbite, and chilblain (pernio).[1,52,136,140,245] Frostbite is the most common of these conditions. Prolonged cold exposure leads to peripheral vasoconstriction. Long exposure to freezing conditions leads to water crystallization with cellular damage in soft tissues and in the endothelial lining of the vessels. Subsequently, edema and ischemic changes occur if the cold stimulus is not removed.[245] This condition can lead to peripheral gangrene. Even when properly managed, the vessels may be sensitized, leading to Raynaud's phenomenon.[101,120,140]

Trenchfoot or immersion foot occurs most commonly in soldiers or in patients with other occupations that result in prolonged exposure to low temperatures with persistent wet foot conditions. Prolonged exposure to wet conditions with temperatures at or near freezing leads to (1) vasoconstriction, (2) increased vessel permeability, (3) vascular injury, and (4) edema and protein loss. Skin maceration, ulceration, and infection follow if the stimulus is not removed and treatment instituted.[1,101]

Chilblain is an uncommon condition in the United States. This cutaneous inflammatory disease is most common in the United Kingdom.[113,136] Young women (15 to 30 years old) are most commonly affected. The symptoms are induced by cold exposure, which leads to raised blue-red lesions of the lower extremities. Pruritus or burning is the most common problem, but ulceration can occur.[101,120,132,134] When lesions heal, there is usually residual pigmentation or cutaneous scarring.[134]

Arterial Occlusive Diseases

Obstruction or occlusion of the small vessels can occur in the foregoing conditions. However, stenosis and occlusion of larger vessels are more commonly associated with arteriosclerosis obliterans (atherosclerosis), thromboangiitis obliterans (Buerger's disease), and thromboembolic diseases.[120,144] The potential causes of the last condition are numerous (Table 8-5). Most of the systemic conditions affect small arteries and arterioles.[2,3,42,132,144,163,186,204]

Arteriosclerosis Obliterans

Arteriosclerosis obliterans is the most common cause of arterial occlusive disease.[45,46,101] Symptoms generally begin between 50 and 70 years of age.[46,120] Men are more commonly affected than women, and the disease typically involves the lower extremities. The superficial femoral, distal aorta and iliac arteries, and popliteal artery are, in order of decreasing frequency, the most common sites of involve-

TABLE 8-5. *Etiology of soft tissue ischemia*

Vascular diseases affecting smooth muscle
  Erythromelalgia
  Raynaud's phenomenon and disease
  Acrocyanosis
  Livedo reticularis
Vascular disease due to hypothermia
  Trenchfoot
  Frostbite
  Chilbain (pernio)
Obstructive vascular diseases
  Arteriosclerosis obliterans
  Thromboangiitis obliterans (Buerger's disease)
  Acute arterial occlusion
  Embolism thrombosis
  Anomalies
Medical and/or other systemic diseases
  Diabetes
  Chronic renal disease (hemodialysis)
  Hyperparathyroidism
  Blue toe syndrome
  Disseminated tuberculosis
  Disseminated intravascular coagulation
  Gout
  Hypercholesterolemia
  Cryofibrinogenemia
  Cryoglobulinemia
  Polycythemia
  Sickle cell disease
  Hemoglobinopathies
  Systemic lupus erythematosus
  Thrombocytosis
  Paroxysmal nocturnal hemoglobinuria

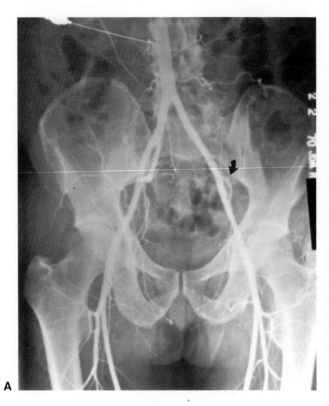

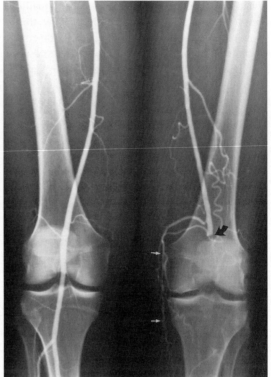

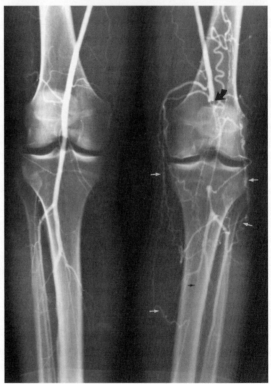

FIG. 8-21. Translumbar aortogram in a patient with left leg pain from arteriosclerosis obliterans. The proximal image (**A**) of the aorta, iliacs, and proximal superficial femoral and profunda arteries is unremarkable except for occlusion of internal iliac branches (*arrow*) on the left. Distal runoff views (**B** and **C**) show occlusion of the popliteal artery on the left (*large arrow*), with numerous collaterals refilling distally (*small white arrows*). A more distal occlusion (*small black arrow*) is seen below the trifurcation on the left.

ment. The pattern of vessel involvement is segmental, with areas of involvement separated by normal vascular segments (Fig. 8-21).[45,46,120,144,163,186]

Patients present with intermittent claudication, but, in more severe cases, pain may be present at rest as well as during periods of exertion. Intermittent claudication is stereotypical, reproducible muscle pain induced by exercise and relieved by rest. Symptoms typically resolve 2 to 5 minutes after activity (usually walking) ceases.[120,132,148] The site of vascular disease correlates consistently with the muscle pain associated with claudication. This information is useful when planning angiographic or MRI procedures. Patients with aortoiliac disease have claudication of the gluteal, thigh, and calf muscles. Common femoral occlusive disease usually causes claudication in the thigh, calf, or both in the involved extremity. Superficial femoral claudication causes muscle pain in the upper two-thirds of the calf, whereas popliteal disease typically results in claudication of the lower calf muscles. More distal disease involving the tibial and peroneal vessels usually presents with claudication symptoms in the lower leg and foot.[43,117,141,160,183] Isolated involvement of the foot and or lower leg is common in patients with thromboangiitis obliterans.[101]

Claudication or claudication-like symptoms have also been reported with vasospastic disorders, popliteal artery entrapment syndrome (Fig. 8-22), amyotrophic lateral sclerosis, muscular dystrophies, and McArdle syndrome.[120,132]

TABLE 8-6. *Conditions associated with claudication*

Arterial occlusive diseases
    Arteriosclerosis obliterans (atherosclerosis)
    Thromboangiitis obliterans (Buerger's disease)
Fibromuscular dysplasia
Thoracic outlet syndrome
Radiation fibrosis
Retroperitoneal fibrosis
Coarctation of the aorta
Ergot toxicity
Primary arterial tumor or tumor compression of arteries
Arteritis
Anomalies

Pseudoclaudication due to spinal stenoses can usually be differentiated from claudication based on history and physical examination. Pseudoclaudication is more variable and is not consistently related to exercise. Moreover, symptoms are often exaggerated by extension of the lumbar spine and are reduced with flexion.[144,163] Table 8-6 summarizes the causes of claudication.

Physical examination reveals diminished or absent peripheral pulses in the involved extremity. The level of pulse deficit is useful for predicting occlusion or stenosis levels. Patients with significant stenosis at the aortoiliac level demonstrate deficits or absent femoral, popliteal, and dorsalis

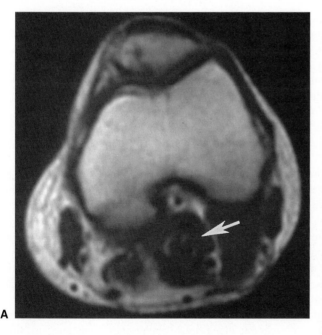

A

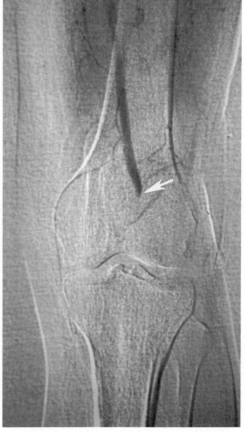

B

FIG. 8-22. MRI and angiogram in a young patient with claudication from popliteal artery entrapment syndrome. **A:** Axial SE 500/11 image demonstrates an anomalous muscle (*arrow*) encasing the popliteal vessels. **B:** Digital subtraction angiogram demonstrates vascular occlusion (*arrow*).

pedis pulses. Femoral pulses are normal when disease involves the femoral popliteal region. Dorsalis pedis pulse deficit may be the only pulse abnormality in patients with tibioperoneal disease.[101,132,144,160] Bruits may also be audible over stenotic lesions. Skin temperature is typically reduced in addition to pallor, hair loss, soft tissue atrophy, and a deep red or red-blue color when the foot is in the dependent position.[101,144,163] Ulcerations and gangrene, when present, are typically located at pressure points on the foot and ankle, especially in diabetes with peripheral neuropathy.[101,120]

Other useful physical findings include the capillary refill test and the ankle-arm or ankle-brachial index.[101,120,135,144] When the capillary bed is compressed and pressure released, there is normally capillary refill in less than 5 seconds. The systolic pressure in the ankle divided by the systolic pressure in the arm is normally greater than or equal to 0.90. When the index is between 0.9 and 0.5, there is usually mild to moderate disease. Patients with severe occlusive disease have an index less than 0.5.[95,101,187] When the index is in the 0.1 to 0.2 range, gangrene is likely to occur.[163] ABI may be misleading and falsely elevated in diabetics and in the elderly in whom the vessels have medial calcinosis and are not compressible. In the patients, pulse volume recording or transcutaneous oximetry may better demonstrate the level of arterial insufficiency.

Histologically, stenotic or occluded areas in the vessels show atheromatous plaques with associated intimal thrombus. These obstructive areas cause decreased flow during exercise or, if severe enough, at rest. Generally, patients are not symptomatic at rest if occlusion is greater than 75%. Obstruction of more than 60% is generally required to cause symptoms during exercise. The extent of collateral development obviously affects the severity of symptoms. Degeneration and calcification of the media are commonly present, especially in diabetic patients. This weakening of the media may lead to aneurysm formation in the popliteal fossa or femoral artery below the inguinal ligaments. Aneurysm formation may also develop in the abdominal aorta and iliac vessels.[144]

In patients with diabetes mellitus, vascular disease is more peripheral, and progression of the disease tends to be more rapid.[144] Arteriosclerosis is the most common cause of morbidity and mortality in diabetic patients.[204] The arteriosclerotic lesions are similar to those of persons without diabetes (Fig. 8-23). Presence of these lesions earlier in diabetic patients may be related to numerous factors associated with hyperglycemia. This list includes (1) abnormal platelet aggregation, (2) abnormal lipid profiles, (3) endothelial damage from elevated low-density lipoprotein, and (4) insulin elevations that can lead to arterial smooth muscle proliferation. Once endothelial damage has occurred, platelet aggregation, lipid deposition, and plaque formation lead to vascular narrowing or occlusion.[132,144,204]

Vascular disease in diabetic patients affects both the major vessels and the microvasculature. Arteriosclerosis obliterans is more marked, progressive, and involves vessels below the knee more commonly than arteriosclerosis in persons who

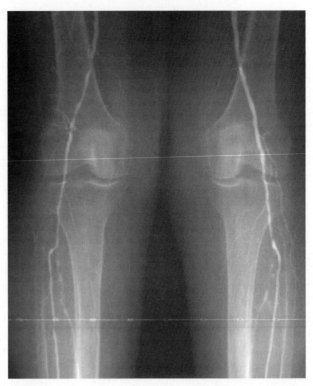

FIG. 8-23. Diabetic with ischemic changes in the feet and claudication. Angiogram reveals segmental stenosis of the superficial femoral, popliteal, and trifurcation arteries with stenosis and occlusions below the trifurcation, predominantly in the peroneal and posterior tibial arteries.

do not have diabetes.[133,204] Ankle and foot ulcerations are probably related to larger vessel disease, but regardless of the type of vessel involvement ulceration, ischemia, gangrene, and infection are significant problems in diabetic patients (see Chapter 7).[48,133] Twenty-five percent of diabetic hospital admissions are for foot problems, and amputations are eventually needed for treatment of ischemic disease in 40% of diabetic patients. Fifty-seven percent of all nontraumatic amputations are in diabetic patients.[48]

Clinical findings are also more complex in diabetic patients. Similar findings may be present with either neurotrophic or ischemic changes. Ulcerations, infections, and evidence of ischemia can be present with neuropathy as well as primary vascular disease. Differentiation of ischemic and neurotrophic ulcers can be accomplished clinically in most cases. Ulcerations are the most common presentation of diabetic neuropathy in the foot. These ulcers are typically painless, are surrounded by thick callus, and are usually located under the metatarsal heads and at the tips of the toes.[48] Ischemic ulcerations have erythematous margins, little if any callus, and are often painful. These ulcers are commonly found along the great toe and fifth metatarsophalangeal joints (pressure points due to footwear) and adjacent to the calcaneus.[48]

Neurotrophic changes can also mimic certain ischemic changes because neuropathy leads to edema as a reult of increased vascular permeability and arteriovenous shunting.[48] Pain can also be present with both diabetic complications. Neuropathy produces random pain that is not related to position. Rest pain due to ischemia usually does not occur unless peripheral pressures are higher than 50 mm Hg. Rest pain tends to awaken patients from sleep and may be improved when the feet are dependent. Claudication is significantly different from rest pain.[48,101,144]

Thromboangiitis Obliterans (Buerger's Disease)

Thromboangiitis obliterans is a disease that primarily affects men in the 20- to 40-year age range. The male-to-female ratio is 9 to 75:1 depending on the source.[2,101,144] Geographically, the disease is more prevalent in Asia, including India, and Israel than in the United States.[2,74,101,133,144]

The cause is unknown, but there is a strong association with cigarette smoking, and because of its geographic distribution, a genetic cause has also been postulated. More recently, the possibility of an autoimmune cause has been entertained. Adar and colleagues[2] demonstrated sensitivity to type I and III collagen, present in the vessel walls. This antibody was noted in 77% of lymphocytes and in the blood of 50% of patients with thromboangiitis obliterans.

Thromboangiitis obliterans affects medium-sized arteries (Fig. 8-24) and veins in a segmental fashion similar to other occlusive vascular diseases (Figs. 8-25 and 8-26). Microscopic evaluation reveals intimal proliferation with inflammatory and giant cells extending into the thrombus. Unlike in arteriosclerosis obliterans, the media is normal. Calcifications and cholesterol deposits are also uncommon.[2,133,144]

Clinical presentation is generally that of a young male smoker with ischemic symptoms in the extremities and a history of thrombophlebitis. Patients may often present with Raynaud's phenomenon, rest pain, and ulceration or gangrenous changes in one or more digits. Peripheral pulses are diminished or absent, similar to other occlusive diseases. Clinical features noted earlier and vascular studies (see later) demonstrating small vessel disease with sparing of larger vessels establish the diagnosis.[101,132]

Acute Arterial Occlusion

Thrombosis, emboli, or acute traumatic transsection may be implicated in acute vascular occlusion. The last condition is not difficult to diagnose and is usually confirmed by clinical and physical findings. Differentiation of occlusion due to thrombosis or emboli can be more difficult.[64,65,80,81,84,86] Table 8-7, based on the study by Hight and Telneyn-Cough,[84] summarizes the findings in thrombotic and em-

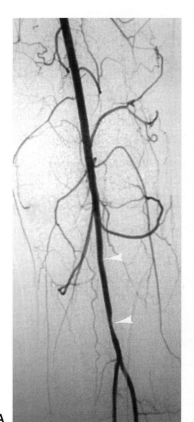 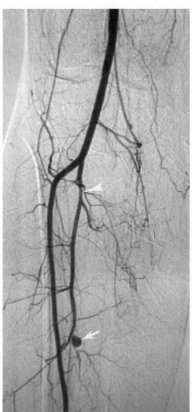 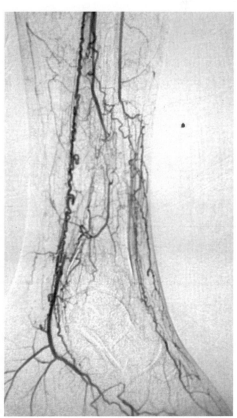

A   **B,C**

FIG. 8-24. Digital subtraction angiogram of the lower extremity in a patient with Buerger's disease. **A:** Image at the distal femoral, popliteal, and trifurcation levels shows segmental narrowing (*arrowheads*). **B:** The anterior tibial fills with narrowing (*arrowhead*) in the proximal posterior tibial artery and an aneurysm distally (*arrow*). **C:** Lateral view distally shows occlusions with multiple tortuous collateral vessels.

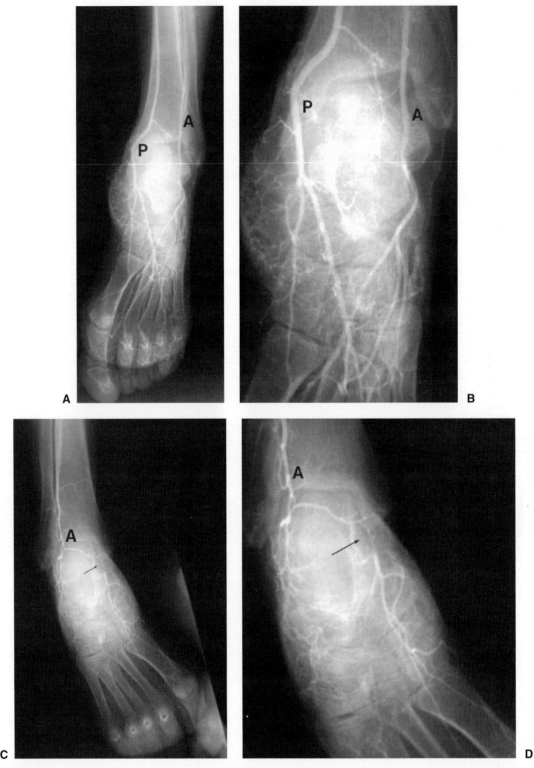

FIG. 8-25. Peripheral angiogram in a patient with thromboangiitis obliterans (Buerger's disease). The left foot and ankle (**A**) and localized view (**B**) show normal caliber anterior (*A*) and posterior (*P*) tibial arteries with good peripheral filling of the branch vessels of the foot. Images of the right foot (**C**) and localized (**D**) show stenosis and collateral vessels in the distal anterior tibial artery at the malleolar level with cross filling of the posterior tibial artery below the ankle because of more proximal occlusion. A stenotic segment (*arrow*) is seen distally.

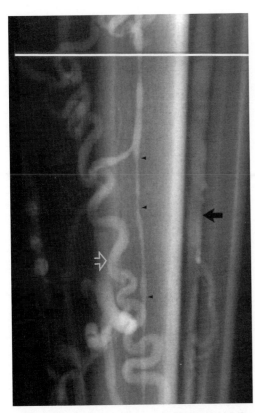

FIG. 8-26. Patient with thromboangiitis obliterans (Buerger's disease) with long-standing thrombophlebitis. The venogram shows multiple varices (*open arrow*), with a normal posterior tibial vein (*black arrow*) and a stenosed or partially recanalized anterior tibial vein (*small black arrowheads*).

TABLE 8-7. *Clinical and radiographic features of thrombosis and embolism in vascular occlusive disease*[a]

Features	Embolism	Thrombosis
Onset	Acute	May be acute
Level of demarcation	Sharp	Vague
History of claudication	Rare	Common
Age	No specific age	40 yrs.
Identifiable sources	Yes	±
Angiographic features	Fewer collaterals, meniscus sign ±, atherosclerosis (see Fig. 8-28)	Atherosclerosis with collaterals common (see Fig. 8-21)

[a] From Hight and Telneyn-Cough, ref. 84, with permission.

bolic occlusion. Both clinical and angiographic features are important in confirming the diagnosis.[84,101,132]

Thromboembolic occlusion may occur with numerous underlying conditions.[49,84,93,130,132,155] Acute occlusion due to thrombosis occurs in approximately 10% of patients with arteriosclerosis obliterans, but it is rare in thromboangiitis obliterans.[132] Cardiac and proximal large vessel arteriosclerosis or aneurysms may serve as sources of emboli (Figs. 8-27 and 8-28). Patients with atrial fibrillation, mitral valve disease, mitral thrombosis, aneurysms, and numerous atheromatous plaques are prone to peripheral emboli.[84,95,101,144] Septic emboli have been reported with bacterial endocarditis, disseminated tuberculosis, and other infections.[96] Soft tissue ischemia, regardless of the cause, can be related to hypoten-

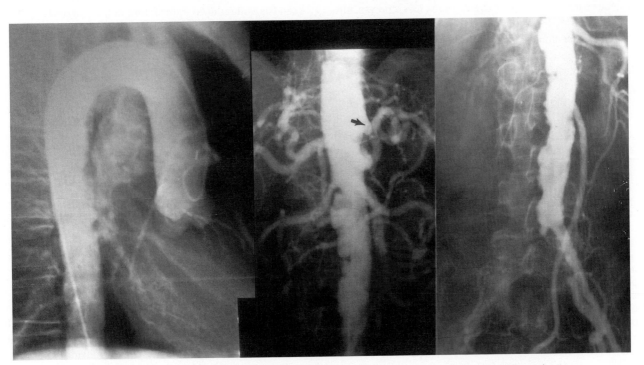

FIG. 8-27. Aortic arch study demonstrating extensive atheromatous change with irregularity and narrowing of the abdominal aorta. The patient has occlusions of the right common iliac and a proximal (*arrow*) major visceral branch. The numerous plaques serve as sources for peripheral small vessel emboli.

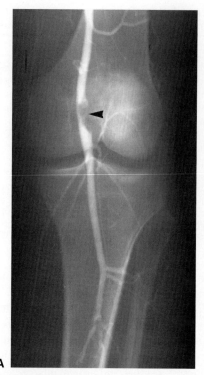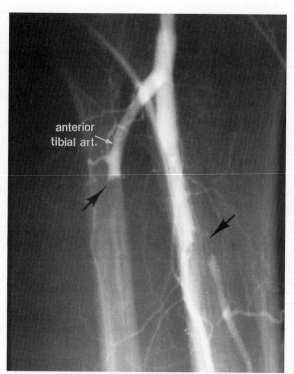

FIG. 8-28. Two patients with acute emboli to the lower extremity. Angiogram in the first patient (**A**) shows a high-grade narrowing (*arrowhead*) from a clot in the popliteal artery. Note the lack of collateral vessels compared with Figure 8-21. The second patient (**B**) demonstrates two sites of acute embolic occlusion below the trifurcation (*arrows*) with a meniscus sign in the anterior tibial artery.

sion, endothelial damage, and complete vascular occlusion.[3, 49,95,101,150,156,189] Intimal damage due to decreased local flow can occur with heart failure, extreme blood loss, and vasculitis.[133] The injured intima serves as a nidus for thrombosis and tissue ischemia. Microvascular occlusion can occur acutely with septic emboli, specifically gram-positive organisms.[74,75] Table 8-8 lists causes of ischemia related to thromboembolic occlusion.

TABLE 8-8. *Etiology of thromboembolic occlusion*[a]

Cardiac and large vessel disease
  Endocarditis
  Mural thrombi
  Atrial fibrillation
  Mitral valve disease
  Mitral thrombosis
  Atheromatous plaques
  Cholesterol emboli
  Aneurysm
Trauma
Septic emboli
Hemoglobinopathies
Disseminated intravascular coagulation
Polycythemia vera
Hyperviscosity
Venous thrombosis (paradoxical emboli)
Vasculitis

[a] Data from references 3, 50, 65, 95, 130, 132, 144, 155, 156, and 189.

Patients with acute thromboembolic disease usually present with acute pain, decreased or absent pulses, pallor, or cyanosis and reduced temperature in the extremity.[58,64] Angiography or MR angiography is necessary to determine the site or sites (multiple emboli) of occlusion (see Figs. 8-27 and 8-28).[15,77]

Diagnostic Techniques

Many soft tissue ischemic diseases can be diagnosed based on history and physical examination.[40,101,144,186] Diagnostic techniques, specifically imaging procedures, are largely used to define vascular anatomy, to determine the likelihood for healing of soft tissue changes (ulcers and necrosis), and to evaluate the most appropriate approach of treatment (medical, surgical, angiointerventional).[40,116–119,132]

Routine Radiography

Routine radiographs provide little, if any, additional information regarding the soft tissues than can be identified by physical examination. Ulcerations, cellulitis, edema, and gangrene can be defined on physical examination. Soft tissue swelling, larger ulcers, and vascular calcification, common in diabetic patients and in patients undergoing dialysis, can be identified.[15,16,189] Routine radiographs predominantly

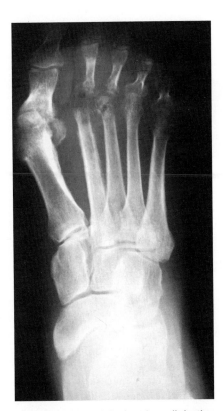

FIG. 8-29. AP view of the right foot in a diabetic patient with soft tissue ulceration. The radiograph demonstrates destruction of the second and third metatarsophalangeal joints with gas in the soft tissues resulting from infection.

TABLE 8-9. *Patterns of thallium uptake in soft tissue ulcers[a]*

Pattern	Early	Delayed	Results
I	+ + +	+ +	All healed
II	+	+ +	22/23 (96%) Healed
III	−	+	5/7 (71%) Healed
IV	−	−	No healing; amputation

+ , positive; ≥ + + , strongly positive; − , no uptake.
[a] From Ohta, ref. 166, with permission.

serve as a screening technique to exclude extension of soft tissue infection to bone (Fig. 8-29). However, isotope studies and MRI are more sensitive in this setting[15,17] (see Chapter 7).

Radioisotope Imaging

Today, radionuclide studies are less frequently used to study flow and healing potential in ischemia of the foot and ankle. Technetium-99m, indium-111, xenon-133, and thallium-201 have all been evaluated as noninvasive imaging techniques.[125,156,166] Lawrance and associates[125] found that three-phase technetium scans were useful in assessing local perfusion and predicting healing of ischemic ulcers. All ulcers studied healed when activity was increased in the region of the ulcer compared with normal tissue background or the normal extremity. Healing was uncommon when uptake was not increased in the ulcerated areas.

Thallium-201 has been used for similar purposes.[167,205] Ohta[167] compared patterns of thallium-201 uptake (a marker of perfusion and tissue viability) in healing and nonhealing ulcers in 36 patients. The pattern of isotope uptake was correlated with hyperemia and inflammation in the ulcer bed. Both early (5 to 15 minutes) and delayed (3 hours) images were obtained after 2 mCi of Thallium 201 was given intravenously. Four patterns of uptake were described (Table 8-

9). All patients with no increase in uptake on either early or delayed studies eventually required amputation.[167] Siegel and colleagues[205] found thallium-201 comparable to Doppler techniques in predicting healing of cutaneous ulcerations.

Platelets labeled with indium-111 have also been employed in studies of patients with soft tissue ischemia. Comerford and associates[32] studied 20 patients using this technique. They noted reduced sensitivity from false-negative studies but found indium-111–labeled platelets useful in predicting healing. In addition, by combining indium-111 with technetium-99m three-phase studies, the results were more accurate. Intradermal xenon-133 injections have also been used to assess cutaneous flow.[125] This technique is more difficult to evaluate and causes more patient discomfort. Thallium-201 studies are accurate but are much more expensive than conventional three-phase technetium studies.[125,137]

Radionuclide studies are useful, but spatial resolution is limited, especially in the lower leg.[132] Therefore, other techniques are more often used at most centers.

Ultrasound

Doppler techniques provide a simple, noninvasive method of assessing peripheral flow.[4,12,33,119,121,133,187] Doppler ultrasound is particularly useful in patients with ischemic disease, diminished peripheral pulses, and reduced peripheral systolic pressures (less than 70 mm Hg).[33] Advantages of Doppler include its low cost, versatility (can be used at the bedside), ease of use, and ability to differentiate occlusive from nonocclusive vascular disease.[12,33,119,121] When used in the 5- to 10-MHz range, the normal arterial pulse is triphasic. During systole, a fast forward pattern is followed by a reversal and a secondary short forward pattern. Distal to occlusions, the pulse is monophasic.[119] In diabetic patients, the reversal portion of the pattern may be absent. In the presence of neuropathy, the flow may be increased up to five times.[11,33,119] This flow abnormality is most likely related to peripheral autonomic neuropathy with dilatation of the vascular bed.[31,33,121,209] Numerous variations in Doppler techniques have been used in an attempt to predict healing of ischemic disease and to evaluate and follow patients with peripheral vascular disease.

Ankle pressure measurements can be obtained when Doppler is used with blood pressure cuffs.[4,119,144,186,204] This allows for detection of low systolic pressures, useful

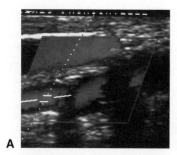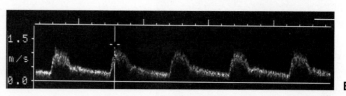

FIG. 8-30. Normal vascular ultrasound demonstrating flow (**A**) and normal arterial waveform (**B**).

information in predicting healing and in determining whether conservative therapy may be helpful.[119,144,186] Healing occurs in 92% of persons who do not have diabetes if ankle pressures are greater than 55 mm of mercury. Seventy-six percent of diabetic ulcers heal at this pressure level. Amputation is likely required when ankle pressures are less than this level.[144,186,204] Toe pressures are more useful in predicting healing in more distal ischemic disease. Doppler is accurate in most situations, but falsely elevated pressures can be seen in diabetic patients or in patients with other diseases that cause extensive vascular calcification.[119,181,189,204] Improved accuracy has been reported using Doppler techniques. Karanfilian and colleagues[104] compared laser Doppler velocimetry with conventional Doppler ankle pressures and transcutaneous oxygen measurements to determine which was most accurate in predicting healing of ischemic ulcers. Transcutaneous Po_2 measurements were most accurate with a sensitivity of 100%, specificity of 88%, and accuracy of 95%. Laser Doppler studies were somewhat less reliable, but compared with Doppler ankle pressure the sensitivities were 79 and 75%, specificities were 96 and 26%, and accuracies were 87 and 52% respectively.[104]

Today, duplex scanning that combines Doppler and B-mode imaging is commonly used to evaluate vascular diseases. This technique allows anatomic evaluation of vessels and flow abnormalities including waveform changes and velocity measurements (Fig. 8-30). Therefore, accurate assessment of stenoses and hemodynamic significance can be accomplished.[119,121,132,133,187]

Low-grade stenoses (less than 20%) have normal waveforms and flow velocity. Stenoses of 20 to 49% demonstrate spectral broadening and more than a 30% increase in flow velocity comparing the prestenotic to poststenotic segment. Stenosis greater than 50% (50 to 100%) demonstrates dramatic spectral broadening and an up to 100% increase in flow velocity to complete reversal of flow (Fig. 8-31).[101,119,121,132]

Duplex scanning has been compared with angiography specifically for accuracy of stenotic lesions of 50% or more. Duplex studies of the lower extremity have sensitivities of 75 to 87%, specificities of 90 to 94%, and positive and negative predictive values of 77 to 80% and 89 to 93%, respectively.[121,133,181] Accuracy ranges of duplex scanning do not permit use of this technique as the sole method of evaluating stenotic lesions, especially multiple segment lesions. Therefore, conventional and MR angiography are frequently required to define lesions more clearly and in some cases to treat patients using angiographic techniques.[132,133,213]

Angiography

Doppler studies are useful and noninvasive,[115] but, to date, angiography (conventional or digital) remains the standard for mapping vascular abnormalities (see Chapter 2). Angiography provides accurate information regarding the extent and sites of stenosis or occlusion, the extent of involvement and collateral circulation, the anatomy of the vessel proximal and distal to the involved segment, prognostic information, and, when indicated, the appropriate level for amputation (see Figs. 8-21 and 8-23 to 8-26).[40,47,66,78,123,188,213,223]

Angiographic techniques also define vascular changes associated with specific disorders such as fibromuscular dysplasia and Buerger's disease (see Figs. 8-24 and 8-25).[24,25,27,86,103,219]

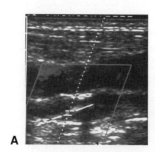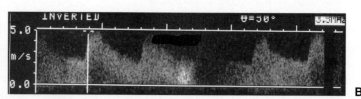

FIG. 8-31. Ultrasound in a patient with stenosis (**A**) and spectral broadening (**B**).

Evaluation of the aorta, iliacs, and major vessels of the lower extremities can be easily accomplished using aortograms with run-off studies of the lower extremities or selective catheterization. However, smaller peripheral vessels in the feet and the pedal arch can be more difficult to identify, especially in the presence of small vessel disease (see Fig. 8-25).[204,213] The pedal arch, for example, is a low-resistance vascular bed with slow flow that can make angiographic filming difficult. Longer filming sequences or vasoactive drugs can be used to define these vessels better.[6,93,167,182,195,215,219]

Magnetic Resonance Angiography

Vascular imaging using MRI has traditionally been performed using special pulse sequences with two-dimensional time-of-flight or phase-contrast techniques.[15] Two-dimensional time-of-flight techniques are most commonly used in the lower extremity.[127] This technique is limited by acquisition time and by multiple artifacts that may decrease image quality. Artifacts (Fig. 8-32) include spin-saturation, turbulence, and step-ladder artifacts from reformatted thin-section images.[76,77,108,127]

Studies using contrast-enhanced techniques provide superior image quality and rapid image acquisition.[76,77,244] Hany and associates[77] compared breath-hold contrast-enhanced

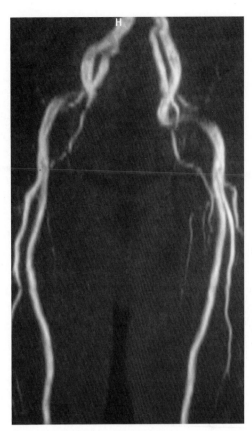

FIG. 8-33. Contrast enhanced bolus-chase image of the iliac and femoral vessels.

MR angiograms (Fig. 8-33) with conventional angiography in 60 abnormal vessels that included stenosis, aneurysms (Fig. 8-34), and occlusions. Using maximum-intensity projection algorithms, accuracy of 96% could be obtained compared with conventional angiography.

Bolus chase MR angiography with subtraction technique (see Fig. 8-33) allows accurate assessment of long segments of the lower extremity similar to conventional angiogram run-off studies. The patient and coils are positioned in several overlapping segments to provide images of the lower aorta and lower extremities.[244] With increased clinical experience, this technique may replace some angiographic procedures. MR angiography may be particularly useful in high-risk patients or in patients who may not tolerate large doses of contrast required for conventional angiography.[77,108,244]

Treatment

Treatment of soft tissue ischemic disorders depends on whether the process is primary or related to a systemic disease. Treatment also differs significantly between occlusive and vasospastic diseases.

Vasospastic Diseases

Patients with vasospastic conditions (see Table 8-5) are usually treated conservatively. For example, patients with

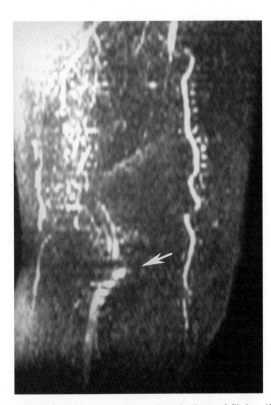

FIG. 8-32. Coronal two-dimensional time-of-flight (*TOF*) image just above the knees in a patient with popliteal artery occlusion. Multiple artifacts are due to slow flow and step-ladder artifacts in the popliteal region (*arrow*).

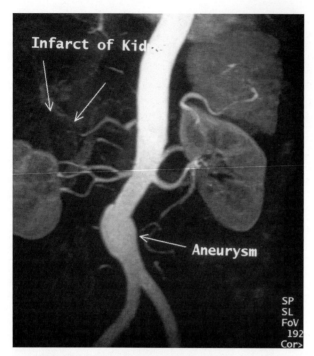

FIG. 8-34. MR angiogram demonstrating an aortic aneurysm and renal artery occlusion (two renal arteries on the right) with an upper pole infarct. (Courtesy of Siemens Medical, Erlangen, Germany.)

Raynaud's phenomenon should be instructed to protect their hands and feet properly in cold weather and to avoid smoking and vasoconstricting substances.[53,100,132] Patients with acrocyanosis and livedo reticularis should also be protected from cold exposure. Sympathetic blocking medications may be required in some patients.[53,132] Some physicians prefer to utilize vasodilators such as prazosin, nifedipine, and phenoxybenzamine. Most patients (90% of patients with Raynaud's) respond and improve with these conservative measures.[98,132]

In some patients, conservative measures are not successful. In this setting, more aggressive therapy may be indicated. Although the role of sympathectomy is unclear, this procedure may be useful in selected cases. Janoff and colleagues[98] noted a successful response to sympathectomy in 10 patients with refractory Raynaud's phenomenon and painful lower extremity vasospasm.

Vascular Occlusive Diseases: Arterial

Treatment of vascular stenosis and occlusion depends on the cause, the location (proximal or large vessel versus distal small or microvascular disease), and the patient's medical status. Therapy generally falls into three categories: conservative, surgical, or percutaneous intervention.[29,158-160,211,212,228]

Conservative therapy is used when possible, especially in patients with small vessel disease, that is, in diabetic patients, or in patients with peripheral ulcers and minor infections. These patients should have ulcers debrided, be given appropriate footwear to reduce pressure on ulcerated areas, and be given appropriate antiseptic or antibiotic therapy.[163,171,181]

Two therapeutic percutaneous techniques may be employed. Percutaneous transluminal angioplasty (PTA) and thrombolysis, either mechanical or chemical, have both proven useful and provide options to bypass surgery.

Treatment of arterial insufficiency in the foot and ankle may be a complex undertaking, especially when atherosclerosis is involved. Because atherosclerosis tends to be a diffuse disease, there is the potential for multiple sequential sites of vascular constriction proximal to the foot and ankle that need to be addressed to optimize therapeutic outcome.[236] Treatment of traumatic lower extremity arterial lesions must be individualized, depending on the physical examination and mode of injury.

Whereas claudication is the main indication directing therapeutic interventions in aortoiliac and femoropopliteal segments involved with atherosclerotic disease, the current consensus among surgeons and those performing PTA is that critical ischemia, characterized by tissue loss or rest pain, should be present before a distal surgical bypass procedure or below-the-knee angioplasty is attempted.[100,117,232–236, 239,248] The primary goal of both of these procedures is to avoid major amputation and to salvage a functioning foot. Although superficially these two techniques (surgery and PTA) appear to be in competition with one another, we, along with others, have found that the patient is best served if a team approach, encompassing physicians proficient in both techniques, is available.[191,192,236,237]

Regardless of whether surgical bypass or PTA is chosen to treat lower leg occlusive disease, important preliminary considerations have an impact on the ultimate success of either therapy. Whereas imaging of the proximal leg vasculature is straightforward, meticulously performed angiography of the tibial arteries and, particularly, the arteries of the foot and ankle is essential in delineating appropriate target sites for distal intervention.[116] This may require selective antegrade catheterization, delayed image acquisition, use of intraarterial vasodilators, and digital subtraction angiography with magnification.[102,116] In addition, the identification of adequate arterial outflow distal to the site of intervention is a major determinant of success for both distal surgical bypass and PTA.[10,23,40,164] This is particularly true for the inframalleolar interventions in which pedal outflow is mandatory for success.[7]

Improvements in surgical techniques have resulted in the development of both a wide diversity of bypass grafts, as well as choices for distal graft target sites and proximal graft origin sites. Consensus opinion is that autologous vein grafts outperform prosthetic grafts for infrapopliteal and inframalleolar surgical bypasses.[7,8,66,134,142,235] Synthetic grafts are reserved mainly for patients in whom autologous conduit is not available. In general, in situ vein grafting has advantages over reversed vein technique for long bypasses to distally located outflow tracts. For distal bypasses, in situ graft early (1 month) patency rates range from 89 to 97%. Primary patency rates at 1 year range from 64 to 87%, and a 5-year patency rate of 73% has been cited.[219] Limb salvage rates at 2 and 5 years of 82 and 81%, respectively, can be expected with patients undergoing in situ distal bypasses.[219]

PTA has become a useful alternative or adjunct to surgical management of occlusive arterial disease of the foot and ankle.[214,217,219,225,239,241,242] development of microcatheters with mounted balloons less than 4 mm in diameter has permitted angioplasty not only of the tibial and peroneal arteries proper, but also of the pedal branches of these vessels (Fig. 8-35). Because of the diffuse nature of atherosclerotic disease of the lower extremities, patient selection based on the anatomy depicted on preliminary arteriography is the critical step in ensuring a successful outcome for tibial and peroneal angioplasty. Most patients with critical lower leg ischemia do not have a disease distribution appropriate for percutaneous management and are better served with operative intervention.[219] Anatomic features predicting a successful outcome to infrapopliteal PTA include the presence of fewer than four to five stenoses or an occlusion less than 6 cm long in a single tibial or peroneal artery. In addition, there should not be significant proximal vessel disease.[235]

Using careful technique in patients with relatively focal infrapopliteal disease and potentially restorable run-off below the site of angioplasty, PTA should result in a technical success rate of greater than 90%.[87,195,235] A limb salvage rate of approximately 80% should be expected.[10,235] Successful limb salvage following PTA is optimized if straight-line flow to the foot is established, the patients are nondiabetic, and gangrene is absent at the time of the procedure.[10,195,235] Good long-term prospective studies comparing PTA with surgery are needed to evaluate PTA below the knee further.

Although approximately 75% of all patients with critical ischemia of the lower legs have lesions that are anatomically better suited for surgical management, PTA sometimes may be more feasible clinically.[235] Because of compromised cardiopulmonary status, some patients may be too unfit clinically to withstand major surgery, and PTA offers a viable alternative. In addition, suitable autologous conduit may not be available because of previous extremity or cardiac bypass. Finally, PTA potentially spares veins for future use in coronary or peripheral applications, in patients expected to require revascularizations in those circulations.[10,39,99,236]

Complications associated with PTA are infrequent, but primarily they include thrombosis and distal embolization. These complications may be readily managed percutaneously using thrombolysis or suction embolectomy. The possibility for procedural complications can be reduced by the periprocedural administration of antiplatelet agents, heparin and vasodilators.[23,235,242] Fortunately, a failed PTA or the occurrence of a procedural complication rarely precludes the performance of bypass graft surgery or alters previously planned surgery.

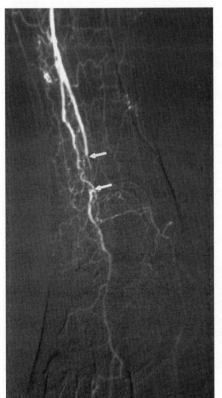
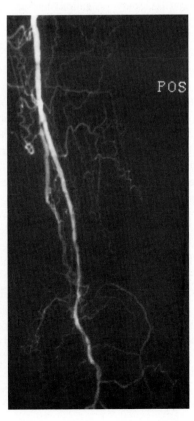

A,B

FIG. 8-35. Angiograms before (**A**) and after (**B**) angioplasty of a short occlusion (*arrows* in **A**) of the anterior tibial artery.

The goal of any infrapopliteal arterial intervention, regardless of whether it is PTA or surgery, is the permanent relief of ischemic symptoms. Unfortunately, some of these patients will develop recurrent ischemic symptoms from failure of these interventions. The failure manifests itself by recurrence of arterial stenosis and ultimately thrombosis. The appearance of thrombosis increases the complexity of interventions necessary to resolve the thrombosis, because mechanical clot removal or thrombolysis may be required. Additionally, in the case of autologous vein graft, the secondary patency rate is significantly reduced once graft thrombosis has occurred as compared with graft revision before thrombosis.[11,247] To detect intervention failure before thrombosis, surveillance is needed. For the most part, noninvasive modalities such as the ankle-brachial index and arterial duplex ultrasound are utilized. Ultrasound is more useful in most situations because it is can enable one not only to diagnose impending intervention failure, but also to identify the actual site responsible for the failure. Surveillance for infrainguinal bypass grafts has become a routine practice in the past few years, whereas surveillance following PTA is more recent but still remains an underused procedure.[208,232]

Graft surveillance is most appropriately performed using ultrasound measurements of flow velocities within the graft. Ultrasound is capable of detecting those grafts with a high likelihood of failure. A peak systolic velocity measurement less than 40 or 45 cm per second within the graft strongly suggests impending graft failure, but it is not specific as to cause.[11,12,90] By using color-flow Doppler sonography, the entire length of the bypass graft may be examined in real time, and sites of suspected stenosis may be identified and quantified using Doppler spectral analysis. The severity of stenoses is graded according to a peak systolic ratio. This is calculated by dividing the peak systolic velocity at the site of suspected stenosis by that measured in the normal graft 2 to 4 cm more proximally. Velocity ratios of 2 or greater correspond to a 50% diameter reduction, whereas ratios of 3 or greater indicate a 75% stenosis.[129,175] Peak systolic velocity ratios greater than 3 generally indicate impending bypass occlusion and warrant intervention.[129,175]

Graft failure occurs for a variety of reasons, depending on the interval that has passed since the operation. Early failures are apparent within 1 month of surgery and are usually ascribed to technical errors. These include suture placement errors, graft kinking, clamp injuries, residual venous side branches, poorly lysed venous graft valves, and poor selection of the anastomotic sites. Intermediate failures occur during the first 1 to 2 years and are attributed to the formation of fibrointimal hyperplasia at the anastomotic sites or within the graft conduit, usually at a venous valve site. Late failures, beyond 2 years, are believed to be a result of the continued atherosclerotic disease process in the native vessels proximal and distal to the anastomosis. The purpose of graft surveillance is to detect intragraft or perianastomotic abnormalities before graft thrombosis can occur.[11,202]

Failed or failing revascularization interventions can be managed in several ways. The method selected depends on the type of revascularization performed, the length of time since intervention, and the cause of the failure.[13,44,47,62,147] Surgical grafts to the lower leg are usually of autologous vein. Early graft failures (less than 30 days postoperatively) usually present with graft thrombosis that is due to a technical problem associated with graft placement. These patients typically return directly to the operating room for a directed graft revision and removal of thrombus. If the precipitating cause of failure is poor outflow, an additional or replacement graft may be required. PTA is not indicated in these patients.[69,82]

Vein graft problems occurring in the intermediate postoperative period (1 to 2 years) are most common and are usually the result of an intrinsic graft lesion, such as fibrointimal hyperplasia at the anastomotic sites or at a venous valve. Stenotic lesions occur in 20 to 30% of grafts.[13,47,50] Various surgical interventions are available and include patch angioplasty, jump graft extension, and excision with either primary reanastomosis or interposition vein graft.[12,219] Excision of the abnormal vein segment with primary anastomosis or interposition grafting restores hemodynamics to a more natural state and may provide the more durable secondary patency.[11]

If a failing graft is identified before thrombosis occurs, a surgical secondary patency rate of approximately 85% can be expected.[11,219] Unfortunately, once graft thrombosis has occurred, surgical secondary patency rates fall precipitously, with 1-year patency rates reported as low as 40%.[11,62,69] Replacement of the clotted vein graft (secondary revascularization) has been advocated by many, with 5-year patency rates of 55 to 65% being achieved when suitable autologous vein is available. Results using synthetic replacement grafts are not as good.[11,21,69,70]

Grafts that fail in the late postoperative period (more than 2 years) may do so because of intrinsic graft lesions, although this is not common. Usually, late failure is due to the progression of atherosclerosis in the native arterial inflow to the graft, at the anastomotic sites, or in the arterial run-off distal to the graft. Arteriographically proven anastomotic narrowings usually benefit from surgical revision, whereas occlusive disease proximal or distal to the graft may require some sort of secondary grafting procedure or PTA.[11,69,70] Percutaneous transluminal interventions (Fig. 8-36) may possess some role in the management of patients with jeopardized lower leg bypass grafts. Because early graft failures are usually technical in nature, there is really no indication for percutaneous therapy in that patient group. The role of percutaneous therapy for grafts failing in the intermediate postoperative period has been examined, with controversial results. Several investigators have had good immediate technical success and long-term patency of graft stenoses treated with PTA.[67,70,208] Midgraft stenoses at valve sites, as opposed to anastomotic stenoses, appear to require higher balloon inflation pressure, longer dilatation times, and overdilatation to achieve success.[208]

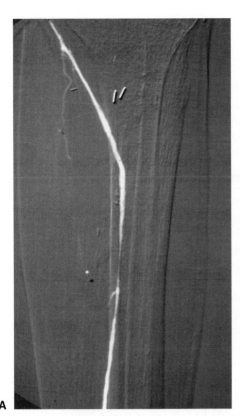 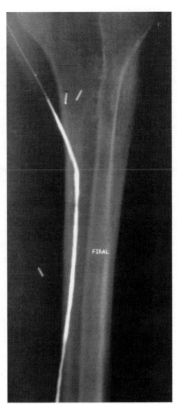 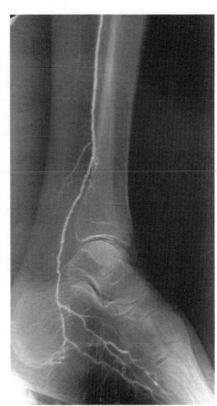

A

B,C

FIG. 8-36. Angiograms before (**A**) and after (**B**) angioplasty for stenosis just distal to a femoroposterior tibial artery vein bypass graft. Lateral images (**C**) of the ankle and hindfoot show the improved run-off distally.

The majority opinion[11,171,173,199–201,239] is that PTA of bypass graft stenoses achieves a high initial technical success rate, but the results are not durable because fibrointimal hyperplasia, unlike atherosclerotic narrowings, exhibits a tendency for elastic rebound following dilatation. Disparate results from these PTA studies may be a reflection of the composition of material causing the graft stenosis. With anastomotic stenoses resulting from progressive atherosclerosis, rather than fibrointimal hyperplasia, angioplasty results may be better than if the stenosis is composed entirely of hyperplastic tissue. Varying combinations of fibrointimal hyperplasia and atherosclerosis have been retrieved from these stenotic sites.[42,44] Percutaneous transluminal directional atherectomy devices have been used to remove the noncompressible material causing graft anastomotic stenoses. The experience is limited, but this technique has generated results superior to those for PTA alone and approaching those reported for surgical revision.[42,44,219] Adjunctive PTA following atherectomy is frequently necessary to achieve optimal results.[42,44]

Perhaps the most important contribution PTA can offer is in patients with grafts that are failed or are failing in the late postoperative period. Because late graft failures are frequently secondary to progressive narrowing of graft in-flow or run-off vessels, PTA (see Fig. 8-36) can be used to extend the life of lower extremity bypass grafts.[11] In addition, percu-

taneous endoluminal procedures may benefit patients who have no suitable veins available for graft revision or replacement. If percutaneous interventions are utilized in intermediate or late graft problems, postprocedure surveillance with ultrasound is critical for continued graft maintenance.[12,219]

Thrombolysis

The discovery of effective thrombolytic agents and the development of sophisticated catheter delivery systems have encouraged increased utilization of nonoperative techniques for treating peripheral vascular occlusive disease.[63,67,68,219] Thrombolytic therapy plays an important role not only as a primary treatment for these vascular occlusions, but also as an adjunct to PTA when tha patient has an underlying focal stenosis. The basis of thrombolysis lies in the ability of exogenously administered agents to dissolve unwanted clot. The action of these agents is targeted toward the lysis of clot fibrin. Fibrinolysis is mediated by the proteolytic enzyme plasmin, which is effective in breaking down fibrin into its inactive degradation products. Plasmin is derived from activation of an inactive proenzyme called plasminogen, which is normally circulating with plasma. Agents capable of activating plasminogen include streptokinase (SK), urokinase (UK), and tissue plasminogen activator (t-PA).[145,146,151,159,169,184,196,228,231]

In the clinical setting, UK is currently the thrombolytic agent of choice in treatment of lower extremity clot. At the time of this writing, UK has been removed from the market and its future status is uncertain. SK is a purified preparation of streptococcal protein that is a foreign protein capable of inducing resistance to its thrombolytic effectiveness as well as precipitating an allergic response. Circulating antibodies from prior streptococcal infection may also inactivate SK, requiring a loading dose of the agent to overcome the antibody effect. In addition, SK may cause depletion of fibrinogen more quickly than UK and is a more potent activator of fibrin and fibrinogen degradation, thus making it more difficult to regulate.[146,147,159,228] UK is an enzyme produced by the kidney and is found in the urine. Therefore, there are no circulating antibodies to cause inactivation, and a loading dose is not necessary. Excessive plasminogen consumption and fibrin/fibrinogen degradation do not occur. UK is not antigenic and does not induce allergic reaction. The half-life of UK is short, averaging 14 minutes.[146,147,159,228]

The newest thrombolytic agent, t-PA, is a proteolytic enzyme that occurs naturally in most tissues and is therefore nonantigenic. At present, this enzyme is manufactured by means of recombinant DNA technology. One theoretic advantage of t-PA over UK appears to be its relative clot specificity. Fibrin-bound t-PA has a much higher affinity for fibrin-bound plasminogen than does freely circulating t-PA for circulating plasminogen. Therefore, t-PA should initiate less systemic effect than UK and more specific clot effect. The half-life of t-PA is approximately 5 minutes.[67,146,151,184]

Although thrombolytic therapy is becoming increasingly accepted, there is some disagreement on the specific thrombolytic agent and the dosages to be used. The cardiology community is principally utilizing SK and t-PA, whereas the radiology community uses UK. Early comparison studies between UK and t-PA demonstrates that t-PA achieves more rapid clot lysis compared with UK.[67,68,151,184,229,238] However, an increase in hemorrhagic complications may be seen with use of t-PA.[151]

UK has repeatedly been shown to be efficacious in thrombolysis of peripheral arterial occlusions.[13,35,47,50,105–107,145–148,220,221,226,228] Because of many factors, including the patient's clinical presentation, the volume of intraluminal clot, patient anatomy, time of day, and hospital policies, numerous techniques for thrombolysis have been spawned. These are well presented in a review article by Kaufman and Bettman.[107] In general, the techniques vary in their method of catheter delivery and in the UK dosing regimen. All techniques involve the placement of the catheter within the targeted clot.[47,50,146]

Two basic catheter delivery schemes are in use, single level and multilevel. With the single-level technique, an end-hole catheter is positioned within the proximal clot and is advanced as lysis progresses.[83,103,106,146] The multilevel technique utilizes catheters with side holes positioned along a varying length of catheter, depending on the length of clot being treated. They are positioned well within the clot,

ideally with the proximal and distal side holes approximating the upper and lower extent of the clot. Multihole catheters are designed for more rapid lysis of clot compared with end-hole catheters.[88,146,219]

Three general UK administration regimens have been described: constant, graded, and pulsatile. Each of these regimens is also linked with a general dosing range of UK. For the most part, low-dose infusions are applied in a constant manner with dosages of 40,000 to 125,000 U/hr being usual.[13,47] Graded infusions are usually associated with an initial high dose of 240,000 U/hr for 2 to 4 hours, and then the dose is reduced to approximately 125,000 U/hr for an additional 2 hours. In some cases, the dose may be lowered again to 60,000 U/hr for the remainder of the infusion.[219,221]

Pulsatile administration of UK utilizes an ultrahigh dose of 25,000 units of UK/ml injected forcefully through the catheter in 5,000 unit aliquots. Approximately 150,000 units are injected over a period of 10 to 20 minutes in 0.2-ml increments. Total required doses typically vary from 100,000 to 600,000 U.[219,221,229] Pulsatile administration is usually restricted to multiple side-hole catheter use; however, constant and graded infusions may also be effective through these catheters. End-hole catheters are usually used only for constant and graded infusions.[107,219,229] The total amount of UK used by the constant and graded infusion techniques, regardless of high- or low-dose technique, ranges from 1 to 3 million U, whereas UK usage with the pulsatile technique is usually less than 1 million U.[107,219] The constant and graded infusion (either high or low dose) are usually preceded by an intraclot bolus injection of between 30,000 and 250,000 units of UK evenly distributed within the clot to hasten the lytic process.[107,219]

No consensus exists in the literature on which thrombolytic technique is superior. The overall success rate for clot lysis approaches 80 to 85% regardless of the therapeutic regimen applied.[13,35,47,88,105–107,123,145–148,219–221,228–231] Because of this, therapy can be customized to the circumstances surrounding the patient at the time of evaluation. At our institution, patients presenting with significant, but not limb-threatening, ischemia undergo a rapid clot lysis regimen using either high-dose graded or ultrahigh-dose pulsatile administration of UK. Patients with lesser degrees of lower limb ischemia also undergo this mode of therapy if they are seen during regular working hours in an attempt to prevent inpatient admission to the intensive care unit. Patients with stable, non–limb-threatening ischemia presenting during the nighttime hours are typically treated with constant low-dose infusion of UK with reevaluation in the morning. Concurrent heparinization during thrombolysis is almost universally performed. The rationale is to prevent both pericatheter thrombosis during therapy and propagation of the targeted clot distally or into side branches.[146,219,228–231]

Long-term patency following thrombolysis of lower extremity occlusions is variable. The longevity of treated proximal occlusions tends to exceed that of more distal occlusions, and grafts exhibit a more durable response than native vessels.[146,148] Vein grafts typically remain patent longer than synthetic grafts.[47,50,219] Most important seems to be correction of the underlying lesion responsible for vessel thrombosis. Long-term patency for lysed vessels with a corrected lesion far exceeds patency of those in which the stenotic lesion remains uncorrected. In the case of grafts, older grafts appear to have greater long-term patency than newer grafts following thrombolysis.[219]

UK is also effective in the treatment of clots that have embolized to the lower extremities. Emboli most commonly originate from the heart, with left atrial appendage clot (secondary to atrial fibrillation) and left ventricular clot (from recent myocardial infarction) being the most common sources.[124,219] Diagnosis is made by a combination of clinical history and angiographic findings. Patients commonly have a history of atrial fibrillation, recent cardioversion, or recent myocardial infarction with no antecedent claudication or lower extremity ischemia. Angiographically, one typically sees multiple branch occlusions in the lower extremities, absent mature collateral vessels, and no underlying flow-limiting stenosis after removal of the embolus.[88] Technical success for lysis of emboli is similar to that encountered in thrombotic occlusions, and limb salvage and survival rates are similar to reports for surgical embolectomy.[88] The age of the embolus does not seem to have a bearing on the success of lysis, as previously thought.[88,219]

Complications associated with the use of UK thrombolysis include bleeding, distal embolization of fragmented thrombus, and pericatheter thrombosis. Major bleeding has been reported in the range of 1 to 25%.[5,47,63,81,88] Most bleeding complications are related to the arterial puncture site; however, infrequent hemorrhage in the brain and retroperitoneum have been seen.[47,63,159,193,219,228] The risk of bleeding seems to be associated with prolonged UK infusions,[63,159,228] the concomitant administration of heparin, and a fibrinogen level of less than 100 mg/dl.[159,224,225,231]

Distal embolization of the thrombus during lysis of a lower extremity clot is one of the most uniformly reported complications and occurs in 5 to 50% of cases.[81,105,228,231] Identification, in most cases, requires careful angiographic evaluation, especially of the ankle and foot vessels. This unavoidable complication fortunately responds well to continuation of thrombolytic infusion.[81,105,228,231] Although emboli may be asymptomatic, dramatic worsening of lower extremity ischemia during treatment should indicate that embolization has occurred. Fortunately, irreversible tissue necrosis and occlusion of distal runoff preventing subsequent surgical reconstruction occur only rarely.[228,231] Percutaneous aspiration thromboembolectomy, using an end-hole catheter, has been found useful in the rapid retrieval of extremity emboli.[218]

Atheroembolus to the lower extremity arterial system is a unique type of occlusive disease in which the source of the embolus, rather than the embolus itself, is of primary therapeutic concern.[176] Aortic aneurysms and occlusive aor-

toiliac disease are the most common sources of atheroemboli.[109–111,219] Plaques in these regions are prone to degeneration with showering of cholesterol, calcium, and thromboembolic debris to the distal circulation. The shaggy aorta, which is lined with irregular, ulcerated plaques, seems to be particularly strongly implicated in atheroembolication.[110] These emboli have a propensity to travel to the small arteries of the foot and ankle, where they may give rise to the classic blue toe syndrome.[20] If allowed to proceed unabated, atheroembolization can result in limb-threatening ischemia. There is no role for percutaneous, nonsurgical interventions in atheroembolic disease. Surgical correction consists of exclusion by bypass or removal of the source by endarterectomy.[111,219]

In the last several years, a technique called percutaneous mechanical thrombectomy (PMT) has garnered considerable interest as a means of treating thrombotic and thromboembolic occlusions of both native vessels and grafts. Development of these devices occurred because of known shortcomings associated with catheter-directed pharmacologic thrombolytic and surgical balloon thrombectomy (e.g., bleeding, prolonged therapy, vessel wall injury, incomplete recanalization). These devices are designed to effect rapid clearing of occlusive thrombus.[199–201]

The more commonly used PMT devices may conveniently be separated into several broad classes: (1) percutaneous aspiration thrombectomy (PAT), in which occlusive thrombus or embolus is manually aspirated through a large-lumen end-hole catheter positioned immediately proximal to the clot; (2) pull-back thrombectomy and clot trapping, in which the thrombus is pulled back with a balloon catheter or basket into a trapping device and removed intact; (3) recirculation mechanical thrombectomy, in which the thrombus is macerated in situ by using devices that generate a hydrodynamic vortex, which is a focus of continuous mixing in which the thrombus becomes captured and pulverized into microscopic fragments by high shear forces; and (4) nonrecirculating mechanic thrombectomy, in which thrombus is shredded using mechanical means without significant hydrodynamic recirculation.[200]

PAT is the simplest, least expensive, and most readily available of the PMT devices. For the most part, its value has been in the retrieval of emboli, either naturally occurring or as a complication of PTA, surgery, or pharmacologic thrombolysis.[30,200,216,217,240] Embolic complications occurring during percutaneous interventions are usually recognized at the time of the intervention, thus permitting PAT to be used as an extension of ongoing procedure. The distal trifurcation arteries of the leg and the foot arteries are common recipients of these procedure-related emboli.[199–201]

Recirculation PMT devices pulverize clot by the creation of hydrodynamic vortices. Two major categories of recirculation devices are currently in use: the rotational recirculation devices, which generate a vortex using a high-speed rotating impeller- and the hydraulic recirculation devices, which generate a vortex using high-speed fluid jets (Venturi effect).[200,201] Recirculation PMT devices are fast and efficient, and they release particulate debris of extremely small average size. These devices, however, are complex, expensive, and can create significant hemolysis.[200] Complications seen in the early experience of these devices in native arteries and grafts include groin hematomas, distal embolization, and device failures.[122,199–201] Emboli can be managed by aspiration thrombectomy or supplemental pharmacologic thrombolysis. The larger size of these PMT devices does not as yet allow their use in the small arteries of the foot and ankle.[199–201]

Nonrecirculating PMT devices, primarily consisting of rotation baskets and brushes, and clot-trapping devices do not have currently significant arterial applications in the United States. The nonrecirculating devices are not as efficient in breaking up clots as the recirculating devices, and the fragment size is considerably larger, making embolization a higher risk when these devices are used in the arterial system. The preferred application of nonrecirculation devices is in the fragmentation of clots in hemodialysis grafts and in venous clots, in which embolization of small clot fragments is less apt to be clinically significant.[199–201]

Management of the Vascular Patient

Considering the wide variety of vascular practice patterns, it is difficult to reach consensus regarding the best means of managing patients presenting with lower leg arterial disease.[56,59,101,216,219,223,233,242,246,249,252–254] However, some general management patterns have evolved. When significant lower leg claudication is the presenting problem and patients are considered appropriate candidates for surgical or percutaneous intervention, a diagnostic arteriogram should be performed to demonstrate the disease extent, morphology, and location. When focal stenosis or occlusions in native vessels are present, PTA may be all that is required to ameliorate symptoms. With more complex disease, including the presence of long stenoses and occlusions or multiple sequential lesions, surgical bypass may be more appropriate. Pharmacologic thrombolysis may be a useful adjunctive procedure in many patients with long occlusions to unmask a more focal atheromatous lesion that may respond to a simpler therapeutic procedure, such as PTA.[66,68]

Failed or failing lower leg grafts also require arteriographic study to determine the cause of their demise. As previously described, the best results with grafts occur with surgical revision if possible. When grafts are thrombosed, pharmacologic or mechanical removal of the clot may be helpful to unmask the nature of the offending lesion and to direct the therapeutic surgical procedure. Adjunctive measures using PTA and directional atherectomy may be appropriate in selected lesions. If distal vessels in the lower leg and foot are inadequate to support run-off, no interventions may be advisable.[66,69]

Acute lower limb ischemia is a threat to both life and limb. Therapeutic time constraints are much narrower than in patients presenting with claudication. Traditional belief states that only a narrow (6- to 8-hour) window is available to perform therapeutic measures before the acutely ischemic leg may not be salvageable; therefore, emergency surgical therapy is mandated. This time frame may, however, be more flexible than previously thought, depending on the extent of collateral circulation available to vessels below the occlusion.[44,45,144,148] Therefore, percutaneous alternatives or adjuncts to surgery may be valuable in properly selected patients. For this reason, treatment of acute ischemia should be based on the sensorimotor examination and the angiographic pattern, rather than on the duration of the symptoms, and should be individualized to the patient's needs.[144,146,148,219]

On rare occasions, a patient may present with acute limb-threatening ischemia necessitating a direct trip to the operating room. Usually, there is sufficient time to obtain an arteriogram to evaluate the lower leg arteries fully before therapeutic decision making. Nontraumatic acute lower leg ischemia is caused by emboli or in situ thrombosis superimposed on critical atherosclerotic vessel narrowings. Surgical management of lower leg emboli makes use of a Fogarty balloon embolectomy catheter to extract the embolus via a small arteriotomy.[219] This procedure works best in normal vessels and those above the trifurcation. Emboli to the distal trifurcation vessels may require separate arteriotomies of those vessels at the ankle to allow clot extraction.[249,250,253] This procedure may be hindered by the presence of significant arteriosclerotic vessel narrowings. Results of balloon catheter clot extraction to treat in situ thrombosis have not been promising and are associated with a higher mortality.[146] In addition, the underlying cause of the thrombosis is usually not addressed.

Pharmacologic treatment of embolic and thrombotic occlusions to lower leg vessels is a viable alternative to surgical techniques, provided the patient's clinical situation permits this approach. UK is used most commonly, and an 80 to 85% response rate for thrombotic and embolic clot lysis can be expected and may be applied to native vessels as well as to grafts.[13,35,47,88,105–107,145–148,219–221,228] Additionally, thrombolysis avoids the potential of endothelial trauma that may be associated with balloon catheter embolectomy and the intimal hyperplasia in native arteries and vein grafts that may result.[43,73] Thrombolysis also demonstrates the underlying cause of acute ischemia and directs further intervention, be it an endovascular therapy such as PTA, or atherectomy, or surgery.

Trauma

Trauma represents the second most common reason for arteriography of the foot and ankle. There is divergent opinion in the literature about the use of arteriography in blunt or penetrating trauma of the lower extremity, much depending on the nature of the individual practices. Generally, patients with definite clinical findings, such as absent pulses, pulsatile hemorrhage, large expanding hematoma, and distal ischemia, proceed directly to emergency surgery.[80,85,86] Emergency arteriography may be employed in these patients if the area of injury is not readily amenable to exploration.[80] Emergency arteriography is frequently reserved for patients with softer clinical findings such as neurologic deficit, stable hematoma, or a history of arterial bleeding.[80] Elective arteriography is indicated when the likelihood of finding significant occult arterial injury is low and the patient has no pulse deficit.[80,185]

The mechanism of injury may predict the likelihood of vascular injury to the foot and ankle and may dictate whether arteriography is appropriate. Tibial and peroneal artery injuries are most commonly encountered with complex fractures of the lower leg (Fig. 8-37).[185] Shotgun injuries and trauma caused by dog bites also have a significant association with vascular injury.[56,59,60] In addition, posterior knee dislocation is an injury likely to result in isolated disruption of the popliteal artery just proximal to the trifurcation and is associated with significant risk of lower extremity amputation.[219]

Injuries to a single lower leg artery may not be apparent clinically because collateral vessels may maintain distal pulses. Arteriography may be critical in determining which patients should undergo surgery in these cases. The amputation rate is 14% when a single tibial artery is injured and 70% if both tibial arteries are injured. Therefore, surgical reconstruction is usually recommended when one or both tibial arteries are injured or when there is injury to the tibial peroneal trunk. It is generally believed that isolated peroneal injuries can be observed.[96,219]

Arteriography and treatment of trauma that does not cause any arterial abnormality on physical examination are controversial. The rate of positive angiography in patients with negative physical examination is low. There is also controversy about what should be done with arteriographically demonstrated, but clinically occult, vascular abnormalities. Although traditional belief is that all arterial abnormalities demonstrated with arteriography should be surgically treated, some reports suggest that many of these lesions may be appropriately managed nonoperatively. Nonocclusive and nonbleeding vascular injuries can generally be managed without immediate surgical repair.[59,60,216] Symptomatic false aneurysms and arteriovenous fistulae have a low probability of spontaneous resolution; however, asymptomatic lesions may resolve over time. Arteriographic follow-up of arterial abnormalities to resolution is important. Those that do not resolve may mandate surgical repair. Observation of appropriate arterial injuries does not appear to increase morbidity or preclude subsequent surgical repair.[96]

Percutaneous management of trauma-related arterial injuries has been advocated as an alternative to surgical repair.[96] Acute bleeding from nonvital branches of extremity arteries can be halted by embolization of the offending branch using a variety of embolic materials.[96] The presence of a rich collateral network in the extremities, however, mandates that the bleeding artery be embolized both proximal and distal to the point of disruption.[96] Posttraumatic arterial pseudoaneurysms and arteriovenous fistulae have also been successfully treated by percutaneous endoluminal placement of covered metallic stent-grafts. Nonoperative therapy may be most appropriate in chronic posttraumatic lesions as well as in acute injuries that are not easily amenable to surgery.[96]

Arteriographically, arterial injuries are classified according to the appearance of the contrast material column. Normal vessels demonstrate a smooth continuous contrast column. Smoothly narrowed vessels showed a diminished contrast column caliber. This appearance denotes arterial spasm, extrinsic compression, or subintimal hematoma. Abrupt termination of the contrast column usually indicates arterial transsection or severe intimal injury with subsequent luminal thrombosis. Pseudoaneurysms are represented by focal widening of the contrast column and are the result of damage to the arterial media. Transmural injury to the artery may manifest itself by the appearance of irregular contrast material extravasation into the adjacent soft tissues or by the formation of an arteriovenous fistula, which is more commonly a late manifestation of trauma. A smooth linear defect within the contrast column is characteristic of an intimal tear, whereas an irregular globular defect in the column is more suggestive of mural thrombus.[80,86,185] These signs may appear alone or in various combinations.

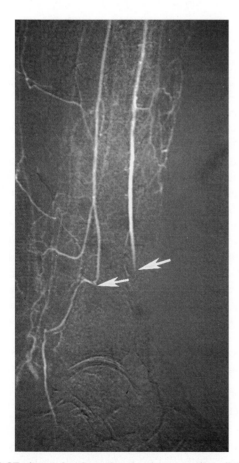

FIG. 8-37. Lateral subtraction angiogram after distal tibial fracture with vascular occlusions (*arrows*) at the fracture level.

Abnormal Arteriovenous Communications

Abnormal arteriovenous communications encompass the conditions known as arteriovenous fistulae and vascular malformations. Arteriovenous fistulae are high-flow single communications between the arterial and venous systems. Although they may be congenital, most fistulae are acquired and result from trauma, infection, or neoplastic disease.[112, 182,183] Clinically, the rapid shunting of arterial blood into the venous system may cause ischemia of tissues distal to the fistula because of a steal phenomenon or congestive heart failure.[178] Larger fistulae create more symptoms clinically.[182,183]

Angiography is necessary to delineate the site and morphology of the fistula accurately. Rapid contrast injection and image acquisition are needed to demonstrate the fistula because of the rapid flow. Although surgical closure of arteriovenous fistulae is usually the treatment of choice, some fistulae are not easily amenable to surgical repair, and percutaneous transcatheter intervention is appropriate. In nonessential vessels or branch vessels, embolic occlusion of the fistula proximal and distal to the communication may be performed using metal coils or detachable balloons.[182,183] Fistulae occurring in essential arteries may be closed using covered endovascular stents.[96]

Vascular malformations are congenital lesions that may be classified as high-flow arteriovenous malformations (AVMs) or low-flow venous malformations. They occur as a local failure of vascular development in utero and most do not become symptomatic.[183] Clinically significant AVMs present as cosmetic deformities, functional disturbances, bleeding, ulceration, or congestive heart failure.[184]

Surgical resection is the treatment of choice of small, localized AVMs. More extensive lesions may be much more difficult to approach surgically, especially when they involve the foot, because of the proximity of essential ligaments and tendons. In these patients, transcatheter embolization is a viable option.[183] Because AVMs represent an tangle of multiple arterial feeding vessels as well as numerous draining veins, devascularization of those lesions is much more difficult than a simple direct arterial venous fistula. Proximal occlusion of the large feeding arteries using balloons, coils, and Gelfoam pledgets is unlikely to provide prolonged benefit because this will lead to the recruitment of other arterial collateral arteries.[183] The result is recurrence of the AVM, with the arterial supply to the lesion being far more complex and much more difficult to access and to treat. Efforts should be directed at permanently obliterating the central nidus of the lesion rather than the feeding arteries. The nidus consists of the web of small arteriovenous communications in the central portion of the AVM. Occluding agents must be capable of reaching this nidus. The agents most likely used include polyvinyl alcohol particles (Ivalon)[183], absolute alcohol[252], and glue-like agents such as isobutyl cyanoacrylate and N-butyl cyanoacrylate that harden into a cast of the blood vessels that they permeate.[219] These agents are delivered

using microcatheters. Some of the best long-term results have been achieved using glues, although they are the most difficult to handle and deliver to the lesion.[183] In certain situations, the AVM cannot be effectively accessed using conventional arterial transcatheter percutaneous approach. This occurs when arterial access to the malformation is limited as a result of prior surgical ligation or proximal embolization of vessels supplying the malformation. In these cases, alternate approaches to the lesions, such as direct puncture of selected arterial or venous components of the malformation, may allow deposition of embolic agents to the target site distal to the proximal occlusions.[96]

Venous malformations are congenital vascular lesions that arise from abnormal vein morphogenesis. Diagnosis of venous malformations is frequently made by MRI, which demonstrates a mass with cavernous or cystic spaces that show little demonstrable flow. Because of the slow flow, arteriography is of little value in evaluating these lesions. The inflow arteries are typically of normal size because there is a normal intervening capillary bed. Late-phase imaging after high-dose contrast material arteriography may, however, reveal subtle staining or puddling within the venous spaces. Venography performed by direct needle puncture of the lesion and contrast material injection is the most effective means of opacifying venous malformations. A significant number of these lesions may also be demonstrated by foot and ankle venography.[183,219]

Therapeutically, venous malformations that are not causing symptoms should be left alone. If treatment is warranted, surgical resection of extremely localized lesions may be curative. Lesions not suitable for surgery may be handled percutaneously. However, only techniques that involve direct puncture of the venous malformation should be used to treat these lesions. Transarterial embolization only thromboses from the capillary bed backward, having minimal effect on the venous abnormality.[183,219] Most commonly, absolute ethanol is used to embolize these lesions percutaneously.[252] This agent causes coagulative necrosis and denaturing of tissues to occlude blood vessels. To limit flow of ethanol to the abnormal venous channels, the application of pneumatic cuffs is often used to restrict flow away from the lesions. Admixture of lipiodol, an oily contrast material to the ethanol, allows direct fluoroscopic visualization of sclerosing agent as it is injected. Large venous malformations may require multiple treatments. Complications of ethanol injection of venous malformations occur in 10% of cases and include skin blisters, sensory nerve injury, motor nerve weakness, superficial cellulitis, deep venous thrombosis, and pulmonary embolism.[219,252]

REFERENCES

1. Abramson DI, Lerner D, Shumacker HB, Hick FR. Clinical picture and treatment of the later stage of trenchfoot. Am. Heart J. 1946; 32: 52–71.
2. Adar R, Papa MZ, Halpern Z, Mozes M, Soshan S, Sofer B, Zinger H,

Dayan M, Mozes E. Cellular sensitivity to collagen in thromboangiitis obliterans. N. Engl. J. Med. 1983; 308:1113–1121.

3. Adeyokunnu AA. Bilateral gangrene of the feet associated with salmonella infection in children with sickle cell anemia. Ann. Trop. Pediatr. 1982; 2:41–43.

4. Allen J, Oates CP, Henderson J, Jago J, Whittingham TA, Chamberlain J, Jones NA, Murray A. Comparison of lower limb arterial assessments using color-duplex ultrasound and ankle/brachial index measures. Angiology 1996; 47:225–232.

5. Altin RS, Flicker S, Naidech HJ. Pseudoaneurysm and arteriovenous fistula after femoral catheterization. Association with low femoral punctures. AJR Am. J. Roentgenol. 1989; 152:629–631.

6. Andros G, Harris RW, Dulawa LB. Need for arteriography in diabetics with gangrene and palpable foot pulses. Arch. Surg. 1985; 119:1260–1263.

7. Andros G, Harris RW, Salles-Cunha SX, Dulawa LB, Oblath RW, Apyan RL. Bypass grafts to the ankle and foot. J. Vasc. Surg. 1988; 7(6):785–794.

8. Ascer E, Veith FJ, Gupta SK. Bypasses to plantar arteries and other tibial branches. An extended approach to limb salvage. J. Vasc. Surg. 1988; 8:434–441.

9. Babb RR, Alacon-Segovia D, Fairbai JF. Erythromelagia. Review of 51 cases. Circulation 1964; 29:136–142.

10. Bakal CW, Sprayregen S, Scheinbaum K, Cynamon J, Veith FJ. Percutaneous transluminal angioplasty of the infrapopliteal arteries. Results in 53 patients. AJR Am. J. Roentgenol. 1990; 154:171–174.

11. Bandyk DF, Bergamini TM, Towne JB, Schmitt DD, Seabrook GR. Durability of vein graft revision. The outcome of secondary procedures. J. Vasc. Surg. 1991; 13:200–210.

12. Bandyk DF, Jorgensen RA, Towne JB. Intraoperative assessment of in situ saphenous vein arterial bypass grafts using pulsed Doppler spectral analysis. Arch. Surg. 1986; 121:292–299.

13. Belkin M, Donaldson MC, Whittemore AD, Polak JF, Grassi CJ, Harrington DP, Mannick JA. Observations on the use of thrombolytic agents for thrombotic occlusion of infra-inguinal vein grafts. J. Vasc. Surg. 1990; 11:289–96.

14. Beltran J, Leigh JH, Bark JM, Zuelzer WA, Clark RN, Lucas JG, Weiss LD, Yang A. Femoral head avascular necrosis. MR imaging with clinical-pathologic and radionuclide correlation. Radiology 1988; 166:215–220.

15. Berquist TH. MRI of the Musculoskeletal System. 3rd Ed. New York, Lippincott-Raven, 1996.

16. Berquist TH. Diagnostic and therapeutic injections as an aid to musculoskeletal diagnosis. Semin. Intervent. Radiol. 1993; 10:326–343.

17. Berquist TH. Imaging of Orthopedic Trauma. 2nd Ed. New York, Raven Press, 1992.

18. Blair H. Comminuted fractures and fracture dislocation of the body of the astralagus. Am. J. Surg. 1943; 59:3743.

19. Bluemke DA, Zerhouni EA. MRI of avascular necrosis of bone. Topics Magn. Reson. Imaging 1996; 8:231–246.

20. Brewer ML, Kinnison ML, Perler BA, White RA. Blue toe syndrome. Treatment with anticoagulants and delayed percutaneous transluminal angioplasty. Radiology 1988; 166:31–36.

21. Brewster DC, LaSalle AJ, Robison JG, Strayhorn EC, Darling RC. Femoropopliteal graft failures. Clinical consequences and success of secondary reconstructions. Arch. Surg. 1983; 118:1043.

22. Brower AC. The osteochondrosis. Orthop. Clin. North. Am. 1983; 14:99–117.

23. Brown KT, Schoenberg NY, Moore ED, Saddekni S. Percutaneous transluminal angioplasty of infrapopliteal vessels. Preliminary results and technical considerations. Radiology, 1988; 169:75–78.

24. Bull PG, Mendel H, Hold M, Schlegl A, Denck H. Distal popliteal and tibioperoneal transluminal angioplasty. Long-term follow-up. J Vasc. Interv. Radiol. 1992; 3:45–53.

25. Campbell WB, Fletcher EL, Hands LJ. Assessment of distal lower limb arteries. A comparison of arteriography and Doppler ultrasound. Ann. R. Coll. Surg. 1986; 68:37–39.

26. Canale ST, Kelly, FB. Fractures of the neck of the talus. J. Bone Joint Surg. Am. 1978; 60:143–156.

27. Casarella WJ. General principles in techniques for percutaneous transluminal angioplasty. Categorical course on interventional radiology. American Roentgen Ray Society, Boston, 1985.

28. Chryssanthow CP. Dysbaric osteonecrosis. Etiologic and pathologic concepts. Clin. Orthop. 1978; 130:94–106.

29. Cisek PL, Eze AR, Comerota AJ, Kerr R, Blake B, Kelly P. Microcirculatory compensation to progressive atherosclerotic disease. Ann. Vasc. Surg. 1997; 11:49–53.

30. Cleveland TJ, Cumberland DC, Gaires PA. Percutaneous aspiration thromboembolectomy to manage the embolic complications of angioplasty and as an adjunct to thrombolysis. Clin. Radiol. 1994; 49:549–552.

31. Clouse ME, Gramm HF, Legg H, Flood T. Diabetic osteoarthropathy. AJR Am. J. Roentgenol. 1974; 121:22–34.

32. Comerford J, Dawsett G, Kennedy J, Ennis J, Bouchler-Hayes D. Ill-Indium labeled platelet scanning in diagnosis of microembolic disease. A prospective study. Irish J. Med. Sci. 1986; 155:121–122.

33. Coni NK. Posture and arterial pressure in the ischemic foot. Age Aging 1983; 12:151–154.

34. Cosgriff TM, Arnold WJ. Digital vasospasm and infarction associated with hepatitis B antigenemia. JAMA 1976; 235:1362–1363.

35. Cragg AH, Smith TP, Corson JD, Nakagawa N, Castaneda F, Kresowik TF, Sharp WJ, Shamma A, Berbaum KS. Two urokinase dose regimens in native arterial and graft occlusions. Initial results of a prospective, randomized clinical trial. Radiology 1991; 178:681–686.

36. Criqui MH, Langer RD, Fronek A, Feigelson HS, Klauber MR, McCann TJ, Browner D. Mortality over a period of 10 years in patients with peripheral arterial disease. N. Engl. J. Med. 1992; 326:381–386.

37. Dahlin DC, Ivins JC. Fibrosarcoma of bone. A study of 114 cases. Cancer 1969; 23:35–45.

38. Dalinka MK, Edeiken J, Finkelstein JB. Complications of radiation therapy in adult bone. Semin. Roentgenol. 1974; 9:29–39.

39. Dardik H, Ibrahim IM, Sussman B, Greweldinger J, Adler J, Kahn M, Dardik I. Morphologic structure of the pedal arch and its relationship to patency of crural vascular reconstruction. Surg. Gynecol. Obstet. 1981; 152:645–648.

40. Darvin HI, King TA. Lower extremity arterial occlusive disease. Clin. Podiatr. Med. Surg. 1992; 9:69–77.

41. Davidson JK. Aseptic Necrosis of Bone. Amsterdam, Excerpta Medica, 1976.

42. deWolf VG. Assessment of circulation in occlusive arterial disease of the lower extremities. Mod. Concepts Cardiovasc. Dis. 1976; 45:91–95.

43. Dobrin PB. Mechanisms and prevention of arterial injuries caused by balloon embolectomy. Surgery 1989; 106:457–466.

44. Dolmatch BL, Gray RJ, Horton KM, Rundback JH, Kline ME. Treatment of anastomotic bypass graft stenosis with directional atherectomy. Short-term and intermediate term results. J. Vasc. Interv. Radiol. 1995; 6:105–113.

45. Dotter CT, Judkins MP. Transcutaneous treatment of atheromatous obstruction. Description of a new technique and preliminary report of applications. Circulation 1964; 30:654–670.

46. Durant JH, Edwards WS. Small vessel occlusion in the extremity after various periods of arterial obstruction. An experimental study. Surgery 1973; 73–240.

47. Durham JD, Geller SC, Abbott WM, Shapiro H, Waltman AC, Walker TG, Brewster DC, Athanasoulis CA. Regional infusion of urokinase into occluded lower extremity bypass grafts. Long-term clinical results. Radiology 1989; 172:83–87.

48. Edmonds ME. The diabetic foot. Pathophysiology and treatment. Clin. Endocrinol. Metab. 1986; 14:889–916.

49. Edwards EA, Cooley MH. Peripheral vascular symptoms as an initial manifestation of polycythemia vera. JAMA 1970; 214:1463–1467.

50. Eisenbud DE, Brener BJ, Shoenfeld R, Creighton D, Goldenkranz RJ, Brief DK, Alpert J, Huston J, Novick A, Krishnan UR. Treatment of vascular occlusions with intra-arterial urokinase. Am. J. Surg. 1990; 160:160–165.

51. Elliot DH, Harrison JAB Bone necrosis occupational hazard of diving. J. R. Nav. Med. Serv. 1970; 56:140–161.

52. Feldaker M, Hines EA, Kierland RR. Livedo reticularis with ulcerations. Circulation 1956; 13:196–216.

53. Feller SR, Docherty GL. Vasospastic disease. Diagnosis and management. Clin. Podiatr. Med. Surg. 1986; 3:463–470.

54. Ficat RF, Arlet J. Ischemia and Necrosis of Bone. Baltimore, Williams & Wilkins, 1980.

55. Fisher DF, Bichek WH, Holley KE, Eilifson RD. Corticosteroid induced aseptic necrosis. Experimental study. Clin. Orthop. 1972; 84:200–206.

56. Fomon JJ, Warren WD. Late complications of peripheral arterial injuries. Arch. Surg. 1965; 91:610–616.

57. Freiberg AH. Infarction of the second metatarsal bone. A typical injury. Surg. Obstet. Gynecol. 1914; 19:191–193.

58. Freiman DB, Spence R, Gatenby R, Gertner M, Roberts B, Berkowitz HD, Ring EJ, Oleaga JA. Transluminal angioplasty of the iliac and femoral arteries. Follow-up results with anticoagulation. Radiology 1981; 141:347–350.

59. Frykberg ER, Crump JM, Dennis JW, Vines FS, Alexander RH. Nonoperative observation of clinically occult arterial injuries. A prospective evaluation. Surgery 1991; 109:85–96.

60. Frykberg ER, Crump JM, Vines FS, McLellan GL, Dennis JW, Brunner RG, Alexander RH. A reassessment of the role of arteriography in penetrating proximal extremity trauma. A prospective study. Trauma 1989; 29:1041–1052.

61. Furcy JG, Ferrell-Torells M, Regan JW. Fibrosarcoma arising at the site of bone infarcts. J. Bone Joint Surg. Am. 1960; 42:802–810.

62. Gardiner GA, Koltun W, Kandarpa K, Whittemore A, Meyerovitz MF, Bettmann MA, Levin DC, Harrington DP. Thrombolysis of occluded femoropopliteal grafts. AJR Am. J. Roentgenol. 1986; 147:621–626.

63. Gardiner GA Jr, Sullivan KL. Complications of regional thrombolytic therapy. In Kadir S, ed. Current Practice of Interventional Radiology. Philadelphia, BC Decker, 1991; pp. 87–91.

64. Gasper MR. Arterial embolism and thrombosis. Major Probl. Clin. Surg. 1981; 4:158–175.

65. Geller SC. Fibrinolytic therapy. Current aspects. Categorical course on interventional radiology. American Roentgen Ray Society, Boston, 1985.

66. Gloviczki P, Morris SM, Bower TC, Toomey BJ, Naessens JM, Stanson AW. Microvascular pedal bypass for salvage of the severely ischemic limb. Mayo Clin. Proc. 1991; 66:243–253.

67. Graor RA, Risius B, Lucas FV, Young, JR, Ruschhaupt WF, Beven EG, Grosshard EB. Thrombolysis with recombinant human tissue-type plasminogen activator in patients with peripheral artery and bypass graft occlusions. Circulation 1986; 74(suppl):15–20.

68. Graor R, Risius B, Young JR, Geisinger MA, Zelch MG, Smith JAM, Ruschhaupt WF. Low dose streptokinase for selective thrombolysis. Systemic effects and complications. Radiology 1984; 152:35–39.

69. Green RM, Ouriel K, Ricotta JJ, DeWeese JA. Revision of failed infra-inguinal bypass graft. principles of management. Surgery 1986; 100:646.

70. Greenspan B, Pillari G, Schulman ML, Badhey M. Percutaneous transluminal angioplasty of stenotic deep vein arterial bypass grafts. Arch. Surg. 1985; 120:492–495.

71. Gregg PJ, Walder DN. Scintigraphy vs. radiography in early diagnosis of bone necrosis. J. Bone Joint Surg. Br. 1980; 62:214–221.

72. Greyson ND, Kassel EE. Serial bone scan changes in recurrent bone infarction. J. Nucl. Med. 1976; 17:184–186.

73. Gruntzig A, Kumpe DA. Technique of percutaneous transluminal angioplasty with the Gruntzig balloon catheter. AJR Am. J. Roentgenol. 1979; 132:547–552.

74. Hallett JW, Greenwood LH, Robinson JG. Lower extremity arterial disease in young adults. Ann. Surg. 1985; 202:647–652.

75. Hallett JW, Yrizarry JM, Greenwood LH. Regional low dose thromboembolic therapy for peripheral arterial occlusions. Surg. Obstet. Gynecol. 1983; 156:148–154.

76. Hands LJ, Payne ES, Bore PJ, Morris PJ, Radda GK. Magnetic resonance spectroscopy in ischemic feet. Lancet 1986; 2:1391.

77. Hany TF, Schmidt M, Davis CP, G(hde S, Debaten JF. Diagnostic impact of four processing techniques in evaluating contrast-enhanced, three-dimensional MR angiography. AJR Am. J. Roentgenol. 1998; 170:907–912.

78. Hausman M. Microvascular application in limb sparing tumor surgery. Orthop. Clin. North Am. 1989; 20:427–437.

79. Hawkins LG. Fractures of the neck of the talus. J. Bone Joint Surg. Am. 1970; 52:991–1002.

80. Hawks SE, Pentecost MJ. Angiography and transcatheter treatment of extremity trauma. Semin. Intervent. Radiol. 1992; 9:19–27.

81. Hess H, Ingrish H, Mietaschk A, Rath H. Local low dose thrombolytic therapy of peripheral arterial occlusions. N. Engl. J. Med. 1982; 307:1627–1630.

82. Hewes RC, White RI, Jr. Murray RR, Kaufman SL, Chang R, Kadir S, Kinneson ML, Mitchell SE, Auster M. Longterm results of superficial femoral angioplasty. AJR Am. J. Roentgenol. 1986; 146:1025–1029.

83. Hicks ME, Picus D, Darcy MD, Kleinhoffer MA. Multilevel infusion catheter for use with thrombolytic agents. J. Vasc. Interv. Radiol. 1991; 2:73–75.

84. Hight DW, Telneyn-Cough, NP. Changing clinical trends in patients with peripheral arterial disease. Surgery 1976; 79:172–176.

85. Hodgson KJ, Summer DS. Non-invasive assessment of lower extremity arterial disease. Ann. Vasc. Surg. 1988; 2:174–184.

86. Hoffer EK, Sclafani SJ, Herskowitz. MM, Scalea TM. Natural history of arterial injuries diagnosed with arteriography. J. Vasc. Interv. Radiol. 1997; 8:43–53.

87. Horvath W, Oertl M, Haidinger D. Percutaneous transluminal angioplasty of crural arteries. Radiology 1990; 177:565–569.

88. Huettl EA, Soulen MC. Thrombolysis of lower extremity embolic occlusions. A study of the results of the STAR registry. Radiology 1995; 197:141–145.

89. Hungerford DS. Early diagnosis of ischemic necrosis of the femoral head. Johns Hopkins Med. J. 1975; 137–270–275.

90. Idu MM, Blankenstein JD, de Gier P, Truyen E, Buth J. Impact of color flow duplex surveillance program on infra-inguinal vein graft patency. A five year experience. J. Vasc. Surg. 1993; 17:42–53.

91. Ilfeld W, Rosen V. Osteochondritis of the first metatarsal sesamoid. A report of 3 cases. Clin. Orthop. 1972; 85:3841.

92. Imhof H, Breitenseher M, Trattnig S, Kramer J, Hoffmann S, Plenk H, Schneider W, Engel A. Imaging of avascular necrosis of bone. Eur. Radiol. 1997; 7:180–186.

93. Imparato AM, Kim GE, Madayag M, Haveson SP. Angiographic criteria for successful tibial arterial reconstruction. Surgery 1973; 74:830–838.

94. Inge GAL, Ferguson AB. Surgery of the sesamoid bones of the great toe. Arch. Surg. 1933; 27:466–489.

95. Itin P, Stalder H, Vischer W. Symmetrical peripheral gangrene in disseminated tuberculosis. Dermatologica 1986; 173:189–195.

96. Jackson JE, Mitchell A. Advanced vascular interventional techniques in the management of trauma. Semin. Intervent. Radiol. 1997; 14:139–149.

97. Jahss MH. The sesamoids of the hallux. Clin. Orthop. 1981; 157:88–97.

98. Janoff KA, Phinney ES, Porter JM. Lumbar sympathectomies for lower extremity vasospasm. Am. J. Surg. 1985; 150:147–152.

99. Jeans WD, Armstrong S, Cole SE, Horrocks M, Baird RN. Fate of patients undergoing transluminal angioplasty for lower limb ischemia. Radiology 1990; 177:559–564.

100. Johnston, KW. Interventional radiology. PTA of peripheral arteries. In Arterial Surgery. New Diagnostic and Operative techniques. New York, Grune & Stratton, 1988.

101. Joyce JW. Examination of patients with vascular disease. In Localzo J, Creager MA, Dzau VJ, eds. Vascular Medicine. 2nd Ed. Boston, Little, Brown, 1996.

102. Karacagil S, Almgren B, Bergquist D. Patterns of atherosclerotic occlusive disease of lower leg and pedal arteries in hypertensive patients undergoing infra-inguinal bypass procedures. Int. Angiol. 1996; 15:57–60.

103. Karacagil S, Almgren B, Bowald S, Eriksson I. A new method of angiographic runoff evaluation in femoro-distal reconstructions. Arch. Surg. 1990; 125:1055–1058.

104. Karanfilian RG, Lynch TG, Ziral JT, Padberg FT, Jamel Z, Hobson RW. The value of laser Doppler velocimetry and transcutaneous oxygen determination in predicting healing of ischemic foot ulceration and amputation in diabetic and nondiabetic patients. J. Vasc. Surg. 1986; 4:511–516.

105. Katzen BT. Technique and results of low-dose infusion. Cardiovasc. Intervent. Radiol. 1988; 11:S41–S47.

106. Katzen BT, van Breda A. Low-dose streptokinase in the treatment of arterial occlusion. AJR Am. J. Roentgenol. 1981; 136:1171–1178.

107. Kaufman JA, Bettman MA. Thrombolysis of peripheral vascular occlusions with urokinase. A review of the literature. Semin. Intervent. Radiol. 1992; 9:159–165.

108. Kaufman JA, McCarter D, Geller SC, Waltman AC. Two-dimensional time-of-flight MR angiography of the lower extremities. Artifacts and Pitfalls. AJR Am. J. Roentgenol. 1998; 171:129–135.

109. Kaufman JL, Stark K, Brolin RE. Disseminated atheroembolism from extensive degenerative atherosclerosis of the aorta. Surgery 1987; 162:63.

110. Kazmier FJ. Shaggy aorta syndrome and disseminated atheromatous

embolization. In Bergan JJ, Yao JS, eds. Aortic Surgery. Philadelphia, WB Saunders, 1989; p. 189.

111. Keen RR, McCarthy WJ, Shireman PK, Feinglass J, Pearce WH, Durham JR, Yao, JS. Surgical management of atheroembolization. J. Vasc. Surg. 1995; 21:773–781.

112. Kent KC, McArdle CR, Kennedy B, Baim DS, Anninos E, Skillman JJ. A prospective study of the clinical outcome of femoral pseudoaneurysms and arteriovenous fistulas induced by arterial puncture. J. Vasc. Surg. 1993; 17:125–133.

113. Kidawa AS. Vasospastic disorders. Clin. Podiatr. Med Surg. 1992; 9:139–150.

114. Köhler A. Ueber eine haufige bisher anscheinende unbekannte Erbronkung einzelner Kurdlicher knocken. Munchen Med. Wochenschr. 1908; 55:1923.

115. Köhler TR, Nance DR, Cramer MM, Vandenburghe N, Strandness DE, Jr. Duplex scanning for diagnoses of aortoiliac and femoro-popliteal disease. A prospective study. Circulation 1987; 76:1074–1080.

116. Kozak BE, Bedell JE, Rosch J. Small vessel leg angiography for distal vessel bypass grafts. J. Vasc. Surg. 1988; 8:711.

117. Kumpe DA, Zwerdlinger S, Griffin DJ. Blue toe syndrome. Treatment with percutaneous transluminal angioplasty. Radiology 1988; 166: 37–44.

118. Kwasnick AM. Limb salvage in diabetics. Challenges and solutions. Surg. Clin. North Am. 1986; 66:305–318.

119. Kwong PK. Applications of Doppler ultrasound to foot and ankle care. Foot Ankle 1982; 2:220–223.

120. Laco JE, Schiller J, Hetherington VJ. Cardiovascular disorders. Diagnostic and therapeutic implications for podiatric medical practice. Clin. Podiatr. 1985; 2:639–652.

121. Lai TM, Glasson R, Grayndler V, Evans J, Hogg J, Etheridge S. Colour duplex ultrasonography versus angiography in the diagnosis of lower extremity arterial disease. Cardiovasc. Surg 1996; 4:384–388.

122. Lang E. A survey of the complications of percutaneous retrograde arteriography. Radiology 1963; 81:257–263.

123. Lang E. Streptokinase therapy. Complications of intraarterial use. Radiology 1985; 154:75–77.

124. Lapeyre AC III, Steele PM, Kazmier FJ, Chesebro JH, Vlietstra RE, Fuster V. Systemic embolism in chronic left ventricular aneurysm. incidence and the role of anticoagulation. J. Am. Coll. Cardiol. 1985; 6:534–538.

125. Lawrance PF, Syverud JB, Disbro MA, Olazraki N. Evaluation of technetium-99m phosphate imaging for predicting skin ulcer healing. Am. J. Surg. 1983; 146:746–750.

126. Lecouvet FE, VandeBerg BC, Maldaque BE, Lebon CJ, Jamart J, Saleh M, Nöel H, Malgehim J. Early irreversible osteonecrosis versus transient lesions of the femoral condyles. Prognostic value of subchondral bone and marrow changes on MR imaging. AJR Am. J. Roentgenol. 1998; 170:71–77.

127. Lee HM, Wang Y, Sostman HD, Schwartz LH, Khilmani NM, Trost DW, Ramirez de Arellano E, Teeger S, Bush HL Jr. Distal lower extremity arteries. Evaluation with two-dimensional MR digital subtraction angiography. Radiology 1998; 207:505–512.

128. Leeson MC, Weiner DS. Osteochondrosis of the tarsal cuneiforms. Clin. Orthop. 1985; 196:260–264.

129. Leng GC, Whyman MR, Donnan PT, Ruckley CV, Gillespie I, Fowkes FG, Allan PL. Accuracy and reproducibility of duplex ultrasonography in grading femoropopliteal stenoses. J. Vasc. Surg. 1993; 17:510–517.

130. Levy LA. Foot and ankle ulcers associated with hematologic disorders. Clin. Podiatr. 1985; 2:631–637.

131. Lionberger DR, Bishop JO, Tullos HS. The modified Blair fusion. Foot Ankle 1982; 3:60–62.

132. Localzo J, Creager MA, Dzau VJ. Vascular Medicine. 2nd Ed. Boston, Little, Brown, 1996.

133. Logerfo FW, Coffmann JD. Vascular and microvascular disease of the foot in diabetics. N. Engl. J. Med. 1984; 311:1615–1619.

134. Londrey GL, Ramsey DE, Hodgson KJ, Barkmeier LD, Sumner DS. Infrapopliteal bypass for severe ischemia. Comparison of autogenous veins, composite and prosthetic grafts. J. Vasc. Surg. 1991; 13:631.

135. Lovett JE, Shestak KC, Makaroun, MS. Analysis of lower extremity bloodflow in the patient with peripheral vascular insufficiency. A guide for plastic surgeons. Ann. Plast. Surg. 1994; 32:101–106.

136. Lynn RB. Chilblains. Surg. Gynecol. Obstet. 1954; 99:720–726.

137. Malone JM, Lecel JM, Moore WS. The gold standard for amputation level selection. Xeron-133 clearance. J. Surg. Res. 1981; 30:449–455.

138. Mann RA. Surgery of the Foot and Ankle. 6th Ed. St. Louis, CV Mosby, 1993.

139. Mann RA. AVN of the metatarsal head following chevron osteotomy. Foot Ankle 1982; 3:125–129.

140. Manusov EG, Lillegard WA, Raspa RF, Epperly TD. Evaluation of pediatric foot problems. Am. Fam. Physician 1996; 54:592–606.

141. Markisz JA, Knowles RJR, Altuk DW, Schneider R, Whalen JP, Cahill PT. Segmental pattern of avascular necrosis of the femoral heads. Early detection with MR imaging. Radiology 1987; 162:717–720.

142. Marks J, King TA, Baele H. Rubin J, Marmen C. Popliteal-to-distal bypass for limb-threatening ischemia. J. Vasc. Surg. 1992; 15:755, 1992.

143. McCauley GK, Koplin PC. Osteochondritis of the tarsal navicular. Radiology 1977; 123:705–706.

144. McGhee SR, Boyko EJ. Physical examination and chronic lower extremity ischemia. Arch. Intern. Med. 1998; 158:1357–1364.

145. McNamara TO. Technique and results of higher-dose infusion. Cardiovasc. Intervent. Radiol. 1998; 11:S48–S57.

146. McNamara TO. Thrombolytic treatment for acute lower limb ischemia. In Strandness DE, van Breda A, eds. Vascular Diseases. Surgical and Interventional Therapy. New York, Churchill Livingstone, 1994; pp. 355–377.

147. McNamara TO, Fischer JR. Thrombolysis of peripheral arterial and graft occlusions. improved results using high-dose urokinase. AJR Am. J. Roentgenol. 1985; 144:769–775.

148. McNamara TO, Bamberger RA, Merchant RF. Intra-arterial urokinase as the initial therapy for acutely ischemic lower limbs. Circulation 1991; 83(suppl I):106.

149. Meilstrup DB. Osteochondritis of the internal cuneiform, bilatera. AJR Am. J. Roentgenol. 1947; 58:329–331.

150. Merino J, Casaneuva B, Piney E, ValBerual F, Rodriguez-Valverde V. Hemiplegia and peripheral gangrene secondary to large and medium sized vessel involvement in CREST syndrome. Clin. Rheumatol. 1982; 1:295–299.

151. Meyerovitz MF, Goldhaber SZ, Reagan K. Recombinant tissue-type plasminogen activators versus urokinase in peripheral arterial and graft occlusions. a randomized trial. Radiology 1990; 175:75–78.

152. Mirra JM, Bullough PG, Marcove RC, Jacobs B, Huvos AG. Malignant fibrous histiocytoma and osteosarcoma in association with bone infarcts. J. Bone Joint Surg. Am. 1974; 56:932–940.

153. Mitchell DG, Ras VM, Dalinka MK, Spritzer CE, Alavi A, Steinberg ME, Fallon M, Kressel HY. Femoral head avascular necrosis. Correlation of MRI, radiographic staging, radionuclide imaging and clinical findings. Radiology 1987; 162:709–715.

154. Mitchell DG, Ras VM, Dalinka MK, Spritzer CE, Axel L, Gefter W, Kricun M, Steinberg ME, Kressel HY. Hematopoeitic and fatty bone marrow distribution in normal and ischemic hip. New observations with 1.5T MR imaging. Radiology 1986; 161:199–202.

155. Moldveen-Gernimus M, Merrian JC. Cholesterol embolization. From pathologic curiosity to clinical entity. Circulation 1967; 35:946–953.

156. Molos MA, Hall JC. Symmetrical gangrene and disseminated intravascular coagulation. Arch. Dermatol. 1985; 121:1057–1061.

157. Mont MA, Schon LC, Hungerford MW, Hungerford DS. Avascular necrosis of the talus treated by core decompression. J. Bone Joint Surg. Br. 1996; 78:827–830.

158. Moshiak A, Soroker D, Pasik S, Mashiah T. Phenol lumbar sympathetic block in diabetic lower limb ischemia. J. Cardiovasc. Risk 1995; 2:467–469.

159. Motarjeme A. Thrombolytic therapy in arterial occlusion and graft thrombosis. Semin. Vasc. Surg. 1989; 2:155–178.

160. Motarjeme A. Thrombolytic therapy in arterial occlusion and graft thrombosis. Semin. Vasc. Surg. 1989; 2:155–178.

161. Mubarak SJ. Osteochondrosis of the lateral cuneiform. another cause of a limp in a child. J. Bone Joint Surg. Am. 1992; 74:285–289.

162. Mulfinger GL, Trueta JC. The blood supply of the talus. J. Bone Joint Surg. Br. 1970; 52:150–167.

163. Nelson JP. The vascular history and physical examination. Clin. Podiatr. Med. Surg. 1992; 9:1–18.

164. Novelline RA. Percutaneous transluminal angioplasty. Newer applications. AJR Am. J. Roentgenol. 1980; 135:893–900.

165. Ogata K, Sugioka Y, Urano U, Chidama H. Idiopathic osteonecrosis of the first metatarsal sesamoid. Skeletal Radiol. 1986; 15:141–145.

166. Ohta T. Non-invasive technique using thallium-201 for predicting ischemic ulcer healing in the foot. Br. J. Surg. 1985; 72:892–895.

167. O'Mara CS, Flinn WR, Neiman HL, Bergan JJ, Yao JS. Correlation of foot arterial anatomy with early tibial bypass patency. Surgery 1981; 89:743–752.

168. O'Mara RE, Weber DA. The osseous system. In Freeman LM, ed. Freeman and Johnson's Clinical Radionuclide Imaging. 3rd Ed. New York, Grune & Stratton, 1984; pp. 1141–1240.

169. Ouriel K, Veith FJ, Sasahara AA. A comparison of recombinant urokinase with vascular surgery in initial treatment for acute arterial occlusion of the legs. N. Engl. J. Med. 1998; 338:1105–11.

170. Ozonoff MB. Pediatric Orthopedic Radiology. 2nd Ed. Philadelphia, WB Saunders, 1992.

171. Panayiotopoulos YP, Tyrrell MR, Arnold FJ, Korzon-Burakowska A, Amiel SH, Taylor EPR. Results and cost analysis of distal (crural/pedal) arterial revascularization for limb salvage in diabetic and nondiabetic patients. Diabet. Med. 1997; 14:214–220.

172. Penny JN, Davis LA. Fractures and dislocations of the neck of the talus. J. Trauma 1980; 20:1029–1037.

173. Perler BA, Osterman FA, Mitchell SE, Burdick JF, Williams GM. Balloon dilatation versus surgical revision of infra-inguinal autogenous vein graft stenoses. long-term follow-up. J. Cardiovasc. Surg. 1990; 31:656–661.

174. Peterson L, Goldie IF. The arterial supply of the talus. A study on the relationship of experimental talar fractures. Acta Orthop. Scand. 1975; 46:1026–1034.

175. Polak JF, Donaldson MC, Dobkin GR, Mannick JA, O Leary DH. Early detection of saphenous vein arterial bypass graft stenosis by color-assisted duplex sonography. A prospective study. AJR Am. J. Roentgenol. 1990; 154:857–861.

176. Ramirez G, O Neill WM Jr, Lambert R, Bloomer HA. Cholesterol embolization. a complication of angiography. Arch. Intern. Med. 1978; 138:1430–1432.

177. Renander A. Two cases of typical osteochondropathy of the medial sesamoid bone of the first metatarsal. Acta Radiol. 1924; 3:521–527.

178. Resnick D. Osteochondroses. In Resnick D, Niwayama G, eds. Diagnosis of Bone and Joint Disorders. 3rd Ed. Philadelphia, WB Saunders, 1995; pp. 3559–3610.

179. Resnick D, Niwayama G, eds. Diagnosis of Bone and Joint Disorders. Philadelphia, WB Saunders, 1995.

180. Resnick D, Pineda C, Trudell D. Widespread osteonecrosis of the foot in systemic lupus erythematosis. Radiologic and gross pathologic correlation. Skeletal Radiol. 1985; 13:33–38.

181. Rhodes GR, Skudder P. Salvage of ischemic diabetic feet. Role of transcutaneous oxygen mapping and multiple configurations of in situ bypass. Am. J. Surg. 1986; 152:165–171.

182. Riles TS, Rosen RJ. Arteriovenous fistulae. In Strandness DE, van Breda A, eds. Vascular Diseases. Surgical and Interventional Therapy. New York, Churchill Livingstone, 1994, pp. 1109–1114.

183. Riles TS, Rosen RJ. Arteriovenous malformations. In Strandness DE, van Breda A, eds. Vascular Diseases. Surgical and Interventional Therapy. New York, Churchill Livingstone, 1994; pp. 1121–1137.

184. Risius B, Graor RA, Geisinger MA, Zelch MG, Lucas FV, Young JR, Grossbard EB. Recombinant human tissue-type plasminogen activator of thrombolysis in peripheral arteries and bypass grafts. Radiology 1986; 160:183–188.

185. Roberts AC, Kaufman JA, Gelles SC. Angiographic assessment in peripheral vascular disease, In Strandness DE, van Breda A, eds. Vascular Diseases. Surgical and Interventional Therapy. New York, Churchill Livingstone, 1994, pp. 201–235.

186. Rockson SG, Cooke JP. Peripheral arterial insufficiency. Mechanisms, natural history and therapeutic options. Adv. Intern. Med. 1998; 43:253–277.

187. Roedersheimer LR, Feins R, Green RM. Doppler evaluation of the pedal arch. Am. J. Surg. 1981; 142. 601–605.

188. Rowe DM, Becker GJ, Rabe FE, Holden RW, Richmond BD, Wass JL, Sequeira FW. Osseous metastases from renal cell carcinoma. embolization and surgery for restoration of function. Radiology 1984; 150:673–676.

189. Rubinger D, Friedlaender MM, Silver J, Kopolovec Y, Czaczkes WJ, Popovtzen MM. Progressive vascular calcification with necrosis of the extremities in hemodialysis patients. A possible role of iron overload. Am. J. Kidney Dis. 1986; 7:125–129.

190. Russell J. A practical essay on the certain disease of bone termed necrosis. Edinburgh, Neill and Co., 1794.

191. Saab MH, Smith DC, Aka PK, Brownlee RW, Killeen JD. Percutaneous transluminal angioplasty of tibial arteries for limb salvage. Cardiovasc. Intervent. Radiol. 1992; 15:211–16.

192. Saddikni S, Sniderman KW, Hilton S. Percutaneous transluminal angioplasty of nonatheromatous lesions. AJR Am. J. Roentgenol. 1980; 135:891–892.

193. Sasahara AA. Fundamentals of fibrinolytic therapy. Cardiovasc. Intervent. Radiol. 1988; 11:S3–S5.

194. Scaglietti O, Struga G, Mizzore W. Plus-variant of the astragalus and subnormal scaphoid space. Two important findings in Koehler's scaphoid necrosis. Acta Orthop. Scand. 1962; 32:499–508.

195. Schwarten DE. Clinical and anatomical considerations for non-operative therapy in tibial disease and the results of angioplasty. Circulation 1991; 83(suppl 1):186–190.

196. Seabrook GR, Mewissen MW, Schmitt DD, Reifsnyder T, Bandyk DF, Lipchik EO, Towne JB. Percutaneous intra-arterial thrombolysis in the treatment of thrombosis of lower extremity arterial reconstructions. J. Vasc. Surg. 1991; 13:646–651.

197. Sever JW. Apophysitis of the os calcis. N. Y. Med. J. 1912; 95: 1025–1029.

198. Shafa MH, Fernandez-Ulloa M, Rost RC, Nyquist SR. Diagnosis of aseptic necrosis of the talus by bone scintigraphy. Clin. Nucl. Med. 1983; 8:50–53.

199. Sharafuddin MJ, Hicks ME. Current status of percutaneous mechanical thrombectomy. Part III. Present and future applications. J. Vasc. Interv. Radiol. 1998; 9:209–224.

200. Sharafuddin MJ, Hicks ME. Current status of percutaneous mechanical thrombectomy. Part II. Devices and mechanisms of action. J. Vasc. Interv. Radiol. 1998; 9:15–31.

201. Sharafuddin MJ, Hicks ME. Current status of percutaneous mechanical thrombectomy. Part I. General principles. J. Vasc. Interv. Radiol. 1997; 8:911–921.

202. Sheridan J, Thompson J, Gazzard S, Birch S, McShane M, Webster J, Chaut T. The role of transluminal angioplasty in the management of femoro-distal graft stenosis. Br. J. Radiol. 1989; 62:564.

203. Shofner CE, Coin CG. The effect of weight bearing on the appearance and development of the secondary calcaneal apophysis. Radiology 1966; 86:201–206.

204. Shuman CR. Foot disorders in the Diabetic. Diabetes 1983; 74: 109–120.

205. Siegel ME, Stewart CA, Kwong P, Sakimura I. 201T1 perfusion study of ischemic ulcers of the leg. Prognostic ability compared with Doppler ultrasound. Int. J. Nucl. Med. Biol. 1982; 143:233–235.

206. Siffert RS. Classification of osteochondroses. Clin. Orthop. 1981; 158: 10–28.

207. Siffert RS, Arkin AM. Post-traumatic aseptic necrosis of the distal tibial epiphysis. J. Bone Joint Surg. Am. 1950; 32:691–695.

208. Sivananthan UM, Browne TF, Thorley DJ, Rees MR. Percutaneous transluminal angioplasty of the tibial arteries. Br. J. Surg. 1994; 81: 1282–1285.

209. Sinha S, Manechoopdappa CS, Kozek EP. Neuropathy in diabetes mellitus. Medicine (Baltimore) 1972; 51:191–210.

210. Smillie IS. Freiberg's infarction (Köhler's second disease). J. Bone Joint Surg. Br. 1957; 39:580.

211. Sniderman KW, Kalman PG, Shewchun J, Goldberg RE. Lower-extremity in situ saphenous vein grafts. Angiographic interventions. Radiology 1989; 170:1023–1027.

212. Sos TA. Percutaneous transluminal renal angioplasty Categorical course on interventional radiology. American Roentgen Ray Society, Boston, 1985.

213. Soulen RL, Tyson RR, Reichle FA, Cohen AM. Angiographic criteria for small vessel bypass. Radiology 1973; 107:513–519.

214. Spence RK, Freiman DB, Gatenby R, Hobbs OL, Barker CF, Berkowitz HG, Roberts B, McLoan G, Oleaga J, Ring EJ. Long-term results of transluminal angioplasty of the iliac and femoral arteries. Arch. Surg. 1981; 116:1377–1386.

215. Spies JB. Complications of diagnostic arteriography. Semin. Intervent. Radiol. 1994; 2:93–101.

216. Stain SC, Yellin AE, Weaver FA, Pentecost MJ. Selective management of nonocclusive arterial injuries. Arch. Surg. 1989; 124: 1136–1141.

217. Staple TW. Modified catheter for percutaneous transluminal treatment of atheromatous obstruction. Radiology 1968; 91:1041–1043.

218. Starck EE, McDermott JC, Crummy AB, Turnipseed WD, Acher CW, Burgess JH. Percutaneous aspiration thromboembolectomy. Radiology 1985; 156:61–66.

219. Strandness DE, van Breda A, eds. Vascular Diseases. Surgical and Interventional Therapy. New York, Churchill Livingstone, 1994; pp. 511–523.

220. Sullivan KL, Gardiner GA Jr, Kandarpa K, Bonn J, Shapiro MJ, Carabasi RA, Smullens S, Levin DC. Efficacy of thrombolysis in infrainguinal bypass grafts. Circulation 1991; 83(suppl 1):I99–105.

221. Sullivan KL, Gardiner GA Jr, Shapiro MJ, Bonn J, Levin DC. Acceleration of thrombolysis with a high-dose transthrombus bolus technique. Radiology 1989; 173:805–808.

222. Sweet DE and Madewell JE. Osteonecrosis. Pathogenesis. In Resnick D, Niwayama G. Diagnosis of Bone and Joint Disorders. Vol. 5. 3rd Ed. Philadelphia, WB Saunders, 1995; pp. 3445–3494.

223. Tegtmeyer CJ, Spinosa DJ, Matsumoto AH. Angiography of bones, joints, and soft tissues. In Baum S, ed. Abrams' Angiography. New York, Little, Brown, 1997; pp. 1179–1821.

224. Terada M, Satoh M, Mitsuzane K, Shioyoyama Y, Tsuda M, Kishi K, Maeda M, Momura S, Yamada R. Short-term intrathrombotic injection of ultrahigh-dose urokinase for treatment of iliac and femoropopliteal artery occlusions. Radiat. Med. 1990; 8:79–87.

225. Thornton MA, Gruentzig AR, Hallman J, King SB, Douglas JS. Coumadin and aspirin in prevention of recurrence after transluminal coronary angioplasty. A randomized study. Circulation 1984; 69:721–727.

226. Totty WG, Gilula LA, McClellan BL, Ahmed P, Sherman L. Low-dose intravascular fibrinolytic therapy. Radiology 1982; 143:59–69.

227. Totty WG, Murphy WA, Guaz WC, Kamor B, Davish WJ, Siegel BA. Magnetic resonance imaging of the normal and ischemic femoral head. AJR Am. J. Roentgenol. 1984; 143:1273–1280.

228. Traughber PD, Cook PS, Micklos TJ, Miller FJ. Intra-arterial fibrinolytic therapy for popliteal and tibial artery obstruction. Comparison of streptokinase and urokinase. AJR Am. J. Roentgenol. 1987; 149:453–456.

229. Valji K, Roberts A, Davis GB, Bookstein JJ. Pulsed-spray thrombolysis of arterial and bypass graft occlusion. AJR Am. J. Roentgenol. 1991; 156:617–621.

230. van Breda A. Regional thrombolysis in the treatment of peripheral arterial occlusions. Appl. Radiol. 1982; 5:63–72.

231. van Breda A, Katzen BT. Thrombolytic therapy of peripheral vascular disease. Semin. Intervent. Radiol. 1995; 2:354–366.

232. Varty K, Bolia A, Naylor AR, Bell PR, London NJ. Infrapopliteal percutaneous transluminal angioplasty. A safe and successful procedure. Eur. J. Vasc. Endovasc. Surg. 1995; 9:341–345.

233. Veith FJ, Gupta SK, Ascer E, White-Flores S, Samson RH, Scher LA, Towne JB, Bernhard VM, Bonier P, Flinn WR. Six-year prospective multicenter randomized comparison of autologous saphenous vein and expanded polytetrafluoroethylene graft in infra-inguinal arterial reconstructions. J. Vasc. Surg. 1986; 3:104–114.

234. Veith FJ, Gupta SK, Samson RH, Flores SW, Janko G, Scher LA. Superficial femoral and popliteal arteries as inflow sites for distal bypasses. Surgery 1981; 90:980.

235. Veith FJ, Gupta SK, Samson RH, Scher LA, Fell SC, Weiss P, Janko G, Flores SW, Rifkin H, Bernstein G, Haimovici H, Gliedman ML, Sprayregen S. Progress in limb salvage by reconstructive arterial surgery combined with new or imposed adjunctive procedures. Ann. Surg. 1981; 194:386–401.

236. Veith FJ, Gupta SK, Wengerter KR, Goldsmith J, Rivers SP, Bakal CW, Dietzek AM, Cynamon J, Sprayregen S, Gliedman ML. Changing arterosclerotic disease patterns and management strategies in lower limb threatening ischemia. Ann. Surg. 1990; 212:402–412.

237. Veith FJ, Panetta TF, Wengerter KR, Martin ML, Rivers SP, Suggs WD, Lyon RT. Femoropopliteal tibial occlusive disease. In Veith FJ, Hobson RW, Wittram RA, Wilson SE, eds. Vascular Surgery. Principles and Practice. 2nd Ed. New York, McGraw-Hill, 1994; pp. 421–446.

238. Verstraete M, Hess H, Mahler F, Mietaschk A, Roth FJ, Schneider E, Baert AL, Verhaeghe R. Femoro-popliteal artery thrombolysis with intra-arterial infusion of recombinant tissue-type plasminogen activator. Report of a pilot trial. Eur. J. Vasc. Surg. 1988; 2:155–159.

239. Vlietstra R, Holmes D. Percutaneous Transluminal Coronary Angioplasty. Philadelphia, FA Davis, 1987.

240. Wagner HJ, Starck EE, Reuter P. Long-term results of percutaneous aspiration embolectomy. Cardiovasc. Intervent. Radiol. 1994; 17:241–246.

241. Walden R, Segaly Y, Rulenstein ZS, Morag B, Bass A, Adar R. Percutaneous transluminal angioplasty. A suggested method for analysis of clinical arteriographic and hemodynamic factors affecting the results of treatment. J. Vasc. Surg. 1986. 3:583–590.

242. Waltman AC. Transluminal angioplasty in the iliac arteries. Categorical course on interventional radiology. American Roentgen Ray Society, Boston, 1985.

243. Wang GJ, Sweet DE, Roger SI. Fat cell changes as a mechanism of avascular necrosis of the femoral head in corticosteroid treated rabbits. J. Bone Joint Surg. Am. 1977; 59:729–735.

244. Wang Y, Lee HM, Khilnani NM, Trost DW, Jagust MB, Winchester PA, Bush HL, Sos TA, Sostman HD. Bolus-chase MR digital subtraction angiography of the lower extremity. Radiology 1998; 207:263–269.

245. Washburn B. Frostbite. N. Engl. J. Med. 1962; 266:974–989.

246. Weaver FA, Modrall JG, Baek S, Harvey F, Siegal A, Rosenthal J, Yellin AE. Syme amputation. results in patients with severe forefoot ischemia. Cardiovasc. Surg. 1996; 4:81–86

247. Wengerter KR, Veith FJ, Gupta SK, Goldsmith J, Farrell E, Harris PL, Moore D, Shanik G. Prospective randomized multicenter comparison of in situ and reversed vein infrapopliteal bypasses. J. Vasc. Surg. 1991; 13:189–197.

248. Whittemore AD, Donaldson MC, Polak JF, Mannick JA. Limitations of balloon angioplasty for vein graft stenosis. J. Vasc. Surg. 1991; 14:340–345.

249. Wilson YG, Wyatt MG, Currie IC, Wakeley CJ, Lamont PM, Band RN. Isolated tibial vessel disease. treatment options and outcome. Panminerva Med. 1996; 38:71–77.

250. Wolf GL. Mechanisms of Angioplasty. Categorical course of interventional radiology. American Roentgen Ray Society, Boston, 1985.

251. Wright DG, Adeloar RS. Avascular necrosis of the talus. Foot Ankle Int. 1995; 16:743–744.

252. Yakes WF, Luethke JM, Merland JJ, Rak KM, Slater DD, Hollis HW, Parker SH, Casasco A, Aymard A, Hodes J. Ethanol embolization of arteriovenous fistulas primary model of therapy. J. Vasc. Interv. Radiol. 1990; 1:89.

253. Youkey JR, Clagett GP, Cabellon S Jr, Eddleman WL, Salander JM, Rich NM. Thromboembolectomy of arteries explored at the ankle. Ann. Surg. 1984; 199:367.

254. Zertler E, Gruntzig A, Schoop W. Percutaneous Vascular Recanalization. Techniques, Applications, and Clinical Results. Berlin, Springer-Verlag, 1978.

Radiology of the Foot and Ankle, Second Edition,
edited by Thomas H. Berquist.
© 2000 by Mayo Foundation.
Published by Lippincott Williams & Wilkins, Philadelphia.

CHAPTER 9

Pediatric Foot and Ankle Disorders

Laura W. Bancroft, Debbie J. Merinbaum, and Alan D. Hoffman

Trauma and infection of the pediatric foot are discussed elsewhere in this text (see Chapters 4 and 7). This chapter focuses on congenital and early acquired abnormalities. Congenital foot abnormalities have been exquisitely discussed previously by Ozonoff,[22] Ritchie and Keim,[24] and Freiberger,[7] and we would like to acknowledge their contributions to this discussion. In this chapter, radiologic techniques and the terminology essential to the understanding of congenital foot disorders are outlined first.

RADIOLOGIC TECHNIQUE

For images to be accurate and reproducible, the radiologic technique for acquiring anteroposterior (AP) and lateral weight-bearing pediatric foot films must be standardized (see Chapter 2). In the infant or the paralyzed or uncooperative child, simulated weight bearing must be provided. The knees are held together, and pressure is applied so the tibia is perpendicular to the cassette.[21] The central radiographic beam is then angled about 15° posteriorly to avoid overlap of the tibia and hindfoot.[1] For the lateral view, a radiolucent

L. W. Bancroft: Mayo Medical School, Mayo Clinic Jacksonville, Jacksonville, Florida 32224.

D. J. Merinbaum: Mayo Foundation, Mayo Medical School, Rochester, Minnesota 55905; Nemours Children's Clinic, Jacksonville, Florida 32207.

A. D. Hoffman: Mayo Medical School, Mayo Clinic Jacksonville, Jacksonville, Florida 32224.

board or block is pressed against the sole to dorsiflex the foot maximally, to simulate weight bearing.

There is no need for oblique views in the foot examination of an infant,[7] but these views can assist in the diagnosis of tarsal coalitions. The Harris or 45° angled view is a tangential view of the heel that is helpful for evaluating the calcaneus and subtalar joints in the evaluation of talocalcaneal coalition. The medial facet projects superiorly and medial to the parallel posterior facet.

Computed tomography (CT) is useful in the evaluation of tarsal coalitions, particularly talocalcaneal coalitions. Subtle joint space narrowing, irregularity, and cystic changes may be appreciated earlier with CT than with routine radiography.

Magnetic resonance imaging (MRI) is excellent for assessing cartilaginous or fibrous tarsal coalitions. MRI is occasionally used for preoperative evaluation of soft tissues in the planning of soft tissue releases for a variety of foot anomalies. The exact position and length of tendons and ligaments can be outlined. Because the navicular can remain unossified until ages 1 to 5.5 years,[22] MRI or sonography can detect exact cartilaginous locations and relation to the other tarsal bones. Furthermore, in the hands of experienced examiners, sonography has proven reliable in the prenatal evaluation of abnormalities of the feet and has led to the diagnosis of associated syndromes.[3]

Terminology

Before congenital foot anomalies can be discussed, one must be familiar with the radiologic terminology:

Talipes: congenital deformity of the foot.
Pes: acquired deformity of the foot.
Valgus: orientation of the bones distal to a joint away from the midline of the body.
Varus: orientation of the bones distal to a joint toward the midline of the body.
Adduction: displacement of the bones or body part in a transverse plane toward the axis of the body.
Abduction: displacement of the bones or body part in a transverse plane away from the axis of the body.
Equinus: fixed plantar flexion of the hindfoot.
Calcaneus: fixed dorsiflexion of the hindfoot.
Cavus: raised longitudinal arch of the foot.
Planus: flattened longitudinal arch of the foot.

NORMAL ANATOMY AND ANGLES

The talus and calcaneus comprise the hindfoot, the remaining tarsal bones make up the midfoot, and the metatarsals and phalanges are the forefoot. For discussion purposes, the talus is considered fixed. Therefore, the relationship of the more distal calcaneus and remaining foot are described by their relative position to the more proximal talus. Multiple angles are derived from the ossified bones on the AP and lateral views (Table 9-1).

On the normal AP view (Fig. 9-1A), extension of a line through the long axis of the talus (midtalar line) should intersect, or be near, the medial base of the first metatarsal, and a line through the long axis of the calcaneus should intersect the base of the fourth metatarsal. The talocalcaneal angle on the AP view (Kite's angle) averages about 40° (range, 25°

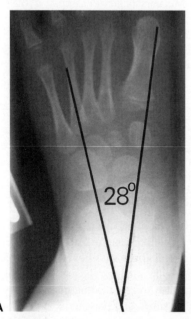

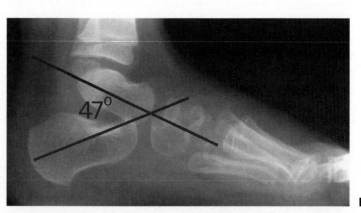

FIG. 9-1. Normal simulated weight-bearing views of the pediatric foot. The talocalcaneal angles on the AP (**A**) (28°) and lateral (**B**) (47°) views are normal. Normal AP angles are 25° to 55°, and lateral are 25° to 55°.

TABLE 9-1. *Normal angles of the foot and ankle*

AP talocalcaneal angle
  Newborn 40° (range, 25–55°)
  Adult 25° (range, 15–35°)
Lateral talocalcaneal angle
  40° (range, 25–55°)
Talo–first metatarsal angle
  Newborn, 20° (range, 9–31°)
  8 years, 5° (range, 10–18°)
Tibiocalcaneal angle
  Newborn, 75°
  6 years, 65°

to 55°) in the newborn and decreases to the adult average of 25° (range, 15° to 35°) by age 9 years (see Fig. 9-1).[27] In the lateral projection (see Fig. 9-1B), the talocalcaneal angle averages 40° (range, 25° to 55°), and is accentuated by dorsiflexion.[21] When the foot is in a neutral position, the talus is plantar flexed and the midtalar line extends through the first metatarsal, except in children less than 5 years old, in whom the midtalar line passes inferiorly to the metatarsal.

When the navicular is ossified, it is normally visualized directly distal to the plane of the talus. When hindfoot varus is present, it is subluxed medially, and when hindfoot valgus is present, it is displaced laterally in relation to the talar axis (Fig. 9-2).

The talar–first metatarsal angle is calculated from lines extending through the long axes of the talus and first metatarsal (Fig. 9-3A). This angle measures about 20° on average at birth and slowly decreases to about 5° at age 8 years on both AP and lateral views. The anterior tibiocalcaneal line (see Fig. 9-3B) measures the relationship between the long axes of the tibia and calcaneus: this has a mean of about 75° in the newborn and 65° at 6 years of age, and then it increases slightly until about 9 years old.[27]

The longitudinal plantar arch is assessed on the lateral film by extending lines along the axis of the calcaneus and the fifth metatarsal and deriving an obtuse angle (Fig. 9-4). This angle normally measures between 150° and 175°. When this angle measures less than 150°, pes cavus is present; when it measures more than 175°, pes planus is present; and when it measure more than 180°, there is a rocker-bottom deformity (see Fig. 9-4). The normal transverse arch is appreciated on the lateral film by the positions of the metatarsals. Normally, the fifth metatarsal is located most inferiorly, and the remaining bones overlap more superiorly.[22,27]

CLASSIFICATION OF ANKLE ABNORMALITIES

Ankle valgus is diagnosed when the tibial plafond is greater than 3° valgus with respect to the tibial diaphysis (normal range, 0° to 3°) (Fig. 9-5). Ankle valgus may exist solely or in conjunction with hindfoot valgus. During childhood and adolescence, multiple conditions can result in relative fibular shortening and ankle valgus. Causes include neurogenic conditions (spina bifida, cerebral palsy, polio, neurofibromatosis), chromosomal abnormalities (Down's

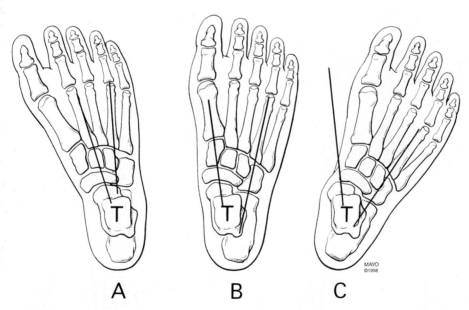

A   B   C

FIG. 9-2. Depiction of AP standing views of hindfoot varus (**A**), a normal foot (**B**), and hindfoot valgus (**C**). The drawings are oriented to emphasize that the talus does not vary in position. On the normal AP view, the midtalar line should intersect, or be near, the medial base of the first metatarsal, and the midcalcaneal line should intersect the base of the fourth metatarsal. When the navicular is ossified, it is normally located distal to the plane of the talus. When hindfoot varus is present, it is subluxed medially, and when hindfoot valgus is present, it is displaced laterally.

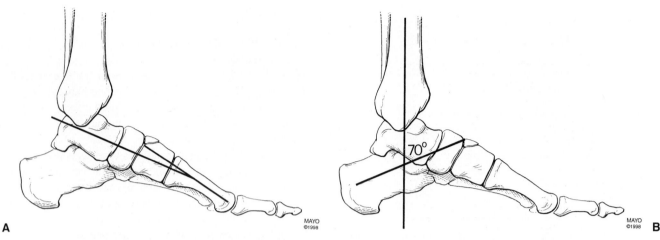

FIG. 9-3. Normal angles. **A:** Illustrations of the lateral talar–first metatarsal angle. In this case the angle is 10°. Normal: newborn, 20° (range, 9° to 31°); 8 years, 5° (range, 10° to 18°). **B:** Illustration of the anterior tibiocalcaneal angle (70°). Normal: newborn, 75°; 6 years, 65°.

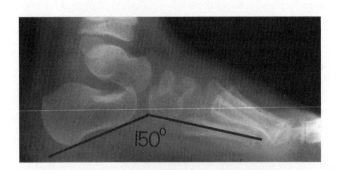

FIG. 9-4. Normal weight-bearing lateral view of the foot. The longitudinal plantar arch is assessed by extending lines along the axis of the calcaneus and the fifth metatarsal and by deriving an obtuse angle. This angle normally measures between 150° and 170°.

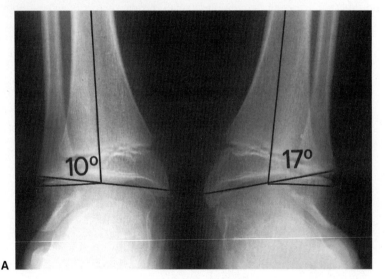

FIG. 9-5. Ankle valgus. **A:** Standing AP views of the ankles in an 8-year old girl. Moderate right and marked left ankle valgus. There is growth retardation of the left distal fibula as demonstrated by the superior position of the growth plate relative to the talar dome. The patient previously had treatment for congenital equinovarus associated with meningocele. **B:** Illustration of the Malhotra classification of ankle valgus: 0, normal, with fibular physis at the level of the plafond; I to III, progressive degrees of valgus related to the fibular physis.

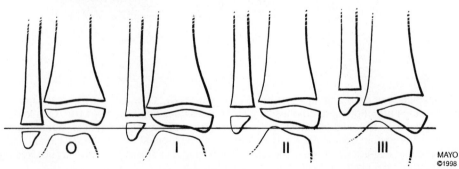

450

syndrome), dysplasias (hereditary multiple exostoses), and congenital conditions (postaxial hypoplasia and clubfeet).[25] Flaccid conditions such as myelomeningocele or polio are treated with fibular-Achilles tenodesis. Otherwise, a varus-producing supramalleolar osteotomy or epiphysiodesis using either medial malleolar staples or a single screw is used for fixation.[25]

CLASSIFICATION OF HINDFOOT ABNORMALITIES

Hindfoot Varus

One large subcategory of congenital foot anomalies is hindfoot varus, which encompasses talipes equinovarus (clubfoot) and certain neuromuscular disorders. In hindfoot varus, the talocalcaneal angle decreases in both the AP and lateral projections, such that the talus becomes more parallel to the calcaneus on lateral views. There is more overlap of the talus and calcaneus on AP views (Fig. 9-6). If the navicular is ossified, it will be displaced medial to the long axis of the talus, and the midtalar line will be displaced lateral to the base of the first metatarsal. Of all the hindfoot varus subtypes, talipes equinovarus is the most common.

Hindfoot Valgus

Hindfoot valgus is a category of disorders in which the calcaneus is abducted and, because of its ligamentous attachments to the midfoot and forefoot, also moves the more distal bones laterally. The talocalcaneal angle is increased on both AP and lateral films, and the midtalar line is displaced medial to the base of the first metatarsal (Fig. 9-7). Lateral displacement of the calcaneus decreases support to the talus, thus resulting in an abnormal talar position on the lateral weight-bearing view. Hindfoot valgus is present in planovalgus, congenital vertical talus, talipes calcaneovalgus, and neuromuscular disorders.[22,27]

Hindfoot Equinus

Plantar flexion or declination of the calcaneus defines hindfoot equinus (Fig 9-8). The tibiocalcaneal angle is greater than 90° on the lateral weight-bearing view. This disorder is associated with talipes equinovarus and congenital vertical talus. Equinus of the entire foot is present in several neuromuscular disorders.[23]

Hindfoot Calcaneus

The calcaneal inclination or pitch is increased in hindfoot calcaneus, resulting in abnormal calcaneal dorsiflexion and occasionally a box-like calcaneal appearance or a constricted or deformed anterior portion (Fig 9-9).[23] The anterior tibiocalcaneal angle is less than 65° in this disorder. Hindfoot calcaneus is frequently associated with pes cavus.[22,23,27]

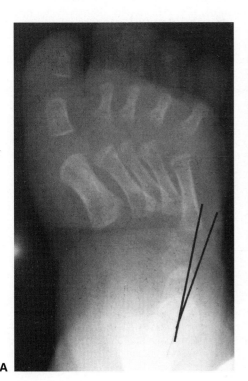

A

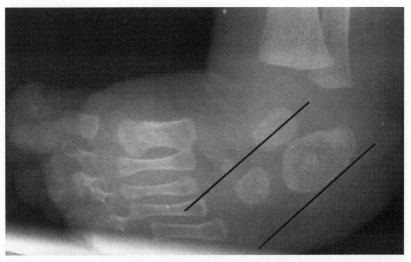

B

FIG. 9-6. Equinovarus. **A:** AP radiograph with simulated weight bearing in a 5-month old male infant with marked changes of equinovarus shows decrease in the talocalcaneal angle (*lines*) with elements of metatarsus adductus. **B:** Lateral simulated weight-bearing view shows equinus deformity of the calcaneus. The long axes of the talus and calcaneus are virtually parallel. There is varus deformity of the forefoot resulting in a stair-step or ladder appearance of the metatarsals (*lines*) with the first metatarsal superior and the fifth metatarsal inferior.

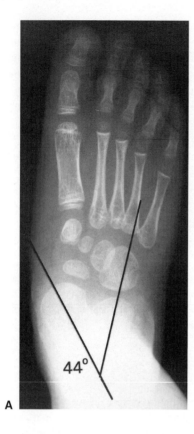

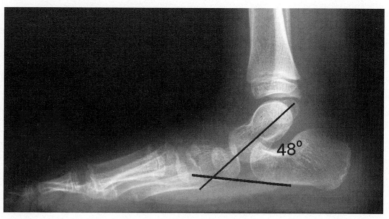

FIG. 9-7. Hindfoot valgus. **A:** AP standing radiograph showing increased talocalcaneal angle and malalignment of the talus with the first metatarsal and lateral displacement of the navicular (which is ossified in this 3-year-old girl) relative to the talus. Note also a pseudoepiphysis of the distal first metatarsal. **B:** Lateral view showing increase of the talocalcaneal angle, malalignment of the midtalar line with the first metatarsal, and decrease in the longitudinal arch of the foot.

CLASSIFICATION OF PLANTAR ARCH ABNORMALITIES

Pes Planus

Pes planus, or flatfoot, exists when the calcaneus does not maintain its normal degree of dorsiflexion (Fig 9-10). The normal longitudinal arch of the foot is lost, whereas the calcaneal–fifth metatarsal angle is greater than 175°. Flatfoot can either be flexible or rigid, in which case it is often associated with tarsal coalition. Rocker-bottom deformity occurs when the calcaneal–fifth metatarsal angle is greater than 180° (Fig. 9-11).[22,27]

Pes Cavus

Pes cavus is an exaggerated longitudinal arch of the foot, characterized by marked dorsiflexion of the calcaneus, plantar flexion of the metatarsals, and flexion of the phalanges (Fig 9-12). The normally straight midtalar–first metatarsal line is angled superiorly. The cavus deformity is more pronounced medially. Pes cavus can be associated with polio, myelomeningocele, and peroneal muscular atrophy (Charcot-Marie-Tooth disease, in which it is acquired and progressive).[23] It can also be associated with pes cavovarus, in which there is adduction of the forefoot or hindfoot varus.[22,23,27]

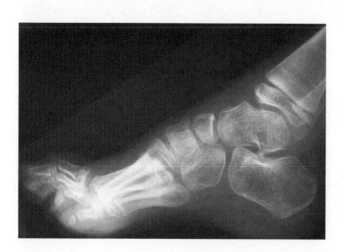

FIG. 9-8. Hindfoot equinus. Lateral non–weight-bearing radiograph shows hindfoot equinus with some element of pes cavus in a 5-year-old girl. The anterior tibiocalcaneal angle is greater than 90°.

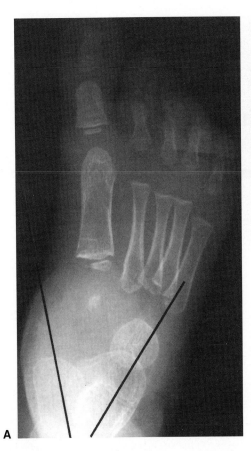

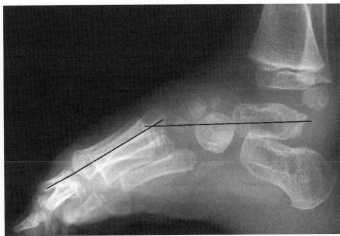

FIG. 9-9. Marked cavus deformity with hindfoot valgus and hindfoot calcaneus. **A:** AP radiograph of a 3-year-old girl shows an increase in the talocalcaneal angle and medial alignment of the talus relative to the base of the first metatarsal. **B:** Lateral image shows the hindfoot calcaneus deformity. Also noted is a prominent longitudinal arch and superior angulation of the midtalar–first metatarsal line.

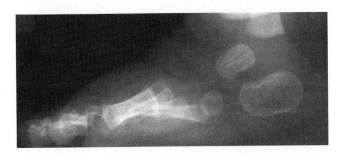

FIG. 9-10. Pes planus deformity. Pes planus exists on this lateral radiograph of a newborn, in whom the calcaneus does not maintain its normal degree of dorsiflexion. The calcaneal–fifth metatarsal angle is greater than 175°. (Courtesy of Dr. Catherine Poole.)

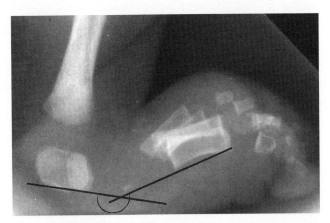

FIG. 9-11. Rocker-bottom deformity. Rocker-bottom deformity occurs when the calcaneal–fifth metatarsal angle is greater than 180° on lateral radiographs.

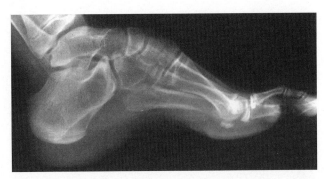

FIG. 9-12. Pes cavus. Non–weight-bearing lateral radiograph demonstrates an exaggerated longitudinal arch of the foot, with marked dorsiflexion of the calcaneus and plantar flexion of the metatarsals. (Courtesy of Dr. George Abdenour.)

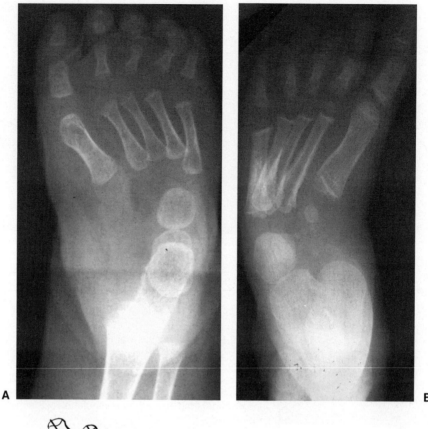

A   B

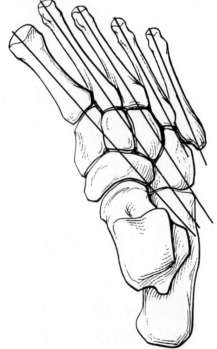

C

FIG. 9-13. Metatarsus adductus. **A** and **B:** Two different patients with differing degrees of metatarsus adductus and hindfoot varus on AP films show medial deviation of the metatarsals. **B:** The second patient also demonstrates proximal metatarsal convergence and forefoot inversion. **C:** Illustration of metatarsus adductus, with *lines* demonstrating the relationships with the tarsal bones.

CLASSIFICATION OF FOREFOOT ABNORMALITIES

Metatarsus Adductus

Adduction of the forefoot or medial deviation of the metatarsals is the most common deformity of the foot in children and may be found in isolation or associated with abnormalities of the midfoot or hindfoot.[10] This condition is generally more apparent clinically than radiographically because the foot is flexible and some degree of correction may occur with positioning for radiographs. Furthermore, because the condition is usually present at birth or in early infancy when the midfoot bones are unossified, radiographic diagnosis may be imprecise. Metatarsus adductus is unilateral in approximately half of cases, and it has no sex predilection.

Patients rarely have symptoms, unless they develop a hallux valgus deformity. Uncomplicated metatarsus adductus usually resolves spontaneously within a few months, and only a few patients require casting or further treatment.

Radiographically, the metatarsals are more convergent proximally than usual, and their convergent rays lie lateral to the calcaneus (Fig. 9-13). A variable degree of varus or inversion may be present in more serious cases.

Skewfoot

Skewfoot, also known as hooked foot, "z foot," or serpentine foot, describes adduction of the forefoot with other associated deformities of the midfoot and hindfoot, such as hindfoot valgus, forefoot varus, or pes cavus (Fig. 9-14).[10]

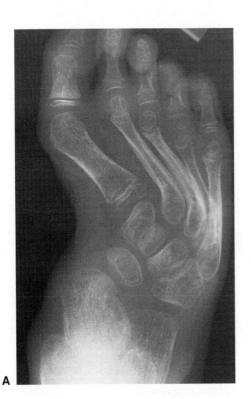

A

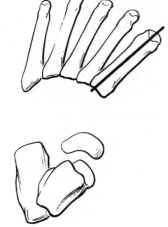

B

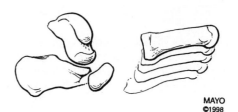

MAYO
©1998

FIG. 9-14. Skewfoot. **A:** AP radiograph shows adduction of the forefoot in a patient with skewfoot deformity, also known as hooked foot, "z foot," or serpentine foot. **B:** Illustration of skewfoot in the AP and lateral views. Note the z configuration of the metatarsal hindfoot anatomy.

TABLE 9-2. *Hallux valgus deformity*

	Mild	Moderate	Severe
Hallux valgus angle	<20°	20–40°	>40°
First-second metatarsal angle	<11°	11–15°	>15°
Percentage of subluxation of lateral sesamoids	<50%	50–75%	>65%

Before the tarsal bones fully ossify in young children, MRI has been shown to be helpful in demonstrating the shapes and positions of the unossified bones. MRI can depict plantar or lateral subluxation of the navicular and medial subluxation of the first metatarsal. [10]

Hallux Valgus

Hallux valgus deformity (Table 9-2) is lateral angulation of the great toe in relation to the first metatarsal (Fig. 9-15). This is typically an acquired deformity, which can affect 22 to 36% of adolescents. [14] Although the precise origin of hallux valgus is uncertain, wearing of narrow shoes, metatarsus primus varus, pes planus, forefoot pronation, and heredity have been implicated. [14,22]

The metatarsophalangeal angle measures more than 20° for mild disease and more than 40° for severe disease. The first-second metatarsal angle measures less than 11° in mild disease and more than 15° in severe disease. This angulation of the first metatarsophalangeal joint results in lateral subluxation of the sesamoids, stretching of the medial collateral ligament and capsule, contraction of the lateral soft tissue structures, plantar subluxation of the abductor hallucis tendon, and development of a sometimes painful bursa over the metatarsal head.

SPECIFIC FOOT DISORDERS

Talipes Equinovarus

Talipes equinovarus, more commonly known as clubfoot, is a three-dimensional deformity composed of hindfoot equinus, hindfoot varus, and forefoot adductus (Fig. 9-16). It occurs in approximately 1 to 1.5 per 1000 live births, with a male-to-female ratio of 2:1. There is an increased incidence of 20 to 30 times the general population in first-degree relatives and 6 times the general population in second-degree relatives.

Clubfoot can be grouped on an etiologic basis into congenital or acquired defects (Table 9-3). [9] The congenital defects can be subdivided into those with idiopathic, neurogenic, myogenic, osteogenic, collagenous, and cartilaginous causes. The idiopathic causes can be divided into intrinsic and extrinsic subtypes. [9] The intrinsic type is the most common subtype, which is composed of a rigid foot with marked fibrosis and abnormal bony relationships. These patients typically require some sort of operative treatment. On the other hand, the extrinsic clubfoot is flexible without marked fibrosis. The normal bony relationships are maintained, and patients cases are frequently treated nonoperatively. The

TABLE 9-3. *Etiologic classification of clubfoot[a]*

I. Congenital
  A. Idiopathic
    1. Intrinsic
    2. Extrinsic
  B. Neurogenic
    1. Open defects: myelomeningocele, meningocele, dermal sinus
    2. Closed defects: diastematomyelia, intraspinal tumor, myelodysplasia, segmentation defects
  C. Myogenic: Abnormal muscle and tendon insertions of anterior tibial, Achilles, peroneal, plantaris, flexor accessorius longus
  D. Osteogenic: tibial hemimelia, primary defect in tarsal bone (esp. talar) development
  E. Collagenous: amniotic bands, arthrogryposis multiplex congenita
  F. Cartilaginous: diastrophic dysplasia
II. Acquired
  A. Neurogenic: poliomyelitis, cerebral palsy, meningitis, sciatic nerve injury
  B. Vascular compromise: Volkmann's paralysis after traction for femoral shaft fracture

[a] From Hersh, ref. 9, with permission.

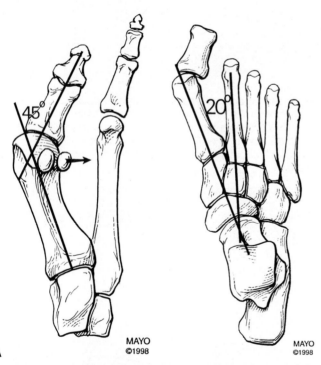

MAYO ©1998

MAYO ©1998

A   B

FIG. 9-15. Hallux valgus **(A)**. Hallux valgus is lateral angulation of the proximal phalanx in relation to the first metatarsal **(B)**. The metatarsophalangeal angle typically measures more than 20° (45° in this illustration). The sesamoids are subluxed laterally (*arrow*).

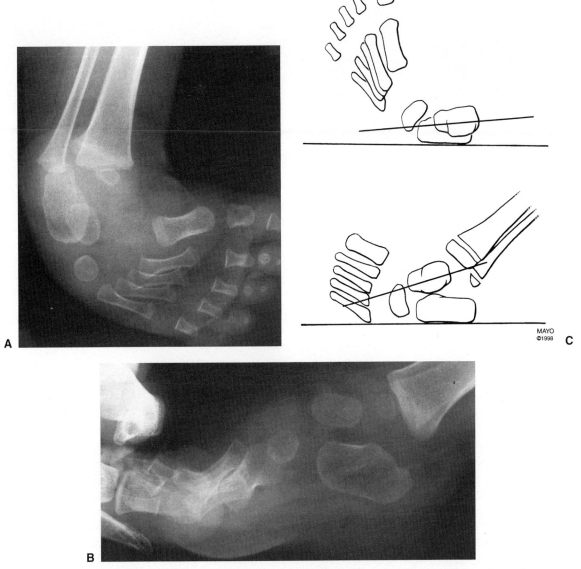

FIG. 9-16. Talipes equinovarus (clubfoot). AP (**A**) and lateral (**B**) views demonstrate the three-dimensional deformity composed of hindfoot equinus, hindfoot varus, and forefoot adductus. (Courtesy of Dr. Christopher Zaleski.) **C:** Illustration of talipes equinovarus, with demonstration of the talocalcaneal angles: AP (*top*) and lateral (*bottom*).

cause of idiopathic clubfoot is still uncertain, but most research supports the theory of polygenic multifactorial inheritance with a sex-linked threshold effect.[2] This theory states that the idiopathic deformity does not occur until the number of abnormal genes exceeds the threshold level, which is higher among females. Because it is proposed that males require relatively fewer defective genes to present with the deformity, the clubfoot defect tends to be less severe and more common in males. In contrast, females tend to have fewer but more severe and resistant cases. Other theories propose extrinsic pressure, including intrauterine compression due to oligohydramnios, as a cause of clubfoot.[2,9]

Certain neurogenic defects commonly result in foot anomalies and should be excluded in patients with clubfoot. About 30% of all children with spina bifida are born with talipes equinovarus.[5] Abnormal muscle and tendon insertions can be detected preoperatively with the assistance of MRI. The reported incidence of clubfoot in patients with constriction bands ranges from 12 to 56%.[1] Arthrogyroposis multiplex congenita is a nonprogressive syndrome characterized by limited motion of multiple joints resulting from muscular fibrosis and thickening and shortening of the periarticular, capsular, and ligamentous tissues. This entity is frequently associated with clubfoot.[4] Finally, acquired causes of clubfoot can be due to poliomyelitis, cerebral palsy, meningitis,

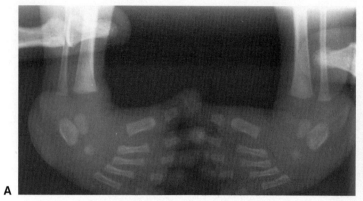

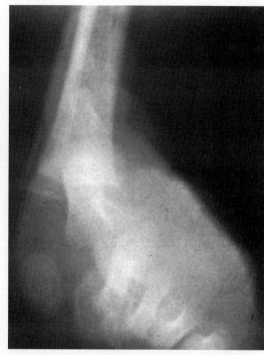

FIG. 9-17. Talipes equinovarus. Bilateral AP (**A**) and lateral (**B**) views of the right foot demonstrate marked clubfoot deformity. Note how the correctly obtained lateral view (**B**) cannot depict the forefoot in its true lateral position. (Courtesy of Dr. Catherine Poole.)

sciatic nerve damage, or vascular compromise, and they may occur after traction for femoral shaft fractures.[9]

The radiologic findings include hindfoot equinus, hindfoot varus, and forefoot adductus (see Fig. 9-16; Fig. 9-17). Hindfoot equinus results in fixed plantar flexion of the calcaneus. Hindfoot varus, once again, results in a decreased talocalcaneal angle on both AP and lateral films, whereas the talus and calcaneus are nearly parallel on lateral views. Forefoot adductus or varus results in medial deviation of the metatarsals and more overlap of their bones on the AP view, and a stair-step arrangement of the metatarsals on lateral view. Consequently, a correctly obtained lateral view cannot depict the forefoot in its true lateral position.

In general, the initial management of the newborn clubfoot is closed, gentle manipulation, redressements, placement of adhesive bands, and serial casting.[2] Only when the defect fails to respond to closed treatment is soft tissue release indicated. There are conflicting opinions regarding the timing, type, and extent of surgical procedures when conservative management is ineffective. Several factors diminish the likelihood of successful correction by conservative methods: (1) marked rigidity of the foot; (2) leg muscular atrophy; (3) small, poorly developed heel; (4) presence of other anomalies; (5) talocalcaneal angles less than 20° on both AP and lateral views; (6) resistant varus deformity; (7) rotational deformity of the leg; and (8) inequality of leg length.[5]

Surgical procedures include complete posterior and medial soft tissue release[30] (Fig. 9-18), lengthening of the Achilles tendon, osteotomies of the tibia and fibula,[19] anterior and posterior tibial tendon transfers, and triple arthrode-

sis.[5] Radiologists should be familiar with the bone grafts, K-wires, and external fixation devices that may be placed.

Decrease in size of the navicular ossification center and flattening, fragmentation, cystic change, and wedging of the navicular can be evident in clinically successful nonoperative cases.[17] Dorsal dislocation of the navicular can be a complication of soft tissue release for equinovarus (Fig. 9-19). Correction of the hindfoot equinus before correcting the hindfoot varus can lead to a rocker-bottom deformity. Undercorrection can lead to residual forefoot adductus, persistent in-toeing, and persistent parallelism of the talus and calcaneus. This problem occurs when forced manipulation compresses the articular surface of the talus, resulting in osteonecrosis, growth disturbances, and flattening of the superior articular surface (Fig. 9-20).[7] Cartilage necrosis of any of the tarsal bones causes long-term incongruity and is closely associated with a cavus foot type.[2] Delayed onset of ossification of the tarsal bones or ossification out of order can also be noted.[16]

Congenital Vertical Talus

Congenital vertical talus is characterized by a dorsal and lateral navicular against the head of the talus, not reducible with maximal plantar flexion confirmed by radiography and a flatfoot.[18] This dislocation locks the talus into an irreducible plantar-flexed position. If the navicular has not yet ossified, dislocation can be inferred by the abnormal relationship between the talus and the third cuneiform and second metatarsal that lie immediately adjacent to the navicular. The disorder can occur as an isolated defect or as part of a syn-

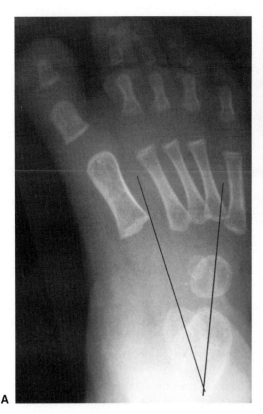

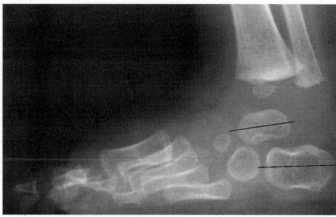

FIG. 9-18. Postoperative release radiographs of a patient with congenital equinovarus. **A:** AP view shows correction of the abnormal talocalcaneal angle. **B:** Lateral radiograph shows persistence of almost parallelism of the talus and the calcaneus. There is marked reduction in the amount of forefoot varus compared with preoperative films.

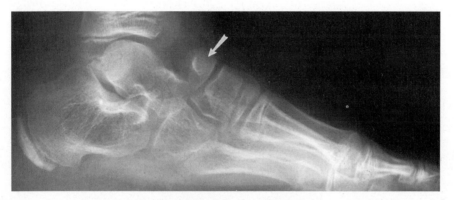

FIG. 9-19. A 9-year-old girl who had previous posterior medial release for equinovarus of the right foot. Lateral standing films show dorsal dislocation of the navicular *(arrow)*.

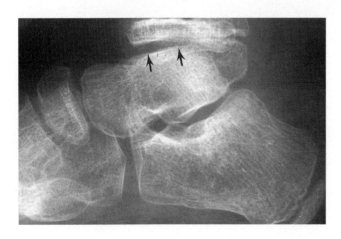

FIG. 9-20. Lateral standing view of the foot of an 8-year-old boy after treatment of equinovarus. There is flattening of the talar dome *(arrows)* from previous compression of the articular surface of the talus, resulting in osteonecrosis.

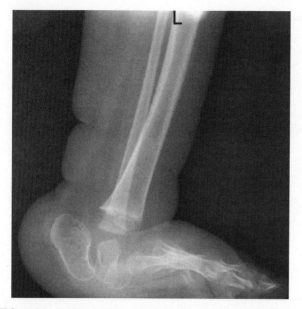

FIG. 9-21. Vertical talus. Lateral image of a 1-year-old boy with a vertical talus demonstrates hindfoot equinus with plantar flexion of both the calcaneus and talus. The forefoot is dorsiflexed, resulting in reversal of the longitudinal arch and a rocker-bottom deformity. The navicular is unossified, but dislocation can be inferred by the abnormal relationship of the talus with the other ossified tarsal bones.

drome. It occurs equally among boys and girls and can be unilateral or bilateral.[23] It is frequently associated with arthrogyroposis or myelomeningocele. On AP images, severe hindfoot valgus and forefoot abduction result in an increased talocalcaneal angle (Fig. 9-21). Lateral images demonstrate an equinus heel with plantar flexion of both the calcaneus and talus. The forefoot is typically dorsiflexed, resulting in reversal of the longitudinal arch and a rocker-bottom deformity.[23] This situation differs from pes planovalgus because of its hindfoot equinus and abnormal position of the navicular. Reports of successful conservative treatment of congenital vertical talus are rare.[29] Surgical treatment can consist of medial, lateral, or posterior soft tissue release, peritalar resection, K-wire fixation, and eventual extraarticular subtalar arthrodesis.[18]

Pes Planovalgus

Pes planovalgus, or flexible flatfoot deformity, is associated with an increase in the talocalcaneal angle, hindfoot valgus, and forefoot adduction. The longitudinal and transverse arches of the foot are flattened, making the metatarsals approximately parallel on the AP film (Fig. 9-22A). On lateral images, the calcaneus and metatarsals are situated horizontally (see Fig. 9-22B). Pes planovalgus is common, generally painless, and a relatively flexible disorder attributed to ligamentous laxity. The disorder is frequently bilateral and has a strong familial predilection. If patients become

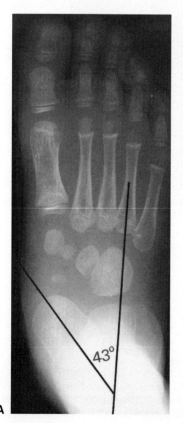

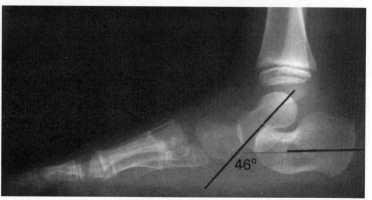

B

FIG. 9-22. Hypermobile flatfoot. **A:** AP standing film of a 5-year-old boy shows an increased talocalcaneal angle with lateral subluxation of the navicular relative to the talus. Forefoot abduction is evident because there is parallelism of the metatarsals rather than the normal proximal convergence. **B:** Lateral standing films show loss of the longitudinal arch, greater declination of the talus than normal, and an increased talocalcaneal angle.

A

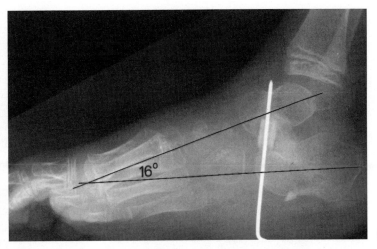

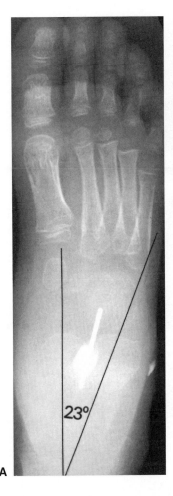

FIG. 9-23. Immediate postoperative Grice procedure in the same patient as in Figure 9-22. Both the AP (**A**) and the lateral (**B**) radiographs show a decrease in the talocalcaneal angle and better alignment of the navicular with the talus. An extraarticular bone graft and a Kirschner wire are seen.

symptomatic, orthotics and conservative management may be helpful. Surgery is reserved for patients who have excessive pain or fatigue that inhibits normal daily activities. One procedure used is the Grice extraarticular arthrodesis (Fig. 9-23).

OTHER DISORDERS INVOLVING THE FOOT AND ANKLE

Tarsal Coalitions

Tarsal coalitions are abnormal bars of fibrous, cartilaginous, or osseous tissue between the tarsal bones. These can either be congenital or acquired as a result of infection, trauma, articular disorders, or surgery.[23] Congenital coalitions are believed to occur because of a failure of differentiation and segmentation of the primitive mesenchyme. Cases can be associated with peroneal spastic flatfoot, vague foot pain, limited subtalar movement, and pes planus.

The most common tarsal coalition involves the calcaneonavicular joint. This coalition can be bilateral (Fig. 9-24), and it may be either asymptomatic or associated with rigid flatfoot. Symptoms are typically less severe than those found in talocalcaneal coalitions. The coalition is best identified in the 45° oblique view, in which findings may include an

osseous bar, eburnation or sclerosis, elongation of the anterosuperior calcaneus (''anteater nose'') (Fig. 9-25A), and joint space narrowing (see Fig. 9-25B). Secondary signs include hypoplasia of the talar head and talar beaking.[23] MRI can confirm a cartilaginous or fibrous union (see Fig. 9-25C and D).

In talocalcaneal coalition, a bar of fibrous, cartilaginous, or osseous tissue is present between the middle facet of the calcaneus and the talus and, much less commonly, between the posterior subtalar joint or anterior facet (Fig. 9-26). This form of coalition is more common in boys and is bilateral in 20 to 25% of cases.[23] Radiographic findings include failure to visualize the middle subtalar joint (Fig. 9-27), talar beaking (Fig 9-28), broadening of the lateral process of the talus, narrowing of the posterior subtalar joint, a concave undersurface of the talar neck, asymmetry of the talocalcaneonavicular joint, and a ball-and-socket joint. Resection of the bar has been recommended for patients with symptoms that persist after cast immobilization or the use of orthotics. Excellent or good long-term results have been achieved in patients in whom the area of coalition measured 50% or less of the cross-sectional area relative to the posterior facet (measured by CT), the hindfoot valgus was less than 16°, and no radiographic signs indicated arthritis of the posterior

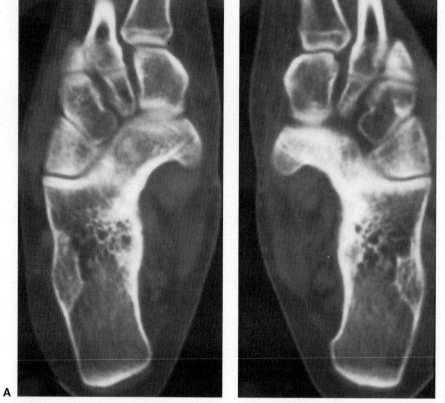

FIG. 9-24. Osseous calcaneonavicular coalitions. **A** and **B:** Axial images through the hindfoot and midfoot regions demonstrate bilateral osseous calcaneonavicular coalitions. This type of tarsal coalition is the most common subtype and can be associated with rigid flatfoot.

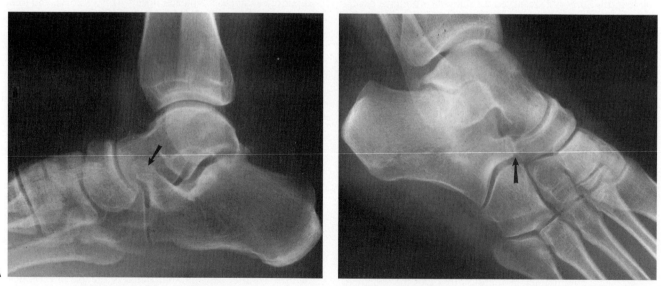

FIG. 9-25. Calcaneonavicular coalition. **A:** Lateral view of the foot demonstrates elongation of the anterosuperior calcaneus ("anteater nose") (*arrow*). **B:** A 45° oblique view demonstrates narrowing of the calcaneonavicular joint (*arrow*). *(continued)*

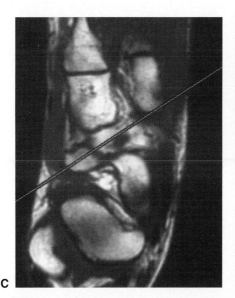 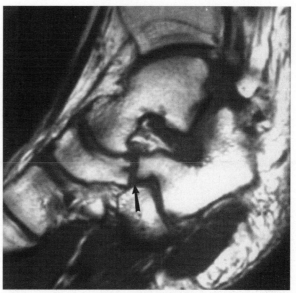

FIG. 9-25. *Continued.* Axial T1-weighted scout view with an oblique sagittal localizer (**C**) and (**D**) T1-weighted oblique sagittal images through the calcaneonavicular joint (*arrow*) demonstrate joint space narrowing, subchondral cyst formation of the navicular, and a prominent anterosuperior process of the calcaneus. Findings are compatible with a fibrous or cartilaginous union.

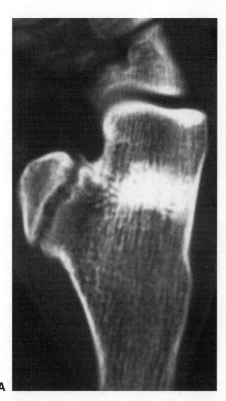 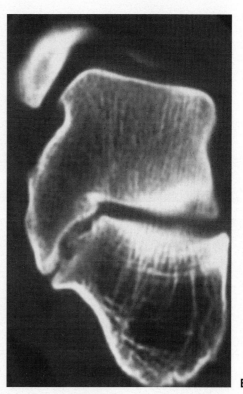

FIG. 9-26. Fibrous talocalcaneal coalition. Axial (**A**) and coronal (**B**) CT images through the left foot demonstrate irregular talocalcaneal joint space narrowing and increased density within the joint, compatible with fibrous tissue. Note the preserved posterior subtalar joint space.

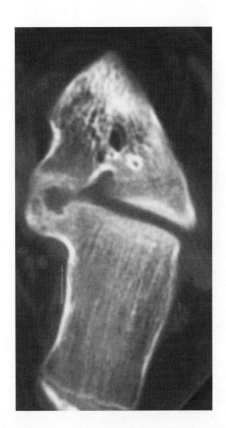

FIG. 9-27. Osseous talocalcaneal coalition. Coronal CT through the middle facet of the calcaneus and talus demonstrates complete osseous coalition.

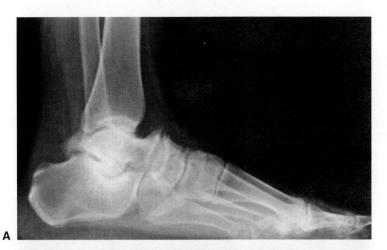

A

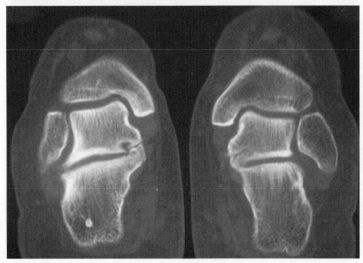

B

FIG. 9-28. Osseous talocalcaneal coalition. **A:** Lateral radiograph fails to demonstrate the middle subtalar joint. Note the prominent talar beaking, which is frequently associated with coalitions. **B:** Coronal CT confirms an osseous talocalcaneal coalition.

subtalar joint.[28] Patients with poor outcomes tend to have persistent painful peroneal spasms and rigid planovalgus, and radiographically they have residual bars, narrowing of the posterior talocalcaneal joint, and impingement of the lateral talar process on the calcaneus. The presence of a talar beak does not impair the clinical outcome and is believed to represent a traction spur rather than an osteoarthritic spur.[28]

Calcaneocuboid coalitions are rare. They can be unilateral or bilateral and may exist with other anomalies. The typical findings of tarsal coalition are present at the joint space and are usually obvious on radiographs. Patients may be symptomatic or may have peroneal spasm.[23]

Isolated first naviculocuneiform coalitions have been reported as extremely rare in the past, but the incidence may be much greater than previously reported. The naviculocuneiform form of coalition presents in an older age range (mean age at onset of symptoms is 31.9 years) than the talocalcaneal and calcaneonavicular forms.[12] This is thought to be a result of the small range of motion of the first naviculocuneiform joint. Patients complain of tenderness over the medioplantar side of the joint, and this type of coalition can be difficult to distinguish clinically from an os externum tibiale. Radiographically, one sees irregularity and severe narrowing of the joint space (particularly medially), occasionally cystic subchondral changes, and a beak-like spur. Some cases have been overlooked or diagnosed as osteoarthritis or bone cysts.[12]

Congenital Constriction Band Syndrome

Congenital constriction band syndrome, also known as amniotic band syndrome, is the end result of mechanical intrauterine deformation and is not a true malformation. This syndrome is believed to occur as a result of early amniotic rupture, followed by temporary oligohydramnios, resulting in intrauterine compression and constriction of the fetal appendages by cords of torn amnion.[6] The typical manifestations of this syndrome are limb reduction (Fig. 9-29), constriction bands (Figs. 9-30 and 9-31), and syndactyly (especially acrosyndactyly). The average patient has three involved limbs with a predilection for the distal, central digits of the upper extremities. Other features include pseudoarthroses (see Fig. 9-31B), peripheral nerve palsies, and skin-tube pedicles. Associated orthopedic diagnoses in patients with congenital constriction band syndrome include clubfoot, metatarsus adductus, tibial torsion, pes planus, metatarsus primus varus, and congenital hip dysplasia.[6]

Child Abuse

Fractures of the feet and ankle in cases of child abuse are unusual, but they may be the only radiographic evidence of abuse (Fig. 9-32). Metatarsal and phalangeal fractures are the most commonly involved bones. Torus fractures predominate, and radiographic findings include buckling of the cor-

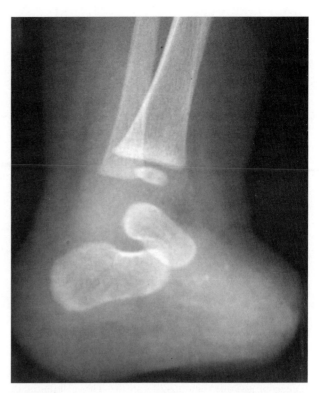

FIG. 9-29. Congenital constriction band syndrome, also known as amniotic band syndrome in a 6-month-old female infant. Lateral film shows congenital absence of the forefoot and tiny ossification centers in the midfoot.

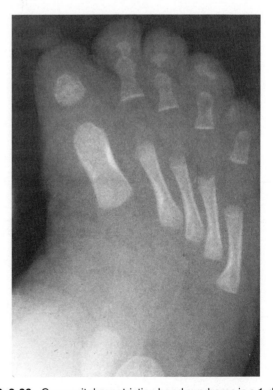

FIG. 9-30. Congenital constriction band syndrome in a 1-day-old male infant. There is soft tissue and osseous involvement of the distal digits. This patient also had involvement of the left foot and right hand.

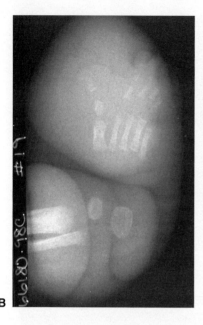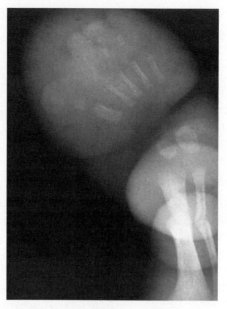

A,B

FIG. 9-31. Congenital constriction band syndrome. Left (A) and right (B) oblique images of the feet and right calf demonstrate multiple constriction bands and marked edematous changes. Also notice the old fracture deformities of the right mid-tibia and fibula, resulting in pseudoarthroses at the level of a constriction band. (Courtesy of Dr. George Abdenour.)

tex, subperiosteal new bone formation, and bony sclerosis.[20] Sclerosis and subperiosteal new bone may mimic the changes of juvenile rheumatoid arthritis. The differential diagnosis of child abuse includes congenital indifference to pain, osteogenesis imperfecta, rickets, other demineralizing disorders, and sickle cell disease.[20]

Syndromes

Chondrodysplasia punctata, Conradi-Hunermann type (Fig. 9-33) is an X-linked disorder with asymmetric, mild shortening of all bones, and punctate calcific deposits in the infantile cartilaginous skeleton, in soft tissues surrounding

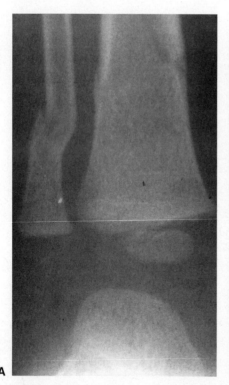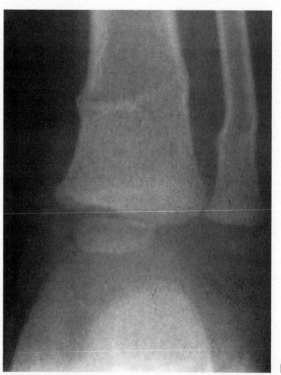

A   B

FIG. 9-32. Child abuse. Right (A) and left (B) AP radiographs of the ankles demonstrate torus fractures of the distal fibulae and the left tibia and a spiral fracture of the distal right tibia. Although fractures of the feet and ankle in cases of child abuse are unusual, they may be the only radiographic evidence of abuse. (Courtesy of Dr. Christopher Zaleski.)

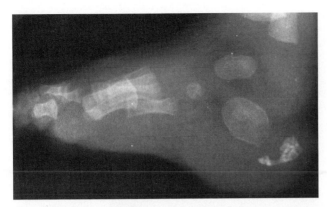

FIG. 9-33. Chondrodysplasia punctata, Conradi-Hunermann type. Lateral radiograph demonstrates multiple punctate calcific deposits in the calcaneal apophysis, classic for this disorder. Stippled calcifications can also be seen in other forms of chondrodysplasia punctata, warfarin embryopathy, alcohol embryopathy, Zellweger's syndrome, and multiple epiphyseal dysplasia. (Courtesy of Dr. Catherine Poole.)

joints, and in epiphyseal centers.[26] Other disorders that may result in stippled calcifications include other forms of chondrodysplasia punctata, warfarin embryopathy, alcohol embryopathy, Zellweger's syndrome, and multiple epiphyseal dysplasia, among others.[26]

Spondyloepiphyseal dysplasia congenita (Fig. 9-34) is an autosomal dominant disorder that can affect the feet and

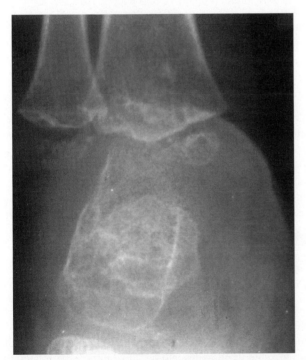

FIG. 9-34. Spondyloepiphyseal dysplasia congenita. AP radiograph of the ankle demonstrates multiple, irregular fibular epiphyseal calcifications. Patients with this disorder can also lack talar or calcaneal ossification centers and may experience marked epiphyseal delay and irregularity of multiple bones. (Courtesy of Dr. Christopher Zaleski.)

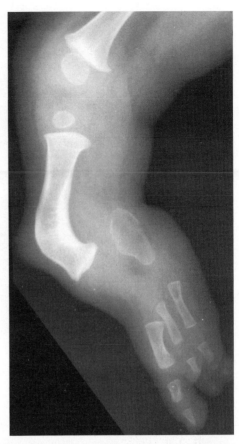

FIG. 9-35. Mesomelic dysplasia and mesomelia (absence of a portion of the foot). Oblique radiograph of the right lower leg and foot in a 1-year-old patient with mesomelic dysplasia and mesomelia. The fibula and fourth and fifth rays are congenitally absent. The tibia is shortened, thickened, and laterally angled.

ankles. Neonates and infants can lack talar or calcaneal ossification centers, and older children can have marked epiphyseal delay and irregularity of multiple bones, including those of the foot.[26]

Mesomelic dysplasia is a heterogenous group of bone dysplasias with disproportionate shortening of the middle segment of the limbs, with or without hand or foot involvement. Characteristics of this disorder include marked shortening and thickening of the tibia and lateral angulation of the tibia (Fig. 9-35).[26]

Overgrowth/Hypoplasia/Aplasia

Macrodactyly

Overgrowth of soft tissue and bones can occur in either focal or generalized distribution. Pedal macrodactyly (Fig. 9-36) is an increase in size of all the structures in one or more digits of the foot. It can be either idiopathic or associated with hemangiomas (Maffucci's and Klippel-Trenaunay-Weber syndromes), arteriovenous malformations, lymphan-

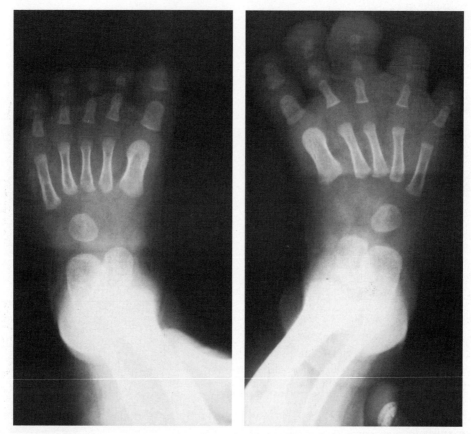

FIG. 9-36. Pedal macrodactyly. AP radiographs of the feet demonstrate increase in size of the right toes. This disorder can be idiopathic or associated with hemangiomas (Maffucci's and Klippel-Trenaunay-Weber syndromes), arteriovenous malformations, lymphangiomas, neurofibromatosis, epidermal nevus syndrome, proteus syndrome, Ollier's disease, and macrodystrophia lipomatosa.

giomas, neurofibromatosis, epidermal nevus syndrome, proteus syndrome, Ollier's disease, and macrodystrophia lipomatosa.[23]

Brachydactyly

Brachydactyly (Fig. 9-37), or abnormal shortening of the fingers or toes, is subdivided by the Temtamy Classification into Types A1-3, B, C, D, and E.[26] Type A1 has short middle phalanges which sometimes fuse with the distal phalanges and short proximal phalanges of the great toes. Type A2 has short middle phalanges of the second toe and triangular or rhomboid shaped middle phalanges. Type A3 has short middle phalanges of the fifth digits. Type B has short middle phalanges, rudimentary or absent terminal phalanges, and deformed great toes. Type C typically involves the hands. Type D has short and broad terminal phalanges of the great toe. Type E has short metatarsals (especially the fourth and fifth), cone-shaped epiphyses, and short phalanges. Brachydactyly can be isolated or associated with a multitude of disorders, including trisomy 13 and 18, fetal alcohol syndrome, fibrodysplasia ossificans progressiva, and mucopolysaccharidoses.[26]

Syndactyly

Syndactyly is the lack of differentiation between two or more digits. This disorder can involve either the soft tissues alone or the soft tissues in combination with the osseous structures. Syndactyly can involve the proximal digit (partial) or the entire digit (complete). Most cases are inherited, although some are sporadic. Males are affected more commonly than females.[23] Syndactyly can be either isolated or associated with a vast array of syndromes, such as Apert's syndrome, Poland's syndrome, mesomelic dysplasia, and amniotic bands.[26]

Polydactyly

Polydactyly is a fairly common congenital deformity involving the foot characterized by supernumerary digits or metatarsals. It has an overall incidence of 1.7 in 1,000 births, occurs equally in males and females, and can be bilateral in 25 to 50% of patients (Fig. 9-38).[13] It is most commonly an isolated condition in which it is generally an autosomal dominant trait with variable penetrance. About 15% of cases of pedal polydactyly are associated with other congenital anomalies, such as polydactyly of the hands, syndactyly, hip

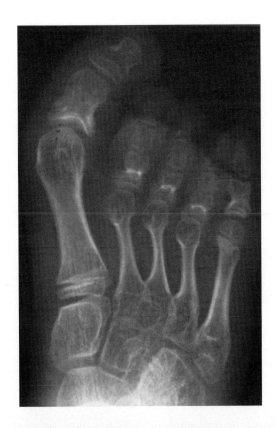

FIG. 9-37. Brachydactyly. AP radiograph of the left foot demonstrates generalized shortening of the second through fourth rays. (Courtesy of Dr. George Abdenour.)

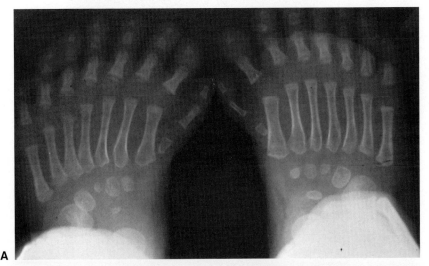

A

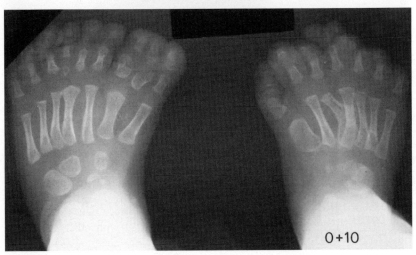

0 +10

B

FIG. 9-38. Polydactyly. Supernumerary digits and metatarsals can be bilateral in 25 to 50% of patients. A and B: AP radiographs of the bilateral feet in two different patients show the variety of duplications involving entire rays or only the phalanges. Notice the diminutive, medially located digits in B.

dysplasia, clubfoot, congenital heart disease, tibial hypoplasia, various trisomies, Ellis–van Creveld syndrome, or Laurence-Moon-Biedl syndrome.[13] Polydactyly is classified into three major groups: preaxial (medial ray or tibial side), central ray, and postaxial (lateral ray or fibular side) (Fig. 9-39). Crossed polydactyly is the coexistence of either preaxial polydactyly in the hand or postaxial polydactyly in the foot or vice versa. Mixed polysyndactyly involves both preaxial and postaxial anomalies. It is termed type A if it is fully

developed with articulating structures and type B if it is rudimentary. Infants with rudimentary digits can often be treated with suture ligation or surgical excision. Treatment ranges from shoe modification to surgery. If osseous components are present, surgery is delayed until the patient is about 1 year old. However, surgical correction should not be delayed much beyond the onset of walking, to allow for maximal remodeling. Generally, the most highly developed, cosmetically attractive digit with the most normal

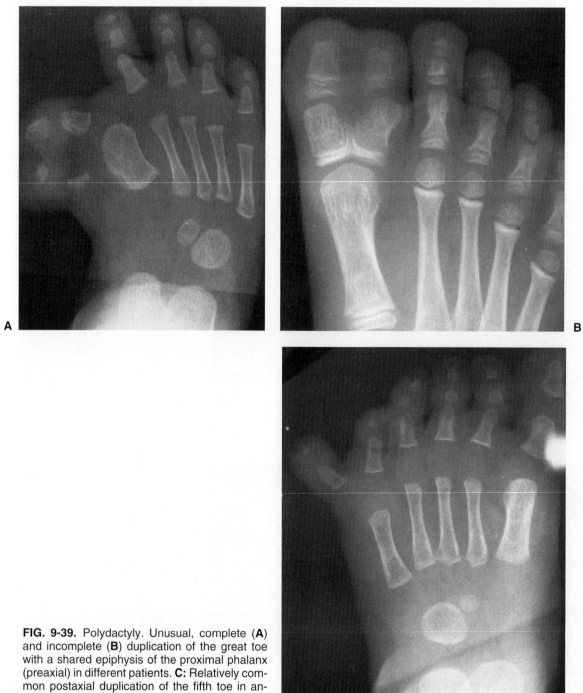

FIG. 9-39. Polydactyly. Unusual, complete (**A**) and incomplete (**B**) duplication of the great toe with a shared epiphysis of the proximal phalanx (preaxial) in different patients. **C:** Relatively common postaxial duplication of the fifth toe in another patient.

metatarsophalangeal joint is spared. Correction of preaxial polydactyly is the most complex, with the poorest results; the most medial digit is usually excised. In postaxial polydactyly, the most lateral digit is excised; long-term results are typically good or excellent.

Delta Phalanx

A delta phalanx (also known as a longitudinally bracketed epiphysis) is a malformation leading to a trapezoidal diaphyseal-metaphyseal unit with an alteration in physeal configuration (Fig 9-40).[23] Delta phalanges typically involve the first rays of either the hand or foot, and they can be an isolated condition or associated with clinodactyly, syndactyly, polydactyly, great toe duplication, tibial hemimelia, Apert's syndrome, Down's syndrome, or Rubinstein-Taybi syndrome.[26]

Osteochondral Lesions of the Foot

Freiberg's Infraction

Freiberg's infraction, otherwise known as posttraumatic osteonecrosis of the metatarsal head, occurs three to four times more often in girls than boys. Patients typically present during late childhood or adolescence, and cases may be bilateral about 10% of the time.[22] A shortened or varus position of the first metatarsal may increase the stress on the more lateral metatarsal heads, leading to Freiberg's infraction. The second metatarsal is most commonly involved, followed by the third and fourth metatarsals. Early radiographic findings include widening of the metatarsophalangeal joint distal to

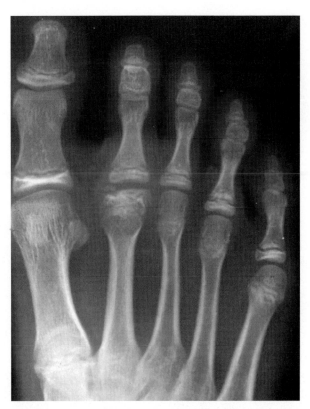

FIG. 9-41. Freiberg's infraction. AP film displays an enlarged, flattened second metatarsal head, which is the result of posttraumatic osteonecrosis.

the involved segment.[22] Next, the metatarsal head may have a mixed lytic and sclerotic appearance and undergoes subchondral cystic change and collapse. Eventually, the metatarsal head remodels, yielding an enlarged and flattened surface (Fig. 9-41).

Köhler's Disease

Köhler's disease is an osteochondrosis of the navicular that usually presents at about 5 years of age, with a 6:1 male-to-female ratio.[22] Patients have local pain, tenderness, swelling, decreased range of motion, and occasionally a preceding history of trauma. It can be difficult to differentiate Köhler's disease radiographically from the varied normal appearances of the navicular during childhood (Fig. 9-42). To diagnose Köhler's disease more definitively, one must identify changes in a once normal navicular, obtain serial radiographic follow-up demonstrating resorption of bone and reossification, or obtain a nuclear bone scan.[22] Skeletal scintigraphy should demonstrate a photopenic defect on initial imaging, followed by increased radiotracer uptake during the reparative phase of avascular necrosis. Köhler's disease has not been well studied with MRI in the literature, but its signal abnormalities typically follow that of osteonecrosis of other areas, such as the hip. The navicular eventually returns to a normal size and trabecular pattern in approxi-

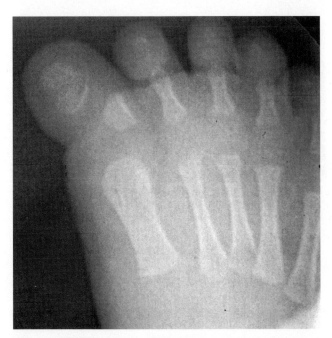

FIG. 9-40. Delta phalanx or longitudinally bracketed epiphysis. The first proximal phalanx has a trapezoidal configuration.

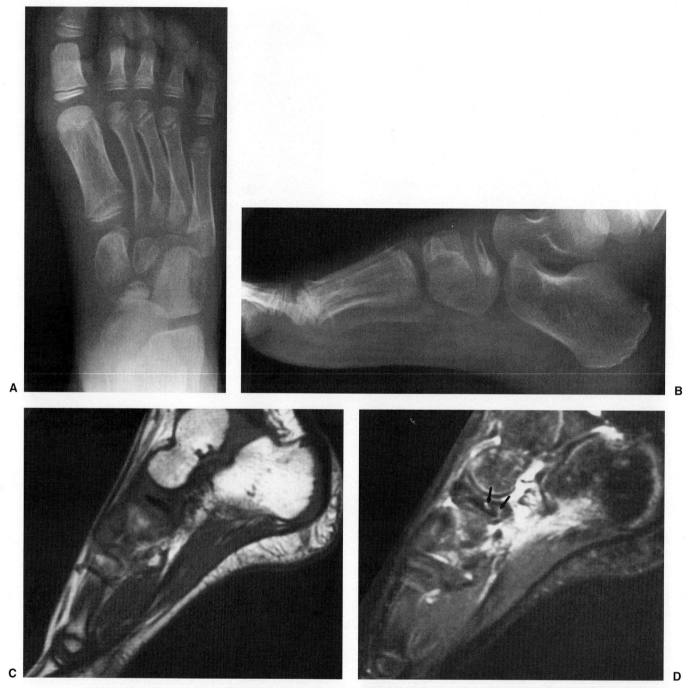

FIG. 9-42. Köhler's disease. **A:** AP radiograph of the foot demonstrates an irregular, sclerotic navicular in a patient with focal pain. **B:** Lateral radiograph taken 4 days later demonstrates progressive collapse of the navicular. **C:** T1-weighted sagittal image demonstrates complete loss of signal of the navicular, consistent with known collapse. **D:** Fast SE T2-weighted fat-suppressed sagittal image shows a hypointense navicular with some focal areas of increased signal (*arrows*).

mately 3 months to 4 years, whether or not the patient is treated.[22]

CONGENITAL VARIANTS

Cleft Calcaneus

The calcaneus generally has two ossification centers. The first one appears in the fourth to fifth fetal month and is often overlooked because of its small size and position. The second site appears in the seventh fetal month, and the two ossification sites fuse during the following month. However, the second center can remain unfused and may be seen separately during the early months of life (Fig. 9-43).[11]

Calcaneal Apophysis

In early infancy, the posterior aspect of the calcaneus is smooth, but it develops an irregular margin just before to the appearance of the apophysis. Between the 6th and 10th years, one or more small ossification centers of the calcaneal tuberosity may appear posterior to the calcaneal border and rapidly fuse, becoming quite dense (Fig. 9-44). This appearance must not be confused with Sever's disease, an overuse syndrome that, contrary to some earlier reports, is not an osteochondrosis and has no radiographic findings.[15] Transverse clefts or grooves remain in the apophysis, which fuses with the body of the calcaneus at around 17 years of age (Fig. 9-45).[11]

Pseudocyst of the Calcaneus

A well-demarcated area of lucency is often seen in the inferior portion of the anterior calcaneus, where there is nor-

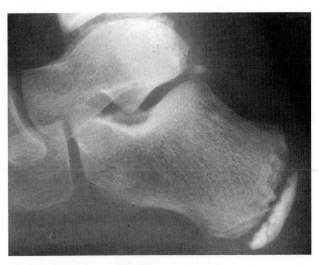

FIG. 9-44. Normal calcaneal apophysis. Between the 6th and the 10th years, one or more small ossification centers of the calcaneal tuberosity may appear posterior to the calcaneal border and rapidly fuse, becoming quite dense.

mally less trabeculation (Fig. 9-46). If this process is too prominent, the differentiation between this variation and a simple bone cyst can be difficult. However, the pseudocyst is usually less lucent than a bone cyst and is not circumscribed by a sclerotic border.[22]

Irregularity of the Navicular

The navicular is the last of the tarsal bones to ossify and it is the least regular, often with multiple ossification centers that are frequently not symmetric bilaterally. This variation in irregularity may make separation of the normal develop-

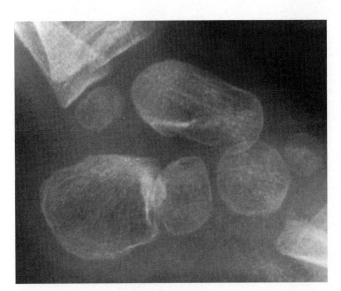

FIG. 9-43. Cleft calcaneus. The calcaneus generally has two ossification centers, which can occasionally remain unfused and may be seen separately during the first few months of life.

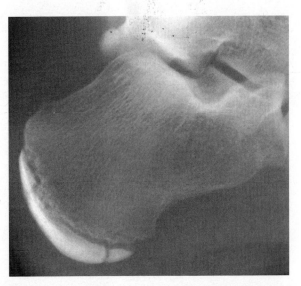

FIG. 9-45. Normal calcaneal apophysis. Transverse clefts or grooves remain in the apophysis, which fuses with the body of the calcaneus at around 17 years of age.

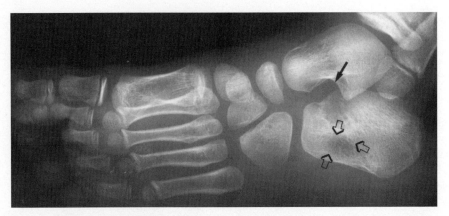

FIG. 9-46. Calcaneal pseudocyst. Oblique radiograph of the foot in a 9-year-old boy. Normal lucency in the anterior calcaneus is due to a relative paucity of trabeculae (*open arrows*). Normal sinus tarsi is also well-demonstrated (*arrow*).

ment from Köhler's osteochondrosis difficult (Fig. 9-47). To make this distinction requires clinical correlation, and often serial filming is necessary. A radionuclide bone scan can be used for differentiation.[11]

Accessory Navicular (Os Tibiale Externum)

The os tibiale externum is present in approximately 10 to 15% of children and is one of the most common accessory ossicles (Fig. 9-48).[11] It is located dorsomedially to the navicular tuberosity and is usually bilateral. It lies within the posterior tibial tendon and is connected by the tendon to the navicular during the first 10 years of life (Fig. 9-49). However, the tendon can insert into this accessory ossicle, rather than normally into the navicular, and can result in pain as a result of loss of appropriate support. A large os tibiale externum can elevate the posterior tibial tendon from its normal insertion to the medial navicular, leading to rotation of the ossicle. Radiographically, a painful accessory navicular is sclerotic, with cystic changes, and occasionally dislocated.[11] If symptoms persist, the ossicle can be excised, and the posterior tibial tendon can be reattached to the navicular.

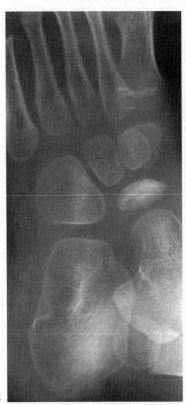
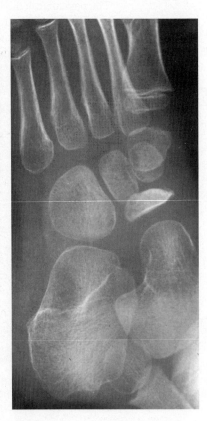

A,B

FIG. 9-47. Normal variations of the navicular. **A** and **B:** Oblique radiographs show normal developmental variations in contour, size, and density of the navicular. Differentiation from Köhler's disease requires clinical correlation and serial imaging or radionuclide studies.

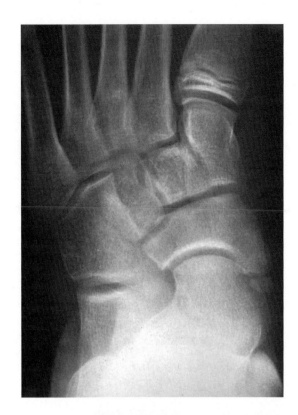

FIG. 9-48. Os tibiale externum. An os tibiale externum (accessory navicular) is present in 10 to 15% of children and is well demonstrated on this oblique film.

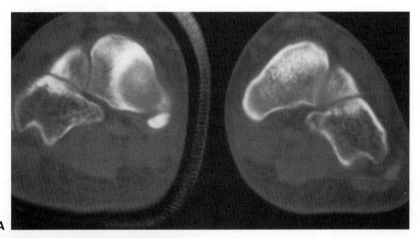

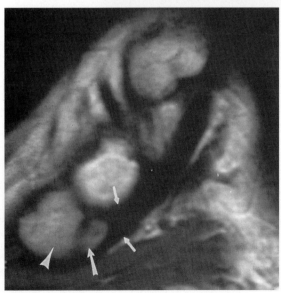

FIG. 9-49. Os tibiale externum. **A:** Coronal CT image of the bilateral midfoot regions demonstrates a sclerotic right accessory navicular in a patient with focal pain and tenderness. Note the fiberglass cast intended to immobilize the foot, decrease motion of the os, and promote healing. **B:** T1-weighted sagittal image through the medial midfoot obtained 5 months after the CT in **A** demonstrates partial fusion of the accessory ossicle (*arrow*) to the navicular (*arrowhead*). Notice the posterior tibial tendon (*small white arrows*) inserting onto the os.

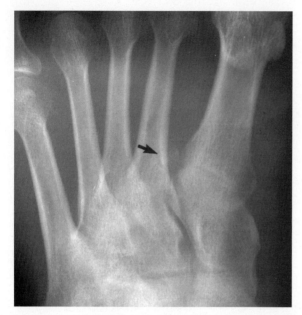

FIG. 9-50. Os intermetatarseum. AP radiograph demonstrates the os intermetatarseum (*arrow*), which is located between the dorsal aspects of the first and second metatarsals.

Variants of Metatarsals and Phalanges

Os Intermetatarseum

The os intermetatarseum is located between the dorsal aspects of the first and second metatarsals and is variable in size, shape, and location. It can appear similar to an os in the accessory tendon of the dorsal interosseous muscle (Fig. 9-50).[11]

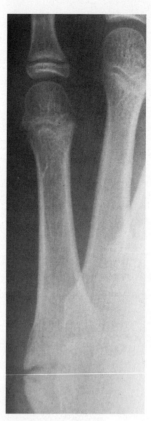

FIG. 9-52. Fracture through the base of the fifth metatarsal. AP radiograph of the left foot in an 11-year-old girl who had an inversion injury while jogging. Transverse fracture is noted at the base of the fifth metatarsal. Compare with Figure 9-51.

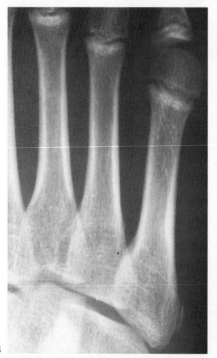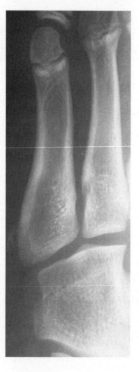

A,B

FIG. 9-51. Ununited apophysis of the fifth metatarsal. AP radiographs of both feet show the normal fifth metatarsal apophysis in the right foot (**A**) but slight separation of the apophysis from the base of the fifth metatarsal on the left (**B**). This separation is of no clinical consequence in this patient, whose symptoms were present on the right.

Apophysis of the Fifth Metatarsal

The normal, united apophysis of the tuberosity of the fifth metatarsal (Fig. 9-51) must be differentiated from a fracture of the base of the fifth metatarsal. The apophysis lies lateral to the metatarsal base and generally consists of one center, but it can be multicentric. It extends in the same longitudinal axis as the metatarsal, unlike the remaining metatarsals, and usually fuses at about 20 years. On the other hand, fractures extend transversely through the metatarsal in the plane perpendicular to the axis of the apophysis (Fig. 9-52).[11]

Cleft Epiphyses

Defects or clefts in the phalangeal epiphyses may be observed in the unfused epiphysis, usually just before puberty (Fig. 9-53). The basal epiphysis of the first proximal phalanx is the most common site, but clefts may occur elsewhere (i.e., distal tibia or calcaneal apophysis). They may be unilateral or bilateral and usually appear as a sharp, lucent line near the central portion or the margin of the epiphysis. The defects occasionally have irregular margins. The origin of epiphyseal cleft is not clear, but it may be the result of a double ossification center. These defects may sometimes be associated with pain, but they are not associated with fracture-related symptoms, and radiographic healing has not been observed.[8]

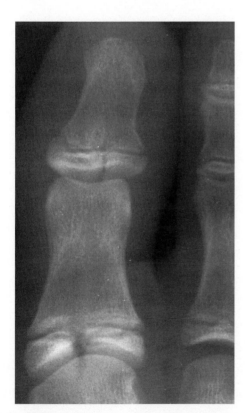

FIG. 9-53. Cleft epiphysis. AP image of the great toe demonstrates cleft epiphyses of the proximal and distal phalanges. The basal epiphysis of the first proximal phalanx is the most common site affected.

REFERENCES

1. Alliongton NJ, Kumar SJ, Guille JT. Clubfeet associated with congenital constriction bands of the ipsilateral lower extremity. J. Pediatr. Orthop. 1995; 15:599–603.
2. Blakeslee TJ, DeValentine SJ. Management of the resistant idiopathic clubfoot. The Kaiser experience from 1980–1990. J. Foot Ankle Surg. 1995; 34:167–176.
3. Bromley B, Benacerraf B. Abnormalities of the hands and feet in the fetus. Sonographic findings. AJR Am. J. Roentgenol. 1995; 165:1239–1243.
4. Chang CH, Hang SC. Surgical treatment of clubfoot deformity in arthrogryposis multiplex congenita. J. Formos. Med. Assoc. 1997; 96:30–35.
5. de Carvalho Neto J, Dias LS, Gabrieli AP. Congenital talipes equinovarus in spina bifida. Treatment and results. J. Pediatr. Orthop. 1996; 16:782–785.
6. Foules GD, Reinker K. Congenital constriction band syndrome. A seventy-year experience. J. Pediatr. Orthop. 1994; 14:242–248.
7. Freiberger RH, Hersh A, Harrison MO. Roentgen examination of the deformed foot. Semin. Roentgenol. 1970; 5:341–353.
8. Harrison BR, Keats TE. Epiphyseal clefts. Skeletal Radiol. 1980; 5:23–27.
9. Hersh A. The role of surgery in the treatment of club feet. Foot Ankle Int. 1995; 16: 672–681.
10. Hubbard AM, Davidson RS, Meyer JS, Mahboubi S. Magnetic resonance imaging of skewfoot. J. Bone Joint Surg. Am. 1996; 78:389–397.
11. Köhler A, Zimmer EA. Borderlands of normal and early pathologic findings in skeletal radiography. 4th Ed. New York, Thieme Medical Publishers, 1993; pp. 773–864.
12. Kumai T, Tanaka Y, Takakura Y, Tamai S. Isolated first naviculocuneiform joint coalition. Foot Ankle Int. 1996; 17:635–640.
13. McCarthy GJ, Lindaman L, Stefan M. Pedal polydactyly. An overview with case report. J. Foot Ankle Surg. 1995; 34:577–582.
14. McDonald MG, Stevens DB. Modified Mitchell bunionectomy for management of adolescent hallux valgus. Clin. Orthop. 1996; 3322:163–169.
15. Micheli LJ, Ireland ML. Prevention and management of calcaneal apophysitis in children. An overuse syndrome. J. Pediatr. Orthop. 1987; 7:34–38.
16. Miyagi N, Iisaka H, Yasuda K, Kaneda K. Onset of ossification of the tarsal bones in congenital clubfoot. J. Pediatr. Orthop. 1997; 17:36–40.
17. Napiontek M. Clinical and radiographic appearance of congenital talipes equinovarus after successful nonoperative treatment. J. Pediatr. Orthop. 1996; 16:67–72.
18. Napiontek M. Congenital vertical talus. A retrospective and critical review of 32 feet operated by peritalar reduction. J. Pediatr. Orthop. 1995; 4:179–187.
19. Napiontek M, Nazar J. Tibial osteotomy as a salvage procedure in the treatment of congenital talipes equinovarus. J. Pediatr. Orthop. 1994; 14:763–767.
20. Nimkin K, Spevak MR, Kleinman PK. Fractures of the hands and feet in child abuse. Imaging and pathologic features. Radiology 1997; 203:233–236.
21. Oestrich AE, Kirks DR. Practical Pediatric Imaging. Diagnostic Radiology of Infants and Children. Boston, Little, Brown, 1991, pp. 315–320.
22. Ozonoff MB. Pediatric Orthopaedic Radiology. Philadelphia, WB Saunders, 1992; pp. 397–460.
23. Resnick D. Diagnosis of Bone and Joint Disorders. 3rd Ed. Philadelphia, WB Saunders, 1995; pp. 4289–4291, 4294–4301, 4313–4314, 4601–4602.
24. Ritchie GE, Keim HA. Major foot deformities. Their classification and x-ray analysis. J Can. Assoc. Radiol. 1968; 19:155–166.

25. Stevens PM, Belle RM. Screw epiphysiodesis for ankle valgus. J. Pediatr. Orthop. 1997; 17:9–12.
26. Taybi H, Lachman RS. Radiology of Syndromes, Metabolic Disorders, and Skeletal Dysplasias. St. Louis, Mosby–Year Book, 1996.
27. VanderWilde R, Staheli LT, Chew DE, Magalon V. Measurements on radiographs of the foot in normal infants and children. J. Bone Joint Surg. Am. 1988; 70:407–415.
28. Wilde PH, Torode IP, Dickens DR, Cole WG. Resection for symptomatic talocalcaneal coalition. J. Bone Joint Surg. Br. 1994; 76:797–801.
29. Wirth T, Schuler P, Griss P. Early surgical treatment for congenital vertical talus. Arch. Orthop. Trauma Surg. 1994; 113:248–253.
30. Yamamoto H, Muneta T, Ishibashi T, Furuya K. Posteromedial release of congenital club foot in children over five years of age. J. Bone Joint Surg. Br. 1994; 76:555–558.

Radiology of the Foot and Ankle, Second Edition,
edited by Thomas H. Berquist.
© 2000 by Mayo Foundation.
Published by Lippincott Williams & Wilkins, Philadelphia.

CHAPTER 10

Reconstructive Procedures: Preoperative and Postoperative Imaging

Thomas H. Berquist and James K. DeOrio

Numerous operative procedures are used to correct deformities and painful arthropathies in the foot and ankle. Appropriate use of imaging procedures and diagnostic injections is essential for planning the surgical approach. Postoperatively, imaging plays an important role in evaluating surgical results and complications.

Fracture reduction and instrumentation are reviewed in Chapter 4. This chapter focuses on other reconstructive procedures commonly used to treat foot and ankle disorders.

ARTHROPLASTY

Ankle Arthroplasty

Ankle pain and instability commonly result in reduced activity. The ankle is one of the most commonly injured joints.[2,12] Degenerative joint disease, pain, and instability are common complications of trauma.[8] Other conditions such as rheumatoid arthritis also frequently involve the ankle.[15,29] Ankle arthroplasty was developed to provide a functional pain-free joint and an alternative to arthrodesis.[5,8,19,22,25,32]

Several procedures have been developed. Resection of tibial or talar osteophytes has been employed as a method to treat anterior impingement secondary to degenerative disease. Anterior degenerative changes are commonly seen in athletes.[12,13] Talar body arthroplasty has been used to treat patients with avascular necrosis or talar crush fractrures.[11] However, most experience has been gained with total ankle arthroplasty. Therefore, this section focuses on preoperative and postoperative imaging of total ankle arthroplasty.

Early experience with total ankle arthroplasty produced unsatisfactory results, with failure rates of 38% and component loosening in 24%.[2,15,16] Since the 1970s, multiple improvements and new component designs have been developed. Components are classified according to design philosophy. Certain systems allow flexion and extension (constrained), whereas others permit some degree of motion in multiple directions (nonconstrained).[2,15,16] Most systems are designed using metal-polyethylene combinations. Ceramic components are also available.[4,8,19,25,30,36,39] Components may be designed to be used with or without cement.[4,5,8,20–22,30,36,39] Currently, no system fully evaluated in the literature has demonstrated significant advantages over another. Newer systems, such as S.T.A.R. (Scandinavian Total Ankle Replacement, Waldeman Link, Hamburg, Germany) may provide improved results. This system allows

---

T. H. Berquist: Mayo Medical School, Mayo Clinic Jacksonville, Jacksonville, Florida 32224.

J. K. DeOrio: Mayo Medical School, Mayo Clinic Jacksonville, Jacksonville, Florida 32224.

free rotation of the tibial component restricted only by the malleoli. This results in neutralizing forces that may induce component loosening.

The Mayo experience with total ankle arthroplasty is comparable to that in other reports.[19,22] Kitaoka and associates[22] reported results on 204 patients who underwent ankle arthroplasty in 1994. Survival of ankle systems at 5, 10, and 15 years was 79%, 65%, and 61%, respectively. Higher failure rates were noted in patients with previous ankle surgery and in patients younger than 57 years of age. Best results were obtained in patients with rheumatoid arthritis or in patients older than 60 years of age who had degenerative disease.[22]

In a more recent review, the same group reported results

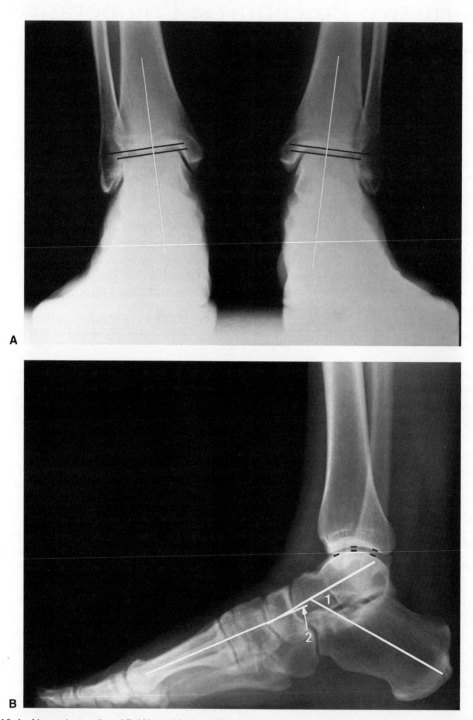

FIG. 10-1. Normal standing AP (**A**) and lateral (**B**) views of the ankle. The AP view shows both ankles for comparison. The ankle joints are congruent (*black lines*) but not parallel to the floor (*white lines*). The standing lateral view (**B**) demonstrates the tibiotalar joint (*broken lines*), tarsal relationships, talocalcaneal angle (*1;* normal, 25° to 30°), and talar–first metatarsal angle (*2;* normal, −4° to + 4°).

using the Mayo total ankle arthroplasty. This series included 160 arthroplasties in 143 patients who were followed for at least 2 years. Results were good in 19%, fair in 34%, and poor in 11%, and there were failures in 36%.[19]

Results of European studies using the S.T.A.R. prosthesis are more encouraging. Survival rates of 87.3 to 96.7% were reported at 7 years.[23,34]

Imaging

Imaging procedures provide valuable data for the orthopedic surgeon preoperatively and postoperatively. Routine radiographs provide essential anatomic information regarding bony relationships, joint congruity, and the degree of osteophyte formation or bone loss (Fig. 10-1).[2,14] Ideally, anteroposterior (AP) and lateral views should be obtained in the standing position to ensure physiologic position of the tibial, fibula, talus, and adjacent tarsal bones (Fig. 10-2).[2,14,33,35]

In some situations, additional studies may be indicated.[2,27,28] Computed tomography (CT) is useful for more detailed evaluation of articular changes such as subchondral cysts and bone deformity (Fig. 10-3).[2] Magnetic resonance imaging (MRI) may be indicated when talar avascular necrosis or soft tissue abnormalities are suspected.[1] However, conventional stress views are usually adequate to evaluate instability. Diagnostic joint injections are useful to localize the source of pain, but this approach is more commonly used in the foot before arthrodesis.[2,18,27]

Postoperative radiographs are important to establish a baseline for evaluating potential complications.[2] We prefer to obtain standing AP and lateral radiographs when the patient is able to tolerate the examination (Fig. 10-4). In some cases, fluoroscopically positioned views are also added to align the component-bone or bone-cement interfaces.[2]

Results of ankle arthroplasty were good to fair in 54% of patients.[19,22] Kitaoka and Patzer[19] defined results as good (19%) when the patients' pain was significantly improved or alleviated, when patients were able to walk six blocks without aids such as a cane, and when there was no radiographic evidence of loosening. Fair results (35%) differed in that a cane was sometimes needed for walking six blocks and pain was improved to a lesser degree. In addition, there was no radiographic evidence of loosening. Patients with poor results (11%) had significant or increased pain compared with preoperative symptoms. Additional walking assistance, such as use of crutches, was required. Thirty-five percent of procedures were considered failures.[19] Complications typically requiring image assistance for evaluation are summarized in Table 10-1.

Serial radiographs remain a valuable tool for evaluating complications of ankle arthroplasty. Component loosening

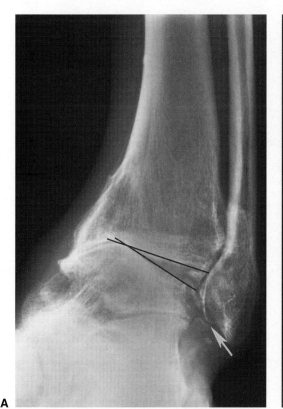 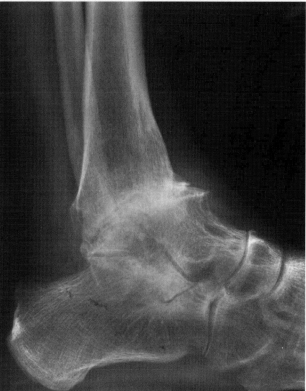

A   **B**

FIG. 10-2. Standing AP (**A**) and lateral (**B**) views in a patient with advanced posttraumatic arthritis. There is tibiotalar and subtalar arthrosis. The tibiotalar joint is asymmetric (*black lines*), and one sees calcaneofibular abutment (*arrow*).

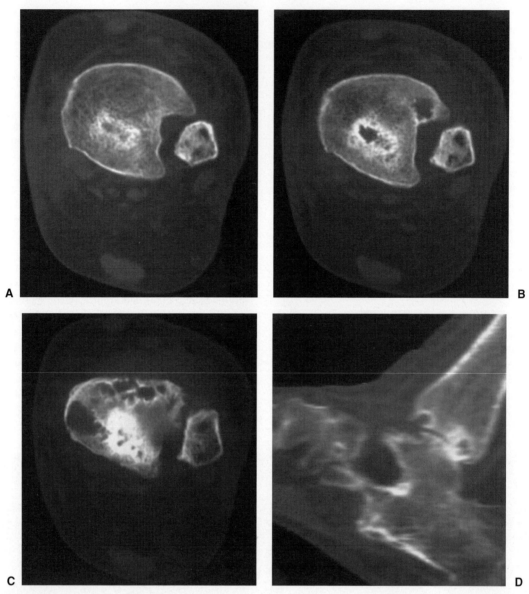

FIG. 10-3. Axial CT images (**A** to **C**) and a reconstructed sagittal image (**D**) demonstrate tibiofibular diastasis and significant bone loss.

can be evaluated by careful evaluation of the interfaces to detect component migration and lucent lines. Lucent lines 2 mm or wider, progression in width, or increase in the extent of lucency about the component are significant. Plain film criteria for loosening have been described as definite when one sees component migration and lucent lines along the entire surface of the component (Figs. 10-5 and 10-6), probable with lucency along the entire surface but no component migration, and questionable if lucent lines extend along only a portion of the component interface.[2,19] Additional studies such as subtraction arthrography and radionuclide scans may provide additional support when loosening is equivocal on radiographs. However, these techniques have not been as well accepted compared with their utility in the hip and knee.

TABLE 10-1. *Ankle arthroplasty complications*[a]

Component loosening
Infection
   Deep
   Superficial
Delayed wound healing
Skin sloughing or ulceration
Malleolar fractures
Impingement
Instability
Heterotopic bone formation

[a] Data from references 8, 19 to 22, 25, and 36.

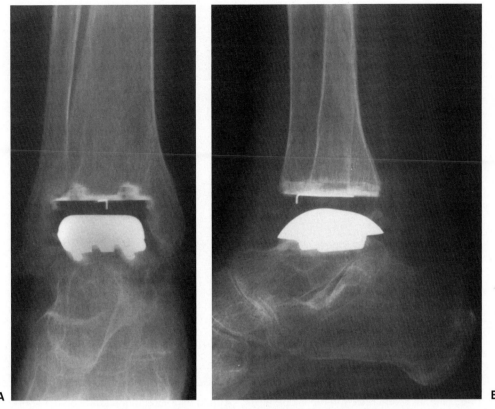

FIG. 10-4. AP (**A**) and lateral (**B**) standing views after ankle arthroplasty. The ankle is fluoroscopically positioned to demonstrate the component cement interfaces optimally.

Stress views after anesthetic injection are useful in selected cases.[2]

The incidence of deep infection ranges from 2.7 to 3.7%.[15,19] The incidence appears to be slightly increased in patients with rheumatoid arthritis.[37] As with arthroplasty in other joints, infection is commonly associated with loosening. When infection is suspected, joint aspiration may be useful to isolate the organism. Radionuclide scans with technetium-99m methylene diphosphonate (MDP) and indium-111–labeled white blood cells may also be useful.[2] Patients with deep infection frequently require component removal and arthrodesis.[20,21]

Impingement, another potential complication, may be a cause of postarthroplasty ankle pain.[2,8,15,19] This condition is usually related to component subsidence (Fig. 10-7).[8,15,19,20] Diagnosis can be suggested on routine standing radiographs. In more subtle cases, stress views may confirm the diagnosis.[2]

Additional complications include malleolar fracture and ankle instability (see Table 10-1).[8,15,19,20,21] Routine radiographs (Fig. 10-8) are usually adequate for diagnosis. Stress views may be required to confirm the extent of instability.

Arthroplasty failures (up to 35% of cases) present a significant problem for orthopedic surgeons. In some cases, revision of the arthroplasty is possible. However, bone loss, subtalar joint arthrosis, and soft tissue abnormalities may make

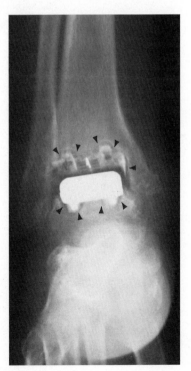

FIG. 10-5. AP radiograph of the ankle demonstrates lucent lines (*arrowheads*) surrounding both the tibial and talar components. Components were not fluoroscopically positioned, so interfaces are not optimally aligned (see Fig. 10-4).

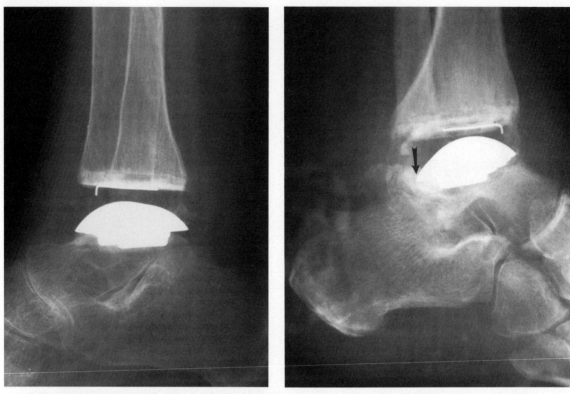

FIG. 10-6. Normal lateral radiograph postoperatively (**A**) and migration of the talar component (*arrow*) with posterior impaction in **B**.

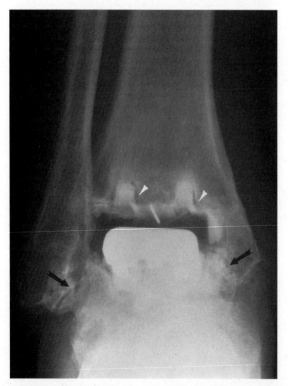

FIG. 10-7. Standing AP view of the ankle demonstrates bi-malleolar impingement (*arrows*). There are also lucent lines at the bone cement interface involving more than 50% of the tibial component (*white arrowheads*).

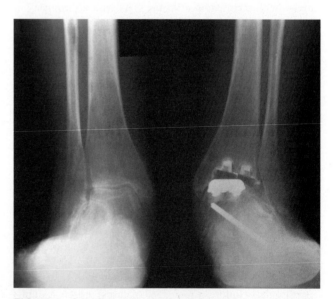

FIG. 10-8. Standing radiographs of the ankles demonstrating instability on the left with asymmetry of the ankle joint. There is a subtalar fusion with pin fixation. (From Berquist, ref. 2, with permission.)

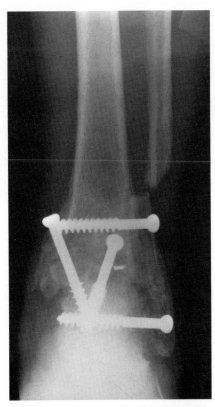

FIG. 10-9. AP radiograph of the ankle after arthrodesis with fibular osteotomy, bone graft, and screw fixation.

revision impossible. Ankle arthrodesis is a potential option in these patients. When considering arthrodesis, it may be necessary to consider subtalar fusion at the same time.[20]

Bone loss and pain localization are important when considering arthrodesis (Figs. 10-9 and 10-10). Selective anesthetic injection of subtalar and adjacent tarsal articulations is useful to localize potential sites for arthrodesis. Injections can be easily performed with fluoroscopic guidance.[2,3,18,27] Bone loss can be evaluated with CT even when implants are in place.[2]

Metatarsophalangeal Arthroplasty

Resection arthroplasty with or without soft tissue interposition, cheilectomy, and arthrodesis have been used for years to deal with disorders of the metatarsophalangeal joints. Most procedures focus on the great toe; however, the lesser toes (2 to 5) have been treated similarly.[10,15–17,26,31,37,38] The Mayo procedure (resection of the first metatarsal head) and the Keller procedure (resection of the proximal phalanx of the first toe) are commonly employed, but both procedures have potential problems.[16,37,38] Disadvantages of resection procedures include recurrent hallux valgus, hallux extensus, loss of flexor strength, and transfer of weight or stress to the lateral metatarsals.[24,37,38]

Joint replacement arthroplasty was developed as an alter-

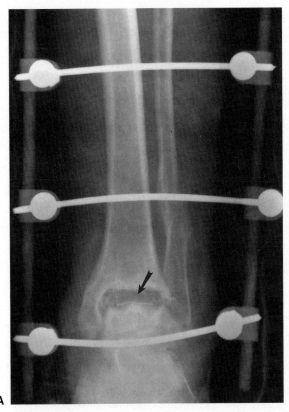

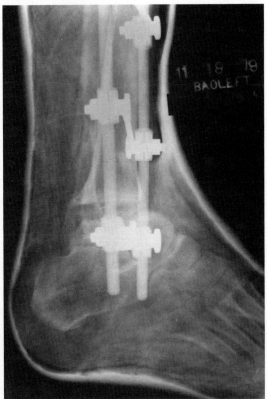

FIG. 10-10. Failed ankle arthroplasty. AP (**A**) and lateral (**B**) radiographs show bone graft (*arrow*) and external fixation.

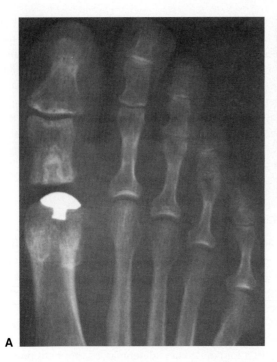

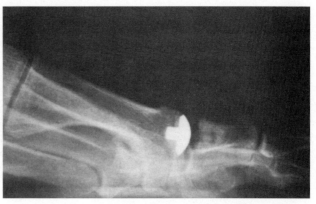

FIG. 10-11. AP (**A**) and lateral (**B**) radiographs of a cemented arthroplasty of the first metatarsophalangeal joint with a metal metatarsal component and polyethylene phalangeal component.

native to the foregoing procedures in an attempt to relieve pain and to improve function.[6,7,24,38] The indications for great toe arthroplasty include hallux valgus, hallux rigidus, degenerative joint disease, rheumatoid arthritis, and failed surgical procedures.[6,7,10,17,26,31,37,38] We emphasize procedures for the great toe. However, the lesser metatarsophalangeal joints have also been treated with arthroplasty for Freiberg's disease, rheumatoid arthritis, subluxation, and bunionette deformities.[2,6,9]

Arthroplasty designs have changed significantly since the 1950s in an attempt to develop better implants. Metal-polyethylene combinations (Fig. 10-11) or single- and double-stemmed silicone implants (Figs. 10-12 and 10-13) are used most frequently. Clinical evaluation considers patient age, activity, and radiographic features.[2,6,7,10] The system se-

lected depends on this assessment, bone stock, patient compliance, and surgical preference. A scoring system (100 points) is used preoperatively and postoperatively to evaluate symptoms and surgical results. Factors considered in the scoring system include pain levels (0, constant pain, to 50, no pain), function (0 to 40 points for conventional footwear, for walking more than 3 blocks, household activity), objective findings (0 to 10 points for calluses, deformity, and point tenderness) and radiographic features.[31]

Imaging

Preoperative radiographs should be obtained using standing posteroanterior (PA) and lateral projections. Numerous features should be assessed on preoperative radiographs. The

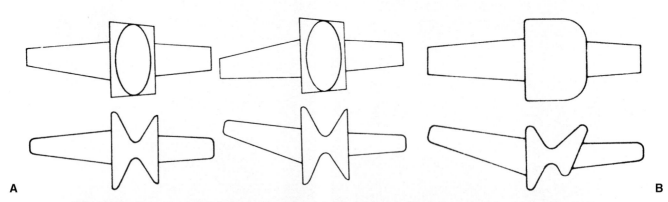

FIG. 10-12. First metatarsophalangeal and lesser toe implants. **A:** Hinged great toe implants with metatarsal stem angled 15° in the sagittal and 10° in the transverse plane to optimize anatomic alignment (LaPorta design). **B:** Hinged great toe implant (Lawrence design). *(continued)*

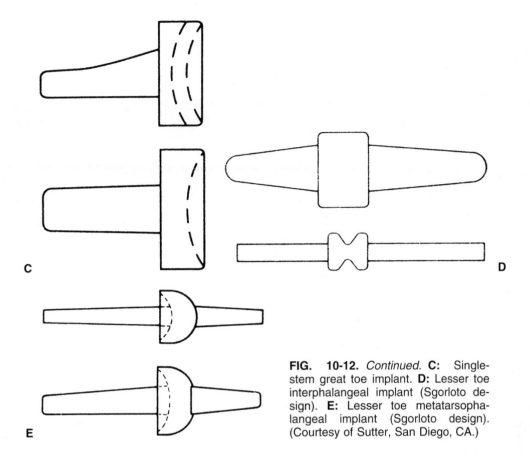

FIG. 10-12. *Continued.* **C:** Single-stem great toe implant. **D:** Lesser toe interphalangeal implant (Sgorloto design). **E:** Lesser toe metatarsophalangeal implant (Sgorloto design). (Courtesy of Sutter, San Diego, CA.)

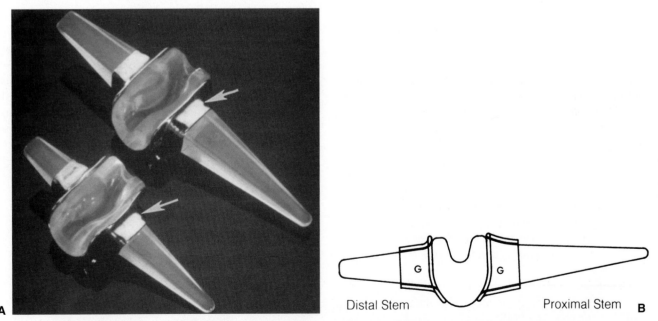

Distal Stem   Proximal Stem   **B**

FIG. 10-13. Swanson Silastic H.P. 100 flexible hinged toe implant with flexible hinge grommet. **A:** The titanium grommet (*arrows*) is designed to shield the bone and silicone portion of the implant. **B:** Sagittal illustration of the distal and proximal stem with grommets (*G*) in place. (Courtesy of Wright Medical Technology, Arlington, TN, and Dr. A.B. Swanson.)

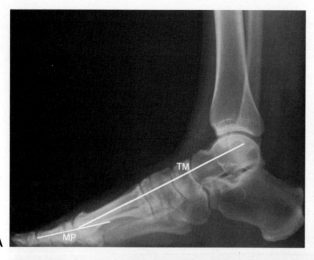

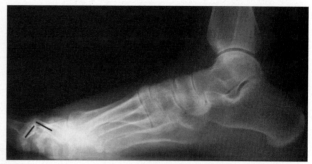

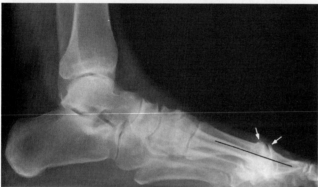

FIG. 10-14. Standing lateral radiographs for preoperative assessment. **A:** The first metatarsal and talus (*TM*, talar–first metatarsal angle) are aligned. The first metatarsophalangeal (*MP*) relationship is defined. **B:** Hallux rigidus. Note the prominent dorsal osteophytes at the first metatarsophalangeal joint (*arrows*). The metatarsal and proximal phalanx are nearly directly aligned (*black line*). Midfoot degenerative joint changes are also noted. **C:** Lateral view demonstrates dorsal swelling with hammer toe (*lines*) deformities of lesser toes.

standing lateral view (Fig. 10-14) should be evaluated for joint alignment including the talar–first metatarsal angle and digital deformities.[2,7,30] Standing AP views (Fig. 10-15) are evaluated to determine the extent of involvement of all metatarsophalangeal joints by degenerative disease, erosive arthritis, subluxation, and angulation. Specific measurements should include the metatarsophalangeal angle, first-second metatarsal angle, phalangeal angles, joint congruency, and position of the sesamoids (see Fig. 10-15).[2,7,30] The sesamoid position can be graded on the AP view by determining the extent of metatarsal coverage. When the lateral sesamoid is completely covered (see Fig. 10-15A, left foot), it is considered in position. When the lateral sesamoid is shifted 10 to 50% and is uncovered by the metatarsal, it is considered subluxed (Fig. 10-15A, right foot). The sesamoid is dislocated when 50% or more is uncovered (see Fig. 10-15B and C).[7]

Additional preoperative imaging studies are required in selected cases. CT may be used to evaluate the articular surfaces and bone loss.[2] MRI is useful for evaluating avascular necrosis, soft tissue changes, and subtle cartilage abnormalities.[1] Joint aspiration or diagnostic injections are not usually required in the forefoot.[3]

Postoperative images are important to serve as a baseline

to evaluate potential complications (Table 10-2). The same clinical scoring system is also used to compare surgical results with the preoperative assessment.[30] Standing AP and lateral radiographs (Fig. 10-16) are generally adequate to serve as a baseline. In certain cases, fluoroscopic positioning may be useful to align the toe for optimal evaluation of the implant bone interface.[2] Radiographs should be evaluated for position of the implant, surrounding lucent zones (see

TABLE 10-2.
Metatarsophalangeal arthroplasty complications[a]

Wound healing
Painful plantar keratosis
Osteophytes around implants
Implant failure (fracture)
Restricted motion
Deep infection
Recurrent deformity
Stress fracture
Transfer metatarsalgia
Synovitis

[a] Data from references 2, 10, 17, 24, 25, and 38.

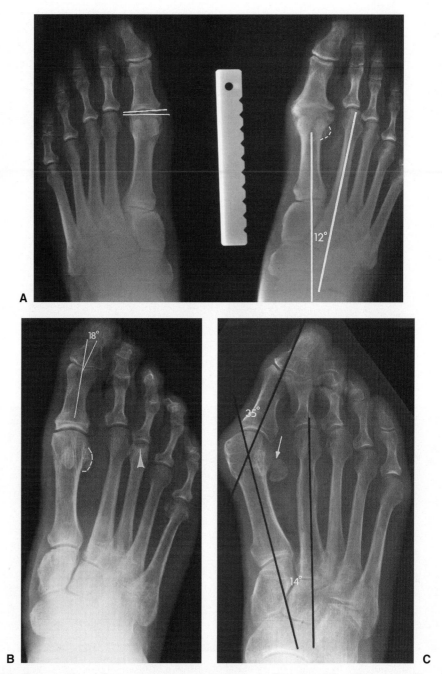

FIG. 10-15. Preoperative AP standing views of the feet. **A:** Standing AP radiographs with advanced hallux rigidus on the right and early joint space narrowing and osteophyte formation on the left. The first-second metatarsal angle (*white lines*) on the right is 12°. The first metatarsophalangeal joint on the left shows mild incongruency (*white lines*). The lateral sesamoid on the left is completely covered by the metatarsal. There is spurring of the right lateral sesamoid (*broken lines*) with 10 to 50% uncovered (subluxation). **B:** Standing AP radiograph in a patient with forefoot pain. There is avascular necrosis (*arrowhead*) of the third metatarsal head. The lateral sesamoid is 50% displaced (*broken lines*). The first phalangeal angle is 18°. **C:** Standing AP radiographs with hallux valgus deformity (angle 35°), first-second metatarsal angle of 14°, and dislocation of both sesamoids (*arrow*). There is an old second metatarsal fracture deformity.

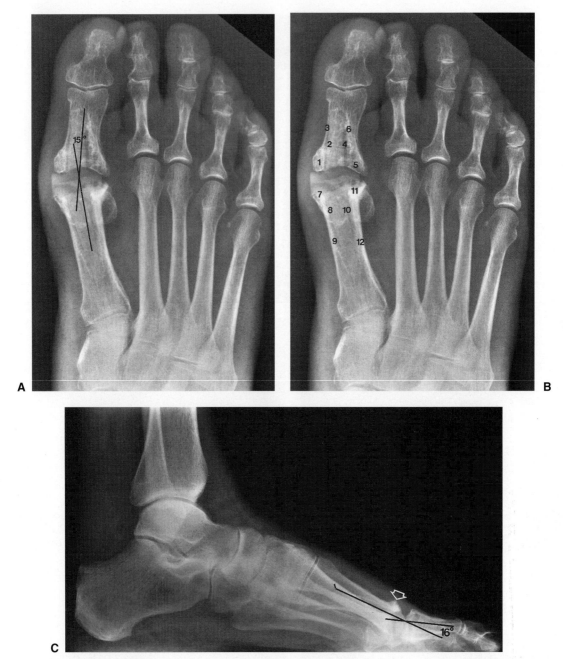

FIG. 10-16. Postoperative evaluation of metatarsophalangeal arthroplasty. **A:** Standing AP radiograph shows a double-stem implant with a metatarsophalangeal angle of 15°. **B:** Same patient as **A** with zones marked that are used to describe lucent areas and osteophyte formation. **C:** Standing lateral radiograph shows slight dorsal sclerosis and osteophyte formation (*open arrow*). The metatarsophalangeal angle is 16°.

Fig. 10-16B), bone scleroses and osteophyte formation (Fig. 10-17), and joint alignment (Fig. 10-18).[2,7,30,37] Lucent zones are evaluated in a similar fashion to other arthroplasty procedures. Lucent zones larger than 2 mm, especially with progression on serial radiographs, may be seen with osteolysis resulting from loosening, synovitis, and infection. Osteophyte formation at the cut metatarsal and phalangeal margins is graded based on encroachment into the cartilage space. Osteophyte formation is slight if visible but only small spurs are identified; it is moderate if there is more than 50% encroachment of osteophytes on the cartilage space; and it is severe if there is more than 50% or complete encroachment.[7]

Complications of metatarsophalangeal arthroplasty are summarized in Table 10-2. Wound healing may be due to early postoperative infection. However, late wound breakdown may also be seen with improperly fitting footwear.[38] Deep infection is unusual. Cracchiolo and associates[7] noted a single deep infection in 88 patients. Imaging of infection

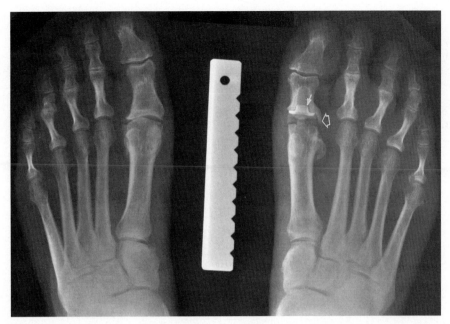

FIG. 10-17. Standing AP radiograph with a Swanson double-stem silicone implant with grommet (*arrow*). The metatarsophalangeal relationship is aligned. A prominent lateral osteophyte extends into the joint region (*open arrow*). There is hallux rigidus on the right.

should begin with routine radiographs. Radionuclide scans may be difficult to interpret in the postoperative period. Subtle periprosthetic bone changes may be more easily appreciated with CT (Fig. 10-19).[2] Infection involving bone or soft

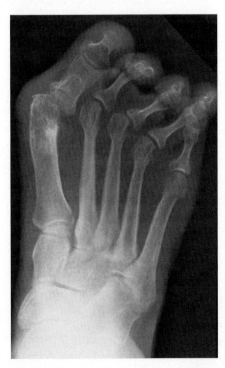

FIG. 10-18. Standing AP radiograph demonstrating loss of joint stability with subluxation. The single-stem phalangeal implant is intact.

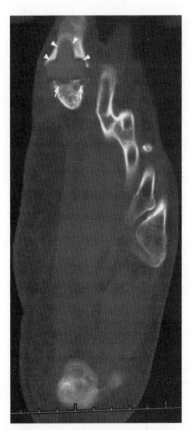

FIG. 10-19. Coronal CT image of the phalangeal stem of a double-stem implant. There is no artifact with silicone implants. The lucent zones around the entire component (*arrowheads*) are easily appreciated. Erosions in the metatarsal (*arrows*) are noted.

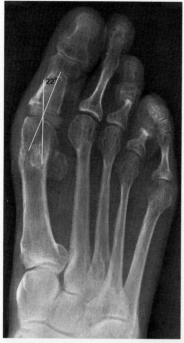
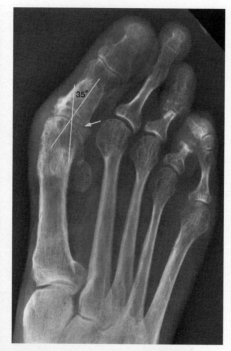
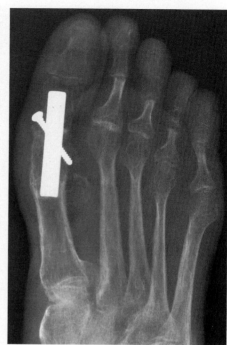

A,B

C

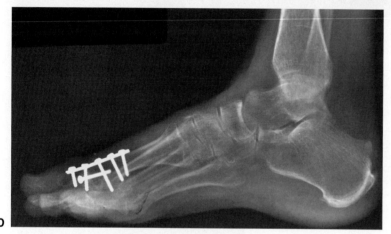

D

FIG. 10-20. Single-stem prosthetic implant with recurrent synovitis, bone erosions, and severe cross under of the fifth toe. **A:** Postoperative standing AP view shows the implant with a metatarsophalangeal angle of 22°. There is a previous second interphalangeal fusion. Clinically, plantar keratosis was noted under the second metatarsal head. **B:** Five years later, the implant has fractured (*arrow*), and the angle has increased to 35°. **C** and **D:** AP (**C**) and lateral (**D**) views after arthrodesis and shortening of the second toe (*arrow*). The crossunder deformity has been corrected.

tissue may be detected with MRI when nonmetallic (silicone) implants are in place.[1]

Lucent zones around the implants may be linear (see Fig. 10-19) or irregular. Thin lucent zones are not unusual and may be evident in up to one-third of patients.[7] Significant lucent zones (larger than 2 mm) or cystic areas may result from an inflammatory process initiated by Silastic or polyethylene shear, synovitis, or infection.[7,30,38] Aspiration of the involved joint is useful to exclude infection.[3]

Angular deformity, progressive hallux valgus, and soft tissue imbalance may also occur (Fig. 10-20). These problems may require soft tissue repair, implant removal, or, in some cases, arthrodesis.[37,38]

Implant fractures (see Fig. 10-20; Fig. 10-21) are seen in 1.9 to 4% of patients.[7,10,38] Implant fractures may be graded as grade 0 (no deformity or fracture), grade 1 (slight deformity or fracture; see Fig. 10-20), or grade 2 (complete de-

struction; see Fig. 10-21).[10] In many cases, implant fractures do not correlate with clinical results. Grade 1 fractures may have a good clinical result.[7,37,38]

In some cases, lateral foot symptoms develop, resulting from overload of the lateral metatarsals because of shortening or reestablished motion in the hallux. Stress fractures and other causes of forefoot pain such as Freiberg's infarction (Fig. 10-22) should be considered.[24]

ARTHRODESIS

Arthrodesis may be used in the ankle or foot as a procedure to restore activity and reduce pain.[40,42,43,45,48,49,56,84] Indications are similar for the ankle, hindfoot, and midfoot and forefoot. However, surgical approaches differ, as do results and complications. Therefore, we discuss clinical and imaging aspects of arthrodesis by region.

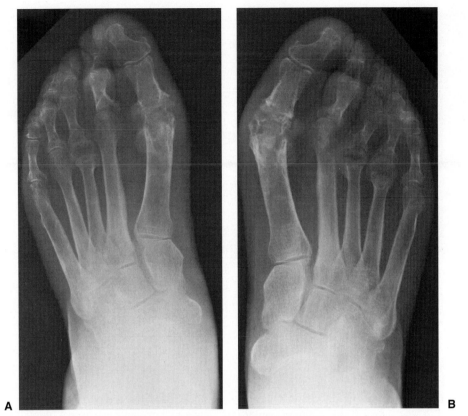

FIG. 10-21. Standing AP radiographs of the left (**A**) and right (**B**) foot in a patient with arthroplasties of the great toes, left third and right third and fourth metatarsophalangeal joints. There is also a bunionette repair on the left. Both great toe implants are fragmented (grade 2).

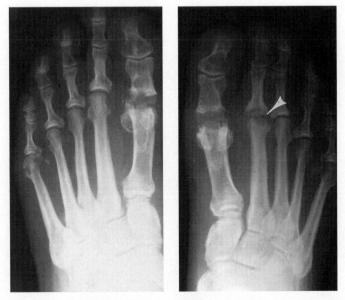

FIG. 10-22. Patient with rheumatoid arthritis and bilateral great toe arthroplasties. There is avascular necrosis of the second metatarsal head on the right (*arrowhead*).

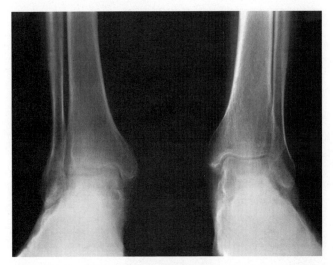

FIG. 10-23. Standing AP radiographs of the ankle with marked joint space narrowing and subchondral sclerosis (grade 2) on the right.

Ankle Arthrodesis

Indications for ankle arthrodesis in adults include osteoarthritis, rheumatoid arthritis, posttraumatic arthritis, infection, selected cases of acute injury, failed arthroplasty, and neoplasms.[38,41,44,47,51,52,54,58,68,80] In children, ankle arthrodesis is most commonly performed for paralytic disorders, congenital deformities, previous sepsis, or severe injury.[69,70,72]

Preoperative decisions are based on clinical and radio-graphic features. Clinical scoring systems have been designed and modified by Mazur and colleagues[70,72] and Kitoaka and associates.[57] Surgical techniques vary depending on patient status, patient compliance, and the surgeon's preference.[56,66] More than 30 procedures have been described for performing ankle arthrodesis, including arthroscopic procedures and external and internal fixation techniques.[40,41,44,46,50,53,55,61,65,67,74–76,82,84]

Preoperative radiographs remain the primary screening examination for evaluating bone changes and alignment of the osseous structures. Standing AP, lateral, and mortise views of the ankle are used to assess changes before surgical treatment. Osteoarthritis is categorized using all three views as grade 1 (joint space narrowing without secondary osteophyte formation and bone scleroses), grade 2 (joint space narrowing with moderate osteophyte formation and sclerosis), and grade 3 (narrowing with severe sclerosis and joint space narrowing) (Fig. 10-23).[41,43,74] All three views should be carefully evaluated. The mortise view is most useful for evaluating the symmetry of the ankle mortise. The standing AP view is used to evaluate the joint space. Several orthopedically significant measurements can be made (Fig. 10-24), including the talocrural angle, talar tilt angle, Shenton's line, and the syndesmotic width.[43,74] The uninvolved ankle can be used for comparison.[41,43] The standing lateral view should be evaluated to assess tibiotalar position, the tibiotalar and subtalar joints, and tarsal alignment.[41,48,74] The talocalcaneal angle, talar–first metatarsal angle, talar height, calcaneal pitch, and tibiocalcaneal angles should all be measured on the standing lateral radiograph (Fig. 10-25).

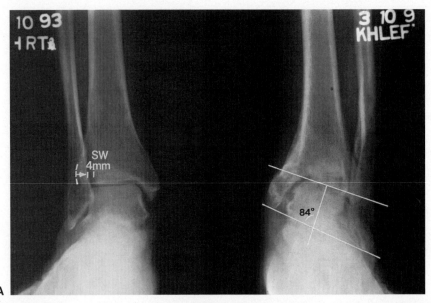

A

FIG. 10-24. Preoperative evaluation of standing AP views of the ankle. **A:** Normal right ankle and posttraumatic arthrosis on the left. The syndesmotic width (SW) (normal, less than 5 mm) is measured 1 cm proximal to the tibial articular surface. In this case, SW is 4 mm (*vertical lines*). The overlap of the tibia (*white broken line*) measured to the medial fibular margin (*arrow*) should not exceed 1 cm. The talocrural angle is measured by a line along the tibial articular surface and a line perpendicular to this and a line along the malleolar tips. This angle is normally 83 ± 4° with a difference of 2° compared with the opposite ankle.[72] *(continued)*

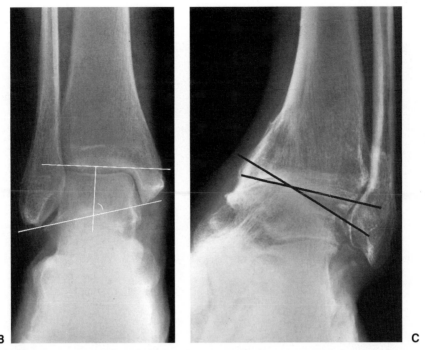

FIG. 10-24. *Continued.* **B:** Lines drawn for measuring the talocrural angle. **C:** Standing AP view with the talar tilt angle demonstrated by lines along the tibial and talar articular surfaces.

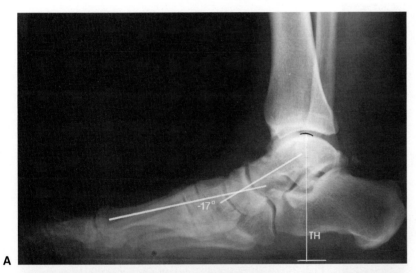

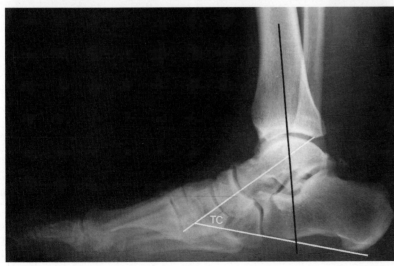

FIG. 10-25. Preoperative evaluation of the standing lateral view. **A:** Standing lateral view of the foot demonstrating talar height (*TH,* talar dome to foot support; normal, 7.3 to 9.5 cm), talar–first metatarsal angle (*TM,* white lines; angle, 17°). The normal talar–first metatarsal angle is 0°, mild deformity is less than or equal to 15°, and severe deformity is more than 15°.[46] **B:** Standing lateral view of the foot demonstrating the talocalcaneal (*TC*) angle, which is measured by lines along the plantar calcaneus and through the talar neck. The tibiotalar and tibiocalcaneal angles can be calculated by a line (*black line*) along the shaft of the tibia that intersects the talar and calcaneal lines.

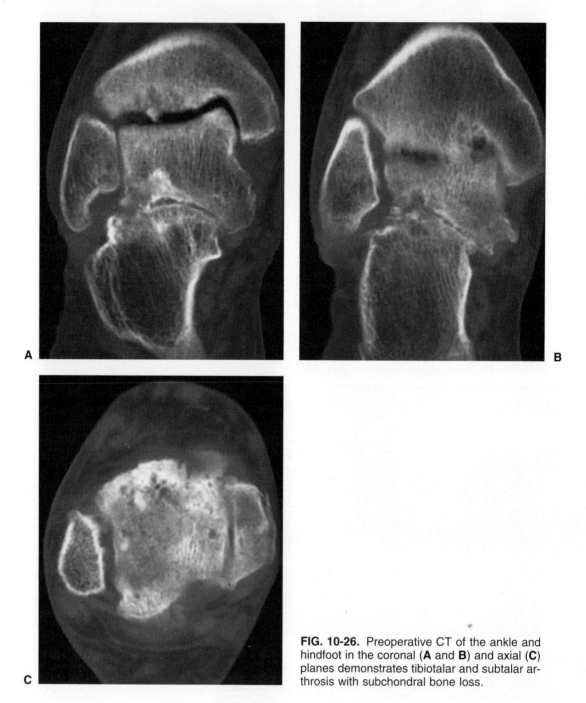

FIG. 10-26. Preoperative CT of the ankle and hindfoot in the coronal (**A** and **B**) and axial (**C**) planes demonstrates tibiotalar and subtalar arthrosis with subchondral bone loss.

In certain cases, CT (bone loss), MRI (avascular necroses, soft tissue integrity), or diagnostic injections may be indicated (Fig. 10-26).[41,42] Diagnostic injections are particularly useful when the exact source of pain is uncertain or when adjacent joints need evaluation to determine whether more extensive surgery may be required.[41,57,66]

As noted earlier, multiple approaches are used for ankle fusion (Figs. 10-27 and 10-28).[40,43,45,50,52,55,60,64,75,76] External fixation can be useful after failed ankle arthroplasty, after failed arthrodesis, or in patients with osteopenia.[51,55,60,67] In patients with rheumatoid arthritis and diminished bone

density, it may be best to use a long intramedullary rod inserted through the calcaneus.[45,75,76] Postoperatively, clinical evaluation including comparison with preoperative scoring and radiographic analysis are used to evaluate the surgical results.

The clinical scoring system evaluates pain, activity, footwear tolerance, and the ability to walk six blocks with or without walking aids. Preoperative and postoperative radiographs (Fig. 10-29) are also compared using the same measurements. On the lateral view (see Fig. 10-29), the foot should be in neutral position, although up to 5° of plantar

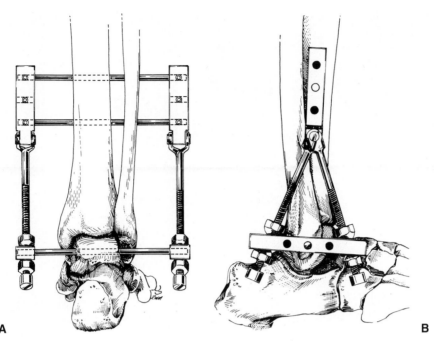

FIG. 10-27. Illustration of external fixation for ankle fusion using the Calandruccio frame seen posteriorly (**A**) and from the side (**B**). (Courtesy of Smith, Nephew, Richards, Inc., Memphis, TN.)

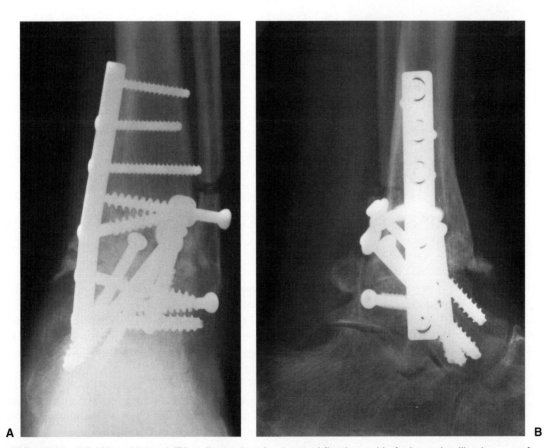

FIG. 10-28. AP (**A**) and lateral (**B**) radiographs after internal fixation ankle fusion using iliac bone graft, fibular osteotomy with lateral screw fixation, and a medial compression plate with screws.

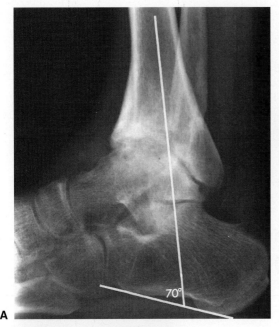

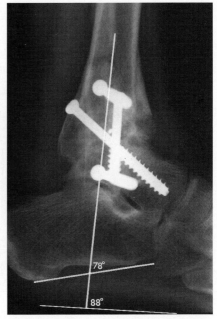

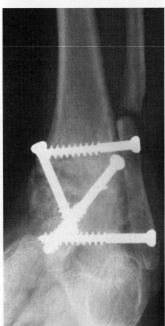

FIG. 10-29. A: Preoperative standing lateral radiograph shows marked posttraumatic arthrosis with a tibiocalcaneal angle of 70°. **B:** Postoperative lateral after internal fixation shows the foot position near neutral (88°) with the tibiocalcaneal angle at 78°. **C:** Standing AP view shows a solid fusion. The foot and ankle are internally rotated, a feature that makes measuring the tibial-hindfoot angle (ideally neutral to 5° hindfoot valgus) difficult to evaluate.

flexion is acceptable.[64,67,69,70–73] Foot motion (dorsiflexion-plantar flexion) can be measured clinically or radiographically.[71,79] Routine radiographs are usually obtained at 3, 6, and 12 months after arthrodesis. Additional studies are indicated when complications are suspected.[41]

Complications

Results of ankle arthrodesis vary depending on multiple factors including the type of procedure and patient compliance. Reports on arthroscopic and external and internal fixation techniques indicate healing rates of about 90%. Healing usually occurs in 3 months, but it may require up to 6 months with revision procedures.[40,45,52,67,75]

Complications also vary significantly. Higher complication rates are reported in patients with previous surgical failures and in patients with rheumatoid arthritis or diabetes mellitus.[45,58,60,76,78,82] Table 10-3 summarizes complications of ankle arthrodesis.

The incidence of nonunion has been reported to vary from 5 to 55%.[40,49,55,75,82] Nonunion following arthroscopic bone grafting and external fixation was noted in 7% by Crosby and colleagues.[48] Moekel and associates[74] compared rates of nonunion using external and internal fixation. Overall

---

TABLE 10-3. *Ankle arthrodesis complications*[a]

Nonunion
Malalignment/loss of position
Infection
  Deep
  Superficial
Wound slough
Fractures
Hardware problems
Subtalar arthrosis

[a] Data from references 40, 46, 48, 51, 58, and 60.

complications were greater with external fixation (61%) compared with internal fixation (28%). The incidence of nonunion was 21% using external fixation techniques (Fig. 10-30) compared with 5% for internal fixation techniques.[75] Serial radiographs provide information concerning healing of fusion sites. Lucent changes about fixation pins or screws used for fixation suggest motion from delayed or nonunion (Fig. 10-31).[41] Stress views, CT, and MRI are useful in selected cases. Injection of the fusion site to determine whether pain has been relieved is also useful.[42]

Infections may be superficial or deep, or they may involve pin tracts when external fixation devices are in position. The incidence of superficial or wound infection is 4 to 18%, that of pin tract infection is 9 to 18%, and that of deep infection is 5 to 60%.[40,53,55,77,78] Infection rates are much higher in patients with diabetes mellitus, rheumatoid arthritis (60%), avascular necrosis, open traumatic injuries, and other major medical disorders.[53,77,78] Nonunion and infection are commonly associated. Therefore, when radiographs suggest nonunion (see Figs. 10-30 and 10-31), infection should also be considered. Additional studies with radionuclide scans or MRI may be useful. However, aspiration of the fusion site or pin tracts may be more definitive.[41]

Serial radiographs provide the necessary information for evaluating most other complications including loss of position, malunion, change in hardware position, and fracture. Stress fractures of the tibia are most common in the medial or distal tibia. Lidor and colleagues[63] noted 12 tibial stress fractures in 167 cases of ankle arthrodesis. When suspected clinically, radionuclide scans correlated with radiographs are definitive.

Hindfoot Arthrodesis

Triple arthrodesis (talonavicular, talocalcaneal, and calcaneocuboid) was initially performed on children with polio or congenital foot deformities. Today, selected fusion of one or more joints is common in adults as well. Indications for arthrodesis include osteoarthritis, rheumatoid arthritis, trauma, congenital deformities, neurotrophic changes, poste-

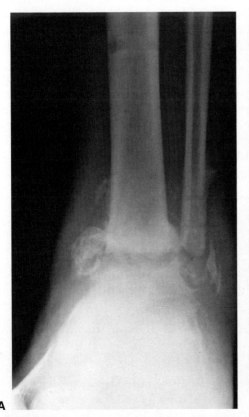 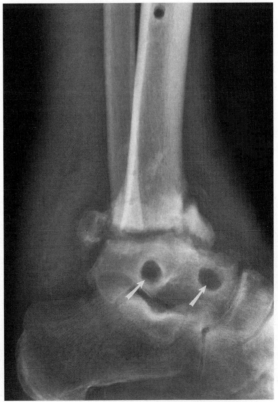

FIG. 10-30. AP (**A**) and lateral (**B**) radiographs of the ankle after removal of the external fixation frame. The talar pin tracts (*arrows*) are expanded because of motion around the pins. Irregularity and sclerosis occur along the fusion site, with no bony union.

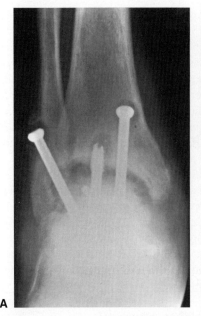
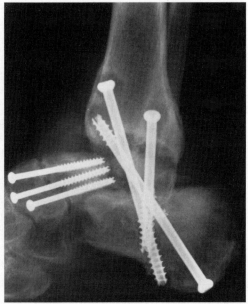

FIG. 10-31. AP (**A**) and lateral (**B**) radiographs after ankle and talonavicular fusion. Obvious lucent zones are seen about the cannulated screws in the tibia and calcaneus resulting from motion and nonunion. Note the lack of bone density in the tibiotalar joint where bone graft was placed. The talar articular surface is barely visible.

rior tibial tendon dysfunction, and other causes of hindfoot pain and instability.[45,46,48,69,81,82,84]

Patients are evaluated clinically using a grading scale similar to that described earlier for the ankle.[60,71,73] Radiographs are evaluated in a similar fashion to that described for ankle arthroplasty (see Figs. 10-24 and 10-25).[41] The talar height, calcaneal pitch angle, tibiocalcaneal angle, and talar-first metatarsal angle are measured on standing lateral views of the foot. The talar height and foot length (distance from posterior calcaneus to the first metatarsal head) are used to calculate the height-to-length ratio. This ratio is compared with postoperative measurements.[47] Joint space congruency and talar tilt can be evaluated on the AP and mortise views.[41,47,68]

Surgical approaches vary. Certain surgeons prefer percu-

taneous pin techniques. However, today internal fixation techniques with staples or cancellous screws and bone grafting are most often preferred.[47,53,80,83] External fixation techniques may be used in selected cases.[50] Subtalar arthrodesis produces the least function loss for the patient, and fusion rates are nearly 100%. Success rates for triple arthrodesis approach 90%.[47,49,68]

Postoperatively, clinical scores and radiographic changes provide data regarding success of surgical procedures. Clinical improvement is based on pain relief, function, and flexibility in use of footwear.[47,68,80] Radiographic measurements are reevaluated and compared with preoperative images (Fig. 10-32). The talocalcaneal and talar–first metatarsal angles are measured on the standing lateral view. Talar height and

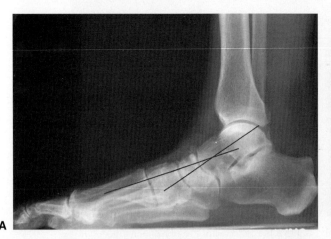
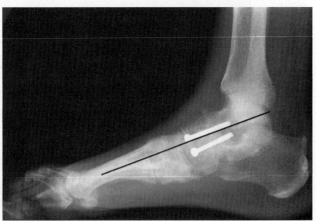

FIG. 10-32. Preoperative and postoperative standing lateral radiographs demonstrating measurements before and after talonavicular arthrodesis for arthrosis. There is improvement (*black lines*) in the talar–first metatarsal angle.

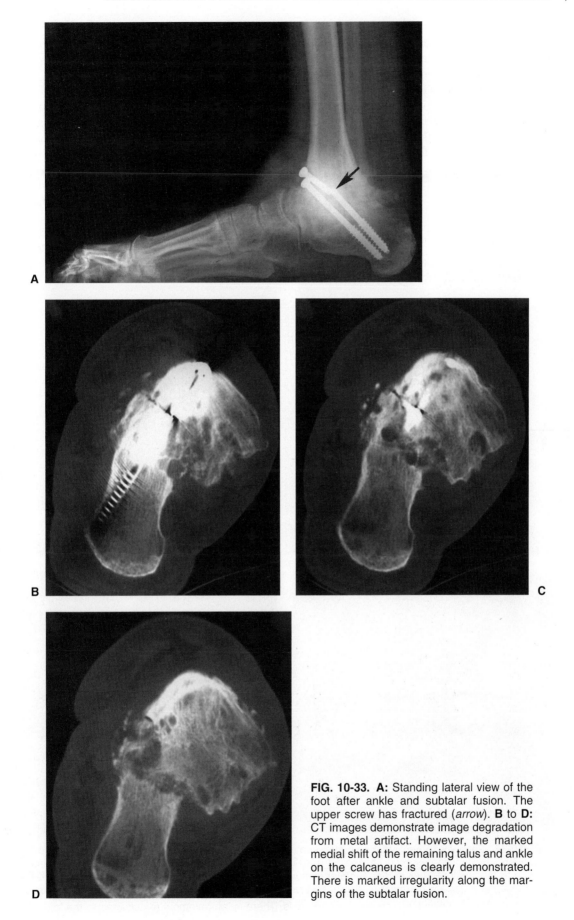

FIG. 10-33. A: Standing lateral view of the foot after ankle and subtalar fusion. The upper screw has fractured (*arrow*). **B** to **D:** CT images demonstrate image degradation from metal artifact. However, the marked medial shift of the remaining talus and ankle on the calcaneus is clearly demonstrated. There is marked irregularity along the margins of the subtalar fusion.

calcaneal pitch or inclination are also measured. The talar-second metatarsal angle, talonavicular congruency, and other measurements (see Chapter 2) are made on the standing AP view of the foot. Changes in preoperative and postoperative measurements vary with the procedure (selected versus triple arthrodesis).[47,53] Graves and colleagues[53] reported improvement in the talocalcaneal angle by an average of 12°, talar-first metatarsal angle by 13°, and 20° improvement in the talar second metatarsal angle of 20° following triple arthrodesis. Cracchiolo and associates[47] noted improvement in these angles and in the height-to-length ratio following hindfoot arthrodesis.

Complications

Complications following hindfoot arthrodesis are similar to those experienced after ankle fusion. Graves and col-leagues[53] reported wound infections in 11%, nonunion in 17%, and talofibular impingement in 5% of patients. Degenerative arthritis in the ankle and nonfused tarsal or tarsometatarsal joints is not uncommon.[46,47,53,57]

Imaging of patients with suspected complications should include serial standing radiographs of the foot and ankle. Infection, nonunion, and other problems such as impingement can often be detected with routine studies (Fig. 10-33). Other imaging procedures may be needed on occasion.[41,62] Selection of the appropriate imaging technique may be complicated by the metal implants (see Fig. 10-33). Both CT and MRI studies may be compromised by metal artifact (Fig. 10-34).[41] Radionuclide scans with combined technetium-99m MDP and indium-111–labeled white blood cell studies may be useful for patients with deep infection. Impingement can usually be identified using routine radiographs. However, in certain cases, stress views may be required.

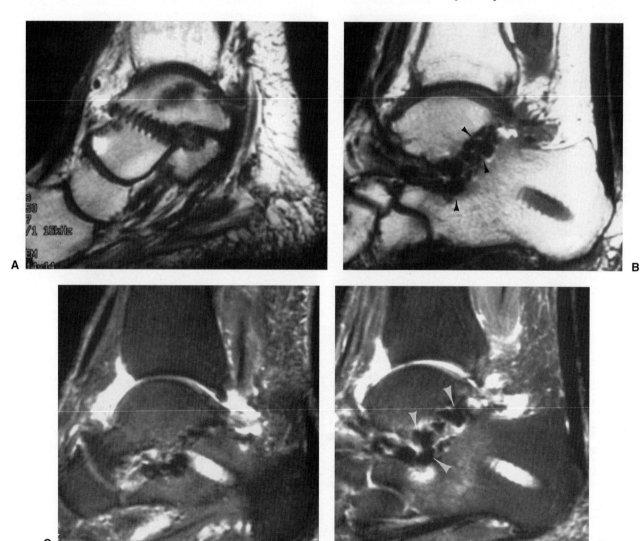

FIG. 10-34. Patient with persistent pain after subtalar arthrodesis MRI scans were obtained to exclude nonunion. Sagittal T1-weighted (**A** and **B**) and T2-weighted (**C** and **D**) images show some artifact related to the screw. However, the subtalar joint space with bone graft seen as areas of low intensity (*arrowheads*) is clearly demonstrated. These are areas of high signal intensity on the T2-weighted images (**C** and **D**), indicating that fusion is not yet solid.

Midfoot and Forefoot Arthrodesis

Indications for midfoot and forefoot arthrodesis are similar to those described in previous sections.[61,68] Intractable pain due to trauma, arthrosis, and other conditions may require arthrodesis. It is not uncommon to correct other conditions such as claw toe or hammer toe deformities simultaneously.[61] Rheumatoid arthritis and hammer toe deformities predominate.[67,68] Forefoot reconstruction is performed when conservative treatment with footwear or orthotics is unsuccessful.

Preoperative imaging includes standing AP and lateral and oblique views of the foot.[41] Comparison with the opposite extremity is often helpful as well (Fig. 10-35). On the standing lateral view, the talar–first metatarsal angle, talocalcaneal angle, and calcaneal inclination are measured. Talar height and foot length can also be evaluated.[46,49,67,68] The hallux valgus angle, talar–second metatarsal angle, and degree of coverage of the talus by the navicular are determined on the standing AP view (see Fig. 10-35).[68] In some cases (Fig. 10-36), preoperative CT studies or diagnostic injections are useful for surgical planning to be sure which joints are affected and may require fusion.[41,62] Diagnostic anesthetic injections are easily performed with fluoroscopic guidance.[42,65]

Postoperatively, images are compared with preoperative measurements (see Figs. 10-35 and 10-36). Evaluation of complications may also require imaging procedures. The type of complications expected depends on the extent of the procedure (Fig. 10-37), the patient's preexisting conditions, and patient compliance.

The most frequent complications after foot arthrodesis include skin slough, infection, nonunion, and malunion.[61,63,67,68] Serial radiographs are often diagnostic for osseous and articular abnormalities. Additional studies such as CT, MRI, radionuclide scans, and bone or joint aspiration and biopsy may be required in selected cases.[41]

HALLUX VALGUS (BUNION)/HALLUX RIGIDUS

Hallux Valgus Deformity

Hallux valgus deformity occurs most frequently in shoe-wearing societies.[87,88] One typically sees lateral deviation of the great toe and varying degrees of medial deviation of the first metatarsal.[97] Although these changes are most obvious, deformity of the interphalangeal joint may also occur. Hypermobility or instability at the medial cuneiform–first metatarsal articulation may be a causative or related problem.[90,98,99]

Although frequently associated with footwear problems, hallux valgus has also been associated with pronation of the hindfoot, pes planus, and increase in the first-second metatarsal angle (Fig. 10-38).[87,89,112] Heredity may also play a role. Hardy and Clapham[93] reported that 63% of patients had a parent with hallux valgus deformity.

A brief review of anatomy critical to this deformity is warranted here. Four muscle groups are involved in the function of the first metatarsophalangeal joint and sesamoids. The extensor hallucis longus and extensor hallucis brevis extend dorsally over the joint (Fig. 10-39). The abductor hallucis is medial and the adductor hallucis muscle lateral

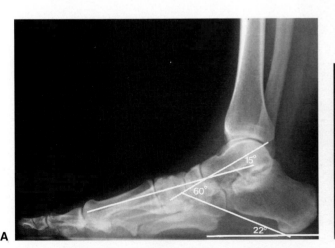
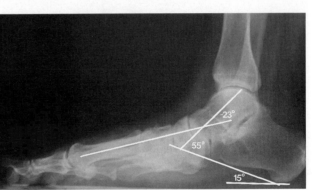

A **B**

FIG. 10-35. A 52-year-old woman with posterior tibial tendon dysfunction, first tarsometatarsal pain, and instability. **A:** Standing lateral views of the asymptomatic foot. The talar–first metatarsal angle is 15°. The talocalcaneal angle is 60°, and the calcaneal inclination is 22°. **B:** Standing lateral view of the involved foot. The talar–first metatarsal angle is −23°, the talocalcaneal angle is 55°, and the calcaneal inclination is 15°. There is obvious tarsometatarsal arthrosis. *(Continued)*

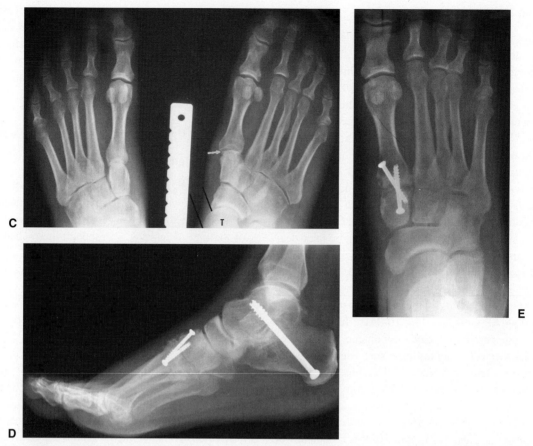

FIG. 10-35. *Continued.* **C:** Standing AP views of the feet demonstrate widening and incongruency of the first tarsometatarsal joint (*arrow*). Note the angular deformity and poor coverage of the talus (*T*) by the navicular (*black lines* mark medial articular margins). There is also an old third metatarsal fracture. **D:** Postoperative nonstanding lateral view after fusion of the subtalar and first tarsometatarsal joints. **E:** Postoperative AP view. Note the improved talonavicular relationship. The talocalcaneal angle is also reduced.

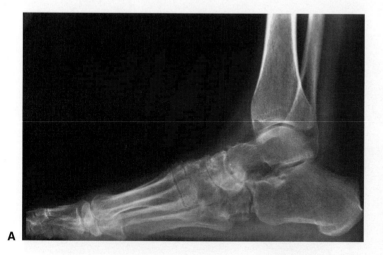

FIG. 10-36. A 40-year-old woman with erosive arthritis involving the left foot. **A:** Standing lateral radiograph demonstrates osteopenia and midfoot erosive changes. *(Continued)*

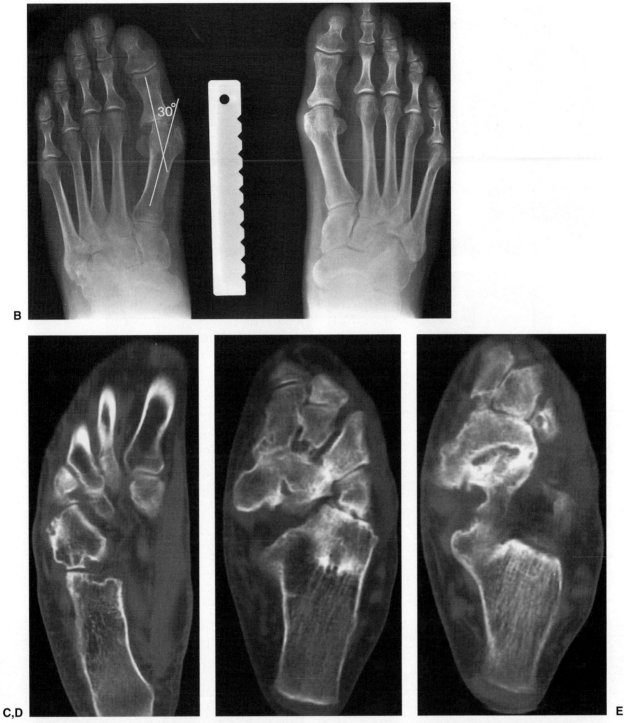

B

C,D   E

FIG. 10-36. *Continued.* **B:** Standing AP view shows narrowed joints in the midfoot with erosive changes, incongruency, and a metatarsophalangeal angle of 30°. **C** to **G:** CT images demonstrate extensive cartilage and bone loss with involvement of multiple tarsal and tarsometatarsal articulations. AP (**H** and **I**), oblique (**J**), and lateral (**K**) views after fusion of the first metatarsophalangeal, talonavicular, calcaneocuboid, navicular cuneiform, and fourth and fifth metatarsal cuboid articulations. *(continued)*

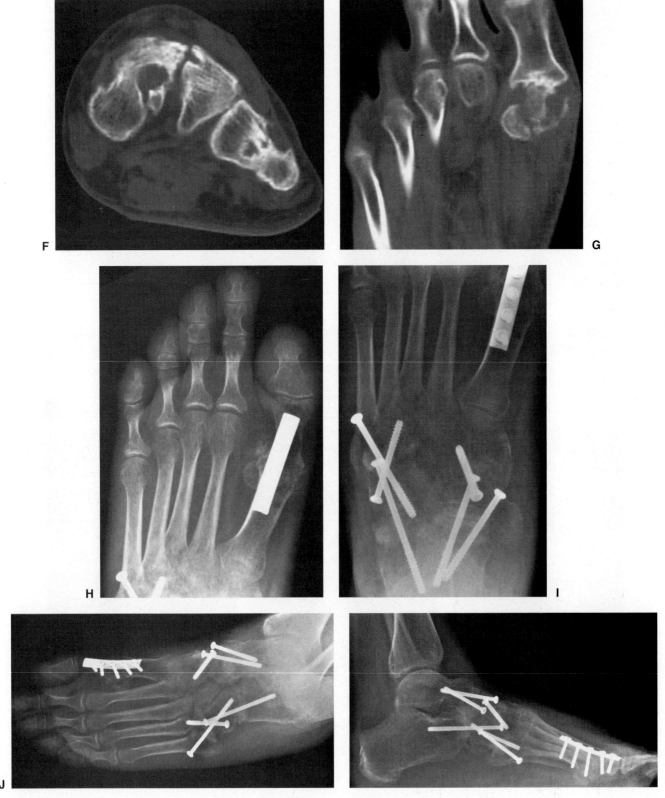

FIG. 10-36. *Continued.*

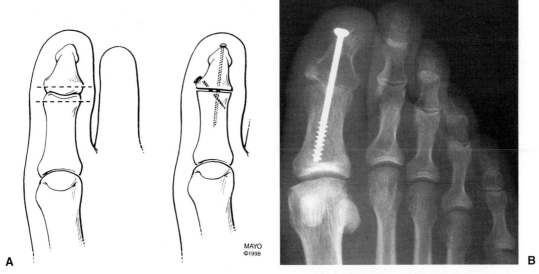

FIG. 10-37. Fusion of the first phalangeal joint with K-wires or a single, partially threaded screw. **A:** Illustration of operative approach and **B:** postoperative AP radiograph.

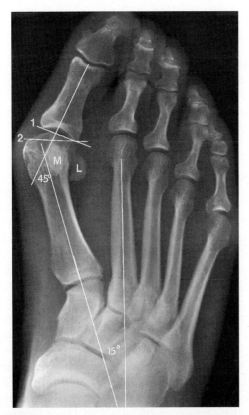

FIG. 10-38. Standing AP radiograph demonstrating a first metatarsophalangeal angle of 45°, a first-second metatarsal angle of 15°, and incongruency of the first metatarsophalangeal joint (*lines 1 and 2*). There is also lateral rotation of the medial (*M*) and lateral (*L*) sesamoids.

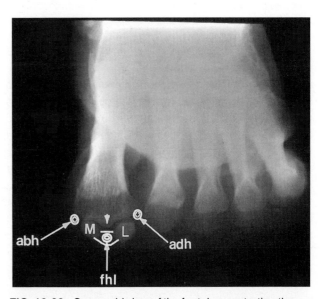

FIG. 10-39. Sesamoid view of the foot demonstrating the medial (*M*) and lateral (*L*) sesamoids separated by the crista (*small arrowhead*). *abh,* abductor hallucis tendon; *fhl,* flexor hallucis longus tendon; *adh,* adductor hallucis tendon.

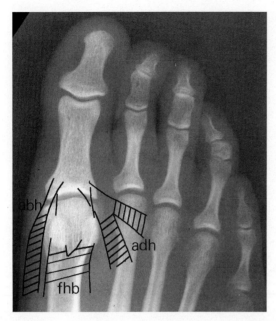

FIG. 10-40. PA radiograph demonstrating the sesamoids and plantar attachments of the abductor hallucis (*abd*), flexor hallucis brevis (*fhb*), and adductor hallucis (*adh*) muscles.

TABLE 10-4. *Hallux valgus (bunion deformity) radiographic assessment[a]*

Standing AP view
  Intermetatarsal (first-second) angle (normal, ≤9°)
  Metatarsophalangeal (hallux valgus) angle (normal, <16°)
  Distal metatarsal articular angle (normal, ≤15°)
  Proximal phalangeal articular angle (normal, <5°)
  Interphalangeal angle (normal, <10°)
  Sesamoid subluxation
  Os intermetatarsareum present or absent
  Joint arthrosis
Standing lateral view
  Talar–first metatarsal angle (normal, 0– ±5°)
  Medial longitudinal arch angle (normal, ≥20°)

[a] Data from references 91, 92, 111, and 112.

required to assist in planning treatment approaches. Oblique views are helpful to assess the degree of arthrosis. Multiple factors and measurements are evaluated on these images. Table 10-4 and Figures 10-41 to 10-44 summarize features that should be evaluated radiographically.

to the great toe (see Fig. 10-39). The sesamoids lie on the plantar aspect of the metatarsal head separated by a notch or crista. The flexor hallucis longus and flexor hallucis brevis pass along the plantar aspect centrally along with the medial and lateral slips of the flexor hallucis brevis, which insert into the medial and lateral sesamoids. The sesamoids are attached to the base of the proximal phalanx by the plantar plate.[97,98,111,112]

In the normally aligned foot, the abductor and adductor hallucis muscles provide major support. The insertion of the adductor hallucis into the base of the proximal phalanx and lateral sesamoid also contributes to the deviation of the proximal phalanx laterally, resulting in hallux valgus deformity. Because of its plantar attachment, the adductor hallucis muscle also pronates the first metatarsal (Fig. 10-40).[111,112]

The approach to treatment of the hallux valgus and associated deformities is based on clinical and radiographic features.[92,97,98,112] Most patients present with pain over the medial aspect of the first metatarsophalangeal joint. Swelling, skin changes, and worsening of symptoms with footwear are also typical. Physical examination permits evaluation of the degree of hallux deformity, metatarsal pronation, and secondary changes such as pes planus and hypermobility of the cuneiform–first metatarsal articulation.[87,88,97,98]

Standing AP, lateral, and, on occasion, sesamoid views are

Treatment

Nonoperative therapy is adequate to relieve symptoms in adolescents and is the first course of action in most adults as well.[87,111,112] Conservative treatment may include changes in footwear and orthotics. Patient compliance is a common problem, especially in young adults and adolescents.[87]

Surgical therapy is reserved for patients with persistent symptoms on conservative programs and for patients with progressive deformity. The goal of surgical therapy is to resolve pain and to restore the articular anatomy of the first metatarsophalangeal joint and other related deformities.[87,97]

Numerous procedures are described in the surgical literature.[85–89,94–112] The procedure selected depends on the symptoms, severity of deformity, and surgical preference. Mann and Coughlin[105] classified deformities as mild, moderate, or severe based on the extent of the hallux valgus angle and other factors (Table 10-5). Mild deformities have a metatarsophalangeal angle (hallux valgus angle) of up to 20° with mild to minimal joint incongruency and slight sesamoid subluxation. The intermetatarsal angle in normal to minimally increased up to 11° (see Fig. 10-42).[105] Moderate hallux valgus deformities have intermetatarsal (first-second) angles of 11° to 18°, a metatarsophalangeal angle of 20° to 40°, and more severe sesamoid subluxation, and the first and second toes are frequently in contact (see Fig. 10-43). Severe deformities have inter-

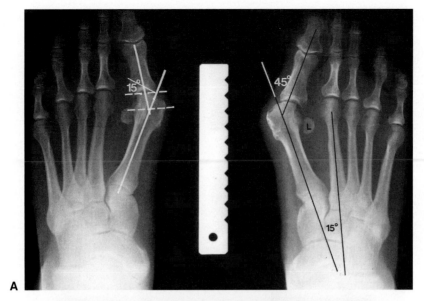

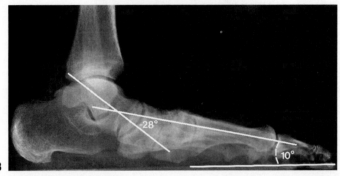

FIG. 10-41. A: Standing AP radiograph demonstrating a first-second intermetatarsal angle on the right of 15° (normal, less than or equal to 9°). The metatarsophalangeal angle is 45° (normal, less than or equal to 16°). The sesamoids are subluxed. The medial sesamoid is under the lateral portion of the metatarsal head, and the lateral sesamoid (L) is completely uncovered. If the lateral sesamoid is 50 to 75% uncovered, subluxation is moderate. In this case, the lateral sesamoid is completely uncovered and the medial sesamoid is lateral. With severe subluxation, this may be the picture, or the medial sesamoid may lie under the lateral sesamoid. On the left, the distal metatarsal articular angle is demonstrated at 15° (normal, less than or equal to 15°). The proximal phalangeal articular angle is also 15° (normal, less than or equal to 5° of valgus). **B:** Standing lateral radiograph demonstrates a talar–first metatarsal angle of −28°. The medial longitudinal arch is 10° (normal, greater than 20°).

metatarsal angles greater than 18°, a metatarsophalangeal angle greater than 40°, and the lateral sesamoid is usually dislocated. Cross-toe deformity is common (see Fig. 10-44).[105,107] The first metatarsal is pronated.[90]

Procedures designed to correct these deformities range from soft tissue repair, osteotomy, and resection arthroplasty to, as described earlier, joint replacement ar-

throplasty.[89,97,98] Mild deformities have been treated using soft tissue repair, distal metatarsal osteotomy (i.e., Chevron), or phalangeal osteotomy (Akin).[89,95–97,100,107,110] These approaches are generally reserved for patients with hallux valgus angles less than 30° and mild increase in the intermetatarsal angle.[89,105,110,112] The Silver repair was modified by McBride[106] and Mann and Coughlin.[104,105] Silver described

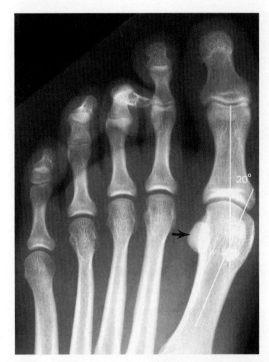

FIG. 10-42. AP radiograph demonstrating mild deformity with a metatarsophalangeal angle of 20° and mild lateral sesamoid subluxation (*arrow*). Note the flexion deformity of the third distal phalangeal joint.

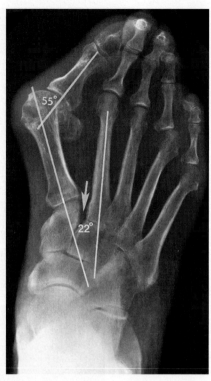

FIG. 10-44. AP radiograph of a severe deformity with a metatarsophalangeal angle of 55°, widening of the first-second metatarsal bases (*arrow*), and an intermetatarsal angle (first-second) of 22°. There is also a cross-toe deformity and sesamoid dislocation.

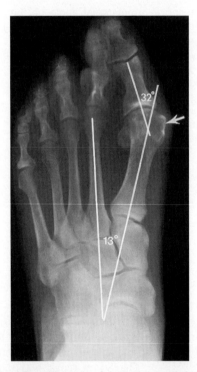

FIG. 10-43. AP radiograph of a moderate deformity with a metatarsophalangeal angle of 32°. The intermetatarsal (first-second) angle is 13°. There is a prominent eminence (*arrow*), and the first and second toes are touching distally.

medial soft tissue repair with resection of the eminence and lateral soft tissue release (Fig. 10-45).[105] McBride[106] modified this procedure adding removal of the lateral sesamoid and transfer of the adductor tendon to the lateral first metatarsal head.[89,106] Later, Mann and Coughlin[105] changed this

TABLE 10-5. *Classification of hallux valgus deformities*[a]

Mild (see Fig. 10-42)
    Metatarsophalangeal angle ≤20°
    Medial eminence
    Joint ± congruent
    Intermetatarsal angle (1–2) ≤11°
    Sesamoids anatomic or <50° subluxation of lateral
      sesamoid
Moderate (see Fig. 10-43)
    Metatarsophalangeal angle 20–40°
    Intermetatarsal angle (1–2) > 11–18°
    ± Contact first–second toes
    Lateral sesamoid subluxed 50–75%
Severe (see Fig. 10-44)
    Metatarsophalangeal angle > 40°
    Intermetatarsal angle (1–2) > 18°
    First–second toes overlap
    Large medial eminence
    Hallux pronated
    Lateral sesamoid dislocated

[a] Data from references 104 and 105.

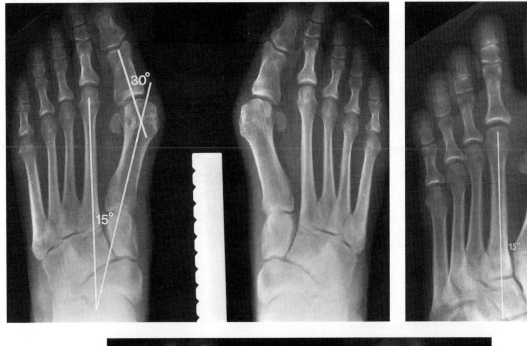

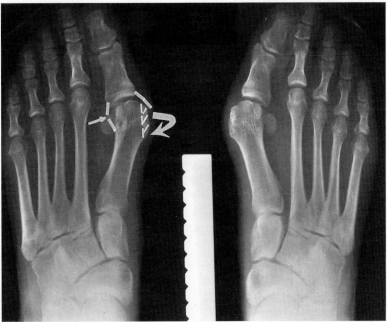

FIG. 10-45. Modified bunion repair. **A:** Preoperative standing AP view of the foot shows a metatarsopha-langeal angle of 30° and a first-second metatarsal angle of 15°. **B:** The medial eminence is resected (*broken line*), the lateral soft tissue is released (*white line, arrow*), and the medial tissues are repaired (*curved arrow*). **C:** Postoperative AP view shows the eminence resection (*arrow*) with a metatarsopha-langeal of 3° (correction of 27°). The intermetatarsal angle (first-second) is 15°.

approach to preserve the lateral sesamoid to avoid hallux varus postoperatively.[105]

The Akin procedure[85] (Fig. 10-46) includes medial eminence resection, medial capsular repair, and a medial closing wedge osteotomy of the proximal phalanx.[85,89] This procedure was designed for patients with mild deformities without significant metatarsus primus varus and mild prominence.[85,97]

The Chevron osteotomy (distal metatarsal osteotomy) is combined with eminence resection and medial soft tissue repair.[95–98,101,104] The Chevron osteotomy (Fig. 10-47) is usually reserved for treatment of patients with mild to moderate hallux valgus deformity (less than 30°) and an intermetatarsal angle less than 13°.[89,95–98] This technique is not designed to correct metatarsal pronation, sesamoid subluxation, or the in-

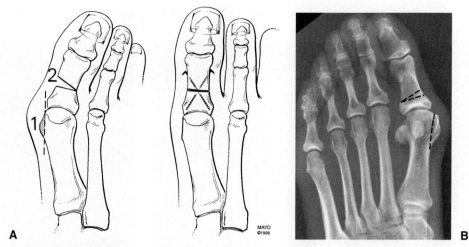

FIG. 10-46. Akin procedure. **A:** Illustration demonstrating resection of the medial eminence (*1*) and a medial closing wedge osteotomy (*2*). **B:** Radiograph with mild hallux valgus deformity demonstrating the Akin procedure (*broken lines*).

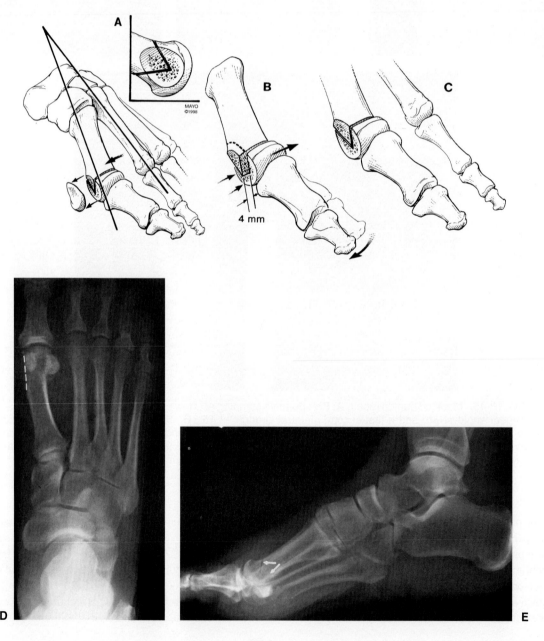

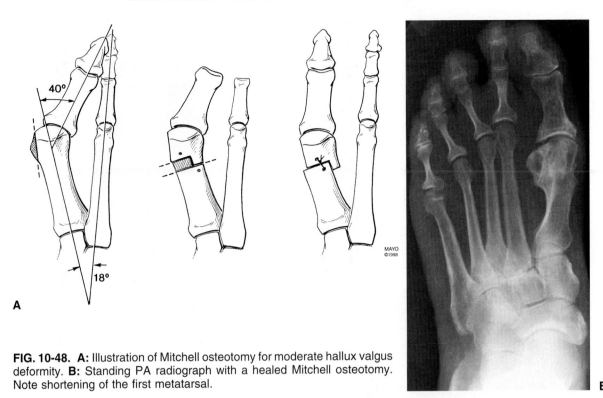

FIG. 10-48. A: Illustration of Mitchell osteotomy for moderate hallux valgus deformity. **B:** Standing PA radiograph with a healed Mitchell osteotomy. Note shortening of the first metatarsal.

termetatarsal angle.[89] The average correction reported for the hallux valgus angle is 12° to 13°.[89,98]

Another approach to distal first metatarsal osteotomy was proposed by Mitchell and others.[107] This procedure (Fig. 10-48) is indicated for moderate hallux valgus (up to 35° to 40°) and intermetatarsal angles less than 18°. The procedure is contraindicated when there is degenerative joint disease, a short first metatarsal, or lateral metatarsalgia.[89,98,107]

Osteotomy of the proximal metatarsal is now a universally acknowledged procedure for moderate to severe hallux valgus (Fig. 10-49) or, in the case of a hypermobile cuneiform–first metatarsal articulation, arthrodesis along with metatarsophalangeal soft tissue repair may be indicated for more severe deformities.[89,98] Arthrodesis of the metatarsophalangeal joint is also reserved for more severe deformities or for patients with rheumatoid arthritis, hallux rigidus, or recurrence after failed bunion repair (Fig. 10-50).[89,98]

Excision or resection arthroplasty (Fig. 10-51) of the proximal phalanx (Keller) is an option for moderate hallux valgus deformity (up to 30°). This procedure is contraindicated in active or young patients or in older patients who require a functioning metatarsophalangeal joint.[89,97,101] Multiple oste-

otomy combinations and soft tissue repairs may be required for severe deformities.[89]

Complications

Postoperative evaluation and complications vary to some degree with the patient's status and the procedure performed. Standing AP and lateral radiographs are essential to measure the degree of correction and to serve as a baseline for recurrence (see Figs. 10-45 and 10-50). Oblique views are useful to assess articular deformity and arthrosis more accurately. The most frequent complications include loss of reduction or recurrent deformity, malunion, nonunion and delayed union, pronation deformity, and pain (Figs. 10-52 and 10-53).[89,110–112] Avascular necrosis of the first metatarsal head was reported in up to 20% of patients after Chevron osteotomy in one series.[89] However, other reports have not noted this complication except on rare occasion.[89] Hallux varus (Fig. 10-54) may occur in up to 11% of patients treated with soft tissue repair and eminence resection (Silver, McBride).[89,106,109,110] Soft tissue slough or superficial wound problems do not require imaging studies for diagnosis.

FIG. 10-47. Chevron repair. **A** to **C:** Illustration of Chevron osteotomy seen from multiple projections. AP (**D**) and lateral (**E**) radiographs after Chevron repair show resection of the eminence (*broken line*). The osteotomy is best seen on the lateral view (*arrows*). Note the V-shaped appearance of the osteotomy.

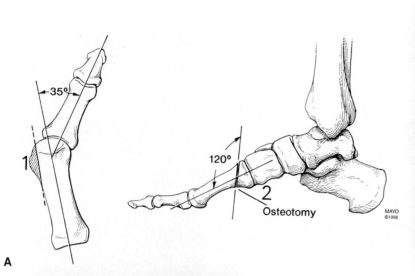
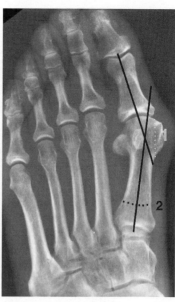
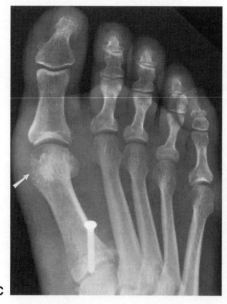
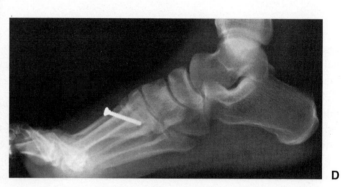

FIG. 10-49. Proximal first metatarsal osteotomy. **A:** Illustration of eminence resection (*1*) and proximal osteotomy (*2*). **B:** AP radiograph demonstrating the eminence resection (*1*) and osteotomy (*2*). AP (**C**) and lateral (**D**) radiographs after eminence resection (*arrow*) and proximal osteotomy with screw fixation.

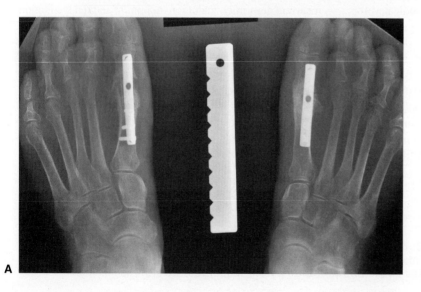

FIG. 10-50. Bilateral first metatarsophalangeal fusions for failed bunion repairs. AP (**A**) and lateral (**B** and **C**) standing views show fusion with dorsal miniplates and screws. There is no residual hallux valgus deformity. The metatarsophalangeal angle is measured on the lateral view. This angle should be 25° to 30°. There are interposition grafts in both metatarsophalangeal joints after removal of silicone implants. *(Continued)*

514

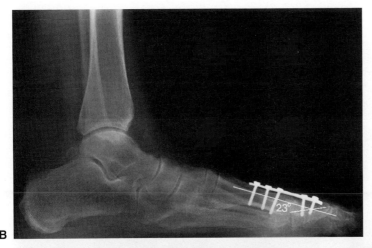

B

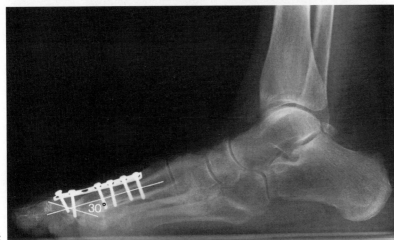

C

FIG. 10-50. *Continued.*

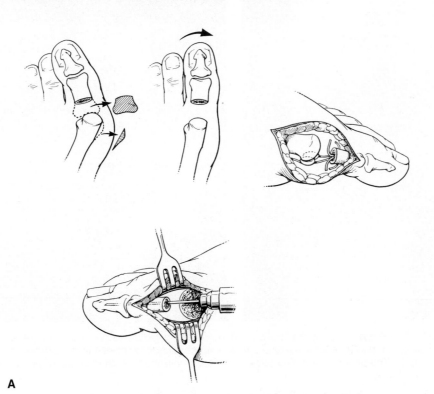

A

FIG. 10-51. Proximal phalangeal resection arthroplasty (Keller). **A:** Illustration of Keller procedure. *(continued)*

515

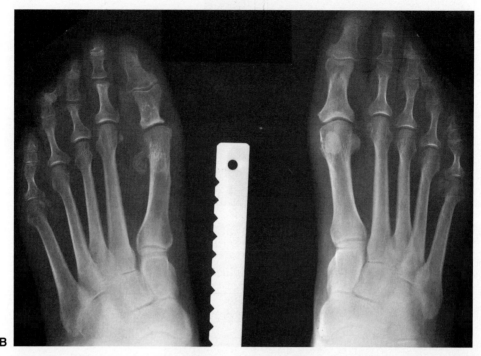

FIG. 10-51. *Continued.* **B:** Standing AP radiograph demonstrating a resection arthroplasty on the left with resection of the eminence. There are also resection arthroplasties of the second and third proximal interphalangeal joints.

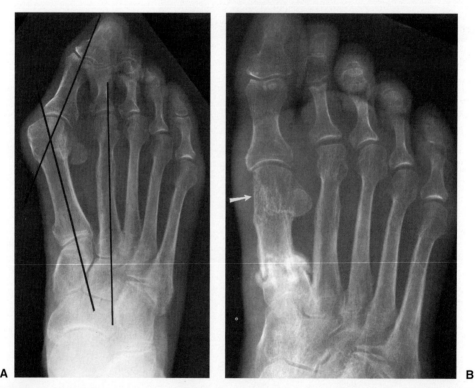

FIG. 10-52. A: AP radiograph preoperatively demonstrating hallux valgus with cross-toe deformity. **B:** AP radiograph 3 months after surgery shows eminence resection (*arrow*) with reduction of the hallux valgus deformity. The proximal first metatarsal osteotomy is irregular, with sclerotic margins suggesting delayed or nonunion.

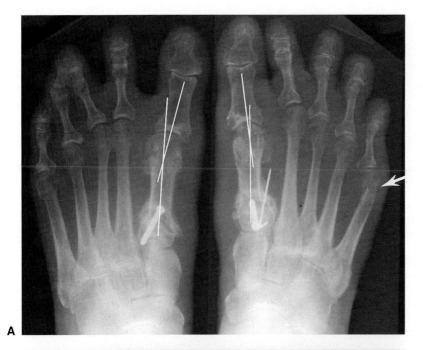

A

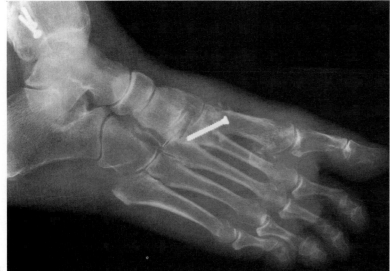

B

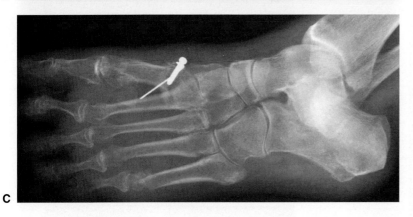

C

FIG. 10-53. Previous bunion repair with proximal first metatarsal osteotomies and pain. **A:** Standing AP radiograph shows irregular callus at both osteotomy sites with hallux varus more marked on the left. There is also a bunionette repair (*arrow*) on the right. **B** and **C:** Bilateral oblique views show soft tissue swelling. The bunionette repair is displaced by design. *(continued)*

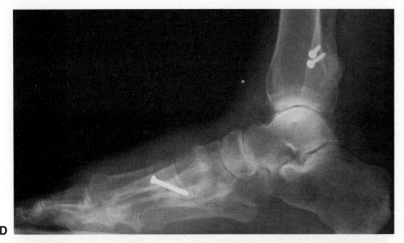

D

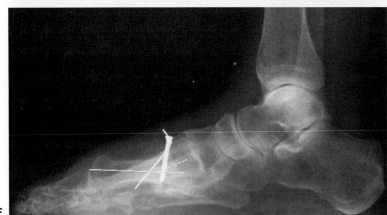

E

FIG. 10-53. *Continued.* **D** and **E:** Standing lateral views show dorsal angulation of the distal first metatarsals, especially on the right (*white lines*). There is dorsal soft tissue swelling bilaterally.

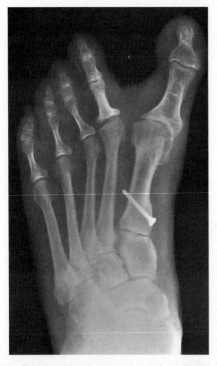

FIG. 10-54. Previous bunion repair on the left with resection of the lateral sesamoid. Severe arthrosis and hallux varus deformity (grade III) are noted.

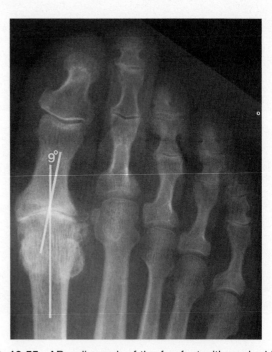

FIG. 10-55. AP radiograph of the forefoot with marked joint space narrowing and osteophyte formation. There is no hallux valgus deformity. The metatarsophalangeal angle is only 9°.

Serial radiographs are usually adequate to image complications and to confirm recurrence. CT may be useful for evaluating bone stock before revision surgery. MRI is useful for evaluating nonunion, tendon shift, and avascular necrosis.[92]

Hallux Rigidus

Hallux rigidus is a painful disorder of the first metatarsophalangeal joint with bone proliferation (osteophytes), diminished range of motion, and no subluxation (Fig. 10-55).[103,104] This condition is the second most common painful condition after hallux valgus deformity. Symptoms are usually unilateral and may be related to previous trauma.[97] Hallux rigidus can be seen in adolescents and adults. Radiographically, the joint space is narrowed with marginal osteophytes. Dorsal osteophytes may cause impingement. Osseous and articular changes are easily identified on AP, lateral, and oblique radiographs (Fig. 10-56).[97,103,104]

Radiographs are used to grade this condition. Grade I changes show mild to moderate osteophytes with a normal or minimally narrowed joint space (Fig. 10-57). Grade II hallux rigidus demonstrates moderate osteophytes with joint space narrowing and subchondral sclerosis. Grade III changes are more severe (see Figs. 10-55 and 10-56) with loss of the joint space and dorsal and plantar osteophytes on the lateral radiograph.[97]

Multiple surgical procedures have been used to correct

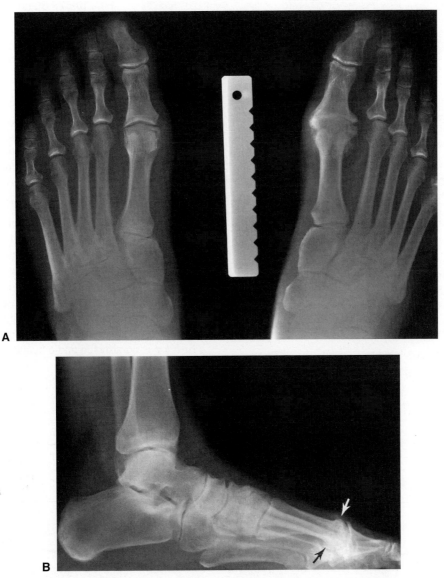

FIG. 10-56. Standing AP (**A**) and lateral (**B**) radiographs demonstrate the typical features of hallux rigidus with prominent marginal osteophytes on the AP view (**A**), and dorsal (*white arrow*) osteophytes and inferior osteophytes (*black arrow*) on the lateral view (**B**) (grade III, hallux rigidus).

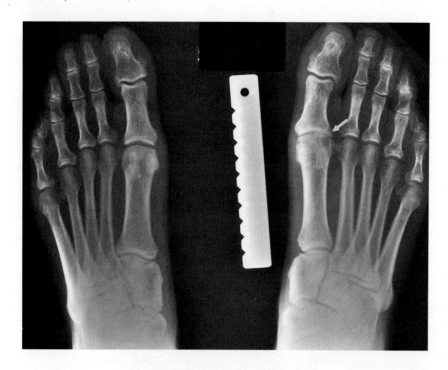

FIG. 10-57. Standing AP radiograph of the left foot. The first metatarsophalangeal joint on the left is normal. The joint on the right is slightly narrowed with an early lateral osteophyte (*arrow*).

this disorder including arthrodesis, resection with soft tissue interposition, and the Keller procedure (see Fig. 10-51B) described earlier.[97,103,104] Joint replacement arthroplasty has been advocated, but this technique has not been consistently successful for hallux rigidus.[88]

Cheilectomy removes 20 to 30% of the dorsal metatarsal head (Fig. 10-58). This technique is useful when, in addition to pain, impingement is the major problem.[97,103,104] The Moberg procedure[108] can occasionally be used to treat hallux rigidus. This technique includes resection of the dorsal eminence and a closing wedge phalangeal osteotomy (Fig. 10-59).[105,108] The phalanx is placed in slight dorsiflexion using a K-wire to secure the osteotomy.[103,108,112]

DEFORMITIES OF THE LESSER TOES

Digital deformities involving the second through fifth toes and metatarsophalangeal joints are usually more easily clas-

sified clinically. Radiographs are often not required except for surgical planning.[114–116,119] Thompson[120] and others have defined these deformities and described treatment approaches.[114,116,118,120] Some deformities are more common in children, whereas others are more commonly seen in adolescents and adults.[119,120] Common conditions and descriptions are summarized as follows:

Curly toe deformities: This is common in children and may be referred to as overlapping toes. The toe is flexed at the proximal interphalangeal joint with lateral rotation and varus deformity. This condition is secondary to shortening of the flexor digitorum brevis and longus muscles.[114,120]

Overlapping fifth toe: This condition is typically bilateral. The deformity is familial and presents with pain and adduction of the fifth toe dorsally over the fourth toe.[120] The fifth toe is dorsiflexed and extended at the metatarsophalangeal joint.[119,120]

Hammer toe: This is a sagittal plane deformity with flexion

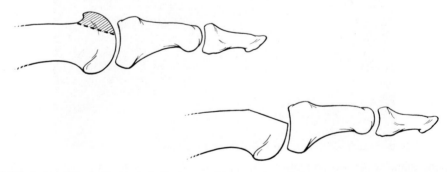

FIG. 10-58. Lateral illustrations of cheilectomy with resection of the dorsal metatarsal head.

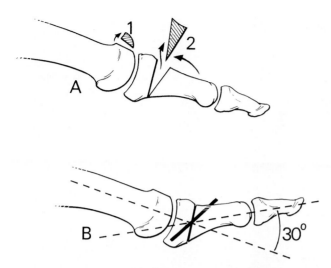

FIG. 10-59. A: Lateral illustration of the Moberg procedure for hallux rigidus. The dorsal eminence is removed (*1*), and a phalangeal wedge osteotomy is performed (*2*). **B:** The osteotomy can be internally fixed with a K-wire with a resulting metatarsophalangeal angle of 20° to 30°.

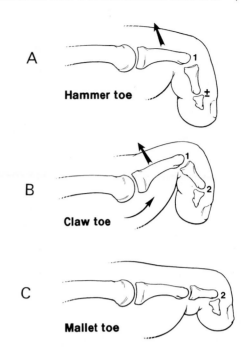

FIG. 10-60. Illustrations of common lesser toe deformities. **A:** Hammer toe: The proximal interphalangeal joint is flexed (*1*). The distal interphalangeal joint may also be flexed (±). Metatarsophalangeal hyperextension (*arrow*) occurring over time may then create a claw toe. The second toe is most commonly affected. **B:** Claw toe: The metatarsophalangeal joint is hyperextended (*arrow*). The proximal interphalangeal joint is flexed (*1*). The distal interphalangeal (*2*) joint is shown flexed but may be uninvolved as well. **C:** Mallet toe: There is a flexion deformity of the distal interphalangeal joint (*2*). The second toes are most commonly affected. There is no hyperextension of the metatarsophalangeal joint or flexion of the proximal interphalangeal joint.

of the proximal interphalangeal joint. The distal interphalangeal joint may also be flexed. The metatarsophalangeal joint eventually hyperextends. This condition is usually bilateral and most often involves the second toe (Fig. 10-60A).[120] The second metatarsal is commonly elongated.[119,120]

Claw toe: There is hyperextension of the metatarsophalangeal joint with flexion deformity of the proximal interphalangeal joint. The distal interphalangeal joint may also be flexed. This condition usually affects all four lesser toes bilaterally and may be associated with pes cavus deformity (see Fig. 10-60B).[119,120] Other causes include neuropathic foot, trauma, and posterior compartment syndrome.

Mallet toe: This condition results in a flexion deformity of the distal interphalangeal joint (see Fig. 10-60C). The cause is believed to be shortening of the flexor digitorum longus.[120] This condition also usually affects the second toe and, like hammer toe deformity, is associated with a long second metatarsal.[114,119,120]

Numerous other conditions are recognized, including polydactyly, syndactyly, and congenital bands. Common pediatric disorders are reviewed in Chapter 9.

Routine radiographs (Fig. 10-61) are usually not required for diagnosis. However, routine studies may be needed to make appropriate measurements and to assess all tarsal and forefoot deformities that may affect the approach to therapy.

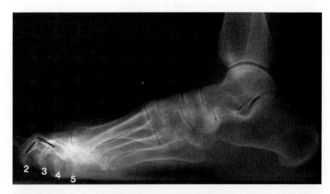

FIG. 10-61. Standing lateral radiograph in a patient with claw toe deformities. The bony overlap compromises the ability to evaluate the toes in the sagittal plane. All four lesser toes (2 to 5) are involved.

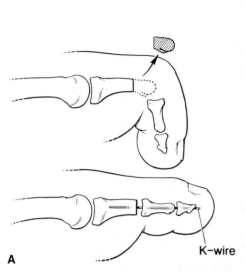
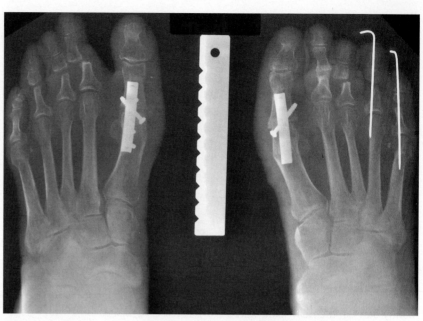

FIG. 10-62. A: Illustration of resection of the distal proximal phalanx with K-wire fixation. **B:** Patient with failed bunion repairs treated with arthrodesis. Resection arthroplasties were performed on the left second to fourth and right second to fifth lesser toes for digital deformities. There is K-wire fixation of the right fourth and fifth toes.

For many of the lesser toe deformities, conservative therapy is ineffective.[114,119,120] Therefore, soft tissue repair with or without resection arthroplasty is usually indicated. K-wire fixation is sometimes required to maintain alignment after resection arthroplasty (Fig. 10-62).[114,120]

Subungual exostosis mimics an osteochondroma. This benign exostosis (Fig. 10-63) is most common in the distal phalanx of the great toe, usually just below the nail bed.[114,118] The lesser toes are less frequently involved.[117] The cause is uncertain, although trauma has been implicated.[118] The condition may be painful and may mimic an ingrown toenail.

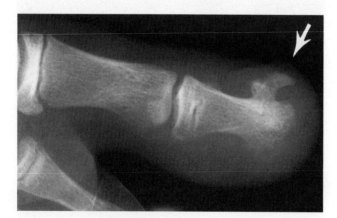

FIG. 10-63. Oblique radiograph of the great toe demonstrating a subungual exostosis (*arrow*).

These lesions require surgical excision when they are symptomatic because conservative therapy is ineffective. Recurrence is possible (11%) after surgical resection.[118]

Bunionette deformities are similar to the more common great toe bunion deformity, but they involve the lateral foot.[113–115,117] There is a painful prominence of the fifth metatarsal head. There may be associated lateral bowing of the distal fifth metatarsal (Fig. 10-64). With more severe deformity, one sees an increase in the fourth-fifth metatarsal angle (normal 6°, range 3° to 11°).[115,117]

Bunionette deformity is related to footwear, especially in females.[113] Patients with increased fourth-fifth metatarsal angles are more often symptomatic (see Fig. 10-64B).[115,117]

Bunionette repair, like bunion repair, may be accomplished with resection of the eminence, an osteotomy, and soft tissue repair (Fig. 10-65). Distal or proximal fifth metatarsal osteotomy may be required for more severe deformities.[115,117,119]

The goals of surgical repair for the foregoing lesser toe deformities are to relieve pain, to correct the deformity, and to improve function and weight-bearing mechanics.[113,117,119] Complications include loss of reduction, overcorrection, and infection.[117,120]

Routine radiographs are usually not required to diagnose these disorders. However, serial radiographs are useful to evaluate complications. In some cases, additional studies such as MRI or aspiration (for suspected infection) may be indicated.

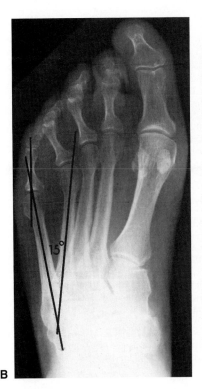
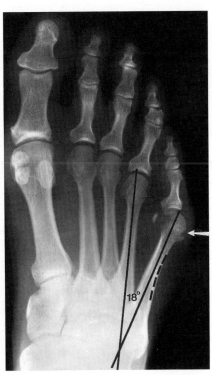

A,B

FIG. 10-64. Bunionette deformities. **A:** Bunionette deformity with a fourth-fifth metatarsal angle of 15°. **B:** More severe bunionette deformity with prominence of the metatarsal head and bone erosion (*arrow*), lateral bowing (*broken line*), and a fourth-fifth metatarsal angle of 18°.

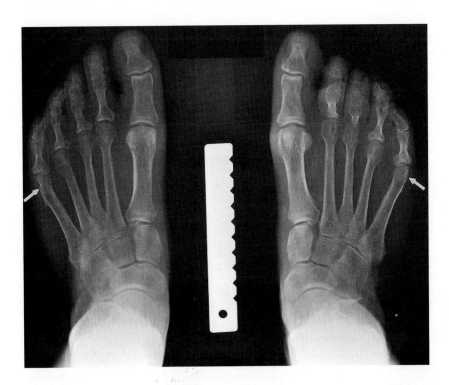

FIG. 10-65. Standing AP views of the feet after bunionette repair with resection of the eminence on the metatarsal heads (*arrows*), resulting in a linear lateral margin.

REFERENCES

Arthroplasty

1. Berquist TH. MRI of the Musculoskeletal System, 3rd Ed. New York, Lippincott-Raven, 1996.
2. Berquist TH. Imaging Atlas of Orthopedic Appliances and Prosthesis. New York, Raven Press, 1995.
3. Berquist TH. Diagnostic and therapeutic injections as an aid to musculoskeletal diagnosis. Semin. Intervent. Radiol. 1993; 10:326–343.
4. Buechel FF, Pappas MJ, Iorio LF. New Jersey low contact stress total ankle replacement. Biomechanical rationale and review of 23 cementless cases. Foot Ankle 1988; 8:279–290.
5. Burge P, Evans M. Effect of surface replacement arthroplasty on stability of the ankle. Foot Ankle 1986; 7:10–17.
6. Craccihiolo A III, Kitaoka HB, Leventen EO. Silicone implant arthroplasty for the second metatarsophalangeal joint disorders with and without hallux valgus deformities. Foot Ankle 1988; 9:10–18.
7. Craccihiolo A III, Weltmer JB, Lian G, Dalseth T, Dorey F. Arthroplasty of the first metatarsophalangeal joint with a double-stem silicone implant. J. Bone Joint Surg. Am. 1992; 74:552–563.
8. Dini AA, Bassett FH III. Evaluation and early result of Smith total ankle replacement. Clin. Orthop. 1980; 146:228–230.
9. Grace DL. The surgical management of the rheumatoid foot. Br. J. Hosp. Med. 1996; 56:473–480.
10. Granberry WM, Noble PC, Bishop JO, Tullos HS. Use of hinged silicone prosthesis for replacement arthroplasty of the first metatarsophalangeal joint. J. Bone Joint Surg. Am. 1991; 73:1453–1459.
11. Harnroongroj T, Vanadurongwan V. The talar body prosthesis. J. Bone Joint Surg. Am. 1997; 79:1313–1322.
12. Hensley JP. Anterior ankle arthroplasty. Clin. Podiatr. Med. Surg. 1991; 8:625–635.
13. Hensley JP, Saltrick K, Le T. Anterior ankle arthroplasty. A retrospective study. J. Foot Surg. 1990; 29:169–172.
14. Hocher K. The skeletal radiology of the distal tibiofibular joint. Arch. Orthop. Trauma Surg. 1994; 113:345–346.
15. Johnson KA. Total ankle arthroplasty. In Morrey BF, ed. Joint Replacement Arthroplasty. New York, Churchill Livingstone, 1991; pp. 1173–1182.
16. Johnson KA, Buck PG. Total replacement arthroplasty of the first metatarsophalangeal joint. Foot Ankle 1981; 1:307–314.
17. Kampner SL. Long-term experience with total joint prosthetic replacement for the arthritic great toe. Bull. Hosp. Joint. Dis. 1987; 47:153–177.
18. Khoury NJ, El-Khoury GY, Saltzman CL, Brandser EA. Intra-articular foot and ankle injections to identify source of pain before arthrodesis. AJR Am. J. Roentgenol. 1995; 167:669–673.
19. Kitaoka HB, Patzer GL. Clinical results after Mayo total ankle arthroplasty. J. Bone Joint Surg. Am. 1995; 78:1658–1664.
20. Kitaoka HB. Salvage of non-union following ankle arthrodesis for failed total ankle arthroplasty. Clin. Orthop. 1991; 268:37–43.
21. Kitaoka HB, Craccihiolo A III. Stress fracture of the lateral metatarsal following double-stemmed silicone implant arthroplasty of the hallux metatarsophalangeal joint. Clin. Orthop. 1989; 239:211–216.
22. Kitaoka HB, Romness DW. Arthrodesis for failed ankle arthroplasty. J. Arthroplasty 1992; 7: 277–2894.
23. Kofoed H. Medium-Term results of cementless Scandinavian Total Ankle Replacement Prosthesis (Link S.T.A.R.) for osteoarthritis. In Kofoed H, ed. Current Status of Ankle Arthroplasty. Berlin, Springer-Verlag, 1998; pp. 116–120.
24. Kofoed H. Cylindrical cemented ankle arthroplasty. A prospective series with long-term follow-up. Foot Ankle Int. 1995; 16:474–479.
25. Laird L. Silastic joint arthroplasty of the great toe. A review of 228 implants using the double-stemmed implant. Clin. Orthop. 1990;255: 268–272.
26. Lucas PE, Hurwitz SR, Kaplan PA, Dussault RG, Mauer EJ. Fluoroscopically guided injections into the foot and ankle. Localization of the source of pain as a guide to treatment-prospective study. Radiology 1997; 204:411–415.
27. Lund PJ, Nisbet JK, Valencia FG, Ruth JT. Current sonographic applications in orthopedics AJR Am. J. Roentgenol. 1996; 166:889–895.
28. Mann RA, Horton GA. Management of foot and ankle in rheumatoid arthritis. Rheum. Dis. Clin. North Am. 1996; 22:457–476.
29. McMaster WC. Total ankle arthroplasty. Adv. Orthop. Surg. 1996; 9:264–272.
30. Moeckel BH, Sculco TP, Alexiodes MM, Dossick PH, Inglis AE, Ranawat CS. The double-stemmed silicone rubber implant for rheumatoid arthritis of the first metatarsophalangeal joint. J. Bone Joint Surg. Am. 1992; 74:564–570.
31. Pappas M, Buechel FF, DePalma AF. Cylindrical total ankle joint replacement. Clin. Orthop. 1976; 118:82–92.
32. Saltzman CL, Brandser EA, Berbaum KS, DeGnore L, Holmes JR, Katcherian DA, Teasdall RD, Alexander IJ. Reliability of standard foot radiographic measurements. Foot Ankle Int. 1994; 15:661–665.
33. Saltzman CL, Nawoczenski DA, Talbot BS. Measurement of the medial longitudinal arch. Arch. Phys. Med. Rehabil. 1995; 76:45–49.
34. Schernberg F. Current results of ankle arthroplasty. European multicenter study of cementless ankle arthroplasty. In Kofoed H, ed. Current Status of Ankle Arthroplasty. Berlin, Springer-Verlag, 1998; pp. 41–46.
35. Scholz KC. Total ankle arthroplasty using biological fixation components compared to ankle arthrodesis. Orthopedics 1987; 10:125–131.
36. Smith EJ, Wood PLR. Ankle arthrodesis in the rheumatoid patient. J. Bone Joint Surg. Br. 1990; 72:530.
37. Stockley I, Betts RP, Getty CJ, Rowley DI, Duckworth T. A prospective study of forefoot arthroplasty. Clin. Orthop. 1989; 248:213–218.
38. Swanson AB, de Groot Swanson G, Mayhew DE, Khan AN. Flexible hinge results in implant arthroplasty of the great toe. Rheumatology 1987; 11:136–152.
39. Takabura Y, Tanaka Y, Sugimoto K, Tamai S, Masahara K. Ankle arthroplasty. A comparative study of cemented metal and uncemented ceramic prosthesis. Clin. Orthop. 1990; 252:209–216.

Arthrodesis

40. Anderson JG, Coetzee C, Hansen ST. Revision ankle fusion using internal compression arthrodesis with screw fixation. Foot Ankle Int. 1997; 18:300–309.
41. Berquist TH. Imaging Atlas of Orthopedic Appliances and Prostheses. New York, Raven Press, 1995.
42. Berquist TH. Diagnostic and therapeutic injections as an aid to musculoskeletal diagnosis. Semin. Intervent. Radiol. 1993; 10:326–343.
43. Bishop AT, Wood MB, Sheetz KK. Arthrodesis of the ankle with free vascularized autogenous bone graft. J. Bone Joint Surg. Am. 1995; 77:1867–1875.
44. Bono JV, Rogers DJ, Jacobs RL. Surgical arthrodesis of the neuropathic foot. Clin. Orthop. 1993; 296:14–20.
45. Carrier DA, Harris CM. Ankle arthrodesis with vertical Steinmann's pins in rheumatoid arthritis Clin. Orthop. 1991; 268:10–14.
46. Cracchiolo A. Surgical arthrodesis techniques for foot and ankle pathology. Instr. Course Lect. 1990; 39:49–63.
47. Cracchiolo A, Pearson S, Kitaoka H, Grace D. Hindfoot arthrodesis in adults utilizing a dowel graft technique. Clin. Orthop. 1990; 257: 193–203.
48. Crosby LA, Yee TC, Ormanek TS, Fitzgibbons TC. Complications following arthroscopic ankle arthrodesis. Foot Ankle Int. 1996; 17: 340–342.
49. Danziger MB, Abdo RV, Decher E. Distal tibial bone graft for arthrodesis of the foot and ankle. Foot Ankle Int. 1995; 16:187–190.
50. Decoster T, Alvarez R, Trevino S. External fixation of the foot and ankle. Foot Ankle 1986; 7:40–48.
51. Dennis DA, Clayton ML, Wong DA, Mack RP, Susman MH. Internal fixation compression arthrodesis of the ankle. Clin. Orthop. 1990; 253:212–220.
52. Frey C, Halikies NM, Vu-Rose T, Ebramzadeh E. A review of ankle arthrodesis. Predisposing factors to non-union. Foot Ankle Int. 1994; 15:581–584.
53. Graves SC, Mann RA, Graves KO. Triple arthrodesis in older adults. J. Bone Joint Surg. Am. 1993; 75:355–362.
54. Helm R. The results of ankle arthrodesis. J. Bone Joint Surg. Br. 1990; 72:141–143.
55. Holt ES, Hansen ST, Mayo KH, Scingeorzan BJ. Ankle arthrodesis using internal screw fixation. Clin. Orthop. 1991; 268:21–28.
56. Khoury NJ, El-Khoury GY, Saltzman CL, Brandser EA. Intra-articular foot and ankle injections to identify source of pain before arthrodesis. AJR Am. J. Roentgenol. 1996; 167:669–673.

57. Kitaoka HB, Alexander JJ, Adelaar RS, Nunley JA, Myerson MS, Sanders M. Clinical rating systems for ankle-hindfoot, midfoot, hallux and lesser toes. Foot Ankle Int. 1994; 15:349–353.

58. Kitaoka HB, Anderson PJ, Morrey BF. Revision of ankle arthrodesis with external fixation for non-union. J. Bone Joint Surg. Am. 1992; 74:1191–1200.

59. Kitaoka HB, Lundberg A, Luo ZP, An K-N. Kinematics of the normal arch of the foot and ankle under physiologic loading. Foot Ankle Int. 1995; 16:492–499.

60. Kitaoka HB, Patzer GL. Arthrodesis for treatment of arthrosis of the ankle and osteonecrosis of the talus. J. Bone Joint Surg. Am. 1998; 80:370–379.

61. Komenda GA, Myerson MS, Biddinger KR. Results of arthrodesis of the tarsometatarsal joints after traumatic injury. J. Bone Joint Surg. Am. 1996; 78:1665–1676.

62. Kuszyk BS, Heath DG, Bliss DF, Fishman EK. Skeletal 3-D CT. Advantages of volume rendering over surface rendering. Skeletal Radiol. 1996; 25:207–214.

63. Lidor C, Ferris LR, Hall R, Alexander IJ, Nunley JA. Stress fracture of the tibia after arthrodesis of the ankle or hindfoot. J. Bone Joint Surg. Am. 1997; 79:558–564.

64. Loder BG, Frascone ST, Wertheimer SJ. Tibiofibular arthrodesis for malunion of the talocrural joint. J. Foot Ankle Surg. 1995; 34:283–288.

65. Lucas PE, Hurwitz SR, Kaplan PA, Dussault RG, Maurer EJ. Fluoroscopically guided injections into the foot and ankle. Localization of the source of pain as a guide to treatment. Prospective study. Radiology 1997; 204:411–415.

66. Malarkey RF, Buiski JC. Ankle arthrodesis with the Calandruccio frame and bimalleolar on lay grafting. Clin. Orthop. 1991; 268:44–48.

67. Mann RA, Horton GA. Management of the foot and ankle in rheumatoid arthritis. Rheum. Dis. Clin. North Am. 1996; 22:457–475.

68. Mann RA, Prieskorn D, Sobel M. Mid-tarsal and tarsometatarsal arthrodesis for primary degenerative osteoarthrosis or arthrosis after trauma. J. Bone Joint Surg. Am. 1996; 78:1376–1385.

69. Mann RA, VanMonen JW, Wapner K, Martin J. Ankle fusion. Clin. Orthop. 1991; 268:49–55.

70. Mauer RC, Cimino WR, Cox CV, Satow GK. Transarticular cross-screw fixation. A technique of ankle arthrodesis. Clin. Orthop. 1991; 268:49-55.

71. Mazur JM, Cummings RJ, McClusky WP, Lovell WW. Ankle arthrodesis in children. Clin. Orthop. 1991; 268:65–69.

72. Mazur JM, Schwartz E, Simon SR. Ankle arthrodesis. Long-term follow-up with gait analysis. J. Bone Joint Surg. Am. 1979; 61:964–975.

73. Miller SD. Late reconstruction after failed treatment for ankle fractures. Orthop Clin. North Am. 1995; 26:313–373.

74. Moekel BH, Patterson BM, Inglis AE, Sculco TP. Ankle arthrodesis. A comparison of internal and external fixation. Clin. Orthop. 1991; 268:78–83.

75. Moore TJ, Prince R, Pochatko D, Smith JW, Fleming S. Retrograde intramedullary nailing for ankle arthrodesis. Foot Ankle Int. 1995; 16:433–436.

76. Moran CG, Pinder IM, Smith SR. Ankle arthrodesis in rheumatoid arthritis. 30 cases followed for 5 years. Acta Orthop. Scand. 1991; 62:538–543.

77. Papa J, Myerson M, Girard P. Salvage with arthrodesis in intractable diabetic neuropathic arthropathy of the foot and ankle. J. Bone Joint Surg. Am. 1993; 75:1056–1066.

78. Paremain GD, Miller SD, Myerson MS. Ankle arthrodesis. Results after mini-arthrotomy technique. Foot Ankle Int. 1996; 17:247–252.

79. Resnick RB, Jahss MH, Choueka J, Kummer F, Hersch JO, Okereke E. Deltoid ligament forces after tibialis posterior tendon rupture. Effects of triple arthrodesis and calcaneal displacement osteotomies. Foot Ankle Int. 1995; 16:14–20.

80. Sangeorzan BJ, Smith D, Vieth R, Hansen ST. Triple arthrodesis using internal fixation in treatment of adult foot disorders. Clin. Orthop. 1993; 294:299–307.

81. Schaap EJ, Huy J, Tonino AJ. Long-term results of arthrodesis of the ankle. Int. Orthop. 1990; 14:9–12.

82. Stranks GJ, Cecil T, Jeffery ITA. Anterior ankle arthrodesis with cross-screw fixation. J. Bone Joint Surg. Br. 1994; 76:943–946.

83. Tisdel CL, Marcus RE, Heiple KG. Triple arthrodesis for diabetic peritalar neuro-arthropathy. Foot Ankle Int. 1995; 16:332–338.

84. vanValburg AA, vanRoermund PM, Lammens J, vanMelkebeek J, Verbout AJ, Lafeber FPJG, Bijlsma JWJ. Can Ilizarov joint distraction delay the need for an arthrodesis of the ankle? J. Bone Joint Surg. Br. 1995; 77:720–725.

Hallux Valgus (Bunion)/Hallux Rigidus

85. Akin OF. The treatment of hallux valgus. A new procedure and its results. Med Sentinel 1925; 33:678–679.

86. Canale PB, Aronsson PD, Lamont RL, Manoli A II. The Mitchell procedure for treatment of adolescent hallux valgus. J. Bone Joint Surg. Am. 1993; 75:1610–1618.

87. Coughlin MJ. Hallux valgus. J. Bone Joint Surg. Am. 1996; 78:932–965.

88. Coughlin MJ. Juvenile bunions. In Mann RA, Coughlin MJ, eds. Surgery of the Foot and Ankle. 6th Ed. St. Louis, Mosby-Year Book, 1993, pp. 341–412.

89. Craccihiolo A III, Weltmer JB, Lian G, Delseth T, Dorey F. Arthroplasty of the first metatarsophalangeal joint with double-stem silicone implant. J. Bone Joint Surg. Am. 1992; 74:552–563.

90. Eustace S, O'Bryne J, Beausang O, Codd M, Stack J, Stephens MM. Hallux valgus, first metatarsal pronation and collapse of the medial longitudinal arch. A radiological correlation. Skeletal Radiol. 1994; 23:191–194.

91. Eustace S, O'Bryne J, Stack J, Stephens MM. Radiographic features enable assessment of first metatarsal rotation: The role of pronation in hallux valgus. Skeletal Radiol. 1993; 22:153–156.

92. Eustace S, Williamson D, Wilson M, O'Byrne J, Bussolari L, Thomas M, Stephens M, Stack J, Weissman B. Tendon shift in hallux valgus: observations at MR imaging. Skeletal Radiol. 1996; 25:519–524.

93. Hardy RH, Clapham JCR. Observations on hallux valgus. Based on a controlled series. J. Bone Joint Surg. Br. 1951; 33:376–391.

94. Hawkins FB, Mitchell CL, Hedwick DW. Correction of hallux valgus by metatarsal osteotomy. J. Bone Joint Surg. Am. 1945; 37:387–394.

95. Horne G, Tantzer T, Ford M. Chevron osteotomy for treatment of hallux valgus. Clin. Orthop. 1984; 183:32–36.

96. Johnson EE, Clanton TO, Baxter DE, Gottlieb MS. Comparison of chevron osteotomy and modified McBride bunionectomy for correction of mild to moderate hallux valgus deformity. Foot Ankle 1991; 12:61–68.

97. Johnson KA. The Foot and Ankle. New York, Raven Press, 1994.

98. Johnson KA, Cofield RH, Morrey BF. Chevron osteotomy for hallux valgus. Clin. Orthop. 1979; 142:44–47.

99. Kelikian H. Hallux Valgus. Allied Deformities of the Foot and Metatarsalgia. Philadelphia, WB Saunders, 1965.

100. Keller WL. The surgical treatment of bunions and hallux valgus. N. Y. Med. J. 1912; 95:696.

101. Kinnard P, Gordon D. A comparison of Chevron and Mitchell osteotomies for hallux valgus. Foot Ankle 1984; 4:241–243.

102. Kleinberg S. Operative cure of hallux valgus and bunions. Am. J. Surg. 1932; 15:75–81.

103. Mann RA, Clanton TO. Hallux rigidus: Treatment by cheilectomy. J. Bone Joint Surg. Am. 1988; 70:400–406.

104. Mann RA, Coughlin MJ. Surgery of the Foot and Ankle. 6th Ed. St. Louis, Mosby-Year Book, 1993.

105. Mann RA, Coughlin MJ. Hallux valgus. Etiology, anatomy, treatment and surgical considerations. Clin. Orthop. 1981; 157:31–46.

106. McBride ED. The McBride bunion hallux valgus operation. Refinements in the successive surgical steps of the operation. J. Bone Joint Surg. Am. 1967; 49:1675–1683.

107. Mitchell CL, Fleming JL, Allen R, Glenney C, Sanford GA. Osteotomy-bunionectomy for hallux valgus. J. Bone Joint Surg. Am. 1958; 40:41–60.

108. Moberg E. A simple operation for hallux rigidus. Clin. Orthop. 1979; 142:52.

109. Piggot H. The natural history of hallux valgus in adolescent and early adult life. J. Bone Joint Surg. Br. 1960; 42:749–760.

110. Silver D. The operative treatment of hallux valgus. J. Bone Joint Surg. 1923; 5:225–232.

111. Tanoka Y, Takabura Y, Kumai T, Samoto N, Tamai S. Radiographic analysis of hallux valgus. A two-dimensional coordinate system. J. Bone Joint Surg. Am. 1995; 77:205–213.

112. Thompson GH. Bunions and deformities of the toes in children and adolescents. J. Bone Joint Surg. Am. 1995; 77:1924–1936.

Deformities of the Lesser Toes

113. Coughlin MJ. Treatment of bunionette deformity with longitudinal osteotomy and distal soft tissue repair. Foot Ankle 1991; 11:195–203.
114. Coughlin MJ, Mann RA. Lesser toe deformities. In Mann RA, Coughlin MJ, eds. Surgery of the Foot and Ankle. 6th Ed. St. Louis, Mosby-Year Book, 1993, pp. 341–412.
115. Fallot LM, Buchholz J. Analysis of tailor's bunion by radiographic and anatomic display. J. Am. Podiatr. Assoc. 1980; 70:597–603.

116. Johnson KA. The Foot and Ankle. New York, Raven Press, 1994.
117. Kitaoka HB, Holiday A. Lateral condylar resection for bunionette deformities. Clin. Orthop. 1991; 278:183–192.
118. Landon GC, Johnson KA, Dahlin DC. Subungual exostosis. J. Bone Joint Surg. Am. 1979; 61:256–259.
119. Mann RA, Coughlin MJ. Surgery of the Foot and Ankle. 6th Ed. St. Louis, Mosby-Year Book, 1993.
120. Thompson GH. Bunions and deformities of the toes in children and adolescents. J. Bone Joint Surg. Am. 1995; 77:1924–1936.

Radiology of the Foot and Ankle, Second Edition,
edited by Thomas H. Berquist.
© 2000 by Mayo Foundation.
Published by Lippincott Williams & Wilkins, Philadelphia.

CHAPTER 11

Miscellaneous Conditions

Thomas H. Berquist and Gina A. Di Primio

Imaging of major diseases involving the foot and ankle is discussed in the preceding chapters. However, numerous conditions (e.g., systemic diseases, metabolic disease) may also affect the foot and ankle. In many cases, imaging of the foot and ankle is not performed for primary diagnostic purposes. However, radiographic changes do occur with these conditions. Therefore, it is important to be aware of the image features associated with these diseases in the foot and ankle.

T. H. Berquist: Mayo Medical School, Mayo Clinic Jacksonville, Jacksonville, Florida 32224; Mayo Foundation, Mayo Clinic, Rochester, Minnesota 55905.
G. A. Di Primio: Mayo Clinic Jacksonville, Jacksonville, Florida 32224.

OSTEOPOROSIS

Osteoporosis is the most common bone disease encountered in clinical practice. The Consensus Development Conference defined osteoporosis as a systemic skeletal disease characterized by low bone mass and microarchitectural deterioration with consequent increase in bone fragility and susceptibility to fracture.[16] Osteoporosis affects 75 million people in the United States, Europe, and Japan and results in about 1.5 million fractures annually in the United States.[13,16] The list of potential causes of osteoporosis is lengthy (Table 11-1). In certain cases, the foot and ankle are not involved. Diagnosis of generalized forms of osteoporosis is usually based on bone mineral density changes in other areas of the skeleton. The lumbar spine, femur, wrist, and calcaneus are most commonly measured.

Osteopenia and osteoporosis have been defined by the World Health Organization based on comparison of bone mineral density of normal young adults (T-score). Normal bone mineral density is greater than -1.0. Osteopenia is defined as T-scores less than -1.0 but greater than -2.5. Osteoporosis is diagnosed when T-scores are less than -2.5.[16,31,35] The radiographic features of osteoporosis vary with the type and extent of skeletal involvement, that is,

TABLE 11-1. *Etiology of osteoporosis*[a]

Generalized
  Senile, postmenopausal osteoporosis
  Endocrine conditions
    Thyroid dysfunction
    Parathyroid dysfunction
    Cushings
    Addison's disease
    Acromegaly
    Pregnancy
    Hypogonadism
    Diabetes mellitus
  Medication
    Steroids
    Heparin
  Chronic liver disease
  Hypoxemia
  Anemias
  Multiple myeloma
  Environmental factors
    Cigarette smoking
    Alcohol abuse
    Physical inactivity
    Thin body habitus
    Low calcium intake
    Nutritional deficiency
  Idiopathic
Localized
  Disuse atrophy
  Sudeck's atrophy (reflex sympathetic dystrophy syndrome)
  Transient regional osteoporosis
  Migratory osteoporosis

[a] Data from references 16 and 31.

TABLE 11-2. *Techniques for evaluating bone mineral density (bone mass)*[a]

Technique	Sites Evaluated
Dual-energy X-ray absorptiometry	Lumbar spine
	Femur
	Forearm
	Total body
Quantitative computed tomography	Spine
	Forearm
Ultrasonography	Calcaneus
	Tibia
	Fingers
	Patella
Magnetic resonance imaging	Distal radius

[a] Data from references 13, 19, 30, and 42.

generalized or local forms. Table 11-2 summarizes methods for measuring bone mineral density.[16,31,42]

Generalized Osteoporosis

Generalized osteoporosis may be related to a long list of disorders (see Table 11-1).[4,8,20,39,50] Generally, foot and ankle images are not required to establish the diagnosis; however, osteopenia of the foot and ankle does occur with these conditions. Therefore, they deserve mention, especially from a differential diagnostic standpoint.

Senile (Postmenopausal) Osteoporosis

Primary (senile) osteoporosis or postmenopausal osteoporosis usually develops in women after the age of 50 years or following menopause. This is the most common cause of generalized osteoporosis.[16,36,52] The risk of fracture in women older than 50 years of age approaches 60% without medical therapy.[35] Similar osteoporotic changes occur in men older than age 60 years.[16,52] Many patients are asymptomatic, but back pain may develop in the presence of early vertebral body compression. Serum calcium (Ca^{2+}), phosphorus, alkaline phosphatase, and acid phosphatase levels are normal. Urine Ca^{2+} and phosphorus values are also generally normal.[16,52]

The exact origin of this condition is unclear, but potential factors include the following: (1) reduced osteocyte and osteoblast activity; (2) dietary insufficiency, especially in the extremely elderly; (3) hormonal imbalance, specifically adrenal and gonadal steroids; and (4) local factors.[16,22,32]

Endocrine Disease

Endocrine disorders are the most common cause of secondary osteoporosis. Osteoporosis may also be related to diseases of the pituitary, adrenal, thyroid, ovaries, testes, and pancreas. The five most common endocrine disorders are hypogonadism, insulinopenia, hyperparathyroidism, hyperthyroidism, and hypercortisolemia.[41] Nonendocrine tumors may also secrete hormone-like substances, thus leading to osteoporosis.[27,41]

Increased levels of cortisol can occur with Cushing's syndrome (adrenal neoplasm or hyperplasia) or exogenous use of steroids. Cushing's disease is due to a corticotropin (ACTH)-producing basophilic adenoma of the pituitary. Similar elevations in cortisol can occur, with ACTH producing extraendocrine neoplasms. The association of these conditions with osteoporosis is well known. Most patients have osteoporosis related to steroid therapy for inflammatory diseases or organ transplants.[29,41] Steroids have direct and indirect effects on bone. Factors include decreased Ca^{2+} absorption, increased osteoclastic activity, decreased matrix formation, and retarded osteoblastic formation.[16,27,41]

Osteoporosis may also occur in hyperthyroidism. Osteopenia is most likely due to an imbalance in osteoclastic and osteoblastic activity. Although both are increased, the osteoclastic response predominates. Patients may have significant elevation of serum alkaline phosphatase and, occasionally, increased serum Ca^{2+}.[41] Parathyroid dysfunction also affects bone remodeling. Hypoparathyroid disorders do not result in osteoporosis. Hyperparathyroidism results in imbalance of bone remodeling that affects areas of the skeleton differently. Although most patients demonstrate osteopenia, osteosclerosis may also occur.[27,41]

Diabetes mellitus is one of the most common endocrine disorders. Patients with type 1 (insulin-dependent) diabetes have diminished bone mineral density in the spine and, to a lesser degree, the extremities. Diabetic osteoporosis may be related to insulin receptors in bone and the action of insulin as a skeletal growth factor. Complications related to diabetes mellitus also play a role in reducing bone mass.[41]

Other causes of generalized osteopenia (see Table 11-1) are also reported. The mechanisms are not always clearly understood.[3, 6,7,16,41]

Radiographic Features

Imaging studies of generalized osteoporosis generally focus on the spine, femur, forearm or wrist, and calcaneus.[2, 5,16,19,31,34,40,47] From 30 to 50% of skeletal mineral must be lost before changes are evident radiographically. Radiographs initially show diminished bone density or a more radiolucent appearance. This is often interpreted as demineralization or osteoporosis. However, radiographs cannot adequately differentiate osteoporosis, osteomalacia, and other causes of reduced bone density. Therefore, when interpreting radiographs, it is more appropriate to use the term osteopenia (poverty of bone).[2] In generalized osteoporosis, the vertebral bodies become osteopenic, and progressive biconcavity of the end plates occurs with or without compression fractures. The appearance is generally not useful in isolating the cause. An exception to this general rule is condensation of end plates associated with steroid-induced osteoporosis.[2,16,21]

Attempts have been made to use the calcaneus as a measure of the degree of osteoporosis.[1,9,15,23,29] Aggarwal and associates[1] studied 200 calcaneal radiographs and correlated

the trabecular pattern with the Singh index in the hips in the same group of patients. In patients with osteoporosis, the calcaneal secondary tensile and compressive trabeculae are resorbed before the primary trabeculae. However, calcaneal radiographs are not commonly used because they are less sensitive, do not correlate well with spine density studies, have an error rate of more than 25%, and are significantly affected by the patient's weight and activity levels.[9,23] There is also a significant variation in observers, thereby making repeated evaluations difficult to correlate.[9] Calcaneal indices have give way to more accurate methods such as dual-energy X-ray absorptiometry (DEXA) and calcaneal ultrasound.[2, 11,19,24,31,42] Although quantitative computed tomography (CT) is effective, DEXA uses less radiation, is more precise (1%), and is easier to use.[2,31] Low bone mineral density and increased fracture risk are well documented. DEXA is used to measure bone mineral density in the lumbar spine (frontal and lateral), femur, and forearm. DEXA has replaced quantitative CT to measure bone mineral density.[31]

Patients' data are compared with age-matched controls (2-score) and young normal subjects (T-scores). Results are considered normal if they are less than 1 standard deviation below the mean (T-score higher than -1.0). T-scores of -1.0 to -2.5 indicate osteopenia (low bone mass), and when scores are lower -2.5, they indicate osteoporosis. This technique is used to evaluate fracture risk and to establish and monitor therapy in patients with osteoporosis.[31,39,42]

More recently, calcaneal ultrasound has been used to evaluate bone density and architecture.[12,14,21,24] Numerous reports have used an Achilles device (LUNAR Corp., Madison, WI) to measure speed of sound (SOS), broadband ultrasound alteration (BUA), and stiffness. The latter is calculated using the mean BUA and SOS ([0.67 × BUA − 0.28 × SOS − 420]).[11,12,14,17,21,24,30,42] This technique has several advantages over DEXA. The equipment is portable, it is more readily available, and the technique is less expensive than DEXA.[16] Therefore, ultrasound is potentially more efficacious as a screening technique for osteoporosis.[16,42] However, to date, precision is reduced compared with DEXA, and values obtained using calcaneal ultrasound correlate moderately with DEXA values in the spine and femur.[12,14,42] Ultrasound may be used as an alternative to screen certain patients before considering DEXA. If results of ultrasound studies are normal, no further studies are required. Equivocal cases can be referred for DEXA studies.

Magnetic resonance imaging (MRI) has also been evaluated as a method for evaluating osteoporosis. Grampp and colleagues[19] compared MRI with quantitative CT and DEXA. Using the section (2-mm) axial images with a repetition time of 67 milliseconds and echo times of 7, 10, 12, 20, and 30 milliseconds and a flip angle of 90° gradient-echo sequence, a T2* map was created to calculate relaxation times. Data correlated well with quantitative CT and DEXA values.[19] This technique may be useful, but it is difficult to imagine that cost and scanner availability will result in common clinical usage of this method.

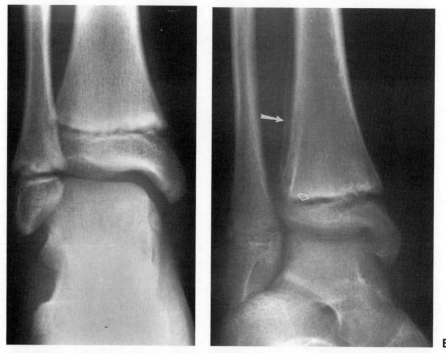

FIG. 11-1. **A:** Normal pediatric ankle showing normal bone density. **B:** Mortise view of the right ankle 4 weeks after cast immobilization demonstrates disuse osteopenia and a healing physeal fracture (*open arrow*) with periosteal new bone (*arrow*).

Regional and Localized Osteoporosis

Osteoporosis may be more localized, affecting single or multiple osseous structures or periarticular regions. These changes typically occur in the appendicular skeleton (see Table 11-1).

Disuse Osteoporosis

Disuse or immobilization osteoporosis is common in the foot and ankle. This condition most frequently follows trauma and develops during cast immobilization and non-weight bearing. The changes are reversible once weight bearing and stress are induced after the period of immobilization.[26]

Radiographic features of disuse osteoporosis occur approximately 8 weeks after immobilization or reduced use of the involved extremity. Osteopenia may be evident sooner in younger patients (less than 20 years of age) and in adults more than 50 years old.[26] In paralyzed patients, bone changes are usually not evident for about 3 months. Several radiographic patterns of disuse osteoporosis have been described. Uniform osteopenia is most common (Fig. 11-1). Other patterns include juxtaarticular osteopenia, small areas of periarticular lucency, subchondral lucency (Fig. 11-2), and lucent areas in the cortex, subperiosteal, and endosteal regions (Fig. 11-3).[26] The last pattern may be difficult to differentiate from infection and neoplasm.[28,39]

Features similar to disuse osteoporosis can be identified with infection and other inflammatory arthropathies. The

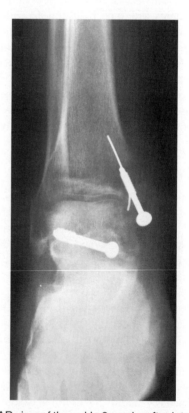

FIG. 11-2. AP view of the ankle 8 weeks after internal fixation of the medial malleolus and talus. Note the patchy metaphyseal osteopenia in the tibia with subchondral lucency at the tibiotalar joint. This feature is absent in the lateral articular aspect of the talus (Hawkins' sign; see Chapter 4) because of early avascular necrosis.

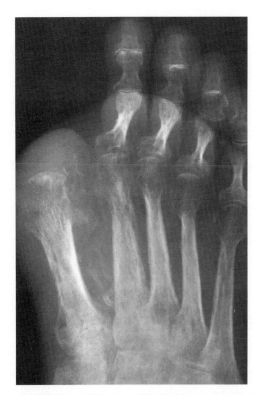

FIG. 11-3. AP view of the foot. The great toe was amputated in this diabetic patient because of ischemia and soft tissue ulceration. Patchy osteopenia and medial cortical involvement in the first metatarsal are noted. There is also cortical thinning in the second metatarsal with juxtaarticular osteopenia of the metatarsophalangeal joints.

cause in these situations is most likely increased bone resorption.[39]

Transient Regional Osteoporosis

Transient regional osteoporosis consists of two major categories: transient osteoporosis of the hip and regional migratory osteoporosis of symptom complexes.[10,15,39,49,51] Regional migratory osteoporosis commonly involves the foot and ankle. Although the cause is unclear, mechanical factors affecting nerve conduction have been described in the foot. Byrd and colleagues[9] demonstrated nerve involvement from tarsal tunnel compression as a cause of regional migratory osteoporosis. Regional migratory osteoporosis frequently affects men (male-to-female ration, 1.7:1) in their forties and fifties. One-third of female patients in the series of Tannenbaum and colleagues[51] were pregnant when symptoms began. Patients present with a rapid onset of pain and swelling of one of the joints of the lower extremity (hip, knee, foot, and ankle). Symptoms typically last 6 to 9 months. When symptoms resolve in the first joint, the adjacent joint typically becomes involved. This may occur immediately or following a symptom-free period of up to 2 years.[3,39] Laboratory studies are usually normal, although slight elevation of the erythrocyte sedimentation rate has been reported.[10,36]

Several variants of regional migratory osteoporosis have been described. Lequesne and associates[32] described a condition they termed partial transient osteoporosis. Two separate categories of this condition were identified. The first, termed the radial form, involved only one or two digits or rays of the hand or foot (Fig. 11-4). The second or zonal

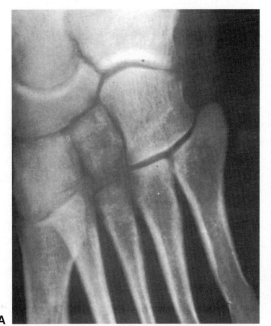
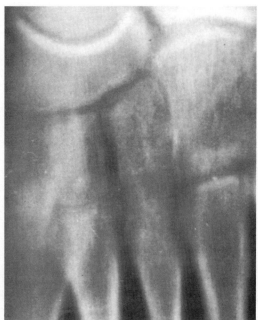

FIG. 11-4. Coned-down AP view (**A**) and tomogram (**A**) of the midfoot that demonstrate osteopenia of the proximal third metatarsal and lateral cuneiform 1 month after pain in this region. The adjacent bones are not involved, and no erosions are present. (From Lequesne, ref. 32, with permission.)

form involved only a portion of the bone or articular surface. For example, when the knee was involved, only one of the femoral condyles could be affected.

Shier and colleagues[45] described a further variant of regional migratory osteoporosis that included the typical migratory changes in the appendicular skeleton and involvement of the axial skeleton in which vertebral compression was also evident.

Radiographic Features

Routine radiographic findings are usually not apparent for 4 to 8 weeks.[15,39] Juxtaarticular osteopenia with extension beyond the epiphysis into the metaphysis and even the diaphysis of the involved skeleton is common. The same patterns of bone involvement noted earlier may be applied in regional migratory osteoporosis. Wavy periosteal reaction may also be noted.[39,48] With the zonal and radial patterns, the distribution of osteopenia is more localized (see Fig. 11-4). In any of the foregoing variants, the joint spaces remain normal, and no erosive changes occur. Although symptoms may subside in 6 to 9 months, the radiographic changes persist longer, particularly when cortical changes are present. Return to normal cortical thickness may take up to 2 years.[15]

Changes can be identified earlier using isotope bone scans. Increased uptake of radionuclide usually extends well beyond the joint, a feature that is useful in differentiating regional or transient osteoporosis from other articular disorders.[33,37,39,43] To date, MRI has not been used extensively in evaluating osteoporosis. Therefore, the image features have been described.[5,39] Marrow signal intensity may be normal or similar to bone marrow edema. In this setting, the signal intensity is decreased on T1-weighted sequences and is increased on T2-weighted sequences (Fig. 11-5).[5]

Reflex Sympathetic Dystrophy Syndrome

Many terms have been used to describe this syndrome including Sudeck's atrophy, causalgia, shoulder-hand syndrome, and posttraumatic osteoporosis.[18,38,39,43,44,46] The accepted term for this symptom complex is reflex sympathetic dystrophy (RSD).[39,44]

This condition is discussed in Chapter 4, but it deserves mention again because the radiographic changes include this process in the causes of regional osteoporosis. RSD usually follows trauma, which may be minor. The syndrome is also noted after myocardial infarction (1 to 20%) and hemiplegia (12 to 20%).[39] The condition has also been described in patients with cardiac disease, degenerative changes in the cervical spine, and neoplasm and after infections.[18,38,39,53] In patients with neoplasms (e.g., lung, ovary, breast, pancreas), the symptoms of RSD may obscure or delay the diagnosis of the primary cause.

Patients typically present with pain, swelling, and reduced range of motion in the foot and ankle. Vasomotor instability,

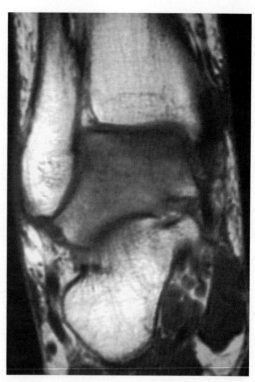

FIG. 11-5. T1-weighted coronal image demonstrates diffuse decreased signal intensity in the talus consistent with local edema or regional osteoporosis.

trophic skin changes, and patchy or aggressive appearing osteopenia are evident (Fig. 11-6).[18] Although the cause is not clear, the vasomotor instability adds to the hypothesis that RSD is due to abnormal neural reflexes.[18,39] The stimulating focus may follow local foot or ankle trauma and acts as the afferent stimulus. The sympathetic nervous system serves as the efferent branch of the reflex.[18] Bone scan findings add to the credibility of this theory because of the marked increase in flow, which is evident using technetium-99m (^{99m}Tc)–pertechnetate methylene diphosphate (MDP) scintigrams.[18,39]

Several conditions radiographically mimic regional osteoporosis. These include infection, septic arthritis, inflammatory arthropathies (such as rheumatoid arthritis), neoplasms, pigmented villonodular synovitis, and synovial chondromatosis (Fig. 11-7) (Table 11-3).[28,39]

Radiographic changes may be nonspecific. However, the osteopenia associated with regional osteoporosis is not associated with bone erosions, which are common with rheumatoid and septic arthritis. The joint space also remains normal in patients with regional osteoporosis.[18,39] Infection, synovial chondromatosis, and pigmented villonodular synovitis are usually monoarticular and involve the large, more proximal joints of the appendicular skeleton.[5,39]

Radionuclide studies may be useful in differential diagnosis. Patients with regional migratory osteoporosis have extension of ^{99m}Tc pertechnetate uptake well into the diaphy-

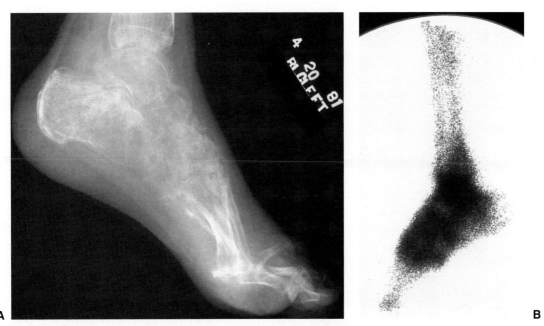

FIG. 11-6. A: Lateral radiograph of the foot demonstrating aggressive patchy osteopenia and soft tissue swelling resulting from reflex sympathetic dystrophy. **B:** Radionuclide scan shows diffuse increased uptake in the ankle, midfoot, and hindfoot.

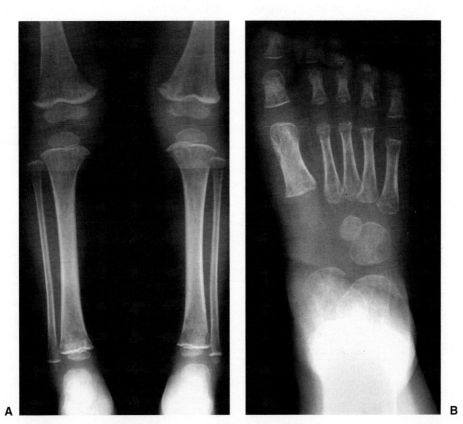

FIG. 11-7. A 2-year-old boy presented with extremity pain and refused to walk. Radiographs of the tibia (**A**) and AP (**B**) and lateral (**C**) views of the feet show mottled osteopenia in the metaphysis with areas of cortical destruction. *(Continued)*

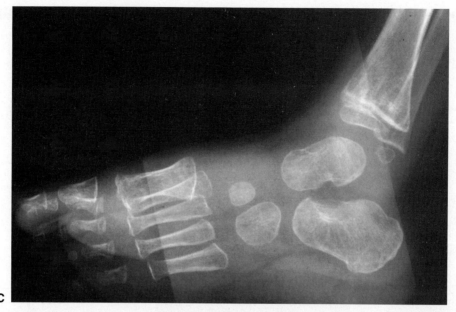

C

FIG. 11-7. *Continued* The distribution was symmetric and involved all extremities. Distribution does not fit migratory osteoporosis. Diagnosis is acute lymphocytic leukemia.

sis. In the other articular and periarticular disorders, the increased uptake is usually confined to the immediate articular region.[39,48]

MRI has also been used to define the cause of osteopenia in the foot and ankle more clearly. MRI may show subtle (Fig. 11-8) or striking changes in signal intensity in patients with RSD and in those with pigmented villonodular synovitis. Patients with pigmented villonodular synovitis usually have joint effusions. The paramagnetic effects of intraarticular hemosiderin in pigmented villonodular synovitis cause areas of low signal intensity in the synovium on T2-weighted images. However, more data are needed before true value of MRI will be evident.[5]

Aspiration of involved joints can be useful in detection of infection and certain inflammatory arthropathies. Synovial fluid cultures and crystal and cell studies can be obtained in this manner. This is especially important if infection is considered clinically. Regional osteoporosis is usually self-limited, unlike the other diseases that may be confused with this condition.[39]

RICKETS AND OSTEOMALACIA

Rickets and osteomalacia are similar histologically. The basic defect is inadequate mineralization of osteoid, although osteoid production is also reduced. Rickets is the term applied to this condition in the growing skeleton, whereas osteomalacia is the term used in the adult skeleton.[72,83] Rickets affects the chondroosseous complex with most obvious changes in the growth plates. Thus, skeletal abnormalities are most obvious in the metaphysis. This feature can have a dramatic effect on linear bone growth. Osteomalacia (literally, bone softening) affects lamellar or mature bone formation. Both can coexist in childhood before growth plate closure.[83,88,94]

Etiology

Numerous diseases are associated with osteomalacia and rickets (Table 11-4).[76,83] The importance of vitamin D in Ca^{2+}-phosphorus balance cannot be understated. Basic knowledge of vitamin D metabolism is necessary in understanding how the diseases of the liver, kidney, and gastrointestinal tract result in osteomalacia or rickets (Fig. 11-9). Vitamin D_2 is a food supplement produced from ergosterol in fungi and yeast. Vitamin D_3 is produced by interaction of ultraviolet light with 7-dehydrocholesterol in the deep layers of the skin. These two inactive forms of vitamin D are hydroxylated in the liver and, to a lesser extent, in the kidney

TABLE 11-3. *Differential diagnosis of regional osteoporosis*[a]

Osteomyelitis
Septic arthritis
Rheumatoid and rheumatoid-like arthridites
Pigmented villonodular synovitis
Hemangiomatosis
Synovial chondromatosis
Neoplasms
Avascular necrosis

[a] Data from references 1, 15, 25, and 39.

MISCELLANEOUS CONDITIONS / 535

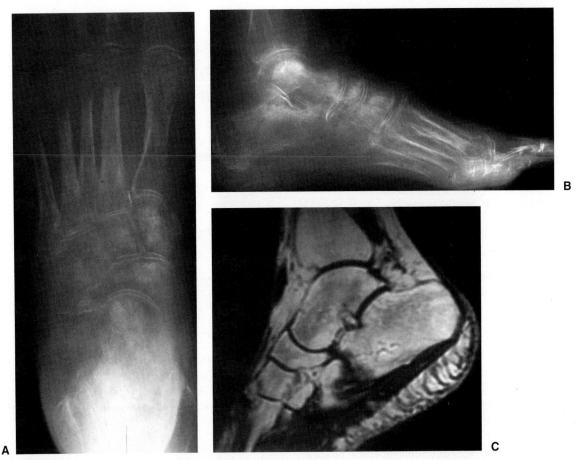

FIG. 11-8. AP (**A**) and lateral (**B**) radiographs demonstrate striking changes of reflex sympathetic dystrophy. Sagittal SE 500/11 image (**C**) demonstrates subtle decreased signal intensity in the calcaneus, talus, and tarsal bones.

TABLE 11-4. *Rickets and osteomalacia*[a]

Neonate and infant
  Hypophosphatasia
  Congenital rubella
  Vitamin D deficiency
  Biliary atresia
  Celiac disease and malabsorption syndromes
Child and adult
  Dietary calcium and phosphorus deficiency
  Hypophosphatemia (vitamin D–resistant)
  Pseudo vitamin D deficiency (vitamin D–dependent
    osteomalacia)
  Sprue
  Pancreatic insufficiency
  Crohn's disease
  Amyloidosis
  Small bowel fistulae
  Small bowel and gastric resection
  Obstructive jaundice
  Chronic liver disease
  Anticonvulsant medication
  Renal tubular disorders
  Hyperparathyroidism
  Axial osteomalacia

[a] Data from references 72, 83, and 94.

and intestine.[72,85] D-25-Hydroxylase is the enzyme required to hydroxylate the 25 position of both compounds resulting in 25-OH-vitamin D_3 and 25-OH-vitamin D_2.[67,68,87] The majority of circulating 25-OH-vitamin D (approximately 85%) is 25-OH-vitamin D_3, a finding suggesting that dietary intake of vitamin D_2 is less significant than vitamin D_3 production.[68,83,86] Hydroxylation of the number 1 carbon position occurs exclusively in the kidney in the presence of 25(OH)D-1-hydroxylase. This results in the active form of vitamin D-1,25(OH)$_2$-vitamin D_3.[55,66,71,97] 1,25(OH)$_2$-Vitamin D_3 is rapidly metabolized, so significant stores are not available. Blood levels are regulated by hormonal feedback systems (serum Ca^{2+}, phosphate [PO_4], and parathyroid hormone levels) and body requirements (Fig. 11-10).[66,72,82,83] 1,25(OH)$_2$-vitamin D_3 acts on the intestine to increase Ca^{2+} and phosphorus absorption. The hormone has two effects on bone (mobilization of Ca^{2+} and phosphorus from mature bone and mineralization of immature bone) that seem opposed, but are not. Although the major effect of 1,25(OH)$_2$-vitamin D_3 is on bone and intestine, evidence also indicates that the hormone affects the kidney and parathyroid glands.[68,70,82] Diseases that affect intestinal absorption and the liver, kidney, and parathyroid result in interruption of

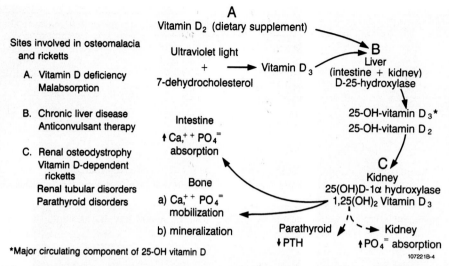

FIG. 11-9. Illustration of vitamin D metabolism and associated diseases that lead to abnormal metabolism and rickets or osteomalacia.

formation of the active form of vitamin D or elevation of parathyroid hormone (see Fig. 11-9A to C). This change results in osteomalacia or rickets.

The interactions of Ca^{2+}, phosphorus, parathyroid hormone, and $1,25(OH)_2$-vitamin D_3 are summarized in Figure 11-10. Low levels of Ca^{2+} and phosphorus cause increased parathyroid hormone, which, in turn stimulates renal production of $1,25(OH)_2$-vitamin D_3. Ca^{2+} and phosphorus levels rise because of the effects of $1,25(OH)_2$-vitamin D_3 on the intestine (increased absorption Ca^{2+} and PO_4) and parathyroid hormone (increased mobilization Ca^{2+} and PO_4) on bone. Because parathyroid hormone causes increased renal PO_4 excretion, the net result is predominantly a rise in serum Ca^{2+}. Low serum PO_4 causes increased active vitamin D_3 formation, which, in turn, reduces parathyroid hormone lev-

els. This results from increased Ca^{2+} levels from the action of $1,25(OH)_2$-vitamin D_3 on the intestine and bone and suppression of the parathyroid glands. Elevated levels of $1,25(OH)_2$-vitamin D_3 cause reduced renal production of the hormone.[83]

Clinical Features

The clinical and laboratory features of osteomalacia can be confusing. Patients generally present with vague discomfort that primarily affects the axial skeleton. Laboratory data depend on the cause and stage of osteomalacia (Table 11-5). Since the advent of vitamin D supplements (vitamin D_2–irradiated ergosterol), the incidence of nutritional osteomalacia and rickets has decreased dramatically. When pres-

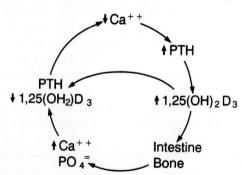

FIG. 11-10. Illustration of calcium, parathyroid hormone, and $1,25(OH)_2$-vitamin D_3 feedback mechanisms.

TABLE 11-5. *Laboratory values in metabolic bone disease[a]*

	Vitamin D Deficiency	Hypophosphatemia	Primary Hyperparathyroidism	Renal Osteodystrophy
Serum Ca^{2+}	Low	Normal	High	Normal-low
Urine Ca^{2+}	Low	Low	Low	High
Serum PO_4	Low	Normal	High	Low
Alkaline phosphatase	High	High	Normal-high	High

[a] Data from references 72 and 83.

ent, a rapid response to vitamin D supplements is easily demonstrated and differentiates this form of osteomalacia from that associated with renal or gastrointestinal disease.[72]

Diseases of the stomach, intestines, hepatobiliary system, and pancreas have also been associated with osteomalacia (see Table 11-3) (Fig. 11-11). In addition, following partial gastric resection, specifically Polya and Bilroth II procedures, up to one-third of patients develop abnormalities in Ca^{2+} metabolism.[64,72] Malabsorption states, especially with steatorrhea, result in Ca^{2+} loss and reduced vitamin D absorption. A similar situation occurs with steatorrhea associated with pancreatic and biliary disease. Parenteral vitamin D may be required to treat bone lesions associated with malabsorption.[72]

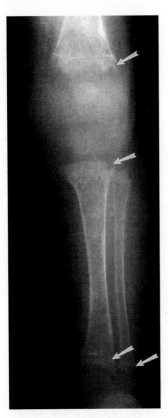

FIG. 11-11. AP view of the lower extremity in a patient with congenital biliary atresia. Noted are marked osteopenia, cortical thinning, and widening and irregularity of the metaphysis (*arrows*).

Rickets and osteomalacia may also occur with inherited disorders. Pseudo-vitamin D deficiency (hereditary vitamin D–dependent rickets) is inherited as an autosomal recessive trait. Male and females are equally affected.[56,61] The clinical and metabolic features resemble those of advanced nutritional rickets.[56,66,92,93] Clinical and radiographic features may be noted by 3 months of age. Serum Ca^{2+} and PO_4 are low, leading to elevated parathyroid hormone. Elevated parathyroid hormone leads to increased urinary PO_4 and aminoaciduria.[66] High doses (greater than or equal to 50,000 U/day) of vitamin D are usually successful in treating this disorder. Although the exact cause is unknown, the response to low doses of 1,25$(OH)_2$-vitamin D suggests that a defect in 25(OH)D-1 hydroxylase may exist.[66,92,93]

A second type of vitamin D–resistant rickets has been described by Brooks and associates.[58] In this setting, one sees a defect in end-organ response to 1,25$(OH)_2$-vitamin D. Therefore, serum levels are markedly increased. Treatment with vitamin D corrects this disorder, but 1,25$(OH)_2$-vitamin D levels remain elevated.

Vitamin D–resistant hypophosphatemic rickets may be inherited as a sex-linked or autosomal dominant abnormality. This condition is associated with a number of generally benign musculoskeletal neoplasms. The tumors are generally more vascular than usual and contain increased amounts of new bone formation.[63,75,83] The list of associated neoplasms includes oteoblastoma, nonossifying fibroma, and giant cell tumors.[63,74] Reduced serum PO_4 and increased alkaline phosphatase are the primary laboratory abnormalities. Serum Ca^{2+} is usually normal. Symptoms may reverse after tumor is removed.[83]

Osteomalacia may also result from treatment with anticonvulsant medications. Hypocalcemia has been demonstrated in up to 25% of patients receiving long-term anticonvulsant medication. Elevated alkaline phosphatase is also generally evident. Bone changes of rickets or osteomalacia are not as common as the laboratory abnormalities. The vitamin D defect is due to interference with hydroxylation of the 25 carbon in the liver. The severity of symptoms is related to dose and duration. Pheneturide, phenytoin, and phenobarbital have been implicated.[72] Osteomalacia has also been described with certain PO_4-binding antacids.[83]

Renal tubular disorders are also associated with rickets and osteomalacia. These disorders are due to defects in either the proximal (resorption of PO_4, glucose, and amino acids) or distal (concentration and acidification) tubules.[60,78] Sex-linked hypophosphatemic rickets is the most common form of renal tubular rickets or osteomalacia. Fanconi's syndrome also affects primarily the proximal tubule.[60,78,83] Changes are essentially related to PO_4 loss and its effect on vitamin D metabolism and the feedback mechanisms involved (see Figs. 11-9 and 11-10).

Axial osteomalacia is an unusual form of osteomalacia that predominantly affects men and involves the axial skeleton.[65] The extremities are spared. Vitamin D is not effective in treating this condition.

Hypophosphatasia is an autosomal recessive condition that resembles rickets and osteomalacia. This condition may be present at birth. These patients have more advanced

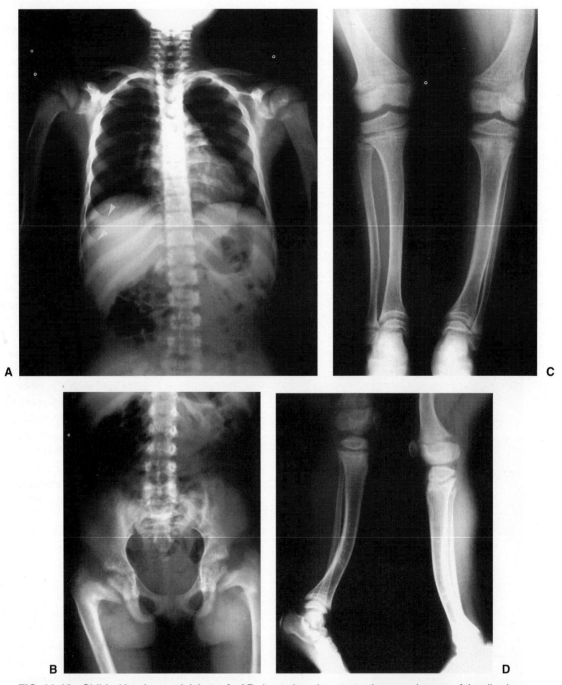

FIG. 11-12. Child with advanced rickets. **A:** AP chest view demonstrating prominence of the ribs (*arrowheads*) at the costochondral junctions (rachitic rosary). The bone density appears increased. **B:** AP view of the pelvis and hips demonstrating marked coxa vara deformity and physeal irregularity. AP (**C**) and lateral (**D**) views of the lower extremities demonstrating widening and irregularity of the growth plates, cupping of the distal tibial metaphysis, and tibial bowing.

radiographic features (dwarfism, fractures, osteopenia, and skeletal deformity) and may die during infancy. A mild form occurs in older children. This group and those who survive the infertile form have many of the features of rickets. Laboratory features include low serum alkaline phosphatase and elevated serum urine phosphoethanolamine levels.[83]

An additional cause of osteomalacia occurs in patients undergoing renal dialysis. Although renal dialysis has improved quality of life for patients with renal insufficiency, the complications associated with this treatment deserve mention.[81] These include encephalopathy, arthropathy, and osteomalacia.[84] Aluminum toxicity is commonly implicated.[81]

Radiographic Features

Radiographic changes vary with age and rate of skeletal development. Rickets primarily involves the growth plate. Changes are most obvious where growth is more highly accelerated, such as the proximal humerus, the distal femur, the distal radius and ulna, and the proximal and distal tibial physis (Fig. 11-12).[72,83] Calcification is diminished in the

zones of the physis. The cartilage continues to proliferate but is less organized and poorly mineralized. Radiographically, this change causes the growth plate to appear widened and irregular (see Figs. 11-11 and 11-12). If changes are not reversed, the metaphysis will progressively widen and develop a cupped appearance. Additional features include cortical thinning and bowing deformities in the tubular bones (see Fig. 11-12). Bowing deformities are generally not evident before weight bearing.[94]

Skeletal changes can be completely reversed if therapy is instituted early (Fig. 11-13). This is especially true if bowing or other types of deformity have not yet appeared. Once deformities have developed, both surgical and medical therapy may be needed to reduce functional impairment (Fig. 11-14).

Three radiographic features are commonly described in the adult with osteomalacia. These are osteopenia, pseudofractures, and bone deformity.[83] Early radiographic diagnosis can be difficult. Generalized lucency resulting from unmineralized trabeculae may be subtle. Remaining mineralized trabeculae may be more prominent, and scattered lucent areas in the cortex may be evident. The presence of pseudofractures is generally believed to be pathogno-

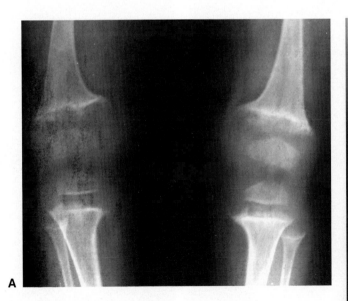

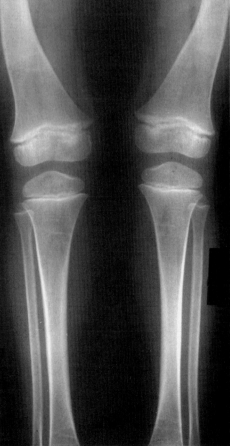

FIG. 11-13. A 1-year-old child with vitamin D–resistant rickets. AP view (**A**) of the knee shows irregularity and widening of the growth plate. Treatment with 10,000 U/day was not successful. Therapy was increased to 50,000 U of vitamin D/day, and follow-up radiographs (**B**) 3 years later (age 4) are essentially normal, except for residual distal femoral bowing.

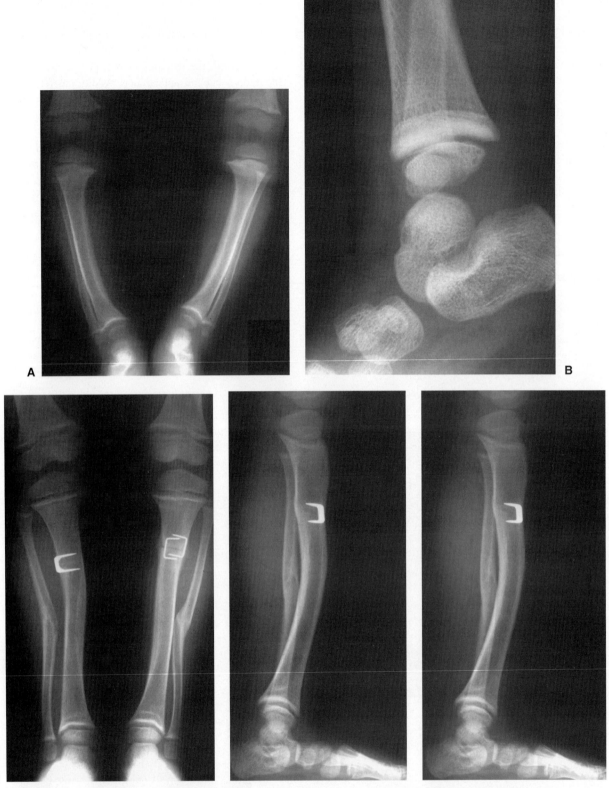

FIG. 11-14. Sequential radiographs on a patient with hypophosphatemic rickets. **A:** AP views of both legs demonstrating metaphyseal change and tibial bowing. **B:** Following medical treatment, a lateral ankle radiograph shows metaphyseal sclerosis. The growth plate is less irregular. **C:** AP views of the legs 3 years later following tibial and fibular osteotomies. Ricketic changes in the growth plates and metaphysis are still noted. **D** and **E:** Lateral views of the legs show residual bowing with hindfoot valgus and vertical talus.

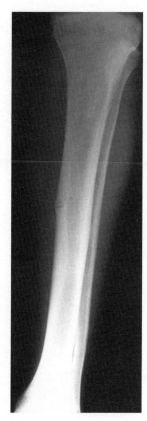

FIG. 11-15. AP radiograph demonstrating a pseudofracture in the midtibia.

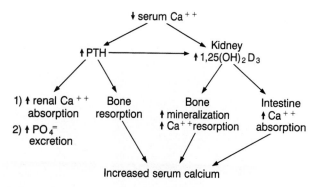

FIG. 11-16. Illustration of effect of decreased serum calcium on parathyroid hormone and vitamin D metabolism.

these levels may exceed those normally seen in primary hyperparathyroidism. Secondary hyperparathyroidism is due to reduced Ca^{2+} levels (Fig. 11-16).[80] Ca^{2+} levels are reduced as renal disease leads to PO_4 retention (therefore, the Ca^{2+}-PO_4 product increases) which in turn reduces $1,25(OH)_2$-vitamin D_3 formation. Thus intestinal absorption of Ca^{2+} is diminished. There also appears to be a reduced skeletal response to parathyroid hormone.[80] The feedback mechanism between parathyroid hormone and $1,25(OH)_2$-vitamin D_3 is also abnormal (see Figs. 11-9 and 11-10). The low levels of the active form of vitamin D result in elevated parathyroid hormone.[80,83]

Abnormalities in vitamin D metabolism are largely due to decreased renal production of the active metabolite ($1,25(OH)_2$-vimatin D_3) and the elevated PO_4 which also leads to reduction in vitamin D hydroxylation in the kidney.[80,83] These changes are most evident in chronic progressive renal disease. This abnormal metabolism is compounded by failure to respond to vitamin D therapy.

Radiographic Features

Radiographic features of renal osteodystrophy generally reflect the two most common factors discussed earlier: secondary hyperparathyroidism and vitamin D deficiency. The radiographic features vary depending on the age of the patient, type of renal abnormality, and treatment regimen. Five basic changes are commonly noted: (1) osteitis fibrosa cystica, (2) osteomalacia or rickets, (3) osteosclerosis, (4) osteoporosis, and (5) avascular necrosis in patients treated with steroids.[70,72,83,89]

Rickets and osteitis fibrosa cystica are prevalent in children (Fig. 11-17). In adults, changes are usually most obvious in the hands. The most obvious features are subperiosteal resorption along the radial aspects of the middle phalanges and resorption of the tufts. Bone resorption can also occur in other subperiosteal regions (Fig. 11-18) and in subchondral locations that cause joint spaces to appear widened.[83]

Osteosclerosis is due to areas of osteoid and mineral redis-

monic (Fig. 11-15). These uncalcified cortical osteoid seams are most common in the femoral necks, pubic symphysis, ribs, and scapula. However, bilateral metatarsal pseudofractures have been described.[54] Unless other areas of the skeleton are involved, radiographically these change could be confused with stress fractures. Osteitis fibrosa cystica may be seen in the presence of secondary hyperparathyroidism.[83]

Radionuclide scans may be normal in early osteomalacia. Later, increased tracer may be evident, although the explanation is controversial. An increased osteoid pool and slow but progressive mineralization have been considered to explain increased uptake of radiotracer in these patients. Secondary hyperparathyroidism may also explain findings on bone scans.[91] Other imaging procedures, such a MRI, provide little additional information in this setting.

RENAL OSTEODYSTROPHY

Bone changes associated with chronic renal disease are not completely understood, but these changes are predominantly due to secondary hyperparathyroidism and abnormal vitamin D metabolism.[80,83,90,91]

Parathyroid hormone levels are significantly increased in patients with renal osteodystrophy and, in certain cases,

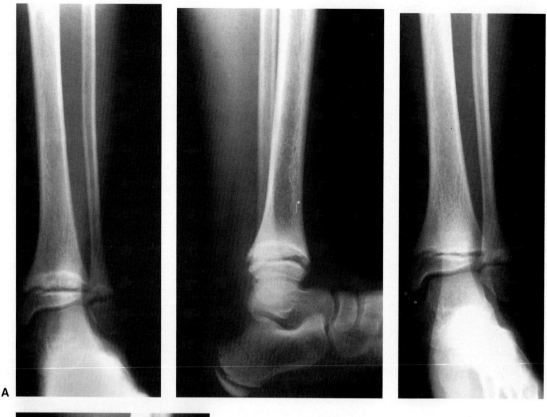

A

B,C

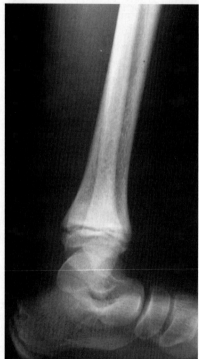

D

FIG. 11-17. An 11-year-old child with chronic renal failure. AP (**A**) and lateral (**B**) views of the ankle with changes of rickets in the distal tibia and fibula. AP (**C**) and lateral (**D**) views or the ankle 1 year after dialysis and vitamin D therapy are near normal.

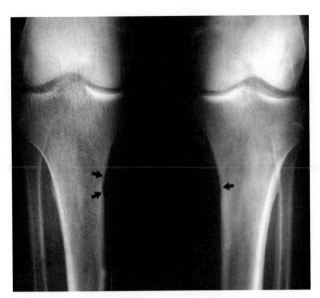

FIG. 11-18. AP views of the knees demonstrating subperiosteal resorption (*arrows*) in the upper tibias.

tribution. It is most commonly seen in the spine (rugger-jersey spine) and metaphyses of long bones (Fig. 11-19).

Osteomalacia occurs with variable frequency. However, Kanis and associates[73] noted histologic changes of osteomalacia in 16% of patients with renal osteodystrophy. Soft tissue calcifications may be periarticular, intraarticular, or vascular. The vascular form is particularly frequent. The foregoing changes can be reversed to some degree with dialysis and vitamin D therapy (see Fig. 11-17).

The radiographic features of osteomalacia, rickets, and renal osteodystrophy overlap and are themselves not useful in defining the underlying cause. Age, clinical symptoms, laboratory data, and response to therapy are all useful in defining the cause.[83]

Radionuclide scans may demonstrate increased radiotracer. In patients undergoing dialysis, aluminum toxicity may cause increased soft tissue uptake and poor quality bone scans because of inhibition of bone uptake.[91,98] MRI may demonstrate nonspecific signal intensity changes in the marrow and physeal regions.

PARATHYROID DISEASE

Parathyroid hormone is essential for proper transport of Ca^{2+} and related ions in the kidney, bone, and intestinal tract.[89,90] Parathyroid hormone affects bone by causing release of Ca^{2+} into the blood and by initiating bone remodeling. Elevation or reduced levels of this hormone have a significant impact on Ca^{2+} metabolism.[89,90]

Hyperparathyroidism falls into three categories: primary, secondary, and tertiary. Primary hyperparathyroidism may be due to parathyroid adenoma, carcinoma, or hyperplasia. Ectopic sites of parathyroid hormone secretion, such as lung and renal carcinoma, have also been reported.[62,74,88,90] Patients have elevated levels of parathyroid hormone, and most have elevated serum Ca^{2+}. In some patients, Ca^{2+} levels may be intermittently elevated or normal.[89]

Secondary hyperparathyroidism may have many causes (Table 11-6). The basic lesion is reduced serum Ca^{2+}, which leads to increased parathyroid hormone secretion. Chronic renal disease with PO_4 retention, depressed intestinal Ca^{2+} absorption, and impaired vitamin D metabolism (failure of $1,25(OH)_2$-vitamin D_3 formation) are, as noted ealier, the most common causes of secondary hyperparathyroidism. Serum Ca^{2+} levels are typically low, and inorganic PO_4 is elevated.[89]

Tertiary hyperparathyroidism develops in patients undergoing renal dialysis and patients with chronic renal

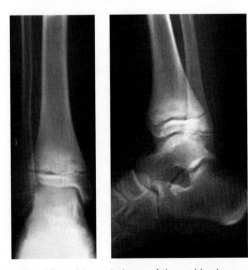

FIG. 11-19. AP and lateral views of the ankle demonstrating metaphyseal irregularity and sclerosis in a patient with renal osteodystrophy.

TABLE 11-6. *Secondary hyperparathyroidism: etiologic factors[a]*

Gastrointestinal conditions
Malabsorption
Decreased intake (rare)
Liver diseases
Chronic liver disease
Hepatitis
Cirrhosis
Alcohol abuse
Renal conditions
Fanconi's Syndrome
Nephrotic Syndrome
Glomerular disease (renal osteodystrophy)
End-organ resistance (Vitamin D–resistant rickets)
Bone and soft tissue tumors
Hemangioma
Osteoblastoma
Giant cell tumor
Hemangiopericytoma

[a] Data from references 75, 83, and 89.

failure or malabsorption.[81,89,91] These patients may have long-standing secondary hyperparathyroidism, which leads to autonomously functioning parathyroid glands that no longer respond to the serum Ca^{2+} control mechanisms.[89,90]

Parathyroid hormone (see Figs. 11-9 and 11-10) primarily affects bone, kidney, and the intestinal tract. The interaction with vitamin D is also important and is discussed previously in the section on osteomalacia and rickets.[69,85,90]

Radiographic Features

Skeletal changes of primary hyperparathyroidism are related to osteoclastic resorption secondary to parathyroid hormone stimulation. Early changes in the subperiosteal cortex are typically seen in the hands, but they also occur in the phalanges of the foot. Resorption of the distal phalangeal tufts may also occur. This phenomenon can also occur in other diseases including psoriatic arthritis, scleroderma, frostbite, leprosy, sarcoidosis, polyvinyl chloride exposure, and hypertropic pulmonary osteoarthropathy. Bony resorption also occurs in cortical, endosteal, and subchondral regions and in sites of ligament and tendon insertions. The calcaneus is the most common site of the latter change in the foot. In children, bone resorption may also occur along the growth plates.[89]

As bone resorption progresses, the process becomes more generalized, giving the skeleton an osteopenic appearance. Pathologic fractures may result in deformities of the metatarsals.

Histologically, osteomalacia, osteoporosis, and areas of vascular fibrogranulation tissue (brown tumor) are evident. Brown tumors (osteoclastomas) may develop following interosseous hemorrhage into areas of resorption. These lytic lesions may be single or multiple and may have an aggressive appearance with expansion of the cortex.

Brown tumors are classically described as occurring with greatest frequency in patients with primary hyperparathyroidism. However, because of the increasing evidence of secondary hyperparathyroidism resulting from chronic renal disorders, they are also seen more commonly in this setting. Osteosclerosis may also be seen in patients with hyperparathyroidism. This feature is most common in patients with secondary hyperparathyroidism or renal osteodystrophy.[89]

Soft tissue calcification, primarily vascular and articular, is more common with secondary hyperparathyroidism. Table 11-7 summarizes the numerous radiographic features associated with hyperparathyroidism.

Hypoparathyroidism

Hypoparathyroidism may be due to surgical excision, such as during thyroidectomy or parathyroid glandular disease, or it may be idiopathic. The idiopathic type usually presents

TABLE 11-7. *Radiographic features of hyperparathyroidism[a]*

Skeletal
Bone resorption
Subperiosteal
Cortical endosteal
Subchondral
Peritendinous or subligamentous
Paraphyseal
Lamina dura about teeth
Osteopenia
Pathologic fractures
Skull
Salt and pepper appearance
Basilar invagination
Brown tumors
Osteosclerosis
Articular calcification
Extraskeletal
Vascular calcification
Nephrolithiasis
Peptic ulcer disease

[a] Data from Resnick and Niwayama, ref. 89.

in childhood.[89] The condition more commonly affects females than males. Patients have neuromuscular symptoms and decreased serum Ca^{2+}.[96]

Radiographic features in hypoparathyroidism and in pseudohypoparathyroidism or pseudo-pseudohypoparathyroidism have some similarities (Table 11-8). Common features include osteosclerosis, calvarial thickening, hypoplastic dentition, and calcification in the basal ganglia. Osteosclerosis is generalized in 9% and more localized in 23% of patients.[77,79,95] Spinal ossification that may resemble ankylosing spondylitis occurs in a small percentage of cases.[89] Changes that may be noted in the foot and ankle include transverse metaphyseal bands, premature epiphyseal fusion, and subcutaneous soft tissue calcification.[77,79,95]

Pseudohypoparathyroidism and Pseudo-pseudohypoparathyroidism

Pseudohypoparathyroidism differs from hypoparathyroidism in that parathyroid hormone levels are normal, with histologically normal or hyperplastic parathyroid glands, but end-organ resistance is noted. This sex-linked dominant condition usually presents in the second decade. Patients are typically short, obese, with round faces, bradydactaly, and mental retardation. Serum Ca^{2+} is decreased, and PO_4 is elevated.[59,89,90]

Radiographic changes (see Table 11-8) may be similar to those of hypoparathyroidism (osteosclerosis and basal ganglia calcification). However, shortening of the metatarsals (Fig. 11-20), metacarpals, and phalanges with widening of tubular bones, exotosis, and cone-shaped epiphysis are useful differential diagnostic features.

TABLE 11-8. *Radiographic features of hypoparathyroidism and pseudohypoparathyroidism[a]*

Radiographic Features	Hypoparathyroidism	Pseudo and Pseudo-pseudohypoparathyroidism
Osteosclerosis	+	+
Soft tissue calcification	subcutaneous	periarticular or ossification
Calvarial thickening	+	+
Basal ganglion calcification	+	+
Hypoplastic dentition	+	−
Spinal calcification	+	−
Exostosis	−	+
Bowing deformities	−	+
Premature epiphyseal fusion	+	+
Shortening of metacarpals, metatarsals, and phalanges	−	+

[a] Data from Lachmann et al., ref. 74.

Pseudo-pseudohypoparathyroidism is often seen in the same family as patients with pseudohypoparathyroidism.[57,95] Both conditions are considered in Albright's hereditary osteodystrophy. The patient's stature and clinical features are similar, but serum Ca^{2+} is usually normal. Radiographic features are similar to those of pseudohypoparathyroidism.[95]

THYROID DISORDERS

Thyroxine and triiodothyronine are predominantly protein bound and are the active forms of thyroid hormone. Diseases of the thyroid gland and resulting changes in levels of these hormones affect protein, fat, and carbohydrate metabolism and mineral turnover. Skeletal changes may be due to primary thyroid disease alone.[89,90] However, other diseases

have been associated with thyroiditis, thereby adding to the radiographic changes. For example, Becker and colleagues[99] reported thyroid fibrositis and thyroiditis in 12% of patients with rheumatoid arthritis. In addition, systemic lupus erythematosus and rheumatoid arthritis have been reported in patients with Hashimoto's thyroiditis.[99,106]

Hyperthyroidism

Hyperthyroidism (elevated thyroxine and triiodothyronine) is most commonly associated with Graves' disease or goiter with active thyroid adenomas.[99] Patients typically present with fatigue, tachycardia, muscle weakness, and exophthalmus. There is increased bone turnover resulting in elevation of serum Ca^{2+} and urine Ca^{2+} and PO_4 in some

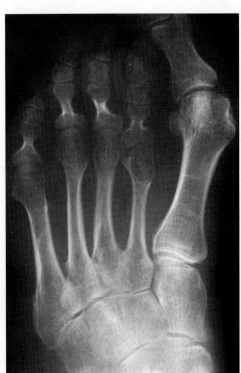

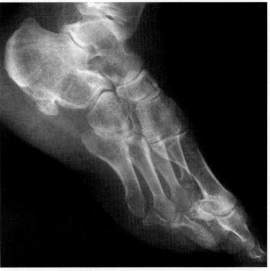

FIG. 11-20. AP (**A**) and lateral (**B**) views of the foot showing shortening of the second and third metatarsals and phalanges of the second toe in a patient with pseudohypoparathyroidism.

patients. Serum alkaline phosphatase and osteocalcin are elevated. Parathyroid hormone and 1,25-dihydroxyvitamin D may be decreased.[107] Bone loss is more common in elderly patients in whom osteoporosis is already occurring.[107,109] Progressive osteopenia may occur over a 1- to 5-year period and may result in vertebral compression fractures. Changes do not differ radiographically from those of idiopathic osteoporosis, except osteopenia in the feet and appendicular skeleton is more common in hyperthyroidism.[99–101,104,105] Changes in the feet include cortical lucent striations and prominent secondary trabeculae, giving the bone a lace-like appearance.[99,100,106] Less frequently, the radiographic changes may be similar to those of osteomalacia with pseu-

dofractures. As noted earlier, changes of rheumatoid arthritis or systemic lupus erythematosus may also be present. These typically mask the more subtle changes of hyperthyroidism. In children, skeletal maturation is accelerated.[106]

Myopathy is common but usually not imaged. Diagnosis is generally based on clinical findings and response to therapy.

Thyroid acropachy is seen in about 1% of patients with thyrotoxicosis.[102,103,106,110] This condition usually appears several years after the initial onset of hyperthyroidism.[106] Patients present with exophthalmus, pretibial edema, and swelling of the digits in the hands and feet (Fig. 11-21). Radiographic features of this condition are distinct in that

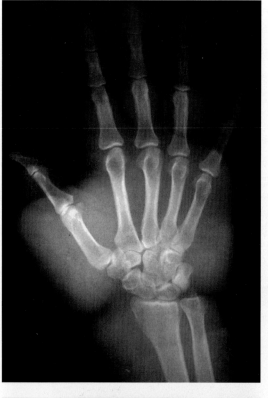
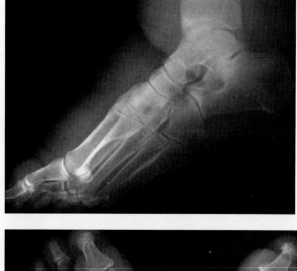
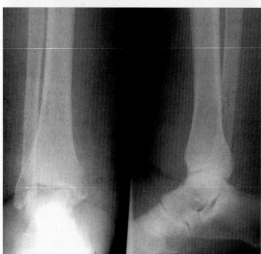
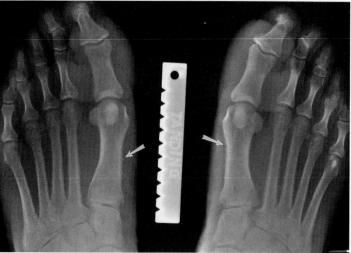

FIG. 11-21. AP view of the hand and wrist (**A**), AP and lateral (**B**) views of the ankle, and lateral views (**C**) of the foot showing dramatic soft tissue swelling. Periostitis has not yet appeared. **D**: Typical soft tissue and periosteal changes (*arrows*) seen with thyroid acropachy.

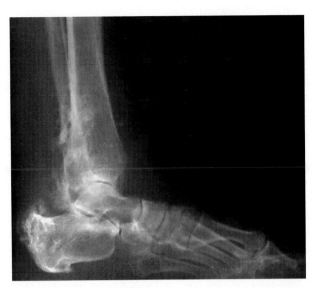

FIG. 11-22. Standing lateral view of the foot and ankle demonstrating shaggy irregular periostitis resulting from pachydermoperiostosis.

swelling with solid or stellate diaphyseal periostitis is demonstrated. The periostitis is asymmetric and involves the metacarpals, metatarsals, and phalanges. Radioisotope studies may demonstrate creased diaphyseal uptake before the appearance of periostitis on radiographs.[108] These periosteal features of thyroid acropachy have several characteristics that differentiate this condition from other disorders associated with periosteal new bone formation. Changes with thyroid acropachy are feathery and do not involve the epiphysis. There is typically no pain associated with the radiographic features. Periosteal reaction with hypertropic osteoarthropathy is more smooth or linear, and patients usually have associated pain. Long bone diaphyseal involvement is most common (tibia, fibula, radius, ulna). Changes may resolve with treatment of the primary disease.

Pachydermoperiostosis (Fig. 11-22) is almost always seen in males and may involve the epiphysis. As with thyroid acropachy, changes do not resolve with therapy.[106,107] Other causes of periostitis include hypervitaminosis A, fluorosis, vascular insufficiency, changes induced by chronic stress, infection, and trauma.[107]

The periosteal reaction differs significantly from other forms of periostitis. In pulmonary hypertropic osteoarthropathy, the periosteal changes are linear, more subtle, and typically involve the tibia, but rarely the feet. Periostitis in pachydermoperiostosis is symmetric. Leukemic periostitis affects the terminal phalanges,[103] and fluorosis most commonly involves the axial skeleton.[106]

The cause of thyroid acropachy is uncertain. Vascular changes were considered to play a role. However, long-acting thyroid-stimulating hormone and human thyroid stimulator may play a more significant role.[101,102,106] Treatment of thyroid disease has little, if any, effect on bone change.[106]

Hypothyroidism

Hypothyroidism and myxedema are the result of reduced serum thyroxine and triiodothyronine.[107] Primary hypothyroidism may be related to any condition (atrophy, radiation or surgical ablation, iodine therapy, and thyroiditis) that reduces the amount of functioning thyroid tissue. Secondary hypothyroidism is due to diminished thyroid-stimulating hormone (pituitary dysfunction).[106,107]

In adults, hypothyroidism is more common in women. Patients present with hoarseness, bradycardia, and dry skin and hair. Skeletal findings, when present, are mild, but increased or decreased skeletal density may be evident. Ca^{2+} levels are usually normal.[106]

In infants (cretinism) and children (juvenile hypothyroidism), clinical and radiographic features are more dramatic. Patients are lethargic, thick tongued, and have delayed dentition, dry skin and hair, hypotonia, and abdominal distension. Radiographic features include remarkably delayed maturation, which is exhibited by delay in appearance and fragmentation of epiphyses. Ca^{2+} retention can also occur, leading to soft tissue calcification.[106]

PITUITARY DISORDERS

Pituitary secretion of growth hormone (somatotropin) is essential for normal musculoskeletal development. Abnormalities can occur with both increased and decreased secretion of growth hormone. However, radiographic abnormalities occur more commonly with the former.[111]

Acromegaly and Gigantism

Hypersecretion of growth hormone is most common with acidophilic and chromophobic adenomas, and it occurs less frequently with pituitary hyperplasia. During the developing years, increased secretion of growth hormone leads to gigantism. Patients are tall and larger than usual but well proportioned. When growth plate closure has occurred, skeletal changes occur more commonly at costochondral junctions and in the periosteal regions. These changes are most obvious in the hands, feet, and mandible (acral skeletal). Therefore, the term acromegaly is applied to this condition.[111,112,114]

Patients with acromegaly have typical physical findings including prominent mandibles, prominent facial features with frontal bossing, and poor dental occlusion. The tongue is often thickened, and the voice is deepened. The digits are broad, and the fingers have a spade-like appearance. Arthropathy may mask the other symptoms of acromegaly in the early stages.[116] Abdominal organs are typically enlarged. There is also increased incidence of associated endocrine disorders. Diabetes has been noted in up to 25% of patients with acromegaly, increased lactation is seen in 4%, and hypercortisolism may also occur. The incidence of islet cell tumors and pancreatic adenomas is also increased in patients with acromegaly. Cardiovascular function is often affected.[111,113]

Radiographic changes result from somatotropin stimulation of endochondral and periosteal bone formation and soft tissue overgrowth. Soft tissue changes of acromegaly are primarily due to skin thickening, increased connective tissue, and edema.[112] Swelling may also occur with other conditions such as congestive heart failure, cellulitis, and venous insufficiency. However, the clinical symptoms and location usually allow these conditions to be differentiated from soft tissue thickening of acromegaly.[118] Soft tissue thickening in acromegaly is most obvious in the scalp, fingers, and toes.[112] Soft tissue thickening has been measured radiographically in an attempt to assist in establishing the diagnosis of acromegaly. Meema and associates[118] measured skin thickness in the forearm using soft tissue technique. Thickness was noted to be 1.1 to 1.8 mm in normal males and 0.9 to 1.7 mm in normal females. Skin thickness in acromegalic patients ranged from 2.0 to 2.8 mm. This technique is not commonly used today.

Measurement of heel pad thickness has also been explored. Using a focal spot distance of 40 inches, Steinbach and Russell[124] evaluated a large group of normal (103 patients) and acromegalic patients. The distance from the plantar aspect of the skin to the most adjacent plantar aspect of the calcaneus was calculated. In normal patients, heel pad thickness varied from 13 to 21 mm, with a mean of 17.8 mm. In acromegalic patients, heel pad thickness ranged from 17 to 34 mm, with a mean of 25.6 mm.[124] Using 21 mm as the upper range of normal, 79% of patients with acromegaly exceeded this measurement, and no normal patients would be included. Although this measurement may be useful, it has been questioned by other investigators. Jackson[115] found that obese patients (more than 200 pounds) frequently had heel pad thicknesses greater than 21 mm (65% of 40 patients weighing more than 200 pounds and 90% of patients weighing more than 275 pounds). Puckette and Seymour[119] found 14% of white males and 40% of black males had heel pad thicknesses that exceeded 21 mm. Overall, their study showed that 26% of normal patients had heel pad measurements exceeding the normal (21 mm) value reported by Steinbach and Russell.[124]

Radiographic changes in the skeleton are most common in the hands, feet, skull, and spine. However, larger joints may also be involved.[117,121–123]

Changes in the skull include thickening of the calvarium, expansion of the sella by the pituitary neoplasm, and, usually more obvious, the enlargement of the frontal sinus, mastoids, prominent occipital spurring, and prominent neck skin folds. Widening of the mandibular angle is also common.[111,120–123]

Up to 50% of patients with acromegaly have significant back pain.[115,120] Hypersecretion of growth hormone leads to increase in the size of vertebral bodies, widening of the disk spaces, and increased appositional bone formation leading to marked anterior spur formation. Posterior scalloping of the vertebral bodies has also been described, although the cause is unclear.[120]

Symptoms in the peripheral joints are evident in 62% of patients. Nearly 20% of patients have symptoms severe enough to evaluate radiographically.[115,120,123] Joint symptoms are related to changes in bone and soft tissue. Synovial thickening and effusion are common. Increased bone formation at sites of tendon and ligament attachment and thickening of the cartilage also occur.[120] Articular abnormalities most commonly occur in the knees, hips, and shoulders. Thickening of the articular cartilage leads to joint space widening (Fig. 11-23). The new bone formation at sites of tendon and ligament attachment results in hypertropic spur formation. Therefore, the appearance of a degenerative joint but with widening of the joint space instead of narrowing is typical in patients with acromegaly. As degeneration of articular cartilage progresses, the joint space narrows, a feature that eventually makes differentiation of acromegaly from osteoarthritis more difficult.[120,123]

Changes in the hands and feet are similar.[113,120] Because of the nature of this text, we emphasize the latter. Soft tissue thickening in the toes and heel pad (see earlier) is common.

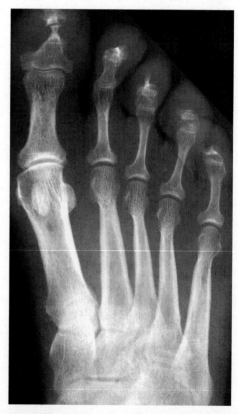

FIG. 11-23. Acromegaly. AP view of the foot with widening of the second through fifth metatarsophalangeal joints, abnormalities in the tufts of the distal phalanges, and square, broad metatarsal heads.

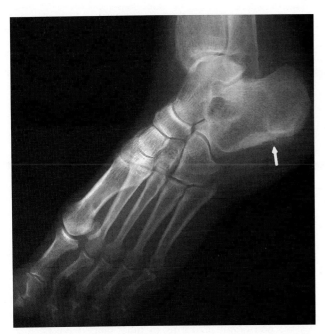

FIG. 11-24. Oblique view of the foot in a patient with acromegaly. Note the periosteal new bone formation at the plantar fascial origin (*arrow*).

Cortical thickening, resulting from stimulation of periosteal bone formation, may result in thickening of the metatarsals and square phalanges.[120,123] Joint space widening because of cartilage thickening is usually most obvious in the metatarsophalangeal joints (see Fig. 11-23). As in the larger joints, one often sees hypertropic beaking at the articular margins and new bone formation at the sites of ligament and tendon attachments giving the appearance of degenerative arthritis. Ligamentous changes are usually most striking in the calcaneus at the insertion of the Achilles tendon and plantar fascial attachments (Fig. 11-24). Prominent tufts (''spade-like'') on the distal phalanges and exostosis are also common.

Sabet and Stark[121] proposed a sesamoid index in diagnosis of acromegaly. The product of the sesamoid length times the width (measured on the anteroposterior [AP] radiograph) was 84 to 122 or mean of 102 in normal males. The normal mean in females was 74. The sesamoid index in acromegaly ranged from 130 to 187, with a mean of 154 in males and 130 in females.

Changes similar to acromegaly have been described with pachydermoperiostosis. However, patient appearance and normal growth hormone levels allow differentiation of this condition from acromegaly.[114]

Hypopituitarism

Reduced pituitary function may follow surgery, infection, vascular insult, or neoplasm. Radiographic features are rarely evident and are generally not an important part of clinical diagnosis. In the developing skeleton, radiographic features include delay of appearance of epiphysis and delayed closure of growth plates.[120,123] These changes are rarely noted in the foot and are not specific because they can occur with other endocrinopathies.

OSTEOLYSIS

Osteolysis or disappearing bone disease can be related to numerous conditions.[128,129,136,137,144,145] Resorption of bone may follow trauma or may be associated with local and systemic conditions such as Sudeck's atrophy, neoplasm, infection, neurologic disorders, gout, rheumatoid arthritis, scleroderma, multicentric reticulohistiocytosis, and leprosy (Table 11-9).[125,132,143,147,148,150,152,153]

Gorham's disease or massive osteolysis is a unifocal disease resulting from bone replacement by hemangiomatous or lymphagiomatous tissue.[131,134,135,138,143] The condition typically involves one bone or one of the larger joints such as the hip or shoulder.[134,135] There are no associated renal or neurologic diseases. Patients may be asymptomatic, except in the presence of a pathologic fracture. Most patients are less than 40 years of age. No familial tendency has been demonstrated.[134,135,143]

Radiographically, the axial or appendicular skeleton may be involved with early findings similar to patchy or diffuse osteoporosis. Over time, one sees progressive bone loss, fragmentation, joint involvement, and involvement of contiguous osseous structures.[134,135,143]

Osteolysis may also be multifocal. Torg and colleagues[148] classified several types of osteolysis that commonly involve the hands and feet (see Table 11-9). Three forms of multifocal (tarsocarpal) acroosteolysis were described. The first form was termed essential osteolysis with nephropathy.[125,130,133,140,141] Although the cause was unclear, these patients have significant renal disease. The osteolysis usually begins in early childhood. Renal disease usually leads to death in the early twenties. The condition does not have familial tendencies, and no histologic changes are evident to define the cause of the osteolysis.[138] Radiographs demonstrate progressive carpal and, to a lesser degree, tarsal bone loss.[143]

The second form of osteolysis is idiopathic hereditary osteolysis. The ankles and wrists may be involved initially. The tarsal and carpal bones are similarly affected. However, there is no associated renal or neurologic disease. Both recessive and dominant patterns of inheritance have been described.[125,126,133,149,151] Onset is usually noted by 3 to 4 years of age. Pain and swelling are the initial symptoms. Erythematous skin lesions and soft tissue nodules have been described with the recessive form.[125,143,148]

The third major category, that charavcterized by miscellaneous patterns (see Table 11-9), does not fit clearly into the previous two groups.[134,135,148] Laboratory studies in all forms are unremarkable, except for increased serum alkaline phosphatase and urinary hydroxyproline resulting from bone

TABLE 11-9. *Osteolysis syndromes: foot and ankle*[a]

Syndrome	Sites	Features
Gorham's osteolysis	Axial and appendicular skeleton	Massive bone loss
Multicentric osteolysis (carpal-tarsal osteolysis)	Carpal and tarsal bones	Local bone loss: hereditary, nephropathic and miscellaneous patterns
Neurogenic osteolysis	Phalanges	Inherited neuropathy and skin ulcerations inherited
Acroosteolysis: Joseph or Shinz	Phalanges	Recessive and dominant inherited, respectively
Winchester's syndrome	Carpal, tarsal bones, and elbow	Infants
Transient phalangeal osteolysis (microgeode disease)	Phalanges	Transient, self-limited

[a] Data from references 125 to 129, 131, 133 to 135, 141, 143, 145, and 148 to 152.

destruction.[139,148] Obviously, in the form associated with nephropathy, renal disease leads to abnormalities in certain serum and urine studies.[148]

Multifocal or tarsocarpal osteolysis usually presents with subtle osteopenia in the wrist or proximal foot. Over a period of months or years, the bones become deformed, and foot deformities such as pes cavus are common (Fig. 11-25).[125,133,148,149] With time, the metatarsals and ankle may also become involved.[141] During the early phases, it may be difficult to differentiate radiographic changes from juvenile rheumatoid arthritis, neurogenic deformity with osteopenia, Sudeck's atrophy, and other causes of osteopenia. However, clinical and laboratory data usually assist in excluding these conditions.[143,146] Other conditions, such as leprosy and frostbite, tend to cause osteolysis of the distal phalanges. Acroosteolysis from occupational conditions, such as polyvinyl chloride exposure, typically involve the hands.[132,152]

Several additional conditions (see Table 11-9) deserve mention. Neurogenic osteolysis is a progressive form of peripheral bone destruction involving the phalanges. Both recessive and dominant forms of inheritance have been described. Patients present in childhood with sensory loss and skin ulcerations on the hands and feet.[139,142,143]

Joseph (recessive inheritance) and Shinz (dominant inheritance) described distal phalangeal osteolysis that was also associated with skin ulcerations. However, patients had no neurologic disease, as described earlier with neurogenic osteolysis.[139,143]

Winchester's syndrome (see Table 11-9) begins in infancy. This disorder presents in infancy with progressive destruction of the carpal and tarsal bones. The condition is inherited (recessive).[143]

Transient phalangeal osteolysis is a self-limited condition. Only 161 cases have been described in the literature.[145] Patients present with swelling and pain in the affected phalan-

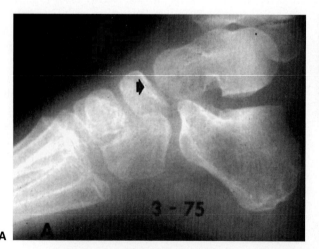
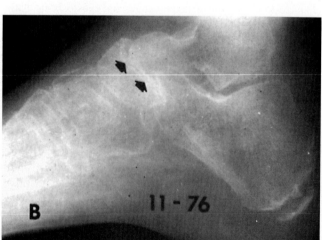

FIG. 11-25. Lateral views of the foot dated 3-75 (**A**) and 11-76 (**B**) show evolving osteolysis with increasing cavus deformity of the foot. (From Whyte et al., ref. 151, with permission.)

ges. Radiographically, one sees small (1-mm) lucent areas in the marrow and cortex of the involved phalanges. The affected phalanx may also appear widened. Radiographic features and symptoms usually return to normal in 6 months. The radiographic features may be confused with those of sarcoidosis or tuberculous osteitis. Tuberculosis more often shows periosteal reaction and cortical destruction, and the middle and distal phalanges are usually involved with tuberculosis. Microgeode disease does not usually involve the distalphalanx. Sarcoidosis is not self-limited and involves multiple organs.[145]

PAGET'S DISEASE

Paget's disease, once considered rare, is a common condition in older patients. The condition is rare in patients younger than 40 years of age, but it occurs in about 3 to 4% of patients older than 40 years and in 10% of patients older than 80 years.[154–157,159] Ninety percent of patients with Paget's disease are more than 55 years old.[159] A geographic distribution has also been reported, with the incidence of Paget's disease higher in the northern United States, England, and Western Europe.[161]

The most common sites of involvement are the axial skeleton, femur, and tibia.[156,159] Collins[156] reported fibular involvement in 4% of patients. The foot, typically considered an uncommon site, may be involved in up to 20% of patients. The calcaneus is involved most commonly. Roughly 10% of patients with foot involvement are symptomatic. This may explain the low incidence of foot involvement previously reported. If patients have no symptoms referable to the foot, radiographs will not be obtained.[156,162]

The cause of Paget's disease is still an unsolved problem. Theories range from inflammation and endocrine disorders to vascular disease and autoimmune abnormalities.[158,159] As recently as 1976, a viral origin was proposed because of the presence of enclusion bodies similar to those produced by paramyxovirus noted using electron microscopy.[159]

As noted earlier, symptoms are frequently absent, especially in the foot. In the report by Rubin and colleagues,[162] only 10% of patients with calcaneal involvement were symptomatic. Symptoms related to axial skeletal involvement are more common.[163] Harris and Krane[157] reported symptoms in up to 80% of patients. Most authors report that nearly two-thirds of patients have no symptoms.[157,159,163]

Although patients may present with pain or deformity in advanced disease, many cases are detected incidentally on radiographs. Laboratory studies may also lead to the diagnosis in asymptomatic patients. Bone resorption causes elevated alkaline phosphatase and increased serum and urine levels of hydroxyproline. Serum Ca^{2+} and PO_4 levels are usually normal.[155,159,162]

Radiographic findings in Paget's disease vary with the stage and histologic changes. Typically, four stages of Paget's disease are described. The initial stage is predomi-

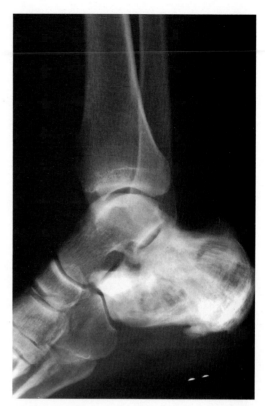

FIG. 11-26. Lateral view of the calcaneus demonstrating marked cortical thickening and prominent trabeculae from Paget's disease.

nantly destructive. This leads to geographic lucent patterns in bone. The characteristic findings are osteoporosis circumscripta in the skull and long lucent lesions with sharp margins (blade of grass or bayonet sign) in the long bones, typically the tibia.[158,159] The trabecular pattern is also coarse during this phase of Paget's disease. As the disease evolves, the sclerotic changes predominate, resulting in a mixed or combined lytic and sclerotic phase (stage 2), and finally a predominantly sclerotic phase (stage 3), which results in cortical thickening, medullary sclerosis, and marked trabecular prominence (Fig. 11-26). When detected radiographically, the disease is usually in the mixed or sclerotic form. A fourth stage, malignant degeneration, is now more commonly recognized. This has been reported in 1 to 10% of patients with Paget's disease (Fig. 11-27).[159]

Skeletal involvement is most often polyostotic, but isolated involvement of a single bone may occur in 10% of cases.[159] The incidence of symptoms is higher in polyostotic disease, and differentiation of Paget's from osteoblastic metastases can be a problem, especially in the spine and pelvis.

Isotope scans may be positive before radiographic features are evident. Radioisotope scans are strongly positive in patients with Paget's disease because of the marked increase in metabolic activity. These studies are also useful to evalu-

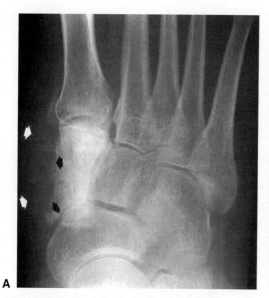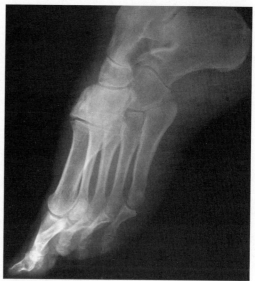

FIG. 11-27. Paget's disease of the medial cuneiform seen on AP (**A**) and oblique (**B**) views of the foot. Soft tissue swelling (*white arrows*) and periosteal irregularity (*dark arrows*) suggest malignant degeneration.

ate the extent of disease and to follow response to treatment (Fig. 11-28).[158,159,163]

CT and MRI are usually not required for detection of Paget's disease.[155,160] In fact, the confusing signal intensity changes presented on MRI (Fig. 11-29) can lead to misdiagnoses. In patients with Paget's disease, routine radiographs should always be correlated with MRI.[155] Paget's disease can be suggested on MRI when the cortex is thickened and irregular and when focal areas of normal marrow are seen within the cortex (Fig. 11-30). MRI is useful to detect soft tissue extension and bone disease in patients with suspected malignant degeneration (see Fig. 11-28).[155]

Complications

Certain complications have been described in patients with Paget's disease. Pathologic fractures are not uncommon because even though excess bone appears to be present, the new bone formation that occurs during the sclerotic phase is disorganized. Therefore, the normal stress lines may be poorly supported, resulting in incomplete or complete fractures and avulsion fractures at sites of ligament or tendon insertions.[155,159]

Malignant degeneration (stage 4) is potentially the most severe complication. Repeat radiographs or other techniques such as CT or MRI (best for soft tissue changes) may be necessary to detect malignant degeneration.[155] Change in symptoms (persistent pain) or the radiographic pattern (see Fig. 11-28) should lead one to consider this possibility. Malignant degeneration can develop in 1 to 10% of patients.[159] The incidence is higher (5 to 10%) when Paget's disease is

widespread compared with patients with localized disease (1%). Patients are usually more than 55 years of age, and men are slightly more commonly affected.[159] The most common malignancy is osteosarcoma, but fibrosarcoma and other types of malignant disease have also been described.[159,161] Up to 25% of osteosarcomas beyond the age of 40 years arise in sites of preexisting Paget's disease.[159]

Other complications include platybasia, cord symptoms (enlargement of vertebral bodies, pedicles, and lamina), cauda equina syndrome, and deafness (enlargement of petrous bone). Increased incidence of hypertension, of congestive heart failure (rare), and of arteriosclerosis has also been noted in patients with Paget's disease.[159,163]

BONE ISLANDS, OSTEOPOIKILOSIS, OSTEOPATHIA STRIATA, AND MELORHEOSTOSIS

These benign sclerotic dysplasias of bone are considered together because of their benign course, similar cause, and the evidence of combinations of these disorders.[179,181]

Bone Islands

Benign sclerotic areas in bone may be single or multiple. Numerous terms have been used to describe these benign sclerotic areas in bone, but bone island and enostosis are most commonly used.[164,179,181] These bone lesions are normally incidentally identified in asymptomatic patients. There is no sex predilection. Lesions may be identified in patients ranging in age from 7 to 78 years.[177]

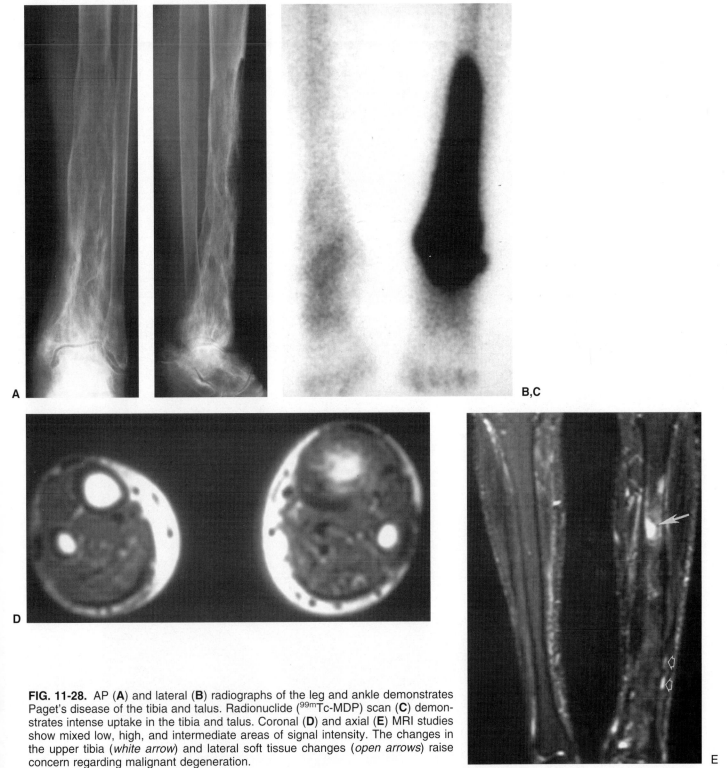

FIG. 11-28. AP (**A**) and lateral (**B**) radiographs of the leg and ankle demonstrates Paget's disease of the tibia and talus. Radionuclide (^{99m}Tc-MDP) scan (**C**) demonstrates intense uptake in the tibia and talus. Coronal (**D**) and axial (**E**) MRI studies show mixed low, high, and intermediate areas of signal intensity. The changes in the upper tibia (*white arrow*) and lateral soft tissue changes (*open arrows*) raise concern regarding malignant degeneration.

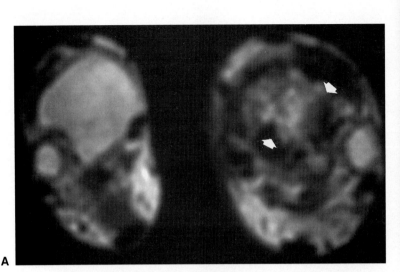
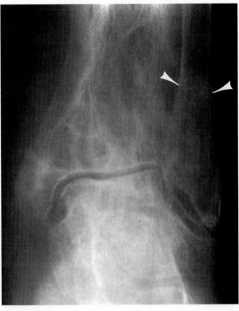

FIG. 11-29. Patient with ankle pain. **A:** Axial MRI demonstrates marked signal abnormality in the tibia at the ankle level (*arrows*). **B:** Routine radiograph demonstrates Paget's disease of the distal tibia and talus. A stress fracture (*arrowheads*) in the fibula was the cause of the ankle pain.

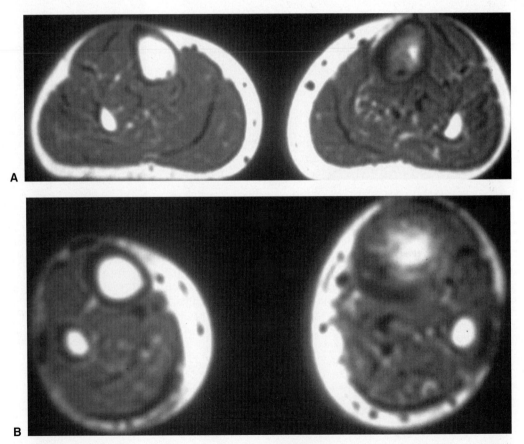

FIG. 11-30. Axial SE 500/11 images of the lower leg demonstrate cortical thickening with residual fatty marrow (**A**) and expansion of the bone and cortical thickening (**B**).

Bone islands are most often detected in the ribs, femora, and pelvis. The epiphysis is the most common site involved in tubular bones. Onitsuka[177] noted that the ankle and foot were involved in more than 10% of 189 patients. Interestingly, 31.9% of bone islands changed in size on subsequent radiographs. This change is probably related to constant resorption and reformation at the medullary margin of the bone island.[177,179]

Histologic examination of bone islands shows that they are round, oval, or spiculated areas of compact bone connected to adjacent trabeculae. This may explain the spiculated appearance of some bone islands. The exact cause is unclear. However, a developmental origin is most likely.[165,173,179]

Radiographically, bone islands are usually round or oval, and 66% are between 0.5 and 1.5 cm in size.[165,173,177] The margins are often spiculated because of the adjacent trabecular incorporation. Although change in size can occur (most enlarge gradually, some become smaller) the rate is much more gradual than in metastatic lesions, there is no history of a primary lesion, and lesions are asymptomatic. Differential diagnosis should also include infarcts, osteopoikilosis, osteoid osteoma, and osteoma.[179]

Other imaging studies such as isotope scans, CT, and MRI are rarely indicated.[168] Tomography may be useful in demonstrating the typical appearance more clearly, but this is rarely indicated. Isotope studies (^{99m}Tc-pyrophosphate) are most often normal in patients with bone islands, but focal increased uptake can occur. This is most likely present in growing bone islands and may also be related to the size, location, and sensitivity of the radiopharmaceutical. When isotope studies are positive, differentiation from metastasis may be difficult.[168,170,181,182]

MRI is not useful in evaluating bone islands or in differentiating these lesions from blastic metastasis. Signal intensity is low (black on image) using both T1- and T2-weighted sequences because of the presence of sclerotic or cortical bone.

Osteopoikilosis

Osteopoikilosis is a sclerotic bone dysplasia that normally begins in childhood.[171,174,179,183] The condition has been noted in all bones except the skull.[164] Lesions are small (2 to 10 mm), oval or spheric, and located in the metaphyses and epiphysis. The oval or elliptic lesions typically are aligned parallel to the long axis to the shaft of the bone.

The condition is generally believed to be a hereditary chondrodysplasia and is probably inherited as an autosomal dominant trait.[179,183] The sclerotic areas are rare before the age of 3 years and may increase in size with development in children. The size of the lesion is usually stable, or lesions may disappear in adults.[165] Patients are usually asymptomatic, although approximately 20% may have pain in the involved joints. Associated dermatologic conditions (derma-

tofibrosis lenticularis disseminata) and a predisposition to keloid formation have also been reported.[179]

Lesions are multiple, usually smaller and better marginated than bone islands, and lesions are confined to the epiphysis and metaphysis of long bones. The appearance is usually so characteristic that differentiation from other conditions is not difficult (Fig. 11-31). However, potential differential diagnostic considerations include tuberous sclerosis, mastocytosis, and, rarely, blastic metastasis. The last diagnosis is particularly uncommon in the foot and ankle.

^{99m}Tc-pyrophosphate scans are typically normal in these patients. Therefore, isotope imaging can be a useful tool if the radiographic appearance is atypical. As with growing bone islands, growing lesions of osteopoikilosis in children can result in positive isotope studies.[182,183]

Osteopathia Striata

Osteopathia striata is a rare condition that is most likely inherited as an autosomal dominant trait.[167,179] This condition was first described by Voorhoeve in 1924.[172] Patients are typically asymptomatic. Radiographs demonstrate linear sclerotic striations in the metaphysis of the long bones. Investigators have suggested the osteopoikilosis and osteopathia striata are related because the former can present with typical rounded areas of sclerosis or more linear striations.[167,179] Patients with either of these conditions are usually asymptomatic, but joint pain can be present with both conditions.

Radiographically, the distinct feature is linear sclerotic metaphyseal bands that run parallel to the shaft of the long bones. The striations typically end at the growth plate but may extend into the epiphysis. Changes are usually bilateral. Striations in the foot are most obvious in the calcaneus and tarsal bones. Changes may be particularly dramatic in the tibia. The skull and ribs, when involved, take on a more uniformly sclerotic appearance that could be confused with osteopetrosis.[167,179] Radionuclide studies are normal, similar to osteopoikilosis.[182]

Melorheostosis

This condition was described by André Leri and J. Joanny in 1922.[166,169,180] The original description was that of an unusual sclerosis of bone involving only one side of the cortex. The appearance reminded the authors of dripping candle wax. Thus the term melorheostosis (from the Greek, meaning limb, flow, bone) was created.[179] The origin of melorheostosis is unclear. However, various causes, including congenital origin, infection, endocrine disease, and vasospasm of subperiosteal angiomas have been postulated.[166,169,175,180] Melorheostosis affects soft tissue and bone. Therefore, muscle atrophy and joint deformities are not uncommon.[176,178,180]

Patients may be asymptomatic or may present with pain in the involved area. Patients range from birth to 63 years

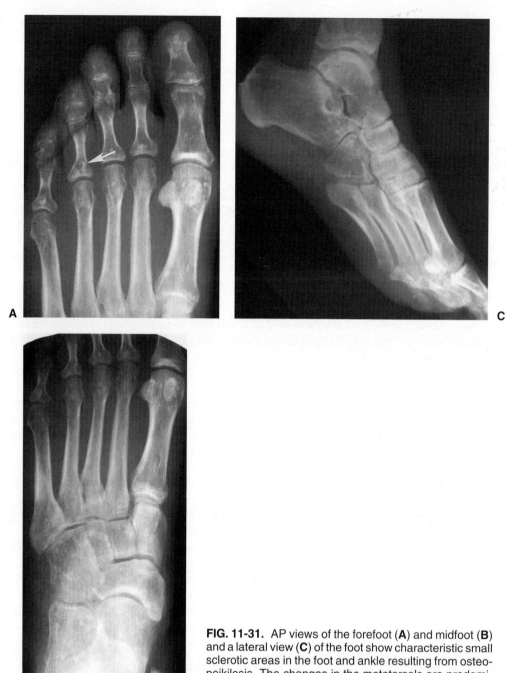

FIG. 11-31. AP views of the forefoot (**A**) and midfoot (**B**) and a lateral view (**C**) of the foot show characteristic small sclerotic areas in the foot and ankle resulting from osteopoikilosis. The changes in the metatarsals are predominantly epiphyseal. Diagnosis was established incidentally when the patient's foot was radiographed for the fracture in the fourth proximal phalanx (*arrow*).

of age (up to 50% present by age 20), and there is no sex predilection.[180] The involved extremity may be shorter or, rarely, longer than the uninvolved side. Bone deformity and muscle atrophy may be present in some patients. The process is most common in the long bones of the extremities and is often unilateral. However, bilateral involvement and in-

volvement of more than one extremity on the same side can occur.[166,179,180,182]

The clinical course is usually slow, with possible symptom-free periods. There is no accepted treatment, although sympathectomy has been used successfully in selected cases. Malignant degeneration has not been reported.[179,180]

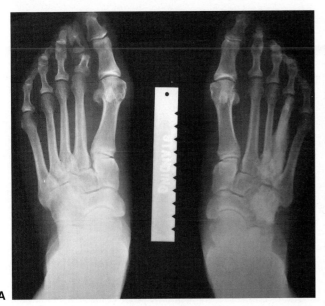
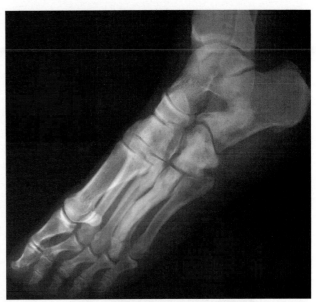

A

B

FIG. 11-32. Melorheostosis. AP (**A**) and oblique (**B**) views of the foot demonstrate irregular cortical thickening of the fourth metatarsal. Sparing of the lateral cortex is evident distally. The calcaneus and cuboid are also involved.

Radiographic features may be evident at birth. In 40 to 50% of patients, changes are persistent by age 20.[169,180] Findings are most characteristic in the tubular bones. There is cortical thickening, usually involving one side of the bone. The pattern resembles dripping candle wax and can be globular or irregular (Fig. 11-32). Typically, the process extends into the metaphysis or epiphysis; however, joint and soft tissue involvement is not unusual. The tarsal bones may develop patchy areas of sclerosis. Unlike osteopoikilosis, radionuclide studies are usually positive in areas involved with melorheostosis.[176,182]

Numerous conditions have been reported in association with melorheostosis. The list includes limb shortening or lengthening, scleroderma, neurofibromatosis, clubfoot deformity, osteopoikilosis, osteopathia striata, and a variety of hemangiomatous conditions.[179,180,182]

OSTEOPETROSIS

Osteopetrosis is a disease of uncertain origin first described by Albers-Schönberg in 1904.[184,188] The condition is related to lysosomal dysfunction in osteoclasts and their precursor cells.[184,189] Multiple forms of this disorder have been described including benign autosomal dominant and more aggressive autosomal recessive categories.[184,187]

The autosomal dominant form is benign with onset in childhood and does not affect life expectancy.[187,189] However, up to 40% of patients have at least one pathologic fracture.[187] Radiographic and clinical features may vary depending on the subtype (Table 11-10). The autosomal recessive forms are more severe (see Table 11-9).[184] Additional features include more severe anemia, short stature, hepatosplenomegaly, and renal disease.[184,185,187]

TABLE 11-10. *Osteopetrosis*[a]

Type	Inheritance	Features
Benign		
Type I	Autosomal dominant	Calvarial and spine sclerosis
Type II	Autosomal dominant	Calvarial, spine, and pelvic sclerosis
Type III	Autosomal dominant	Calvarial, hand, foot sclerosis
Malignant		
Lethal	Autosomal recessive	Generalized sclerosis, failure to thrive, deafness and blindness, hepatosplenomegaly
Renal tubular acidosis	Autosomal dominant	Skeletal sclerosis, renal tubular acidosis, cerebral calcification
Intermediate type	Autosomal dominant	Short stature fractures, anemia, hepatomegaly

[a] Data from references 184, 185, 187, and 189.

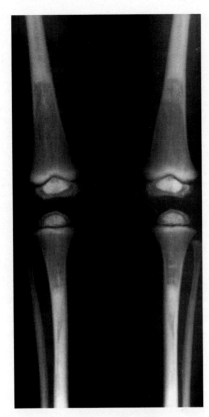

FIG. 11-33. AP views of the lower extremities in a child with osteopetrosis. There is dense sclerosis in the diaphysis of the femurs, tibia, and fibulas. Transverse dense bands are most obvious in the distal femoral metaphysis. Note the epiphyseal bone-within-a bone appearance.

Bone changes are similar in all clinical forms of osteopetrosis. Transverse metaphyseal bands and longitudinal sclerotic bands are common with progression to larger areas of dense bone and a bone-within-a-bone appearance (Fig. 11-33). Facial bone density is frequently increased in the infantile form. Sclerotic or underdeveloped sinuses are also common.[189]

In the delayed form, the skeleton is usually normal at birth. Radiographic changes develop during childhood. Erosions in the tufts of the hands and feet and early degenerative arthritis have been reported in addition to the usual findings. Facial changes are less obvious.[186,190–192] Complications of osteopetrosis include fractures, deformities, and osteomyelitis.[186,190,193]

Pyknodysostosis can present with features similar to those of autosomal recessive osteopetrosis. Patients present with osteosclerosis and short stature, but in addition they have radiographic features of occipital bossing, small facies, and short broad hands.[189] The bones of the feet are sclerotic, short, and hypoplastic, and there is usually osteolysis of the distal phalanges (pencil point).[189] The last finding may be confused with acroosteolysis. Patients with pyknodysostosis do not present with anemia, which is seen with osteopetrosis.

VITAMINOSIS

Vitamins are essential catalysts in bone development, especially in the growth plate regions. Vitamins A, C, and D are particularly critical. Vitamin A is essential for chondrogenesis and normal longitudinal bone growth. Vitamin C is required for collagen and matrix formation. Vitamin D (see the section on osteomalacia and rickets) is essential for Ca^{2+} and phosphorus balance.[202] With today's nutritional standards, bone abnormalities due to hypovitaminosis and hypervitaminosis are unusual.

Vitamin A

Hypervitaminosis A can produce clinical and radiographic abnormalities in adults and children.[199,200,204] Acute vitamin A intoxication is rare today, but it has been reported following overdoses or ingestion of polar bear, shark, and chicken liver, which contain massive amounts of vitamin A.[196,200] In the acute setting, adults present with symptoms of increased intracranial pressure. Headache and vertigo have been reported. Children may develop acute symptoms after overdosage of vitamin drops. Drowsiness, emesis, and bulging of fontanels in infants have been described. Symptoms in adults and children clear quickly when vitamin A is withdrawn.[196,197]

Clinical presentation in chronic vitamin A poisoning is significantly different, and skeletal changes are more likely to be evident radiographically. In children, the clinical presentation is usually delayed several months after vitamin A administration is initiated. The onset of symptoms is dose related, so a shorter latent period is noted with higher doses.[194] Patients present with a variety of symptoms and physical findings including anorexia, pruritus, tender subcutaneous nodules over the long bones, coarse hair, and fissuring of the legs and bleeding.[199] Hepatosplenomegaly and clubbing of the fingers have also been reported.[200] Vitamin A levels (normal, 50 to 130 IU) are elevated, a finding that establishes the diagnosis.[199]

Radiographic features of hypervitaminosis A are confined to the growing skeleton. Periosteal new bone formation with a smooth, wavy pattern is common along the ulna and metatarsals. This may be evident on isotope scintigraphy before radiographic changes are evident.[198] Hyperostosis and metaphyseal abnormalities also occur. The former may have radiographic features similar to those of infantile cortical hyperostosis (Caffey's disease). Differentiation of these two conditions is based on clinical and radiographic features. Caffey's disease commonly involves the mandible, and vitamin A levels are normal. The mandible is not involved in hypervitaminosis A, and onset is usually about 1 year of age compared with infantile cortical hyperostosis, which occurs in the first 6 months of life.[197,200,203] Metaphyseal deformities occur with central growth plate closure resulting in continued peripheral growth, so the epiphysis appears drawn into the metaphysis.

Spine and long bone deformities are not usually evident with vitamin A poisoning. However, Ruby and Mital[201] noted scoliosis and bowing deformities in patients with chronic vitamin A intoxication. Radiographic features are usually absent in hypovitaminosis.[200]

Vitamin C

Excessive levels of serum vitamin C are rare. Vitamin C is excreted by the kidneys. In addition, gastrointestinal absorption decreases when oral intake of the vitamin is increased. Therefore, excessive amounts of circulating vitamin C are unusual.[200]

Vitamin C deficiency is uncommon today, but it can result in skeletal changes in both adults and children. Radiographic changes are most common in children and usually involve the proximal extremities. The foot and ankle are rarely involved.

As originally described, the deficiency commonly occurred following boiling of milk before feeding. Boiling destroys vitamin C. This technique is unusual with today's milk products and feeding techniques. Infants present initially with failure to thrive. Petechiae and more dramatic hemorrhagic episodes (e.g., extremity swelling, melena, hematuria, bleeding gums) occur later. Bleeding tendencies are probably related to reduced levels of intercellular cement in capillaries.[200] Symptoms in infants do not usually present until approximately 1 year of age because a lag period of 4 to 10 months occurs between the time of reduced vitamin C intake and the onset of symptoms.

The most dramatic radiographic changes of vitamin C deficiency occur in infants and children. The most obvious and specific changes occur in the growth plate, metaphysis, and epiphysis. Reduced matrix formation, collagen production and osteoblastic activity lead to disorganization of the growth plate.[200] Several characteristic changes result. The zone of provisional calcification becomes thick and sclerotic, demonstrated as a dense metaphyseal band radiographically (Fig. 11-34). A lucent zone is evident on the metaphyseal side of this band. This lucent zone (scurvy line) is due to reduced trabecular bone. In addition, one sees beak-like metaphyseal extension, marginal lucent metaphyseal changes (corner sign) (see Fig. 11-34), and periosteal elevation. Hemorrhage in these areas is responsible for many of the radiographic features, especially the marked elevation of the periosteum.[200] The epiphyses of the tubular and tarsal bones also have dense provisional zones of calcification at their margins with lucent centers (Wimberger's sign).[200]

Articular involvement, primarily from hemarthrosis, is unusual. When this does occur, the larger joints are most commonly involved. The feet are usually spared. Growth disturbances are also common in treatment if it is not instituted before significant growth plate damage has occurred.

Following treatment, radiographic changes may revert to

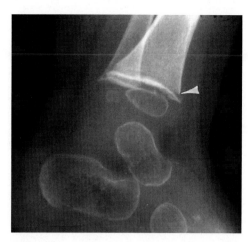

FIG. 11-34. Lateral radiograph of the ankle in a young child with scurvy. A lucent metaphyseal line and corner sign are present (*arrowhead*) in the distal tibia.

normal, or residual dense lines may develop in the lucent metaphyseal region (scurvy line). Cortical thickening may be evident in areas where periosteal elevations were evident.

Radiographic features in adults are rare. When they occur, they are usually in malnourished elderly patients, so the osteopenia of vitamin C deficiency is difficult to separate from senile osteoporosis.[200]

Vitamin D

Vitamin D deficiency is discussed earlier in this chapter with regard to osteomalacia and rickets. High levels of vitamin D can also result in clinical symptoms in adults and children.[195,200] Vitamin D intoxication has been reported in children treated for skeletal disorders and in adults with Paget's disease.[200]

Both acute and chronic forms of intoxication occur. Systemic symptoms are common with both. Anorexia, vomiting, fever, and abdominal and musculoskeletal pain are common presenting complaints. Renal failure may occur eventually if sufficient metastatic calcification occurs in the kidneys.[200]

The most obvious radiographic features may be related to hypercalcemia and metastatic calcification. Calcifications can involve the vasculature, periarticular regions (Fig. 11-35), or abdominal viscera. These features are not specific and can be noted with a variety of other disorders (Table 11-11).[200,203]

Skeletal abnormalities include dense metaphyseal bands resulting from increased Ca^{2+} deposits and a variety of bone density changes. Some patients have cortical thickening from periosteal bone mineral increase or areas of sclerosis, and in some cases cortical thinning and osteopenia are evident.[200]

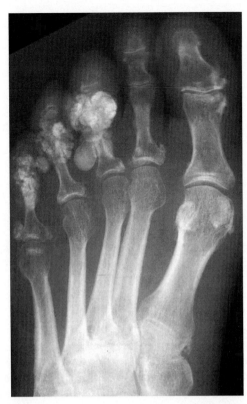

FIG. 11-35. AP view of the foot demonstrating dense areas of amorphous calcification in the periarticular soft tissues. Juxtaarticular osteopenia is also present. The diagnosis is vitamin D intoxication.

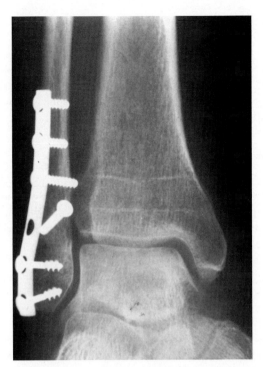

FIG. 11-36. Adult with recent ankle fracture and plate and screw fixation of the fibula. Two transverse bands ("growth arrest lines") are seen in the tibial metaphysis.

TABLE 11-11. *Conditions associated with soft tissue calcification*[a]

Metastatic (Calcium-phosphorus metabolism)
   Hyperparathyroidism
   Hypervitaminosis D
   Sarcoidosis
   Multiple myeloma
   Metastasis
   Milk-alkali syndrome
   Renal osteodystrophy
Calcinosis (normal calcium metabolism)
   Collagen vascular disease
   Tumoral calcinosis
   Calcinosis universalis
   Dermatomyositis
Dystrophic calcification (normal calcium metabolism)
   Trauma
   Neoplasms
   Inflammatory

[a] Data from references 199 and 202.

HEAVY METAL DISORDERS AND TRANSVERSE METAPHYSEAL BANDS

Sclerotic transverse bands are commonly noted on extremity radiographs. These dense linear bands are commonly referred to as growth arrest lines.[208,213,214] This term is a misnomer because the transverse lines are more likely recovery lines that remain after periods of transient reduced or retarded growth.[213,214]

Although their exact origin is unclear, investigators have theorized that these lines develop as osteoblasts build a transverse trabecular structure along the growth plate. When growth continues, this template remains and is seen radiographically as a transverse sclerotic band (Fig. 11-36).[213–215] The location of these bands (diametaphyseal) and their minimal thickness serve to differentiate them from the thicker juxtaphyseal metaphyseal bands associated with heavy metal intoxication and other conditions.

Disorders related to metals such as lead, aluminum, and copper can also lead to skeletal abnormalities.[205,206,209,212,215] Lead intoxication has received the most attention in the radiographic literature. Lead intoxication occurs in neonates of mothers with lead intoxication, or it may be acquired by ingestion of lead-containing paints or inhaling lead-containing fumes.[209,210,215] Clinical symptoms may be acute, with patients complaining of abdominal pain, seizures, and other neurologic symptoms. Chronic or more subtle symptoms such as fatigue, muscle weakness, and anemia may

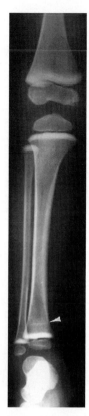

FIG. 11-37. AP radiograph of the lower extremity in a child with lead poisoning. Note the dense transverse metaphyseal bands in the metaphysis at the knee and ankle. A growth arrest line (*arrowhead*) is present in the distal tibia.

also occur.[210] Increased urine porphyrin and hematologic smears are the useful diagnostic screening studies in patients with suspected lead toxicity. Radiographic changes occur late and are less useful. Routine radiographs reveal thick sclerotic bands adjacent to the growth plate (Fig. 11-37). The sclerosis was originally believed to be primarily due to lead deposits. Although small amounts of lead can be demonstrated, most of the density is due to excessive amounts of Ca^{2+}.[207,210] This finding is not specific and can also be noted in healthy persons, healing rickets, leukemia, scurvy, hypothyroidism, vitamin D intoxication, and transplacental infections.[215] Other heavy metal disorders may have similar radiographic findings.

Patients undergoing dialysis or taking aluminum hydroxide to reduce PO_4 absorption may develop aluminum toxicity. Radiographs are of little value because osteomalacia can be seen with aluminum toxicity and renal osteodystrophy. Histologic bone evaluation is the most accurate method of diagnosis.[206,212]

Copper deficiency has been reported in infants receiving total parenteral therapy. Radiographic findings are nonspecific. Osteopenia, metaphyseal cupping, periostitis, and wide, irregular growth plates (similar to rickets) have been reported.[205,211]

HEMOGLOBINOPATHIES AND ANEMIA

Fetal hemoglobin (HbF) constitutes 60 to 90% of hemoglobin at birth. Adult hemoglobin (HbA) usually replaces HbF by 4 months of age. Normal HbA consists of paired polypeptide chains. There are two alpha chains with 141 amino acids and two beta chains with 146 amino acids. Variations in the amino acids on either the alpha or beta chains lead to a spectrum of clinical conditions including sickle cell disease and thalassemia.[217,218,220,235]

Before discussing clinical and image aspects of hemaglobinopathies and anemia, it is important to review the normal progression of red and yellow marrow. Marrow is composed of bony trabeculae, hemopoeitic cells, and fat.[241] Red marrow is composed of the active hemopoietic cells, and yellow marrow primarily consists of fat cells. Red marrow is about 40% water, 40% fat, and 20% protein. Yellow marrow has lower water content (15%), 80% fat, and 5% protein.[241] This composition results in different appearances on MRI.[240,241]

Conversion of red to yellow marrow occurs with a predictable pattern during skeletal development. At birth, nearly the entire skeleton is red marrow. Conversion of red to yellow marrow occurs from the peripheral to the axial skeleton (Fig. 11-38). In long bones (see Fig. 11-38), progression is from diaphysis to metaphysis. Epiphyses and apophyseal ossification centers contain yellow marrow. Adult marrow distribution is usually achieved by 25 years of age (see Fig. 11-38). Marrow conversion can result from many factors, including anemias and hemaglobin disorders discussed within section. Marrow conversion occurs in reverse of the normal progression from red to yellow marrow. Therefore, the axial skeleton converts to red marrow first, followed by the proximal and then the distal extremities.[240,241]

Sickle Cell Anemia

Sickle cell disease has different clinical and radiographic features depending on the configuration of the hemoglobin molecule. Sickle cell anemia is the homozygous form (HbS-S). In this setting, the alpha-hemoglobin chain is normal, but valine replaces glutamic acid on the beta chain. This condition is evident in up to 1.3% of American blacks.[229,230,235]

The heterozygous form (HbA-S) or sickle cell trait is less significant clinically, and radiographic changes are essentially nonexistent. This form of sickle cell anemia occurs in 7% of black Americans.[235] Sickle cell HbC is an intermediate form of sickle cell disease. This heterozygous form of hemoglobin (HbC-S) occurs when the S gene is inherited from one parent and the C gene from another.[217] This condition occurs in 1.3% of American blacks. A fourth variant, sickle cell thalassemia, occurs when one S gene and one thalassemia gene are inherited.[229,236]

Clinical symptoms in sickle cell disorders are most severe in the homozygous form, with milder symptoms in patients

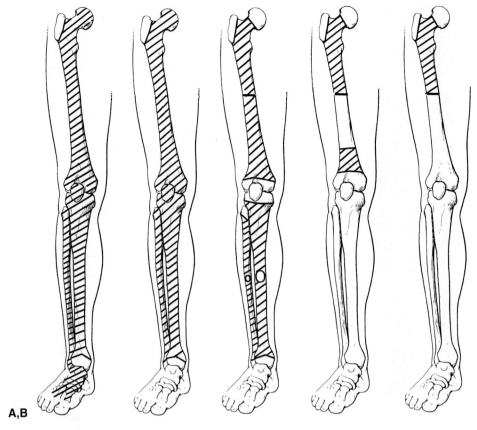

A,B

C,D,E,

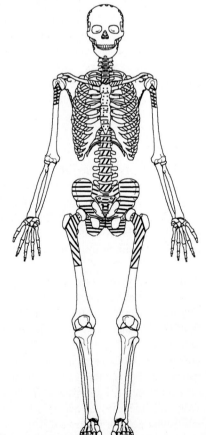

F

FIG. 11-38. Illustrations of red (*black lines*) and yellow (*white areas*) marrow distribution during skeletal development (**A** to **E**) and in the adult skeleton (**A**). Yellow marrow replaces red marrow beginning in the periphery of the extremities. **A:** At birth, the peripheral skeleton is almost entirely red marrow, except for the distal tibia and greater trochanteric apophysis. **B:** Age 7 years. **C:** Age 14 years. **D:** Age 21 years. **E:** Age 28 years. **F:** Illustration of the adult skeleton with red marrow (*black lines*) in the calvarium, axial skeleton, ribs and proximal femurs, and humeri, except in the epiphysis, greater trochanters, and humeral epiphyses and tuberosities.

with sickle cell trait, sickle cell HbC, and sickle cell thalassemia.[217,224,225,229,235] Symptoms are rare during the first 6 months of life because of the presence of HbF. Painful swelling of the hands and feet (dactylitis) can occur between 6 months and 2 years of age. Sickle cell crises are usually associated with bone necrosis, resulting in pain in the joints and extremities. Fever, anemia, and abdominal pain from visceral involvement are also common. These episodes are usually evident by 20 to 30 years of age. Symptom-free periods occur between episodes.[236,237]

Physical examination may reveal enlargement of the liver and spleen. Leg ulcerations are common, especially over the malleoli. Adenopathy may also be noted. Other associated conditions include osteomyelitis, cholelithiasis, peptic ulcer disease, hematuria, and priapism.[217,236,237]

Radiographic findings are predominantly related to bone infarction, marrow hyperplasia, and complications such as osteomyelitis (Fig. 11-39).[227,233,235] Chronic anemia leads to a hypercellular response in the red marrow. In adults, this is evident in the axial skeleton. In infants, red marrow is also present in the hands and feet, but regression axially occurs during childhood. Therefore, radiographic features of marrow hyperplasia are common in the foot and ankle in young children, but they may not be evident in older patients (see Fig. 11-39E).[235] Radiographically, this hypercellular response leads to cortical thinning, osteopenia, and fewer but more prominent trabeculae in spongy bone.[217,235] These changes may be identified in the skull, spine, and appendicular skeleton. In the skull, the diploic space widens and both tables are thinned. This finding is less common in patients with sickle cell variants. Only 25% of patients with sickle cell HbC have typical changes in the skull. The vertebral bodies are osteopenic, with ballooning of the disk spaces (see Fig. 11-39B and C) and flattened vertebral end plates centrally.[235,240]

Vascular occlusion leads to bone infarction in the diaphysis, metaphysis, and epiphysis (Fig. 11-40). Radiographic features vary with the patient's age and type of hemoglobin. Changes in children occur most often with sickle cell anemia (HbS-S). From 10 to 20% of children, commonly between 6 months and 2 years of age, develop dactylitis in the metatarsals and metacarpals. These patients present with pain, swelling, and periosteal new bone radiographically.[235] Infarcts may also develop in the larger tubular bones, where diaphyseal involvement is most common in the femur and upper tibia (see Fig. 11-39D). Epiphyseal osteonecrosis is most common in the femoral and humeral heads and is usually bilateral (see Fig. 11-39A).[217,235] Although radiographic findings are usually more common in sickle cell anemia (HbS-S), the incidence of avascular necrosis of the femoral and humeral heads may be higher in sickle cell HbC disease. Hill and colleagues[229] reported an incidence of 8% in homozygous sickle cell anemia compared with 17% for sickle cell HbC disease. This finding was possibly related to the increased viscosity of blood in the latter.

Ischemic changes involving the growth plates and adjacent epiphysis and metaphysis can result in growth deformity. Epiphyseal deformities such as cone-shaped epiphyses are particularly common in the hands and feet. These changes are not specific for sickle cell anemia, but they can also be seen following trauma and infection. Premature epiphyseal closure can lead to leg-length discrepancy or, when asymmetric closure occurs, joint deformity. Talar tilt is an example of the latter. This was originally believed to be a common feature of sickle cell anemia.[222,231] Shaub and associates[238] reported this finding in 39% of patients with sickle cell anemia. Others believe that this finding is less common (3.6%). In addition, tibiotalar tilt is also evident in patients with juvenile rheumatoid arthritis, hemophilia, and epiphyseal dysplasia.[216,217]

Deformity of the vertebral bodies from end-plate ischemia leads to a typical central depression giving the vertebra an H-type configuration (see Fig. 11-39B and C). This finding is also seen in thalassemia, Gaucher's disease, and hereditary spherocytosis.[219,220,228]

Arthropathy can be associated with sickle cell anemia, usually the homozygous (HbS-S) variety. Typically, patients have mild, nonerosive arthritis with transudative synovitis.[235,238] However, Rothschild and Sebes[237] reported erosive changes in 14% of 100 patients with sickle cell anemia. Erosions involved the tarsal bones and metatarsal heads in 5 patients, and 9 patients had erosions in the superior calcaneal cortex near the anterior insertion of the Achilles tendon. Calcaneal involvement was bilateral in 5 patients and unilateral in 4 patients. All but 1 patient had HbS-S. Sickle cell thalassemia was present in 1 patient. Similar findings can be seen in rheumatoid arthritis, psoriatic arthritis, ankylosing spondylitis, Reiter's syndrome, and inflammatory bowel disease.[235,239]

Radiographs are usually not positive initially in patients with sickle cell disease and its variants. Early changes of bone infarction are identified more readily using ^{99m}Tc methylene diphosphonate (MDP) scans and marrow scans using ^{99m}Tc sulfur colloid.[235,239] More recently, MRI studies have been more commonly used to detect subtle bone changes and infarction. MRI studies are more sensitive, and often the appearance of infarction is more specific than with radionuclide studies.[234,235]

Complications of sickle cell disease include fractures and osteomyelitis. The former may occur with minor trauma. The increased susceptibility to fracture is related to marrow hyperplasia and cortical thinning.[221,235] The incidence of osteomyelitis in patients with sickle cell disease is 100 times that of the healthy population. Several explanations exist for the increased incidence, including bone infarction, reduced splenic function, bowel infarction leading to vascular seeding, and more frequent hospitalization of patients with sickle cell anemia. Over 50% of infections are due to *Salmonella*. *Staphylococcus* is the second most common organism, followed by *Escherichia coli, Haemophilus,* and other organisms.[235] Diaphyseal involvement is more common in patients with sickle cell disease.[222,224] Radionuclide studies

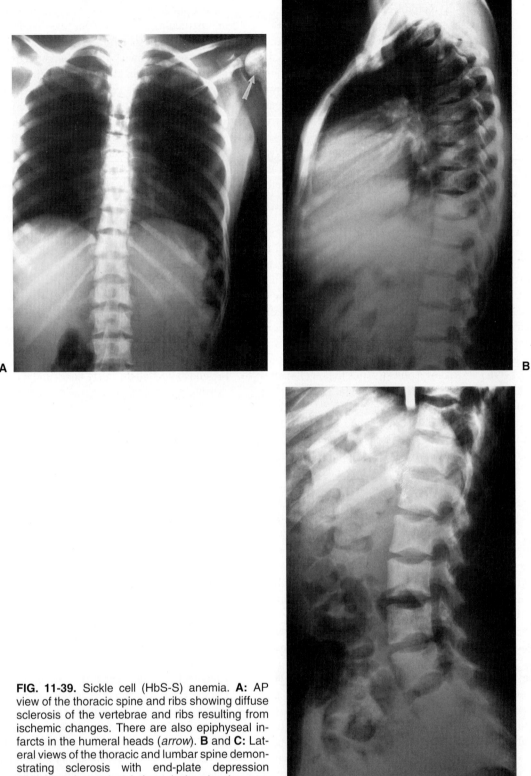

FIG. 11-39. Sickle cell (HbS-S) anemia. **A:** AP view of the thoracic spine and ribs showing diffuse sclerosis of the vertebrae and ribs resulting from ischemic changes. There are also epiphyseal infarcts in the humeral heads (*arrow*). **B** and **C:** Lateral views of the thoracic and lumbar spine demonstrating sclerosis with end-plate depression ("H"shaped vertebrae) from ischemic changes. *(continued)*

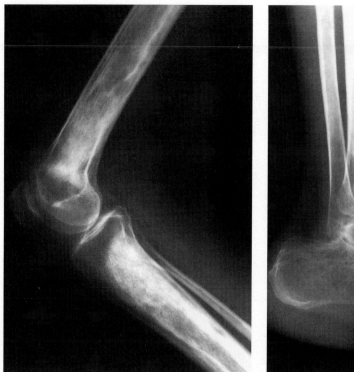
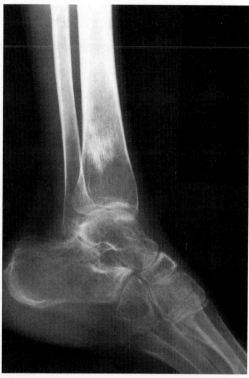

D

E

FIG. 11-39. *Continued.* **D:** Lateral view of the knee demonstrates diffuse, predominantly diaphyseal infarction in the femur and tibia giving nearly a bone-within-a-bone appearance. **E:** Lateral view of the ankle demonstrating an area of infarction in the distal tibia with marrow hyperplasia replacing the trabeculae in the foot. This is most evident in the calcaneus.

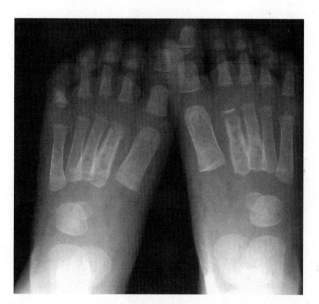

FIG. 11-40. AP views of the feet in a child with sickle cell anemia and infarction with periosteal new bone formation in the second and third metatarsals.

(combined technetium and indium-111–labeled white blood cells) and MRI may be helpful in selected cases. However, MRI features are often nonspecific.

Thalassemia

Thalassemia, sometimes referred to as Cooley's anemia, was first described by Cooley and Lee in 1925.[220] The term thalassemia is derived from the Greek work for sea because the original group of patients was of Mediterranean origin. As in sickle cell anemia, several forms of thalassemia are recognized. The basic disorder is an inherited abnormality in hemoglobin synthesis. Two main forms of anemia exist. Alpha-thalassemia occurs with abnormal alpha-chain synthesis and beta-thalassemia with beta-chain abnormalities. The clinical and radiographic features are most dramatic with the homozygous form (thalassemia major or Cooley's anemia) and are less severe with thalassemia minor. The disease is still more common in the Mediterranean regions, but can also occur in other regions and in Native Americans and blacks.[218]

Thalassemia major (either alpha or beta) is diagnosed early, and life expectancy is significantly reduced. Patients with alpha-thalassemia major have complete absence of the alpha chain. Alpha-thalassemia is the most severe form and is a cause of hydrops fetalis and in utero death. Beta-thalas-

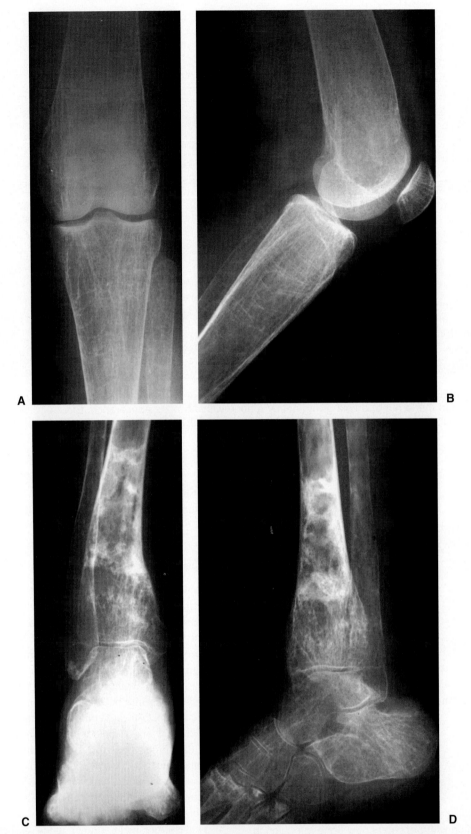

FIG. 11-41. Thalassemia major. AP (**A**) and lateral (**B**) views of the knee show marrow hyperplasia with sparse prominent trabeculae and cortical thinning. Erlenmeyer's flask deformity of the distal femur (**A**) is present. AP (**C**) and lateral (**D**) views of the ankle show similar marrow hyperplasia with sclerosis in the distal tibia resulting from infarction.

semia is diagnosed in infancy or early childhood. Patients have severe anemia and hepatosplenomegaly and typically do not live beyond their teens. Patients with thalassemia minor have mild anemia and may have slight splenomegaly.[218,233,235,236]

Radiographic features are similar to those of other forms of severe chronic anemia. The major finding consists of marrow hyperplasia, which leads to medullary bone expansion, sparse trabeculae, and cortical thinning (see Fig. 11-38). In the foot and ankle, this is most obvious in the distal tibia and tarsal bones (see Fig. 11-38C and D). Changes in the foot and ankle are most evident in young children before regression of red marrow from the peripheral appendicular skeleton.[218,233,235] Erlenmeyer's flask deformity in the metaphysis is typical of thalassemia but not specific, because other marrow expanding disorders, such as Gaucher's, produces similar changes (Fig. 11-41A and B). Peripheral marrow changes are often more prominent in thalassemia, which is useful in differentiating this disease from other anemias.[233,235]

Changes in the skull may be similar to those of sickle cell anemia, with widening of the diploic space and thinning of the inner and outer table. An important differential diagnostic feature is the hair-on-end appearance, resulting from bone proliferation in the outer table. Facial involvement, from osseous expansion of the facial bones, is also more common in thalassemia major.[233,235] The H-shaped vertebra characteristic of sickle cell anemia is rarely seen in thalassemia.[235]

Growth deformities and pathologic fractures can develop.[221,223] Fractures have been described in one-third of patients, typically in the spine and lower extremities.[223,226]

Arthropathy may develop related to secondary hemachromatosis from numerous transfusions. This feature can also occur in other severe anemias such as hereditary spherocytosis.[232,235]

TABLE 11-12. *Conditions associated with periostitis[a]*

Localized
Trauma
Infection
Neoplasms
Neurogenic
Diffuse or Generalized
Primary hypertropic osteoarthropathy
Secondary hypertropic osteoarthropathy
Mesothelioma
Bronchogenic carcinoma
Benign fibrous tumor of the pleura
Bronchiectasis
Cystic fibrosis
Lung abscess
Congenital heart disease (cyanotic)
Chronic active hepatitis
Bile duct carcinoma
Primary biliary cirrhosis
Portal cirrhosis
Ulcerative colitis
Regional enteritis
Hodgkin's disease
Gastrointestinal polyps
Thyroid acropachy
Vascular insufficiency
Hypervitaminosis A
Caffey's disease
Syphilis (congenital)
Leukemia
Neuroblastoma
Rickets
Scurvy
Histiocytosis X
Neurofibromatosis
Diffuse idiopathic hyperostosis
Fluorosis
Acromegaly

[a] Data from references 243, 244, 252, 254, and 255.

PERIOSTITIS

Periosteal reaction and ossification occur in numerous local and systemic conditions (Table 11-12). Many of the conditions, especially localized periostitis (Fig. 11-42), are discussed in the previous chapters. Therefore, this discussion concerns the more diffuse forms of periostitis in which foot and ankle involvement may be evident.

Primary Hypertropic Osteoarthropathy (Pachydermoperiostosis)

Primary hypertropic osteoarthropathy is inherited as an autosomal dominant condition with variable penetrance. This form of diffuse periostitis is less common (3 to 5%) than secondary hypertropic osteoarthropathy. The origin remains a mystery, although histologic studies suggest that periosteal vascular changes may be the cause.[243,253]

Clinical presentation is variable, although the typical syndrome includes clubbing of the hands and feet, enlargement of the extremities due to periosteal bone thickening, soft tissue swelling, and swelling in the periarticular regions. Dramatic skin thickening (pachydermia) may also occur.[243,247,253] Cortical thickening may become so extensive that marrow failure and extramedullary hematopoesis develop.[250]

The syndrome is more common in males than females, and blacks are more commonly affected than whites. Symptoms tend to progress over a period of approximately 10 years and then cease spontaneously. Primary hypertropic osteoarthropathy is usually a painless periostitis, in contrast to secondary hypertropic osteoarthropathy.[253]

Radiographic features vary with the patient's age and duration of symptoms. However, the periosteal changes can be distinctive, a feature that is useful in differentiating primary from secondary and other forms of periostitis (Table 11-13).Primary hypertropic osteoarthropathy most commonly

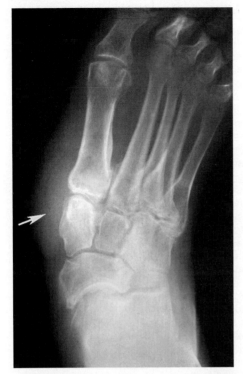

FIG. 11-42. Diabetic patient with neurotrophic arthropathy and ischemic disease. AP view of the foot shows a large neurotrophic ulcer (*arrows*) medially with smooth periosteal new bone formation along the lateral margin of the first metatarsal.

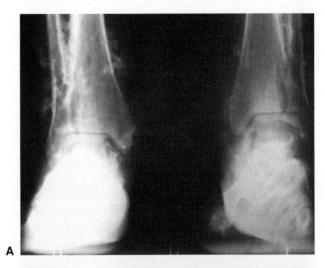

A

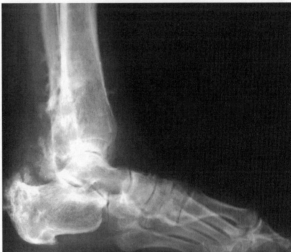

B

FIG. 11-43. Pachydermoperiostitis. AP (**A**) radiograph of the ankle and lateral (**B**) radiograph of the foot demonstrating marked irregular periostitis with extensive changes adjacent to the superior calcaneus near the Achilles tendon insertion. The diaphysis, metaphysis, and epiphysis are all affected.

TABLE 11-13. *Periostitis*[a]

Condition	Radiographic Features
Primary hypertrophic osteoarthropathy (pachydermoperiostitis)	Tibia, fibula, tarsal, metatarsal diaphysis, metaphysis, epiphysis, shaggy periostitis, ligament ossification
Secondary hypertropic osteoarthropathy	Tibia, fibula; tarsal metatarsal uncommon; diaphysis and metaphysis smooth periostitis
Thyroid acropachy	Metatarsals, phalanges spiculated periostitis (hands metacarpals and phalanges more common than feet)
Venous insufficiency	Tibia, fibula, metatarsals phalanges, diaphysis, metaphysis smooth undulating periostitis
Hypervitaminoses A	Tibia, fibula, metatarsals, diaphysis undulating periostitis

[a]Data from references 241, 243, 245, and 251 to 253.

involves the tibia, fibula, radius, ulna, and hands and feet. Periostitis commonly extends into the epiphyseal regions, in addition to the diaphysis and metaphysis, and is much more irregular and shaggy in appearance than other forms of periostitis (Fig. 11-43).[243,248,253] In some cases, this pattern does not occur. Instead, a more generalized, irregular cortical thickening is evident (Fig. 11-44).[253]

Arthropathy occurs less frequently in primary than secondary hypertropic osteoarthropathy. When present, the clinical and radiographic features are nonspecific.[247] However, ligament ossification adjacent to the calcaneus, patella, and olecranon is a useful differential diagnostic feature.[253] Acroosteolysis has also been reported.[248]

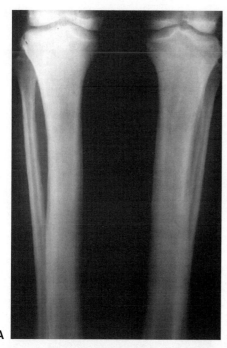
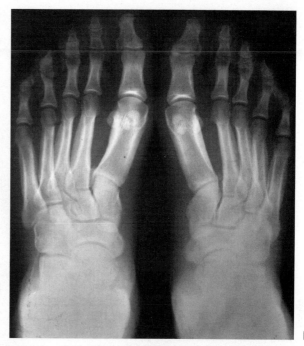

FIG. 11-44. AP (**A**) radiographs of the tibia and fibula and both feet (**B**) in a patient with pachydermoperiostitis. There is diffuse cortical thickening with smooth periosteal changes in the metatarsals.

Secondary Hypertropic Osteoarthropathy

Secondary hypertropic osteoarthropathy is a more useful term than pulmonary osteoarthropathy because numerous nonpulmonary disorders are also associated with osteoarthropathy (see Table 11-12). Pulmonary disorders are commonly associated with secondary osteoarthropathy. This feature is noted in up to 50% of patients with mesotheliomas or benign fibrous tumor of the pleura and in up to 12% of patients with bronchogenic carcinoma (Fig. 11-45).[253] Other pulmonary diseases (cystic fibrosis, lung abscess), congenital heart disease, and numerous gastrointestinal disorders (see Table 11-12) have also been associated with secondary hypertropic osteoarthropathy.[244,252,253,255,256]

Joint symptoms are common and may be the presenting complaint. Thirty-four percent of patients have joint symptoms at some point during their clinical course. These symptoms are increased with activity and tend to be increased at night, as opposed to many arthropathies, which present with early morning pain and stiffness.[253]

The origin of secondary hypertropic osteoarthropathy is unknown. Humoral, neurogenic, and vascular changes may play a role in this disorder.[244,256]

Periostitis is the prominent radiographic feature of secondary hypertropic steoarthropathy. Changes occur most commonly in the distal tibia, fibula, radius, and ulna. Foot involvement is less common than in primary hypertrophic ostosteoarthropathy (see Table 11-13).[253] Several patterns of periostitis have been described. The most common pattern is subtle linear or laminated periostitis involving the diaphysis and metaphysis (see Fig. 11-45).

Greenfield and associates[244] also described three other patterns: irregular, localized periostitis; solid, wavy periosteal thickening; and diffuse cortical thickening (Fig. 11-46). These patterns are also seen in primary osteoarthropathy and vascular insufficiency.[244,253]

Radioisotope scintigraphy is sensitive in early detection of any type of osteoarthropathy. Increased uptake is usually most obvious along both sides of the diaphysis, but it follows the pattern that evolves radiographically (Fig. 11-47).[253,254]

MRI may also demonstrate increased signal intensity in the juxtacortical region on T2-weighted axial images. This technique is rarely required to detect periostitis, and features are not specific for the causes described in Table 11-13.

Vascular Insufficiency

Vascular disease, particularly venous stasis, is also commonly associated with lower extremity periostitis. Sparing of the upper extremities is a useful differential diagnostic feature. Changes occur most frequently along the diaphysis and metaphysis of the femur, tibia, fibula, and metatarsal, and phalanx (see Table 11-13).[249,253]

Other vascular conditions, including arterial disease, periarteritis nodosa, and malformations such as Klippel-Trenaunay-Weber syndrome, may also be associated with periostitis.[253]

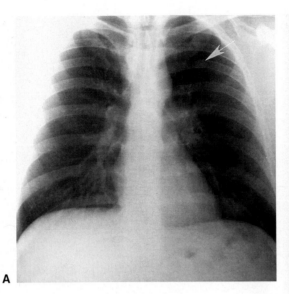

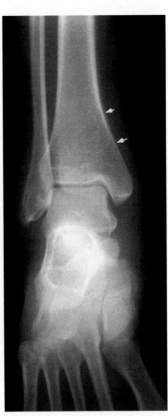

FIG. 11-45. Secondary hypertrophic osteoarthropathy associated with carcinoma of the lung. PA (**A**) view of the chest demonstrating a small carcinoma in the left upper lobe (*arrow*). AP (**B**) view of the ankle demonstrating subtle laminated periostitis (*arrows*) along the medial tibial diaphysis and metaphysis. The epiphysis is not involved.

Periostitis of venous stasis is typically wavy and is thicker than secondary hypertropic pulmonary osteoarthropathy. However, this feature is not specific (Figs. 11-48 and 11-49). Additional features such as pleboliths, soft tissue ossification, edema, and penetrating ulcers are useful in defining the cause of the periostitis more clearly.[249]

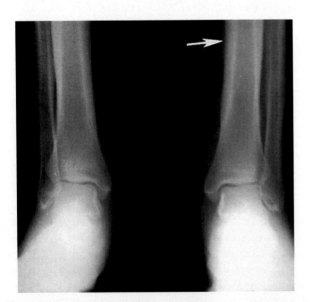

FIG. 11-46. AP views of the ankles in a patient with secondary hypertrophic osteoarthropathy associated with cystic fibrosis. The patient has irregular cortical thickening in the diaphysis of the tibias and fibulas with subtle periostitis (*arrow*).

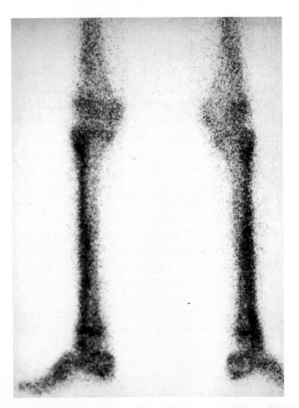

FIG. 11-47. Technetium-99m–methylene diphosphonate (MDP) scans of the lower extremities showing diffuse cortical uptake in both legs from hypertrophic osteoarthropathy.

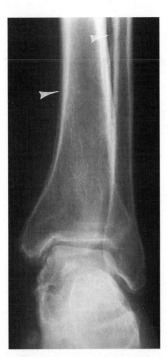

FIG. 11-48. AP radiograph of the ankle demonstrating thick, slightly irregular periostitis along the distal tibia and fibula (*arrowheads*) in a patient with soft tissue ulcerations and vascular insufficiency.

Differential Diagnosis

Differentiation of the various causes (see Table 11-13) of periostitis may not be possible based solely on routine radiographic features. However, the patient's age, location of bone involvement, duration of symptoms, history of trauma, infection, diabetes mellitus, and laboratory findings are all useful.[253]

Changes in Caffey's disease (infantile cortical hyperostosis) (Fig. 11-50) are almost always evident by 5 months of age. Involvement of the foot can occur; however, the mandible is involved in 80% of cases.[246,251] Deformity and marked cortical thickening are usually more dramatic than in the more subtle and linear periostitis associated with leukemia, neuroblastoma, or congenital infections (e.g., syphilis, rubella).[246,251]

Thyroid acropachy (see the earlier discussion in this chapter on thyroid disorders) involves the hands and feet most commonly. Soft tissue swelling is dramatic, even on radiographs (see Fig. 11-21). Periostitis is generally irregular or spiculated, and results of thyroid studies are typically abnormal.

Fluorosis typically involves the axial skeleton with associated ligament ossification. Patients with acromegaly have abnormal pituitary hormone levels, characteristic skull findings, and extremity changes and a typical clinical appearance. The periostitis (Fig. 11-51) is more irregular than in

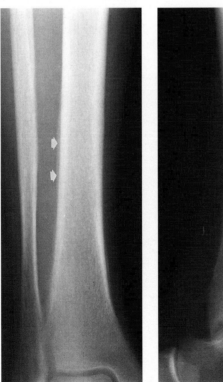
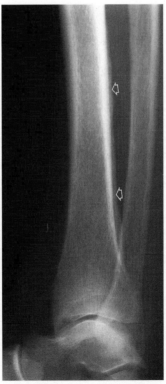

A   **B**

FIG. 11-49. AP (**A**) and lateral (**B**) radiographs of the lower leg in a young male patient with secondary hypertrophic osteoarthropathy from chronic pulmonary disease. The periostitis is wavy along the lateral posterior aspect of the tibia (*open arrows*). Changes are more linear along the medial tibia (*closed arrows*).

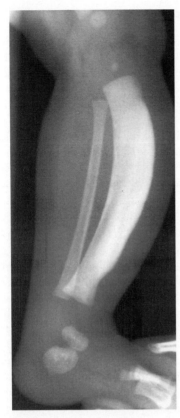

FIG. 11-50. Lateral view of the leg in an infant with Caffey's disease. Note the marked cortical thickening and bowing deformity.

secondary hypertropic osteoarthropathy but is not specific. Other conditions, such as fibrous dysplasia, which cause expansion of the normal tubular shape of long bones, are less difficult to differentiate from periostitis (Fig. 11-52).

SOFT TISSUE CALCIFICATION AND OSSIFICATION

Soft tissue calcifications can be noted in many locations with varying radiographic appearances. In certain cases, the location and appearance are useful in defining the nature of the patient's systemic or regional disease process. In other cases, the appearance of the Ca^{2+} deposit is nonspecific and may be difficult to differentiate from ossification.[274,292,296,304,306,311]

The list of conditions leading to soft tissue calcification is extensive. Both local and systemic conditions are implicated (Table 11-14). Greenfield described three categories of soft tissue calcifications.[274] Metastatic calcification occurs when there is imbalance in the Ca^{2+}-PO_4 product. Conditions included in this type of soft tissue calcification include hyperparathyroidism, renal osteodystrophy, hypervitaminosis D (see Fig. 11-35), milk-alkali syndrome, sarcoidosis, and massive bone destruction such as multiple myeloma or diffuse metastasis.[273,285,296,302] Generalized calcinosis, the second category, includes conditions that lead to calcification in the presence of normal Ca^{2+} and phosphorus metabolism. Calcinosis interstitiales universalis is a condition of unknown origin that results in subcutaneous calcifications initially. Soft tissue calcifications spread to involve deeper tis-

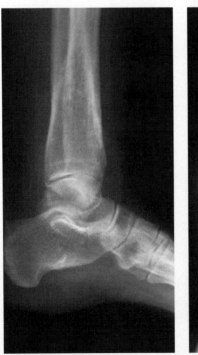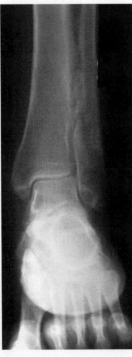

A

FIG. 11-51. AP and lateral (**A**) views of the ankle and oblique (**B**) views of the foot in a patient with acromegaly and irregular periostitis involving the lower tibia and fibula. *(continued)*

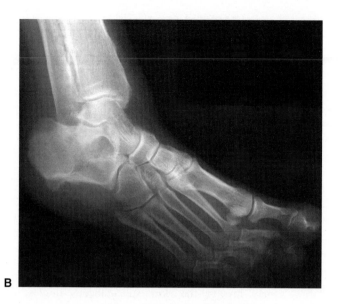

B

FIG. 11-51. *Continued.* There are no other radiographic changes in the foot and ankle to define the nature of the periosteal changes.

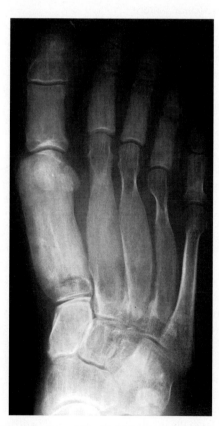

FIG. 11-52. AP view of the foot shows expansion of the first through fourth metatarsals and the first through fourth proximal phalanges with a ground-glass appearance resulting from fibrous dysplasia. The cortex is thin, especially in the second through fourth metatarsals, thus allowing easy differentiation from cortical thickening and periostitis.

sues over time. Calcinosis circumscripta presents with more focal Ca^{2+} deposits offer in the hands and wrists. This form of soft tissue calcification is usually seen in collagen diseases such as scleroderma.[262,268,275,296,303] Dystrophic calcification, the third category, occurs in devitalized or necrotic tissue. This category includes the inflammatory, traumatic, and neoplastic conditions.[274]

Differential Diagnosis

The radiographic appearance of soft tissue calcification is often nonspecific. However, the distribution (localized, periarticular, generalized), configuration (mass-like, linear, reticular, circular), involvement of specific tissues (vessels,

TABLE 11-14. *Etiology of soft tissue calcification*[a]

Metastatic Calcification
    Hyperparathyroidism
    Renal osteodystrophy
    Hypoparathyroidism
    Hypervitaminosis D
    Milk-alkali syndrome
    Sarcoidosis
    Skeletal metastasis
    Multiple myeloma
Calcinosis
    Collagen vascular disease
    Calcinosis universalis
    Tumoral calcinosis
Dystrophic
    Trauma
    Inflammation
    Neoplasm

[a] Data from references 273, 291, 295, 297, 298, 306, and 307.

nerves, fascial, fat), and clinical setting when taken together can be useful in defining the disease process more clearly.[274, 296] Generalized calcinosis occurs with a number of systemic diseases including scleroderma, collagen vascular diseases, dermatomyositis, and idiopathic calcinosis universalis.[274]

Idiopathic calcinosis universalis occurs in infants and children. The cause is unknown. Calcification is usually seen initially in the subcutaneous fat. Therefore, this condition is more typical in infants. An unusual differential diagnostic consideration is infantile subcutaneous fat necrosis. This diffuse condition regresses over a period of 15 months and requires no treatment.[299] Calcinosis universalis progresses during childhood to involve the muscles and other connective tissue. At this stage, the radiographic appearance is similar to that of dermatomyositis. However, muscle enzymes are not elevated in calcinosis universalis. With further progression, large, mass-like collections of Ca^{2+} occur in calcinosis universalis. This feature is not useful because this finding also occurs in dermatomyositis, tumoral calcinosis, and other connective tissue diseases.[274,296,299]

Dermatomyositis is included in a group of inflammatory myopathies. Soft tissue calcinosis is most common in childhood dermatomyositis (Fig. 11-53 and Table 11-15).

TABLE 11-15. *Classification of polymyositis[a]*

Type	Incidence (%)
I Typical polymyositis	35
II Typical dermatomyositis	25
III Dermatomyositis with malignancy	15–20
IV Dermatomyositis of childhood[b]	10
V Acute myolysis	
VI Polymyositis with Sjögren's syndrome	5

[a] Data from Ozonoff and Flynn, ref. 292.
[b] Radiographically demonstrable. Calcification most common.

Calcification occurs in more than 40% of patients and may involve the skin, subcutaneous tissues, and muscles.[262,293,295] Blane and colleagues[262] described four patterns of calcification: (1) deep nodular or calcaneal masses, (2) superficial calcaneal masses, (3) deep linear deposits, and (4) lacy or reticular subcutaneous calcification (Fig. 11-54). The prognosis is more guarded in patients with the reticular pattern.[262,269]

Tumoral calcinosis (calcifying collagenosis, lipocalcinogranulomatosis, lipocalcinogranulomatosis bursitis, lipocalcinosis) was first described in 1899.[258-260,266,277,278,286,305] The cause is unknown, although 30 to 40% of cases are familial.[261,311] Other etiologic considerations include fat necrosis, chronic renal disease, and local trauma.[274,278,307,309]

Symptoms are usually evident by the second decade. The condition is more common in blacks than whites.[261] Patients present with pain, decreased range of motion in the involved joint or joints, and swelling.[278] The largest joints (shoulder, elbow, hips) are most commonly affected. The lateral aspect of the foot is involved less commonly. Serum Ca^{2+} is normal, but elevated serum PO_4 has been reported.[261,309,311]

Radiographs demonstrate nodular, mass-like calcifications about the involved joints that vary from 1 to 20 cm in size (Fig. 11-55). Ca^{2+} fluid levels have been described on routine radiographs and CT.[273,274,281] Prognosis is excellent if the disorder is diagnosed before long-standing joint and muscle effects occur. Surgical resection is generally successful, and recurrence at the site of previous surgery is unusual.[278]

Tumoral calcinosis may be similar to hypervitaminosis D, milk-alkali syndrome, renal osteodystrophy, and calcaneal dermatomyositis radiographically. Elevated serum Ca^{2+} and calcification in other structures (e.g., vessels, subcutaneous fat) away from the involved joint are useful in differentiating these conditions from tumoral calcinosis, which is usually localized to the periarticular region.[274,278,296] Generalized soft tissue calcification in adults is more common in scleroderma and collagen vascular disease (Fig. 11-56).[296]

Isotope scintigraphy (^{99m}Tc-MDP) is not useful in differ-

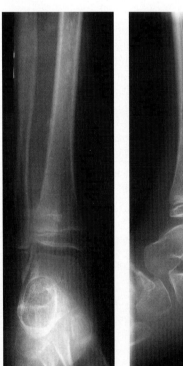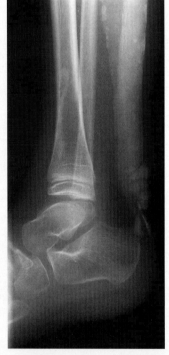

FIG. 11-53. AP and lateral radiographs of the ankle in a child with dermatomyositis. There is dense calcification in the Achilles tendon and superficial muscles of the posterior compartment.

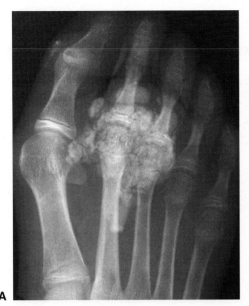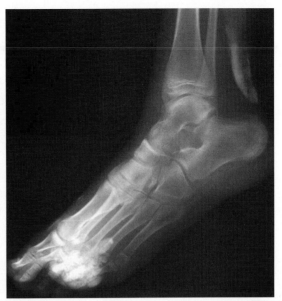

A   B

FIG. 11-54. Young teenager with dermatomyositis. The AP (**A**) view of the foot shows deep periarticular mass-like calcifications. The oblique view of the foot (**B**) shows sheet-like calcification in the muscles posteriorly in addition to the mass-like calcifications in the foot. The change in **A** would be difficult to differentiate from hypovitaminosis D in Figure 11-35. If the muscle changes were not present tumoral calcinosis could also be considered. The latter condition typically involves the larger, more proximal joints.

ential diagnosis. Increased vascularity, increased capillary permeability, or possibly some unknown metabolic reaction can result in increased soft tissue uptake in the presence of inflammation and calcification, as well as when heterotopic bone formation has occurred (Fig. 11-57).[264,266,267,276,284,302] CT is useful in certain cases. MRI is rarely used to evaluate soft tissue calcifications.

More localized soft tissue calcification is commonly associated with trauma, neoplasm, or a chronic infectious or inflammatory process (Fig. 11-57).[274,306] For example, calcification, with a shelf-like configuration, has been described in patients with chronic compartment syndrome.[308]

In some cases, the tissue involved and the radiographic appearance are more useful in defining the underlying cause of soft tissue calcification. Phleboliths have a characteristic radiographic appearance and suggest venous insufficiency or, if they are multiple and localized, hemangioma. Circular calcification in muscles can occur with parasitic infestations such as cysticercosis. Neural calcification has been described in patients with leprosy. Subcutaneous reticular calcification is commonly noted in the earlier stages of childhood dermatomyositis.[274,296]

Ossification

Soft tissue ossification may occur with a variety of conditions.[263,277,296] However, the differential diagnostic considerations are fewer than in soft tissue calcification (Table 11-16).[263,272,283,288–290,294,296] Frequently, sequential radiographs or CT studies are required to detect evolving ossification.[265,269,300] In the early stages, it may be difficult to differentiate calcification from ossification. The distinction may be difficult until a definite trabecular pattern is evident (ossification). Features noted with MRI may be confusing, espe-

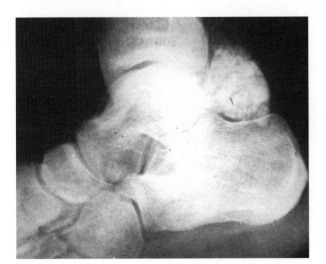

FIG. 11-55. Oblique view of the ankle demonstrating tumoral calcinosis posterior to the talus. (From Hacihanefioglu, ref. 275, with permission.)

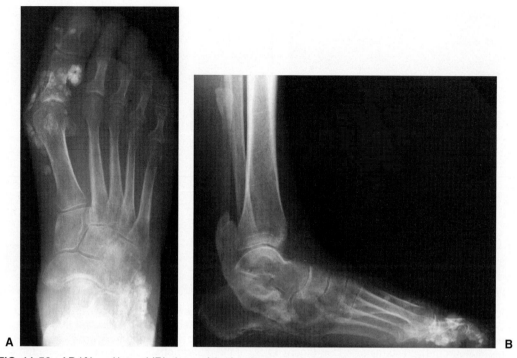

FIG. 11-56. AP (**A**) and lateral (**B**) views of the foot in an adult with scleroderma demonstrating periarticular and tendinous calcification.

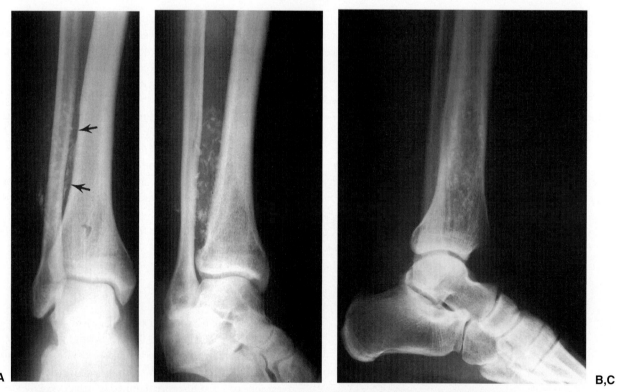

FIG. 11-57. Extraarticular synovial chondromatosis. AP (**A**), oblique (**B**), and lateral (**C**) radiographs demonstrate calcifications in the interosseous membrane with slight scalloping of the tibia (*arrows*). *(continued)*

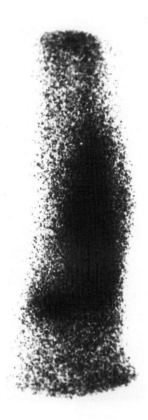

FIG. 11-57. (*Continued*) Technetium-99m–methylene diphosphate scan (**D**) shows intense uptake in the leg.

cially when radiographs or CT are not available for comparison.[282,296]

Myositis Ossificans

Myositis ossificans may be confused with malignancy both radiographically and histologically.[257,272,277,291] Myositis ossificans was categorized into four groups by Noble and Paterson.[290,294] Myositis ossificans progressiva, also known as fibrodysplasia ossificans progressiva, is a rare inherited disorder (autosomal dominant) that presents shortly after birth.[263,280,304] Progressive ossification of skeletal muscle and connective tissue cause pain and disability.[263] Additional findings include shortening of the first metatarsal (70%), microdactaly of the toes (90%), and phalangeal fu-

TABLE 11-16. *Conditions associated with soft tissue ossification*[a]

Paralysis
Trauma
Burns
Venous insufficiency
Neoplasm
Myositis ossificans
Melorrheostosis
Previous surgery
Diffuse idiopathic skeletal hyperostosis

[a] Data from references 262, 269, 273, 286, 287, 293, and 295.

sion (Fig. 11-58).[263,290,294] Microdactaly of the hallux is rarely associated with dermatomyositis.[310] The second category was typical posttraumatic myositis ossificans, and the third type of myositis ossificans associated with burns, paralysis, and chronic infections (see Table 11-16). From 60 to 75% of cases of localized myositis may clearly be related to trauma.[272,274,296] The last or fourth group includes localized myositis ossificans with no history of trauma or any associated etiologic factors (Fig. 11-59). In this setting, differentiation from malignancy is particularly difficult. This condition has been called pseudomalignant osseous tumor of soft tissue.[272,282,296] All the categories except myositis ossificans progressiva are more localized.[263, 274,288,297]

Histologically, Ackerman[257] described myositis ossificans as a zonal process. The central zone consists of fibroblasts with areas of necrosis and hemorrhage. Just peripheral to the central zone is a surrounding area of osteoblasts and immature bone. The most peripheral zone consists of more mature bone.[257]

Radiographic, CT, and MRI features of myositis ossificans reflect these histologic changes.[263,282,296] Soft tissue swelling may be the only feature initially. As the ossification evolves, soft tissue calcification may be noted (4 to 8 weeks).[265] This is followed by mature bone formation peripherally with a lucent line separating the area of myositis from the adjacent bone. Lesions are most commonly adjacent to the diaphysis (see Fig. 11-59), and volume may actually decrease on sequential radiographs. These features are useful in differentiating myositis ossificans from osteosar-

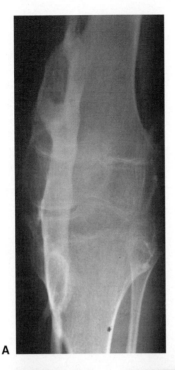

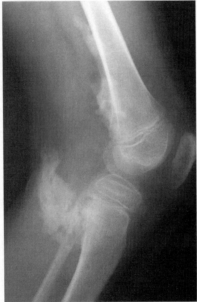

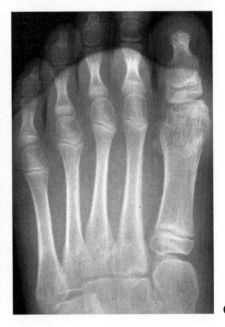

FIG. 11-58. Myositis ossificans progressiva. AP (**A**) and lateral (**B**) views of the knee demonstrating soft tissue ossification. AP view of the foot (**C**) shows shortening of the first metatarsal and microdactaly.

coma and other malignancies. In addition, myositis ossificans tends to occur in younger patients. Soft tissue osteosarcomas occur in elderly patients.[263,270]

Myositis ossificans can also be demonstrated by soft tissue uptake on ^{99m}Tc-MDP and gallium-67 citrate scintigrams.[263,275,282,288] However, findings are not specific. The peripheral mature ossification (Fig. 11-60E) is easily defined using CT.[265,296] MRI displays different signal intensity depending on the stage of development and pulse sequences. The central region of proliferating fibroblasts is typically inhomogeneous and of high signal intensity. The peripheral zone is typically of low intensity on T1-and T2-weighted sequences. A zone of edema at the margins (high intensity on T2-weighted sequences) is common during the first few months. Once mature, the MRI appearance may resemble that of bone marrow with low-intensity cortical bone at the peripheral margins (see Fig. 11-60C and D). Central fluid-fluid levels have also been reported.[282,296] Because CT is more sensitive in detecting soft tissue calcification and the peripheral ossification is easily appreciated, this method is preferred in patients with suspected myositis ossificans (see Fig. 11-60).

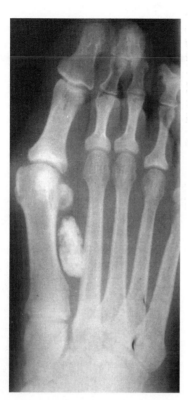

FIG. 11-59. AP view of the foot demonstrating myositis ossificans between the first and second metatarsal. (From Mandracchia et al., ref. 287, with permission.)

Ossification in Other Sites

Soft tissue ossification has also been described in ligaments and tendons and in association with chronic venous insufficiency.[283,296,301,310]

Ghormley[271] described 21 patients with ossification in the Achilles tendon. The condition was four times more common in males than in females. Although etiologic theories include embryonic rests, sesamoid bone formation, neoplasm, and infection, 30% of patients had a history of significant trauma (Figs. 11-61 and 11-62). When ossification occurs, further trauma can lead to fracture.[286]

Ossification of tendons and ligaments is also common in patients with diffuse idiopathic skeletal hyperostosis (DISH). Although changes are most common in the axial skeleton, the foot is also commonly involved.[270]

DISH is most common in men older than 55 years of age. The cause is unknown, laboratory studies are normal, and although the true incidence is unknown, the condition has been reported in 12% of autopsies.[270,296] Diagnosis is based on three criteria: (1) flowing hyperostosis in the anterior longitudinal ligament of at least four contiguous vertebrae; (2) preservation of vertebral disk height and lack of degenerative disk disease; and (3) absence of sacroiliac joint ankylosis.[297]

The feet are involved in 70% of patients with DISH. Poste-

rior calcaneal spurring is particularly common, and pain is reported in 23% of these patients. Thickening of the tarsal bones and sesamoids is also common (Fig. 11-63).[270]

Ossification or calcification in the precalcaneal and retrocalcaneal bursae may be difficult to differentiate from calcaneal spurring. In most cases, this differentiation is not important clinically. However, in patients with significant pain, one should be aware of potential injection or surgical techniques that may benefit patients (Fig. 11-64). Invasive retrocalcaneal bursitis is such a condition. Radiographs demonstrate squaring of the posterior superior calcaneus and ossification in the bursa (see Fig. 11-64). Patients respond well to surgical resection.[279]

SARCOIDOSIS

Sarcoidosis is a granulomatous disease of unknown origin.[312,321] The presence of noncaseating granulomas suggests infection as a likely cause. However, although tuberculosis, fungal disease, and viral infections have been searched for, no organism has been isolated to date. Geographic and familial factors have been reported. The highest incident has been reported in Sweden.[320] Autoimmune abnormalities have also been considered.[312,315,316,320] Males outnumber females, and blacks are more often affected than whites. Clinical symptoms are most common from the second through fourth decades. Multiple organs can be involved in sarcoidosis; however, the lung, cutaneous tissues, and eyes are most commonly affected.[312,317]

Patients with pulmonary involvement may be asymptomatic, with bilateral hilar and right paratracheal adenopathy noted on chest radiographs taken for screening purposes. In some cases, patients are referred for chest radiographs because of cough or chest pain. Other common presenting features include uveitis, iritis, iridocyclitis, and discrete erythematous skin rash.[320] Patients may have erythema nodosum during the acute stages.

Additional physical findings may include adenopathy and hepatosplenomegaly.[312] Laboratory abnormalities include eosinophilia, elevated serum Ca^{2+} in 25%, and in 80% of acute pulmonary cases angiotensin-converting enzyme is elevated.[320]

Radiographic Features

Musculoskeletal involvement may lead to muscle weakness (caseating granulomas in 50 to 80%), arthropathy, and lucent and sclerotic skeletal lesions.[320] The exact incidence of skeletal abnormality is difficult to assess because many skeletal lesions are asymptomatic. However, the literature reports an incidence of about 5%.[316,317] Patients with cutaneous lesions appear to have an increased incidence of skeletal lesions.[320]

Radiographs of the axial skeleton may reveal nonspecific osteopenia or scattered sclerotic areas. Characteristic radiographic findings are usually more obvious in the hands and, less frequently, the feet.[318-320,322] Well-margined cystic le-

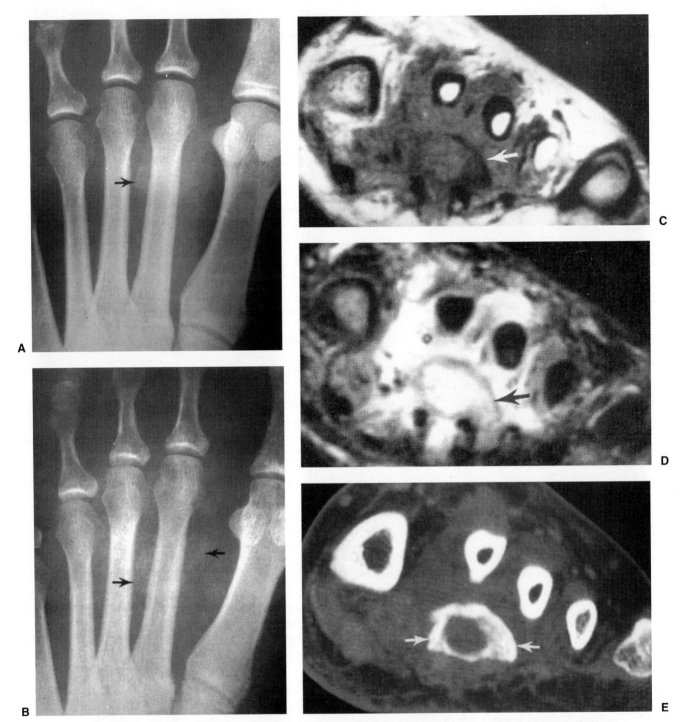

FIG. 11-60. A: AP radiograph of the left foot demonstrates a density (*arrow*) adjacent to the second metatarsal. **B:** Repeat radiograph 2 months later shows an enlarging density (*arrows*). T1-weighted (**C**) and T2-weighted (**D**) MRI studies demonstrate a low-intensity margin (*arrow*) with low intensity centrally on T1-weighted (**C**) and high intensity on T2-(**D**) weighted images. There is surrounding edema on the T2-weighted image (**D**). CT image (**E**) demonstrates the peripheral ossification (*arrows*). (From DeMaeseneer et al., ref. 264, with permission.)

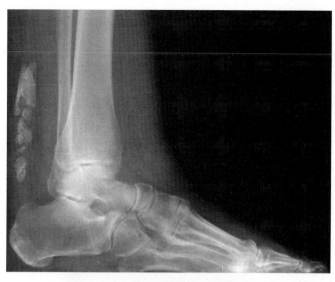

FIG. 11-61. Lateral view of the ankle in a patient with post-traumatic ossification in the Achilles tendon.

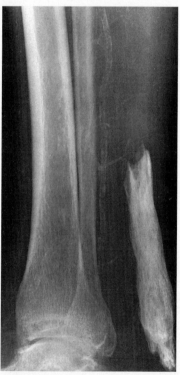

FIG. 11-62. Lateral view of the ankle demonstrates dense ossification in the Achilles tendon. This patient with hyperparathyroidism has vascular calcification.

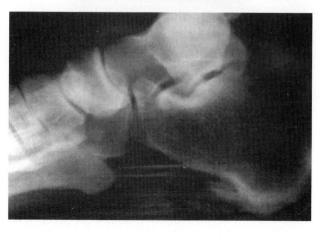

FIG. 11-63. Lateral view of the foot in a patient with diffuse idiopathic skeletal hyperostosis demonstrating ossification in the plantar fascia at the calcaneal attachment. There is also hyperostosis at the base of the fifth metatarsal. (From Garber and Silver, ref. 269, with permission.)

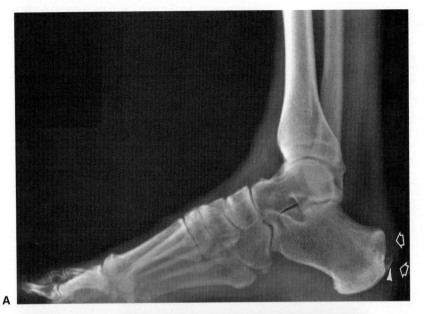

A

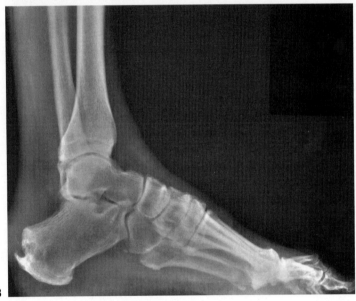

B

FIG. 11-64. A: Lateral radiographs in a patient with retro-Achilles bursitis shows swelling (*open arrows*) and bursal calcification (*arrowhead*). **B:** Lateral radiograph of the other foot demonstrates swelling and erosive pre-Achilles or retrocalcaneal bursitis.

sions (also seen in healthy persons) (Fig. 11-65) and honeycomb lytic areas are most common (Figs. 11-66 and 11-67).[314,320] When the area of the abnormal trabecular pattern becomes sufficiently large, pathologic fractures may occur (Fig. 11-68). This may be the only evidence of skeletal involvement because many lesions may be asymptomatic. Periostitis in the absence of fracture is unusual.[314,320]

Acrosclerosis, particularly in the tufts of the hands and feet, has also been described in patients with sarcoidosis.[318,322] This finding has been reported in 31 to 54% of patients with sarcoidosis. These changes are not specific and have also been noted in healthy persons and in patients with scleroderma, rheumatoid arthritis, and systemic lupus erythematosus.[314,318,320]

Radiographic features of joint changes are nonspecific. Soft tissue swelling and joint space narrowing may occur.[314,320] Involvement of large joints is not common.[313]

Generally, more complex imaging techniques such as radionuclide scans, CT, and MRI are not useful in defining skeletal involvement.[319,321] MRI may show inflammatory changes in muscles in patients with severe muscle weakness. However, to date, inflammatory changes on MRI do not allow specific histologic correlation.

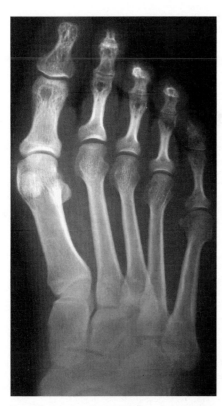

FIG. 11-65. AP radiograph of the foot in a patient with sarcoidosis. Note the well marginated lucent ("cystic") lesions in the distal aspects of the proximal phalanges of the great toe and middle phalanges of the second through fourth toes. There are also typical lace-like trabecular changes in the distal phalanges of the great toe.

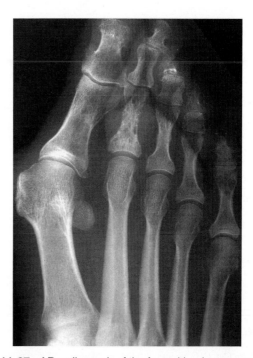

FIG. 11-67. AP radiograph of the foot with a honeycomb trabecular pattern in the second proximal phalanx resulting from sarcoidosis.

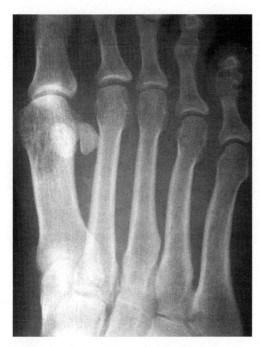

FIG. 11-66. Subtle lucent area in the distal first metatarsal in a patient with sarcoidosis. The pattern is not yet typical.

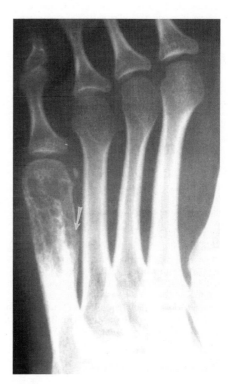

FIG. 11-68. Sarcoidosis involving the distal fifth metatarsal. The patient had been asymptomatic before the pathologic fracture (*arrow*).

REFERENCES

Osteoporosis

1. Aggarwal ND, Singh GD, Aggarwal R, Kaur RP, Thapar SP. A survey of osteoporosis using the calcaneum as in index. Int. Orthop. 1986; 10:147–153.
2. Ahmed AIH, Ilic D, Blake GM, Rymer JM, Fogelman I. Review of 3,530 referrals for bone mineral measurements of spine and femur. Evidence that radiographic osteopenia predicts low bone mass. Radiology 1998; 207:619–624.
3. Arnstein, AR. Regional osteoporosis. Orthop. Clin. North Am. 1972; 3:585–600.
4. Asher JD, Nichols G. Heparin stimulation of bone collagenase. Fed. Proc. 1965; 24:211.
5. Berquist TH. MRI of the Musculoskeletal System. 3rd Ed. New York, Lippincott–Raven, 1996.
6. Bloom RA. A comparative estimation of combined cortical thickness of various bone sites. Skeletal Radiol. 1980; 5:167–170.
7. Bordier PJ, Miravet L, Hisco D. Young adult osteoporosis. Clin. Endocrinol. Metab. 1973; 2:277–292.
8. Burrows HJ, Graham G. Spinal osteoporosis of unknown cause. Ann. Rheum. Dis. 1947; 6:129–145.
9. Byrd JW, Riccardi JM, Jung BI. Regional migratory osteoporosis and tarsal tunnel syndrome. Clin. Orthop. 1981; 157:164–169.
10. Calvo E, Alvarez L, Fernandez-Yruegas D, Vallejo C. Transient osteoporosis of the foot. Acta Orthop. Scand. 1997; 68:577–580.
11. Cepollaro C, Gomelli S, Pondrelli C, Martini S, Montagnani A, Rossi S, Gennari L, Gennari C. The combined use of ultrasound and densitometry in the prediction of vertebral fracture. Br. J. Radiol. 1997; 70:691–696.
12. Cheng XG, Nicholson PHF, Boonen S, Lowet G, Brys P, Aerssens J, Van der Perre G, Dequeher J. Prediction of vertebral strength in vitro by spinal bone densitometry and calcaneal ultrasound. J. Bone Miner. Res. 1997; 12:1721–1728.
13. Cockshott WP, Occleshaw CJ, Webber C, Walter SD, O'Brien K. Can a calcaneal morphologic index determine the degree of osteoporosis. Skeletal Radiol. 1984; 12:119–122.
14. Cunningham JL, Fordham JN, Hewitt TA, Speed CA. Ultrasound velocity and attenuation at different skeletal sites compared with bone mineral density measured using dual energy x-ray absorptiometry. Br. J. Radiol. 1996; 69:25–32.
15. Duncan H, Frame B, Fronst H, Arnstein AR. Regional migratory osteoporosis. South. Med. J. 62:41–44.
16. Eastell R. Treatment of post menopausal osteoporosis. N. Engl. J. Med. 1998; 338:736–746.
17. Fournier B, Chappared C, Rouji C, Berger G, Laugier P. Quantitative ultrasound imaging at the calcaneus using an automatic region of interest. Osteoporosis Int. 1997; 7:363–369.
18. Genant HK, Kozin F, Beherman C, McCarty DJ, Sims J. The reflex sympathetic dystrophy syndrome. Radiology 1975; 117:21–32.
19. Grampp S, Majumdar S, Jergas M, Newitt D, Lang P, Genant HK. Distal radius. In vivo assessment with quantitative MR imaging, peripheral quantitative CT and dual x-ray absorptiometry. Radiology 1996; 198:213–218.
20. Griffith GC, Nicols G, Asher JD, Flanagan B. Heparin osteoporosis. JAMA 1965; 193:91–94.
21. Hans D, Dargent-Molina P, Schott AM, Sebert JL, Cornier C, Kotzki PO, Delmas PD, Ponelles JM, Breart G, Meunier PJ. Ultrasonographic heel measurements to predict hip fracture in elderly women. The DRIDOS prospective study. Lancet 1996; 348:511–514.
22. Hurley DL, Khosla S. Update on primary osteoporosis. Mayo Clin. Proc. 1997; 72:943–949.
23. Jackson WPU. Osteoporosis of unknown cause in younger people: Idiopathic osteoporosis. J. Bone Joint Surg. Br. 1958; 40:420–441.
24. Jaworski M, Lebiedowshi M, Lorenc RS, Trempe J. Ultrasound bone measurement in pediatric subjects. Calcif. Tissue Int. 1995; 56:368–371.
25. Jharmaria NL, Lal KB, Udawat M, Manerji P, Kabras SG. The trabecular pattern of the calcaneus as an index of osteoporosis. J. Bone Joint Surg. Br. 1983; 65:195–198.
26. Jones G. Radiological appearances of disuse osteoporosis. Clin. Radiol. 1969; 20:345–353.
27. Jowsey J, Riggs LB. Bone formation in hypercortisonism. Acta Endocrinol. 1970; 63:21–28.
28. Keats TE, Harrison RB. A pattern of post-traumatic demineralization of bone simulating permeative neoplastic replacement. A potential source of misinterpretation. Skeletal Radiol. 1978; 3:113–114.
29. Lane JM, Vigorita VJ. Osteoporosis. J. Bone Joint Surg. Am. 1983; 65:274–278.
30. Langton CM, Ballard PA, Bennett DK, Purdie DW. A comparison of sensitivity and specificity of calcaneal ultrasound measurements in the clinical criteria for bone densitometry (DEXA) referral. Clin. Rheumatol. 1997; 16:117–118.
31. Lanchik L, Sartoris DJ. Current concepts in osteoporosis. AJR Am. J. Roentgenol. 1997; 168:905–911.
32. Lequesne M, Kerboull M, Bensasson M, Perez C, Dreiser R, Forest A. Partial transient osteoporosis. Skeletal Radiol. 1977; 2:1–9.
33. Longstreth PC, Malinak LR, Hill CS. Transient osteoporosis of the hip in pregnancy. Obstet. Gynecol. 41:563–569.
34. Mazess RB. Os calcis results questioned. Am. J. Obstet. Gynecol. 1986; 155:1144.
35. Miller PD, Bonnick SL, Rosen CJ. Clinical utility of bone mass measurements in adults. Consensus of an International panel. Semin. Arthritis Rheum. 1996; 25:361–372.
36. Naides SJ, Resnick D, Zvaifler NJ. Idiopathic regional osteoporosis: A clinical spectrum. J. Rheumatol. 12:763–768.
37. O'Mara RE, Pinals RS. Bone scanning in regional migratory osteoporosis. Radiology 1970; 97:579–581.
38. Poplawski ZJ, Wiley AM, Morry JF. Post-traumatic dystrophy of the extremities. J. Bone Joint Surg. Am. 1983; 65:642–655.
39. Resnick D, Niwayama G. Osteoporosis. In Resnick D, Niwayama G, eds. Diagnosis of Bone and Joint Disorders. 3rd Ed. Philadelphia, WB Saunders, 1995; pp. 1783–1853.
40. Roberts JG, Ditomosse E, Weber CE. Photon scattering measurements of calcaneal bone density. Invest. Radiol. 1982; 17:20–28.
41. Rosen CJ: Endocrine disorders and osteoporosis. Curr. Opin. Rheumatol. 1997; 9:355–361.
42. Rosenthall L. Selective supplementation of calcaneal ultrasound densitometry with dual energy x-ray absorptiometry of the spine and femur for population screening. Can. Assoc. Radiol. J. 1997; 47:38–41.
43. Ryan PJ, Fogelman I. Bone scintigraphy in matabolic bone disease. Semin. Nucl. Med. 1997; 27:291–305.
44. Schutzer SF, Gassling HR. The treatment of reflex sympathetic dystrophy syndrome. J. Bone Joint Surg. Am. 1984; 66:625–629.
45. Shier CK, Ellis BI, Kleerekoper M, Jurisson ML. Disseminated migratory osteoporosis: An unusual pattern of osteoporosis. J. Can. Assoc. Radiol. 1987; 38:56–59.
46. Simpson S. An unusual case of post-traumatic decalcification of the bones of the foot. J. Bone Joint Surg. 1937; 19:223–227.
47. Singh M, Magrath AR, Maini PS. Changes in the trabecular pattern of the upper end of the femur as an index of osteoporosis. J. Bone Joint Surg. Am. 1970; 52:457–467.
48. Steiner RM, McKeever C. Regional migratory osteoporosis. J. Can. Assoc. Radiol. 1973; 24:70–75.
49. Swerzey RL. Transient osteoporosis of the hip, foot and knee. Arthritis Rheumatol. 1970; 13:858–868.
50. Swislocki ALM, Barnett CA, Darnell P, Noth RH. Hyperthyroidism. An unappreciated cause of diffuse bone disease. Clin. Nucl. Med. 1998; 23:241–243.
51. Tannenbaum H, Esdaile J, Rosenthall L. Joint imaging in regional migratory osteoporosis. J. Rheumatol. 1980; 7:237–244.
52. Thompson DL, Fame B. Involution osteopenia. Current concepts. Ann. Intern. Med. 1976; 85:780–803.
53. Turpin S, Taillefer R, Lambert R, Leverlle J. Cold reflex sympathetic dystrophy in an adult. Clin. Nucl. Med. 1996; 21:94–97.

Osteomalacia, Rickets, and Parathyroid and Related Disorders

54. Bhargava SK, Gupta R, Loheal BS, Ikranullah AM, Salum F. Unusual radiological changes in the metacarpals, metatarsals, and phalanges in rickets. J. Indian Med. Assoc. 1983; 81:175–176.
55. Birtwell WM, Magsaman BF, Fenn PA, Torg JS, Toutellottes D, Martin JH. An unusual hereditary osteomalacia disease. Pseudo vitamin D deficiency. J. Bone Joint Surg. Am. 1970; 52:1222–1228.

56. Blunt JW, DeLuca HF, Schnoes HK. 25-hydroxycholecalciferol. A biologically active metabolite of vitamin D. Biochemistry 1968; 7: 3317–3322.

57. Bronsky D, Kushner DS, Dubin A, Snapper I. Idiopathic hypoparathyroidism and pseudohypoparathyroidism. Medicine 1958; 37:317–352.

58. Brooks MH, Bell NH, Love L, Stern PH, Orfei E, Queener SF, Hamstra AJ, DeLuca HF. Vitamin D dependent rickets type II. N. Engl. J. Med. 1979; 298:996–999.

59. Burnstein MI, Kottainaser SR, Pettifor JM, Sochett E, Ellis BI, Fram B. Metabolic bone disease in pseudohypoparathyroidism. Radiology 1985; 155:351–356.

60. Dent CE. Rickets (and osteomalacia), nutritional and metabolic (1919–1969). Proc. R. Soc. Med. 1970; 63:401–408.

61. Dent CE, Friedman M, Watson L. Hereditary pseudo vitamin D deficiency rickets. J. Bone Joint Surg. Br. 1968; 50:708–719.

62. Doppman J. Multiple endocrine syndromes. A nightmare to the endocrine radiologist. Semin. Roentgenol. 1985; 20:7–63.

63. Drezner MK, Feinglos MN. Tumor induced 1,25 dehydroxycholicalciferal deficiency. A cause of oncogenic osteomalacia. Clin. Res. 1977; 25:31A.

64. Eddy RL. Metabolic bone disease after gastrectomy. Am. J. Med. 1971; 50:442–449.

65. Frame B, Frost HM, Ormond RS, Hunter RB. A typical osteomalacia involving the axial skeleton. Ann. Intern. Med. 1961; 55:632–639.

66. Fraser D, Scriver CR. Familial forms of vitamin D resistant rickets revisited. X-linked hypophosphatemia and autosomal recessive vitamin D dependency. Am. J. Clin. Nutr. 1976; 29:1315–1329.

67. Frolik CA, DeLuca HF. 1, 25 dehydroxycholecalciferol. The metabolite of vitamin D reasonable for increased intestinal calcium transport. Arch. Biochem. Biophys. 1971; 147:143–147.

68. Haddad JG, Hahn TJ. Natural and synthetic sources of circulating 25-hydroxyvitamin D in man. Nature 1973; 244:515–516.

69. Harris WH, Heaney RP. Skeletal renewal and metabolic bone disease. N. Engl. J. Med. 1969; 280:193–202.

70. Harrison HE, Harrison HC. Rickets then and now. J. Pediatr. 1975; 87:1144–1151.

71. Holick MF, Schnoes HK, DeLuca HF, Suda T, Cousins RJ. Isolation and identification of 1, 25 dehydroxycholecalciferol. A metabolite of vitamin D active in intestine. Biochemistry 1971; 14:2799–2804.

72. Jawarski ZFG. Pathophysiology, diagnosis and treatment of osteomalacia. Orthop. Clin. North Am. 1972; 3:623–652.

73. Kanis JA, Adams ND, Earnshaw M, Heyner G, Ledingham JGG, Oliver DO, Russell RGG, Woods CG. Vitamin D, osteomalacia, chronic renal failure. In Vitamin D. Biochemical, Chemical, and Clinical Aspects Related to Calcium Metabolism. Proceedings of the 3rd Workshop on Vitamin D, Asilomar, Pacific Grove, CA. New York, Walter de Gruyter, 1977; p. 671.

74. Lachmann M, Kricune ME, Schwartz EE. Case report. Skeletal Radiol. 1985; 13:248–252.

75. Linovitz RJ, Resnick D, Keissling P, Kondon JJ, Sehler B, Nejdl RJ, Rowl JH, Deftos LJ. Tumor induced osteomalacia and rickets. A surgically curable syndrome, report of two cases. J. Bone Joint Surg. Am. 1976; 58:419–423.

76. Long RG, Skinner RK, Meinhard E, Wills MR, Sherlock S. Serum 25-hydroxy vitamin D values in liver disease and hepatic osteomalacia. Gut 1976; 17:824.

77. Malter IJ, McAlister WA. Pseudohypoparathyroidism and myositis ossificans progressiva in the same patient. J. Can Assoc. Radiol. 1972; 23:27–32.

78. Mankin HJ. Rickets, osteomalacia, and renal osteodystrophy. Part II. J. Bone Joint Surg. Am. 1974; 56:352–386.

79. Mann J, Alterman S, Hels AG. Albright's hereditary osteodystrophy comprising pseudohypoparathyroidism and pseudopseudohypoparathyroidism. Ann. Intern. Med. 1962; 56:315–342.

80. Massry SG, Ritz E. Pathogenesis of secondary hyperparathyroidism of renal failure. Is there a controversy. Arch. Intern. Med. 1978; 138: 853–854.

81. Netta P, Kessler M, Gaucher A, Bannworth B. Does aluminum have a pathologic role in dialysis associated arthropathy. Ann. Rheum. Dis. 1990; 49:573–575.

82. Norman AW, Henry H. The role of the kidney and vitamin D metabolism in health and disease. Clin. Orthop. 1974; 90:258–287.

83. Pitt MJ. Rickets and osteomalacia. In Resnick D, Niwayama G, eds. Diagnosis of Bone and Joint Disorders. 3rd Ed. Philadelphia, WB Saunders, 1995; pp. 1885–1922.

84. Parkinson IS, Ward MK, Kerr DNS. Dialysis encephalopathy, bone disease and anemia. The aluminum intoxication syndrome during regular hemodialysis. J. Clin. Pathol. 1981; 84:1285–1294.

85. Ponchon G, Kennan AL, DeLuca HF. Activation of vitamin D by the liver. J. Clin. Invest. 1969; 48:2032–2037.

86. Preece MA, Tomlinson S, Ribot CA, Pietrek J, Korn HJ, Davies DM, Ford JA, Dunnigan MG, O'Riordan JLH. Studies of vitamin D deficiency in man. Q. J. Med. 1975; 44:575–589.

87. Puschett JB, Moranz J, Karnick WJ. Evidence for diet action of cholecalciferol and 25-hydroxycholecalciferol on the renal transport of phosphate, sodium and calcium. J. Clin. Invest. 1972; 51:373–385.

88. Rasmussen H, Bordier P, Kurokawa K, Nagata N, Ogata E. Normal control of skeletal and mineral homeostasis. Am. J. Med. 1974; 56: 751–758.

89. Resnick D, Niwayama G, eds. Diagnosis of Bone and Joint Disorders. 3rd Ed. Philadelphia, WB Saunders, 1995.

90. Rosen CJ. Endocrine disorders and osteoporosis. Curr. Opin. Rheumatol. 1997; 9:355–361.

91. Ryan PJ, Fogelman I. Bone scintigraphy and metabolic bone disease. Semin. Nucl. Med. 1997; 27:291–305.

92. Scriver CR. Rickets and the pathogenesis of tubular transport of phosphates and other solutes. Am. J. Med. 1974; 57:43–49.

93. Scriver CR. Familial hypophosphatemia. The dilemma of treatment. N. Engl. J. Med. 1973; 389:531–532.

94. Steinbach HL, Noetzli M. Roentgen appearance of the skeleton in osteomalacia and rickets. AJR Am. J. Roentgenol. 1964; 91:955–972.

95. Steinbach HL, Radhe U, Jonsson M, Young DA. Evaluation of skeletal lesions in pseudohypoparathyroidism. Radiology 1965; 85:670–676.

96. Steinberg H, Waldron BR. Idiopathic hypoparathyroidism. Analysis of 52 cases including a report of a new case. Medicine 1952; 31: 133–154.

97. Steinmetz PR, Balko C, DeLuca HF. The kidney as an endocrine organ for production of 1, 25 dehydroxyl vitamin D_3, a calcium mobilizing hormone. N. Engl. J. Med. 1973; 389:359–365.

98. Vanherweghem JL, Schoutens A, Bergmann P. Usefulness of 99m-Tc pyrophosphate bone scintigraphy in aluminum bone disease. Trace Elements Med. 1984; 1:80–83.

Thyroid Disorders

99. Becker KL, Ferguson RH, McConahey WM. The connective tissue diseases and symptoms associated with Hashimotos thyroiditis. N. Engl. J. Med. 1963; 268:277–280.

100. Doyle FH. Radiographic assessments of endocrine effects on bone. Radiol. Clin. North Am. 1967; 5:289–301.

101. Follis RH. Skeletal changes of hyperthyroidism. Bull. Johns Hopkins Hosp. 1953; 92:405–421.

102. Gimlette TMP. Thyroid acropachy. Lancet 1960; 1:22–24.

103. Glatt W, Weinstein A. Acropachy in lymphocytic leukemia. Radiology 1969; 92:125–126.

104. Meema HE, Schatz DL. Simple radiographic density of cortical bone loss in thyrotoxicosis. Radiology 1970; 97:9–15.

105. Meunier RJ, S-Bianchi GG, Edouad CM, Bernard JC, Courpron P, Vignon GE. Bony manifestations of thyrotoxicosis. Orthop. Clin. North Am. 1972; 3:745–775.

106. Resnick D. Thyroid disorders. In Resnick D, Niwayama G, eds. 3rd Ed. Diagnosis of Bone and Joint Disorders. Vol. 4. Philadelphia, WB Saunders, 1995; pp. 1995–2011.

107. Rosen CJ. Endocrine disorders and osteoporosis. Curr. Opin. Rheumatol. 1997; 9:355–361.

108. Siegal RS, Thrall JH, Sasson JC. 99m-Tc pyrophosphate scans plus radiographic correlation in thyroid acropachy. J. Nucl. Med. 1976; 17:791–793.

109. Swislocki ALM, Barnett CA, Darnell P, Noter RH. Hyperthyroidism. An unappreciated cause of diffuse bone disease. Clin. Nucl. Med. 1998; 23:241–243.

110. Torres-Reyes E, Staple TW. Roentgen appearance of thyroid acropachy. Clin. Radiol. 1970; 20:95–100.

Pituitary Disorders

111. Detenbeck LC, Tressler HA, O'Duffy JD, Randall RV. Peripheral joint manifestations of acromegaly. Clin. Orthop. 1973; 91:119–127.

112. Doyle FH. Radiologic assessment of endocrine effects on bone. Radiol. Clin. North Am. 1967; 5:289–302.

113. Duncan TR. Validity of the sesamoid index in diagnosis of acromegaly. Radiology 1975; 115:617–619.

114. Harbison JB, Nice CM. Familial pachydermoperiostitis presenting as an acromegaly-like syndrome. AJR Am. J. Roentgenol. 1971; 112: 532–536.

115. Jackson DM. Heel pad thickness in obese persons. Radiology 1968; 90:129.

116. Lacks S, Jacobs RP. Acromegalic arthropathy. A reversible rheumatic disease. J. Rheumatol. 1986; 13:634–636.

117. Lang EK, Bessler WT. The roentgen features of acromegaly. AJR Am. J. Roentgenol. 1961; 86:321–328.

118. Meema HE, Shappard RH, Rapoport A. Roentgenographic visualization and measurement of skin thickness and its diagnostic application in acromegaly. Radiology 1964; 82:411–417.

119. Puckette SE, Seymour EQ. Fallibility of the heel pad thickness in diagnosis of acromegaly. Radiology 1967; 88:982–983.

120. Resnick D. Pituitary disorders. In Resnick D, Niwayama G, eds. Diagnosis of Bone and Joint Disorders. 3rd Ed. Vol. 4. Philadelphia, WB Saunders, 1995; pp. 1971–1994.

121. Sabet D, Stark AR. Sesamoid index of the foot in acromegaly. J. Am. Podiatr Assoc. 1981; 71:625–627.

122. Shore RM, Mazers RB, Bargman GJ. Bone mineral status in growth hormone deficiency. J. Pediatr. 1980; 96:393–396.

123. Steinbach HL, Feldman R, Goldberg MB. Acromegaly. Radiology 1959; 72:535–549.

124. Steinbach HL, Russell W. Measurement of heel pad as an aid to diagnosis of acromegaly. Radiology 1964; 88:982–983.

Osteolysis

125. Amin PH, Exons ANW. Essential osteolysis of the carpal and tarsal bones. Br. J. Radiol. 1978; 51:539–541.

126. Brower AC, Culver JE, Keats TE. Diffuse cystic angiomatosis of bone. AJR Am. J. Roentgenol. 1973; 118:456–463.

127. Cheney WD. Acro-osteolysis. AJR Am. J. Roentgenol. 1965; 84: 595–607.

128. Destuet J, Murphy WA. Acquired acro-osteolysis and osteonecrosis. Arthritis Rheum. 1983; 26:1150–1154.

129. Elias AN, Anderson HC, Gould LV, Streeten DHP. Hereditary osteodysplasia with acro-osteolysis (The Hadju-Cheney Syndrome). Am. J. Med. 1978; 65:627–636.

130. Erickson CM, Hirshberger M, Steckler GB. Carpal-tarsal osteolysis. J. Pediatr. 1978; 93:779–782.

131. Fornasier VL. Hemangiomatosis with massive osteolysis. J. Bone Joint Surg. Br. 1970; 52:444–451.

132. Gama C, Meira JB. Occupational osteolysis. J. Bone Joint Surg. Am. 1978; 60:86–90.

133. Gluck J, Miller JJ. Familial osteolysis of the carpal and tarsal bones. J. Pediatr. 1972; 81:506–510.

134. Gorham LW, Stout AP. Massive osteolysis (acute spontaneous absorption of bone, phantom bone, disappearing bone). J. Bone Joint Surg. 1955; 37:985.

135. Gorham LW, Wright AW, Shulta HH, Moxon FC JR. Disappearing bones. A rare form of massive osteolysis. Am. J. Med. 1954; 17:674–.

136. Hajdu N, Kauntze R. Cranio-skeletal dysplasia. Br. J. Radiol. 1948; 21:42–48.

137. Joseph B, Chacks V. Acro-osteolysis associated with hypertrophic pulmonary osteoarthropathy and pachydermoperiostitis. Radiology 1985; 154:343–344.

138. Kery L, Wouters HW. Massive osteolysis. J. Bone Joint Surg. Br. 1970; 52:452–459.

139. Kohler E, Babbitt D, Huizenga B, Good TA. Hereditary osteolysis. Radiology 1973; 108:99–105.

140. Lagier R, Rutishauser E. Osteoarticular changes in a case of essential osteolysis. J. Bone Joint Surg. Br. 1965; 47:339–353.

141. Lemaitre L, Smith M, Nuyts JB, Cousin J, Farine MO, Debeugny P. Carpal and tarsal osteolysis. Pediatr. Radiol. 1983; 13:219–226.

142. MacPherson RI, Walter RD, Korvall MH. Essential osteolysis with neuropathy. J. Can. Assoc. Radiol. 1973; 24:98–103.

143. Resnick D, Niwayama G. Osteolysis and chondrolysis. In Resnick D, Niwayama G, eds. Diagnosis of Bone and Joint Disorders. Vol. 6. Philadelphia, WB Saunders, 1995; pp. 4467–4490.

144. Resnick D, Weisman M, Goergen TG, Feldman PS. Osteolysis with detritic synovitis. A new syndrome. Arch. Intern. Med. 1978; 138: 1003–1005.

145. Sato K, Sugiura H, Aoki M. Transient phalangeal osteolysis (microgeode disease). J. Bone Joint Surg. Am. 1995; 77:1888–1890.

146. Stefano PD, Pignatti CB, Bails C, Young LW. Carpal tarsal osteolysis. Am. J. Dis. Child 1985; 139:793–794.

147. Stout AP. Tumors of blood vessels. Texas State J. Med. 1944; 40: 362–365.

148. Torg JS, DiGeorge AM, Kirkpatrick JA, Trujillo MM. Hereditary multicentric osteolysis with recessive transmission. A new syndrome. J. Pediatr. 1969; 75:243–252.

149. Tyler T, Rosenbaum HD. Idiopathic multicentric osteolysis. AJR Am. J. Roentgenol. 1976; 126:23–31.

150. White AA. Disappearing bone disease with arthropathy and severe scarring of the skin. J. Bone Joint Surg. Br. 1971; 53:303–309.

151. Whyte MP, Murphy WA, Kleerehoper M, Tertelbaum SL, Avioli L. Idiopathic multicentric osteolysis. Arthritis Rheum. 1978; 21: 367–376.

152. Wilson RH, McCormick WE, Tatum CF, Creech JL. Occupational acro-osteolysis. JAMA 1967; 201:577–581.

153. Winchester P, Grossman H, Lin WN, Dones BS. A new acid mucopolysaccharidosis with skeletal deformities simulating rheumatoid arthritis. AJR Am. J. Roentgenol. 1969; 106:121–128.

Paget's Disease

154. Barry HC. Paget's Disease of Bone. Baltimore, Williams & Wilkins, 1969.

155. Berquist TH. MRI of the Musculoskeletal System. 3rd Ed. New York, Lippincott–Raven, 1996.

156. Collins DH. Paget's disease of bone. Lancet 1956; 271:51–57.

157. Harris ED, Krane SM. Paget's disease of bone. Bull. Rheum. Dis. 1968; 81:506–511.

158. Lavender JP, Imogen MA, Arnst R, Bowring S, Doyle FH, Joplin GF, MacIntyre I. A comparison of radiography and radioisotope scanning in detection of Paget's disease and in the assessment of response to human calcitonin. Br. J. Radiol. 1977; 50:243–250.

159. Resnick D, Niwayama G. Paget's disease. In Resnick D, Niwayama G, eds. Diagnosis of Bone and Joint Disorders. 3rd Ed. Vol. 4. Philadelphia, WB Saunders, 1995; pp. 1923–1968.

160. Roberts MC, Kressel HY, Fallon MD, Zlatkin MB, Dalinka MK. Paget's disease. MR image findings. Radiology 1989; 177:341–345.

161. Rosenbaum HD, Hanson DJ. Geographic variation in prevalence of Paget's disease of bone. Radiology 1969; 92:959–963.

162. Rubin RP, Adler JJ, Adler DP. Paget's disease of the calcaneus. J. Am. Podiatr. Med. Assoc. 1983; 73:263–267.

163. Winfield J, Stamp TCB. Bone and joint symptoms in Paget's disease. Ann. Rheum. Dis. 1984; 43:769–773.

Bone Islands, Osteopoikilosis, Osteopathia Striata, and Melorhesotosis

164. Albers-Schönberg H. Eine seltene, bisher nicht bekannte Struktornamolie des skelettes. Fortschr. Geb. Roentgen St. Nuklearmed. 1916; 23:174–175.

165. Blank N, Lieber A. The significance of growing bone islands. Radiology 1965; 85:508–511.

166. Campbell CJ, Papadeinetriou T, Bonfigio M. Melorheostosis. J. Bone Joint Surg. Am. 1968; 50:1281–1304.

167. Fairbank HAT. Osteopathia striata. J. Bone Joint Surg. Br. 1950; 32: 117–125.

168. Genant HK, Bautovich GJ, Singh M, Lathrop KA, Harper PV. Bone seeking radionuclides. An in vivo study of factors affecting skeletal uptake. Radiology 1974; 113:373–382.

169. Green AE, Ellowood WH, Collins JR. Melorheostosis and osteopoikilosis. AJR Am. J. Roentgenol. 1962; 87:1096–1117.

170. Hall FM, Goldberg RP, Davies JAK, Fainsurger MH. Scintigraphic assessment of bone islands. Radiology 1980; 135:737–742.

171. Holly LE. Osteopoikilosis. A five 5-year study. AJR Am. J. Roentgenol. 1936; 36:512–517.

172. Hurt RL. Osteopathia striata. Voorhoeve's disease. J. Bone Joint Surg. Br. 1953; 35:89–96.

173. Kim SK, Barry WF Jr. Bone islands. Radiology 1968; 90:77–78.
174. Ledoux-Lebard R, Chabaneix S, Desane. L ostéopoecille; forme nouvelle d'ostéite condensante généralisée sans symptomes cliniques. (Fig. de radiol. et d'électral). 1916–1917; 2:133–134.
175. Morris JM, Samilson RL, Corley CL. Melorheostosis. J. Bone Joint Surg. Am. 1963; 45:1191–1206.
176. Mudge I, Hughes K, Fitzgibbons T, McMullen S, Stolarskyj A. Melorheostosis of the foot. A case report and review of the literature. Nebr. Med. J. 1996; 81:18–21.
177. Onitsuka H. Roentgen aspects of bone islands. Radiology 123: 607–612.
178. Pollock JL. Melorheostosis and sclerodermatoid skin changes. Mayo Clin. Proc. 1996; 71:318.
179. Resnick D, Niwayama G. Enostosis, hyperostosis, periostitis. In Resnick D, Niwayama G, eds. Diagnosis of Bone and Joint Disorders. 3rd Ed. Vol. 6. Philadelphia, WB Saunders, 1995; pp. 4396–4466.
180. Rozencwaig R, Wilson MR, McFarland GB. Melorheostosis. Am. J. Orthop. 1997; 26:83–89.
181. Sickles EA, Genant HK, Hoffer PB. Increased localization of ^{99m}Tc-pyrophosphate in a bone island. J. Nucl. Med. 1976; 17:113–115.
182. Whyte MP, Murphy WA, Siegel BA. ^{99m}Tc-pyrophosphate bone imaging in osteopoikilosis, osteopathia striata and melorheostosis. Radiology 1978; 127:439–443.
183. Wilcox LF. Osteopoikilosis. AJR Am. J. Roentgenol. 1933; 30: 615–617.

Osteopetrosis

184. Al-Rasheed SA, Al-Mohrij O, Al-Jurayyan N, Al-Herbish A, Al-Mageiren M, Al-Shallouin A, Al-Hussain M, El-Desouk M. Osteopetrosis in children. Int. J. Clin. Pract. 1998; 52:15–18.
185. Breighton D, Hamersma H, Cremin BJ. Osteopetrosis in South Africa. The benign, lethal, and intermediate forms. S. Afr. Med. J. 1979; 55: 659–665.
186. Cameron HU, Dewar FP. Degenerative arthritis associated with osteopetrosis. Clin. Orthop. 1977; 127:148–149.
187. Kovacs CS, Lambert RGW, Lavoie GJ, Suminoski K. Centrifugal osteopetrosis. Appendicular sclerosis with relative sparing of the vertebrae. Skeletal Radiol. 1995; 24:27–29.
188. Kovanlikaya A, Loro ML, Gilsanz V. Pathogenesis of osteosclerosis in autosomal dominant osteopetrosis. AJR Am. J. Roentgenol. 1977; 168:929–932.
189. McAlister WH, Herman TE. Osteochondrodysplasia, dysostoses, chromosomal aberrations, mucopolysaccharidosis, and mucolipidosis. In Resnick D, Niwayama G, eds. 3rd Ed. Vol. 5. Diagnosis of Bone and Joint Disorders. Philadelphia, WB Saunders, 1995; pp. 4163–4244.
190. Moss AA, Mainzer F. Osteopetrosis. An unusual cause of tuft erosion. Radiology 1970; 97:631–632.
191. Otsuka N, Fukkanaga M, Ono S, Morita K, Nagai K. Bone marrow scintigraphy and MRI in a patient with osteopetrosis. Clin. Nucl. Med. 1991; 16:443–445.
192. Roitberg D, Vitte RA, Maslack MM. Osteopetrosis. Appearance on three-phase bone scintigraphy. Clin. Nucl. Med. 1997; 22:858–859.
193. Shapiro F, Glimcher MJ, Holtrop ME, Toshjian AH, Brinckley-Passons D, Kenyara JE. Human osteopetrosis. J. Bone Joint Surg. Am. 1980; 62:384–399.

Vitaminosis

194. Caffey J. Chronic poisoning due to excess vitamin A. Pediatrics 1950; 5:672–688.
195. Holman CB. Roentgen manifestations of vitamin D intoxication. Radiology 1952; 59:805–816.
196. Mahoney CP, Margolis T, Knaiss TA, Labbe RF. Chronic vitamin A intoxication in infants fed chicken liver. Pediatrics 1980; 65:893–896.
197. Melton JB, Leonard JC, Fraser JJ, Stuemky JH. Hypervitaminosis A. Pediatrics 1982; 69:112–113.
198. Miller JH, Hayon II. Bone scintigraphy in hypervitaminosis A. AJR Am. J. Roentgenol. 1985; 144:767–768.
199. Pickup JD. Hypervitaminosis A. Arch. Dis. Child. 1956; 31:229–232.
200. Resnick D. Hypervitaminosis and hypovitaminosis. In Resnick D, Niwayama G, eds. 3rd Ed. Vol. 5. Philadelphia, WB Saunders, 1995; pp. 3343–3352.
201. Ruby LK, Mital MA. Skeletal deformities following chronic hypervitaminosis A. J. Bone Joint Surg. Am. 1974; 56:1283–1287.
202. Seffert RS. The growth plate and its affections. J. Bone Joint Surg. Am. 1966; 48:546–563.
203. Stewart VL, Herling P, Dalinka MK. Calcification in the soft tissues. JAMA 1983; 250:78–81.
204. Toomey JA, Morrisette RA. Hypervitaminosis A. Am. J. Dis. Child. 1947; 73:473–480.

Heavy Metal Disorders and Transverse Metaphyseal Bands

205. Allen TM, Manoli A II, Lamont RL. Skeletal changes associated with copper deficiency. Clin. Orthop. 1982; 168:206–210.
206. Andreoli SP, Smith JA, Bergstern JM. Aluminum bone disease in children: Radiographic features from diagnosis to resolution. Radiology 1955; 156:663–667.
207. Blickman JG, Wilkinson RH, Graef JW. The radiologic lead band revisited. AJR Am. J. Roentgenol. 1986; 146:245–247.
208. Garn SM, Silverman FN, Hertzog KP, Rohmann CG. Transverse lines with tibia. Med. Radiol. Photogr. 1968; 44:58–89.
209. Greengard J. Lead poisoning in childhood. Signs, symptoms, current therapy, clinical expressions. Clin. Pediatr. 1966; 5:269–276.
210. Leone AJ. On lead lines. AJR Am. J. Roentgenol. 1968; 103:165–167.
211. Levy J, Berdon WE, Abramson SJ. Epiphyseal separation simulating pyarthrosis secondary to copper deficiency in infants on prolonged total parenteral nutrition. Br. J. Radiol. 1984; 57:636–638.
212. McCarthy JT, Kurtz SB, McCall JT. Elevated bone aluminum content in dialysis patients with osteomalacia. Mayo Clin. Proc. 1985; 60: 315–320.
213. Park EA. The imprinting of nutritional disturbances on the growing bone. Pediatrics 1964; 33:815–562.
214. Park EA, Richter CP. Transverse lines in bone. The mechanism of their development. Bull. Johns Hopkins Hosp. 1953; 93:234–248.
215. Resnick D. Heavy metal poisoning. In Resnick D, Niwayama G, eds. Diagnosis of Bone and Joint Disorders. 3rd Ed. Vol. 5. Philadelphia, WB Saunders, 1995; pp. 3353–3364.

Anemia and Hemoglobinopathies

216. Barrett-Connor E. Bacterial infection and sickle cell anemia. An analysis of 250 infections in 166 patients and a review of the literature. Medicine 1971; 50:97–112.
217. Booker CB, Scott RB, Ferguson AD. Studies in sickle cell anemia. XXII. Clinical manifestations during the first two years of life. Clin. Pediatr. 1964; 3:111–115.
218. Caffey J. Cooley's anemia. A review of roentgenographic findings in the skeleton. AJR Am. J. Roentgenol. 1957; 78:381–391.
219. Chung SMK, Alavi A, Russell MO. Management of osteonecrosis in sickle cell anemia and its genetic variants. Clin. Orthop. 1978; 130: 158–174.
220. Cooley TB, Lee P. A series of splenomegaly in children with anemia and peculiar bone changes. Trans. Am. Pediatr. Soc. 1925; 37:29.
221. Currarino G, Erlandson ME. Premature fusion of the epiphysis in Cooley's anemia. Radiology 1964; 83:656–664.
222. Diggs LW. Bone and joint lesions in sickle cell anemia. Clin. Orthop. 1967; 52:119–144.
223. Dines DM, Canole VC, Arnold WD. Fractures in thalassemia. J. Bone Joint Surg. Am. 1976; 58:662–666.
224. Engh CA, Hughes JL, Abrams RO, Bowermans JW. Osteomyelitis in the patient with sickle cell disease. Diagnosis and management. J. Bone Joint Surg. Am. 1971; 53:15.
225. Espinosa LR, Spilbert I, Osterland CK. Joint manifestations of sickle cell disease. Medicine 1974; 53:295–305.
226. Finstenbush A, Farber I, Mogle P, Goldfarb A. Fracture patterns in thalassemia. Clin. Orthop. 1985; 192:132–136.
227. Golding JSR, MacIver JE, Went LN. The bone changes in sickle cell anemia and its genetic variants. J. Bone Joint Surg. Br. 1959; 41: 711–717.
228. Hansen GC, Gold RH. Central depression of multiple vertebral endplates. A pathognomonic sign of sickle hemoglobinopathy in Gaucher's disease. AJR Am. J. Roentgenol. 1977; 129:343–344.
229. Hill MC, Oh KS, Bowerman JW, Siegelman SS, James AE Jr. Abnor-

mal epiphysis in sickle cell disorders. AJR Am. J. Roentgenol. 1975; 124:34–43.

230. Karayalcin G, Rosner F, Kim KY, Chandra P, Aballi AS. Sickle cell anemia. Clinical manifestations in 100 patients and a review of the literature. Am. J. Med. Sci. 269:51–69.

231. Leichtman DA, Bigongiari LR, Wicks JD. The incidence and significance of tibiotalar slant in sickle cell anemia. Skeletal Radiol. 1978; 3:99–101.

232. Loiacono PJ, Reeder MM. An exercise in radiologic pathologic correlation. Radiology 1969; 92:385–394.

233. Mosely JE. Skeletal change in the anemias. Semin. Roentgenol. 1974; 9:169–184.

234. Rao VM, Fishman M, Mitchell DG, Steiner RM, Ballas SN, Axel L, Dalinka MK, Gefter W, Kressel HY. Painful sickle crisis. Bone marrow patterns observed with MR imaging. Radiology 1986; 161: 211–215.

235. Resnick D. Hemoglobinopathies and other anemias. In Resnick D, Niwayama G, eds. Diagnosis of Bone and Joint Disorders. 3rd Ed. Vol. 4. Philadelphia, WB Saunders, 1995; pp. 2107–2146.

236. Reynolds J, Pritchard JA, Ludders D, Mason RA. Roentgenographic and clinical appraisal of sickle cell beta-thalassemia disease. AJR Am. J. Roentgenol. 1973; 118:378–400.

237. Rothschild BM, Sebes RI. Calcaneal abnormalities and erosive bone disease associated with sickle cell anemia. Am. J. Med. 1981; 71: 427–430.

238. Shaub MS, Rosen R, Boswell W, Gordonson J. Tibiotalar slant. A new observation in sickle cell anemia. Radiology 1975; 117:551–552.

239. Valdez VA, Jacobsteen JG. Decreased bone uptake of technetium-99m polyphosphate in thalassemia major. J. Nucl. Med. 1980; 21: 47–49.

240. Vande Berg BC, Malghem J, Lecouvet FE, Maldague B. Magnetic resonance imaging of normal bone marrow. Skeletal Radiol. 1998; 27:471–483.

241. Vogler JB, Murphy WA. Bone marrow imaging. Radiology 1988; 168:679–693.

Periostitis

242. Dannels EG, Nashel DJ. A manifestation of venous disease and skeletal hyperostosis. J. Am. Podiatr. Assoc. 1983; 73:461–464.

243. Fam AG, Shin-Saug H, Ramsey CA. Pachydermoperiostitis. Scintigraphic, thermographic, plethysmographic, and capillaroscopic observations. Ann. Rheum. Dis. 1983; 42:90–103.

244. Greenfield GB, Schorsch HA, Shkolnik A. The various roentgen appearances of pulmonary hypertrophic osteoarthropathy. AJR Am. J. Roentgenol. 1967; 101:927–931.

245. Grogan DP, Martinez R. Transient idiopathic periosteal reaction associated with dysproteinemia. J. Pediatr. Orthop. 1984; 4:491–494.

246. Harris VJ, Romilo J. Caffey's disease. A case originating in the first metatarsal and review of 12 years experience. AJR Am. J. Roentgenol. 1978; 130;335–337.

247. Jajic I, Pacina M, Krstulovic B, Kovacevia D, Spaventi S. Primary hypertrophic osteoarthropathy and changes in joints. Scand. J. Rheum. 1980; 9:89–96.

248. Joseph B, Chacko V. Acro-osteolysis associated with hypertrophic pulmonary osteoarthropathy and pachydermoperiostitis. Radiology 1985; 154:343–344.

249. Lippman HI, Goldin RR. Subcutaneous ossification of the legs with chronic venous insufficiency. Radiology 1960; 74:279–288.

250. Neiman HL, Gompels BM, Mortel W. Pachydermoperiostitis with bone marrow failure and gross extramedullary hematopoesis. Radiology 1974; 110:553–554.

251. Newberg AH, Tampas JP. Familial infantile cortical hyperostosis. An update. AJR Am. J. Roentgenol. 1981; 137:93–96.

252. Oppenheimer DA, Jones HH. Hypertrophic osteoarthropathy of chronic inflammatory bowel disease. Skeletal Radiol. 1982; 9: 109–113.

253. Resnick D, Niwayama G. Enostosis, hyperostosis, and periostitis. In Resnick D, Niwayama G, eds. Diagnosis of Bone and Joint Disorders. 3rd Ed. Vol. 6. Philadelphia, WB Saunders, 1995; pp. 4396–4466.

254. Rosenthal L, Kush J. Observations in the radionuclide imaging in hypertrophic osteoarthropathy. Radiology 1976; 120:359–362.

255. Segal AM, McKenzie AH. Hypertrophic osteoarthropathy. A 10 year retrospective analysis. Semin. Arthritis Rheum. 1982; 12:220–231.

256. Simpson EL, Dalinka MK. Association of hypertrophic osteoarthropathy and gastrointestinal polyps. AJR Am. J. Roentgenol. 1985; 144: 983–984.

Soft Tissue Calcification and Ossification Soft Tissue Calcification and Ossification

257. Ackerman LV. Extraosseous localized non-neoplastic bone and cartilage formation. So called myositi ossificans. J. Bone Joint Surg. Am. 1958; 40:279–298.

258. Ballina-Garcia FJ, Queiro-Silva R, Fernandez-Vega F, Fernandez-Sanchez J, Weruaga-Rey A, Perez-Del Rio MJ, Rodrigez-Perez A. Diaphysitis in tumoral calcinosis syndrome. J. Rheumatol. 1996; 23: 2148–2151.

259. Barton DL, Reeves RJ. Tumoral calcinosis. Report of 3 cases and review of the literature. AJR Am. J. Roentgenol. 1961; 86:351–358.

260. Bishop AF, Destouet JM, Murphy WA, Gilula LA. Tumoral calcinosis. Case report and review of the literature. Skeletal Radiol. 1982; 8:269–274.

261. Black JR, Sladek GD. Tumoral calcinosis in the foot and hand. J. Am. Podiatr. Assoc. 1983; 73:153–155.

262. Blane CE, White SJ, Braunstein EM, Bowyer SL, Sullivan DB. Patterns of calcification in childhood dermatomyositis. AJR Am. J. Roentgenol. 1984; 142:397–400.

263. Bridges AJ, Hsu K-C, Singh A, Churchill R, Miles J. Fibrodysplasia (myositis) ossificans progressiva. Semin. Arthritis Rheum. 1994; 24(3):155–164.

264. Brown MC, Thrall JH, Cooper RA, Kun YC. Radiography and scintigraphy in tumoral calcinosis. Radiology 1977; 124:757–758.

265. DeMaeseneer M, Jasvisidha S, Lenchik L, Vaughan LM, Russack U, Sartoies DJ, Resnick D. Myositis ossificans of the foot. J. Foot Ankle Surg. 1997; 36:290–293.

266. Duret MH. Tumeurs multiples et singulaires des bourses sereuses. Bull. Mem. Soc. Ant. Paris 1899; 74:725–731.

267. Epstein DA, Solar M, Levin EJ. Demonstration of long-standing metastatic calcification by ^{99m}Tc diphosphonate. AJR Am. J. Roentgenol. 1977; 128;145–147.

268. Fam AG, Pritzker KPH. Acute calcificperiarthritis in scleroderma. J. Rheumatol. 1992; 19:1580–1585.

269. Fishel B, Dramant S, Papo I, Yaron M. CT assessment of calcinosis in a patient with dermatomyositis. Clin. Rheumatol. 1986; 5:242–244.

270. Garber EK, Silver S. Pedal manifestations of DISH. Foot Ankle 1982; 3:12–16.

271. Ghormley JW. Ossification of the tendo Achilles. J. Bone Joint Surg. 1938; 20:153–160.

272. Goldman AB. Myositis ossificans circumscripta. A benign lesion with a malignant differential diagnosis. AJR Am. J. Roentgenol. 1976; 126: 32–40.

273. Gordon LF, Arger PH, Dalinka MK, Coleman BG. Computed tomography of soft tissue calcification layering. J. Comput. Assist. Tomogr. 1984; 8:71–73.

274. Greenfield GB. Radiology of Bone Diseases. 5th Ed. Philadelphia, JB Lippincott, 1990.

275. Gülaldi NCM, Elahi N, Sasani J, Erbargi G. Tc-99m MDP scanning in a patient with extensive fibrodysplasia ossificans progressiva. Clin. Nucl. Med. 1995; 20:188–190.

276. Hacihanefioglu U. Tumoral calcinosis. A clinical and pathologic study of 11 reported cases in Turkey. J. Bone Joint Surg. Am. 1978; 60: 1131–1135.

277. Hudson TM. Radiologic-Pathologic Correlation of Musculoskeletal Lesions. Baltimore, Williams & Wilkins, 1987.

278. Inclan A. Tumoral calcinosis. JAMA 1943; 121:490–495.

279. Ippolito E, Ricciardi-Pollini PT. Invasive retrocalcaneal bursitis. A report of 3 cases. Foot Ankle 1984; 4:204–208.

280. Kaplan FS, McCluskey W, Hahn G, Tabas JS, Muenke M, Zasloff MA. Genetic transmission of fibrodysplasia ossificans progressiva. J. Bone Joint Surg. Am. 1993; 75:1214–1220.

281. Kolwavole TM, Bohrer SP. Tumoral calcinosis with fluid levels in the tumoral masses. AJR Am. J. Roentgenol. 1974; 120:461–465.

282. Kransdorf MJ, Meis JM, Jelinek JS. Myositis ossificans. MR appearance with radiologic-pathologic correlation. AJR Am. J. Roentgenol. 1991; 157:1243–1248.

283. Kumar R, Roper PR, Guinto FC. Subcutaneous ossification in the

leg in chronic venous stases. J. Comput. Assist. Tomogr. 1983; 7: 377–378.

284. Lafferty FW, Reynolds ES, Pearson OH. Tumoral calcinosis. A metabolic disease of obscure etiology. Am. J. Med. 1965; 38:105–188.

285. Leistyma JA, Hassan AHI. Interstitial calcinosis. Am. J. Dis. Child. 1964; 107:96–101.

286. Lotbe PA. Ossification of the Achilles tendon. J. Bone Joint Surg. Am. 1970; 52:157–160.

287. Malhotra CM, Lally EV, Buckley WM. Ossification of the plantar fascia and peroneus longus tendons in diffuse idiopathic skeletal hyperostosis. J. Rheumatol. 1986; 13:215–218.

288. Mandracchia V, Molran KT, Pruzanky J, Uricchio JN. Myositis ossificans. A report of a case in the foot. J. Am. Podiatr. Assoc. 1983; 73: 31–33.

289. Moreno AJ, Yedinak MA, Spicer MJ, Turnbull GL, Byrd BF, Brow TJ. Myositis ossificans with Ga 67 uptake. Clin. Nucl. Med. 1985; 10:40–41.

290. Noble TP. Myositis ossificans: A clinical and radiologic study. Surg. Gynecol. Obstet. 1924; 39:795–802.

291. Norman A, Dorfman HD. Juxtacortical circumscribed myositis ossificans. Evolution and radiographic features. Radiology 1970; 96: 301–306.

292. Orlow SJ, Watsky KL, Bolognia JL. Skin and bones. J. Am. Acad. Dermatol. 1991; 25:205–221.

293. Ozonoff MB, Flynn FJ. Roentgenographic features of dermatomyositis of childhood. AJR Am. J. Roentgenol. 1973; 118:206–212.

294. Paterson DC. Myositis ossificans circumscripta. Report of 4 cases without history of injury. J. Bone Joint Surg. Br. 1970; 52:296–301.

295. Pearson CM. Polymyositis. Ann. Rev. Med. 1976; 1&?–82.

296. Resnick D, Niwayama G. Soft tissues. In Resnick D, Niwayama G, eds. Diagnosis of Bone and Joint Disorders. 3rd Ed. Philadelphia, WB Saunders, 1995; pp. 4491–4622.

297. Resnick D, Shapiro RF, Wiener KB, Niwayama G, Utsinger PD. Diffuse idiopathic skeletal hyperostosis. Semin. Arthritis Rheum. 1978; 7:153–157.

298. Samuelson K, Coleman S. Nontraumatic myositis in healthy individuals. JAMA 1976; 235:1132–1133.

299. Schacheford GD, Barton LL, McAlister WH. Calcified subcutaneous fat necrosis in infancy. J. Can. Assoc. Radiol. 1975; 26:203–207.

300. Schätte HE, Vander Heul RO. Pseudomalignant, non-neoplastic osseous soft tissue tumors of the hand and foot. Radiology 1990; 176: 149–153.

301. Simon DB, Ringel SP, Sufet RL. Clinical spectrum of fascial inflammation. Muscle Nerves 1982; 2:525–537.

302. Steinfeld JR, Thorne NA, Kennedy TF. Positive ^{99m}Tc-pyrophosphate bone scan in polymyositis. Radiology 1977; 122:168.

303. Stewart UL, Herling P, Dalinka MK. Calcification in soft tissues. JAMA 1983; 250:78–81.

304. Tabas JA, Zasloff M, Fallou MO, Gannon FIT, Cohen RB, Kaplan FS. Enchondroma in a patient with fibrodysplasia ossificans progressiva. Clin. Orthop. 294:277–280.

305. Thompson JG. Calcifying collagenosis (tumoral calcinosis). Br. J. Radiol. 1966; 39:526–532.

306. Tibrewal SB, Iossifidis A. Extra-articular synovial chondromatosis of the ankle. J. Bone Joint Surg. Br. 1995; 77:659–660.

307. Verness B, Malik MOA, El-Hassan AM. Tumoral lipocalcinosis. A clinical-pathologic study of 20 cases. J. Pathol. 1976; 199:113–118.

308. Viau MR, Pederson HE, Salciccioli GE, Manoli A II. Ectopic calcification as a late sequel of compartment syndrome. Clin. Orthop. 1983; 176:178–180.

309. Wilker JF, Slatopolsky E. Hyperphosphatemia and tumoral calcinosis. Ann. Intern. Med. 1968; 68:1044–1049.

310. Young SWR, Hovey PJ. Case report 314. Skeletal Radiol. 1985; 13: 318–321.

311. Zeev A, Rozner I, Rosenbaum M. Tumoral calcinosis: A case report and review of the literature. J. Dermatol. 1996; 23:545–550.

Sarcoidosis

312. Bacharach T. Sarcoidosis. A clinical review of 111 cases. Am. Rev. Respir. Dis. 1961; 84:12–16.

313. Bjarnason DF, Forrester DM, Swezey RL. Destruction within large joints. A rare manifestation of sarcoidosis. J. Bone Joint Surg. 1973; 55:618–622.

314. Bonakdapour A, Levy W. Osteolytic changes in sarcoidosis. AJR Am. J. Roentgenol. 1971; 113:646–649.

315. Gunter B. Sarcoidosis. Orthopedics 1995; 18:214–218.

316. James DG, Neville E, Carstairs LS. Bone and joint sarcoidosis. Semin. Arthritis Rheum. 1996; 6:53–81.

317. Mayock RL, Bertrand P, Morrison CE, Solt JH. Manifestations of sarcoidosis. Analysis of 145 patients with a review of 9 series selected from the literature. Am. J. Med. 1963; 35:67–89.

318. McBrune CS, Fisher MS. Acrosclerosis in sarcoidosis. Radiology 1975; 115:279–281.

319. Requiato AJ, Schiappoccasse V, Guzzman L, Clause H. ^{99m}Tc pyrophosphate in bone sarcoid. J. Rheumatol. 1976; 3:426–436.

320. Resnick D. Sarcoidosis. In Resnick D, Niwayama G, eds. Diagnosis of Bone and Joint Disorders. 3rd Ed. Vol. 6. Philadelphia, WB Saunders, 1995; pp. 4333–4352.

321. Sartoris DJ, Resnick D, Resnick C, Yaghmai I. Musculoskeletal manifestations of sarcoidosis. Semin. Roentgenol. 1985; 20:376–386.

322. Young DA, Laman ML. Radiodense skeletal lesions in Boeck's sarcoid. AJR Am. J. Roentgenol. 1972; 114:553–558.

Subject Index